Canadian Community as Partner

THEORY & MULTIDISCIPLINARY PRACTICE

Canadian Community as Partner

THEORY & MULTIDISCIPLINARY PRACTICE

SECOND EDITION

Ardene Robinson Vollman, PhD, RN
Adjunct Associate Professor, Faculties of Nursing and Medicine
Department of Community Health Sciences
University of Calgary
Calgary, Alberta

Elizabeth T. Anderson, DrPH, RN, FAAN
Professor (ret)
The University of Texas Medical Branch
School of Nursing
Galveston, Texas

Judith McFarlane, DrPH, RN, FAAN
Parry Chair in Health Promotion and Disease Prevention
Texas Women's University
College of Nursing
Houston, Texas

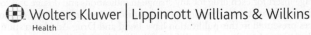

Wolters Kluwer | Lippincott Williams & Wilkins
Health
Philadelphia · Baltimore · New York · London
Buenos Aires · Hong Kong · Sydney · Tokyo

Senior Acquisitions Editor: Margaret Zuccarini
Managing Editor: Michelle Clarke
Editorial Assistant: Season Evans
Production Project Manager: Cynthia Rudy
Director of Nursing Production: Helen Ewan
Senior Managing Editor / Production: Erika Kors
Design Coordinator: Holly McLaughlin
Manufacturing Coordinator: Karin Duffield
Production Services / Compositor: Aptara, Inc.

2nd edition

9 8 7 6 5 4 3

Printed in China

Library of Congress Cataloging-in-Publication Data

Vollman, Ardene Robinson.
    Canadian community as partner : theory & multidisciplinary practice / Ardene Robinson Vollman, Elizabeth T. Anderson, Judith McFarlane. — 2nd ed.
        p. ; cm.
      title: Community as partner
    Canadian version of: Community as partner / Elizabeth T. Anderson, Judith McFarlane. 5th ed. Wolters Kluwer/Lippincott Williams & Wilkins, c2008.
    Includes bibliographical references and index.
    ISBN-13: 978-0-7817-8426-9
    ISBN-10: 0-7817-8426-3
  1. Community health nursing—Canada. 2. Community health nursing—Canada—Case studies. I. Anderson, Elizabeth T. II. McFarlane, Judith M. III. Anderson, Elizabeth T. Community as partner. IV. Title.
V. Title: Community as partner.
    [DNLM: 1. Community Health Nursing—Canada —Case Reports. 2. Community Health Planning—methods—Canada—Case Reports. 3. Consumer Participation—Canada—Case Reports. 4. Health Promotion—Canada—Case Reports. 5. Models, Nursing—Canada. WY 106 V924c 2008]
    RT98.V64 2008
    610.73′430971—dc22
                                                                                                                    2007028795

Care has been taken to confirm the accuracy of the information presented and to describe generally accepted practices. However, the authors, editors, and publisher are not responsible for errors or omissions or for any consequences from application of the information in this book and make no warranty, expressed or implied, with respect to the currency, completeness, or accuracy of the contents of the publication. Application of this information in a particular situation remains the professional responsibility of the practitioner; the clinical treatments described and recommended may not be considered absolute and universal recommendations.

The authors, editors, and publisher have exerted every effort to ensure that drug selection and dosage set forth in this text are in accordance with the current recommendations and practice at the time of publication. However, in view of ongoing research, changes in government regulations, and the constant flow of information relating to drug therapy and drug reactions, the reader is urged to check the package insert for each drug for any change in indications and dosage and for added warnings and precautions. This is particularly important when the recommended agent is a new or infrequently employed drug.

Some drugs and medical devices presented in this publication have Food and Drug Administration (FDA) clearance for limited use in restricted research settings. It is the responsibility of the health care provider to ascertain the FDA status of each drug or device planned for use in his or her clinical practice.

RRS1001

Dedication

To Marie des Anges Loyer-DaSilva, RN, PhD
Outstanding leader in public health and nursing,
scholar, educator, volunteer, philanthropist.

Inspiration, mentor and friend.

Contributors

Robert C. Annis, PhD
Rural Development Institute
Brandon University
Brandon, Manitoba

Antonia Arnaert, MBA, PhD, RN
Assistant Professor
McGill University, School of Nursing
Montreal, Quebec

Simon Carroll, PhD (c)
Associate Director
Community Health Promotion Research
University of Victoria
Victoria, British Columbia

Dana S. Edge, PhD, RN
Associate Professor
School of Nursing
Faculty of Health Sciences
Queen's University
Kingston, Ontario

Roxanne Felix, BSc, MSc
Manager
Health and Community Initiatives
Edmonton Mennonite Center for Newcomers
Edmonton, Alberta

Laurie Fownes, BSW, MSc
Program Consultant
Public Health Agency of Canada (PHAC)
Alberta/NWT Region
Calgary, Alberta

Jim Frankish, PhD
Senior Scholar, Michael Smith Foundation for
    Health Research
Acting Director, Institute of Health Promotion
    Research
Associate Professor, College for Interdisciplinary
    Studies
University of British Columbia
Vancouver, British Columbia

Donna Pierrynowski Gallant, PhD, RN
Assistant Professor
Saint Francis Xavier University
Antigonish, Nova Scotia

Tracy Halbert, MScN, RN
Performance & Data Manager
Health Systems and Portfolio Performance
Southeast Community Portfolio, Calgary Health
    Region
Calgary, Alberta

Donna Hardy-Cox, EdD
Memorial University of Newfoundland
School of Social Work
St. John's College
St. John's, Newfoundland

Gwen K. Healey, BSc, MSc
Executive Director
Arctic Health Research Network – Nunavut
Iqaluit, Nunavut

Marcia Hills, PhD, RN
Centre for Community Health Promotion Research
University of Victoria
Victoria, British Columbia

Truc Huynh, PhD(c), RN
Clinical Nurse, La Montagne Health Centre
Montreal, Quebec

Annette Johns, MSW, RSW
Memorial University of Newfoundland
St. John's, Newfoundland

Jenean Johnson, BSc, RDH
Public Health
David Thompson Health Region
Red Deer, Alberta

Candace Lind, PhD, RN
Assistant Professor
University of Calgary
Faculty of Nursing
Calgary, Alberta

Gail MacKean, PhD
Consultant, Knowledge into Action Department
Calgary Health Region
Adjunct Assistant Professor, Faculty of Medicine
Department of Community Health Sciences
University of Calgary
Calgary, Alberta

Aliyah Mawji, BN, MPH, RN
Instructor, Faculty of Nursing
University of Calgary
Calgary, Alberta

Heather McElroy, RDH
Employee Health
David Thompson Health Region
Red Deer, Alberta

Mary Ann Murray, MScN, PhD(c), CON(C), GNC(C), CHPCN(C), RN
Doctoral Candidate
University of Ottawa
School of Nursing
Ottawa, Ontario

Dorothy Nicolaou, MSW
Human Relations Agent
Childhood & Family Team
CSSS de la Montagne
Montreal, Quebec

Karoline Philipp, BN, RN
Director Population Health
Chinook Health
Lethbridge, Alberta

Frances E. Racher, PhD, RN
Associate Professor, School of Health Studies
Research Affiliate, Rural Development Institute
Brandon University
Brandon, Manitoba

Irving Rootman, PhD
Co-chair, CPHA Expert Panel on Health
  Literacy
Adjunct Professor and Chair of the Health and
  Learning Knowledge Centre
University of Victoria
Victoria, British Columbia

Catherine M. Scott, PhD
Adjunct Assistant Professor, Faculty of Medicine
Department of Community Health Sciences
University of Calgary
Director, Knowledge Into Action Department
Calgary Health Region
Calgary, Alberta

Malcolm Shookner, MA
Project Coordinator
Rural Communities Impacting Policy
Atlantic Health Promotion Research Centre
Dalhousie University
Halifax, Nova Scotia

Sheilah Sommer, MSc, RN
Past President, Canadian Public Health Association
Chief Executive Officer, Orion Health
Calgary, Alberta

Monique Stewart, MN, RN
Director
First Nations and Inuit Health Branch
Health Canada
Ottawa, Ontario

Michelle Sullivan, PhD, RSW
Assistant Professor
School of Social Work
Memorial University of Newfoundland
St. John's, Newfoundland

Nancy Sullivan, MSW, PhD, RSW
Associate Professor
School of Social Work
Memorial University of Newfoundland
St. John's, Newfoundland

Wilfreda E. Thurston, PhD
Professor
University of Calgary
Department of Community Health Sciences
Calgary, Alberta

Lewis Williams, PhD
Director, Prairie Region Health Promotion
  Research Centre
Department of Community Health and
  Epidemiology
Director, Community Development and Health
  Promotion Programs
University of Saskatchewan
Saskatoon, Saskatchewan

Sharon Yanicki, BSN, MSc, RN
Lecturer
University of Lethbridge
School of Health Sciences
Lethbridge, Alberta

Reviewers

Barbara Campbell, BN, MN, PhD(c), RN
University of Prince Edward Island
School of Nursing
Charlottetown, Prince Edward Island

L. Elizabeth Hood, BScN, MSN, PhD, RN
Grande Prairie Regional College
Grande Prairie, Alberta

Anne Judith Kearney, BN, MHSc, PhD, RN
Coordinator of Research Office, Faculty Member
Centre for Nursing Studies
Memorial University of Newfoundland
St. John's, Newfoundland

Judith C. Kulig, DNSc, RN
Professor
School of Health Sciences, University of
    Lethbridge
Lethbridge, Alberta

Jean M. Langdon, BSN, MN
Sessional Instructor, Assistant Professor Emeritus
University of Calgary
Calgary, Alberta

Marilyn Ziemian Mardiros, PhD, RN
Associate Professor
University of British Columbia–Okanagan
Kelowna, British Columbia

Judith G. Moody, MN, RN
Assistant Professor
School of Nursing
Memorial University of Newfoundland
St. John's, Newfoundland

Elaine Schow, BScN, NM, RN
Faculty
Mount Royal College
Calgary, Alberta

Patricia Seaman, BN, MN
Senior Instructor
Faculty of Nursing
University of New Brunswick
Fredericton, New Brunswick

Bonnie Seim, BSCN, RN
Nursing Instructor
Keyano College
Fort McMurray, Alberta

Cheryl Zawaduk, BSN, MS
Assistant Professor
Thompson Rivers University
Kamloops, British Columbia

Foreword

It is a pleasure to be asked to write a Foreword for the second edition of *Canadian Community as Partner: Theory & Multidisciplinary Practice*. The first edition has made an important contribution to the education of community health professionals and to the people they serve. This book, based on the Ottawa Charter for Health Promotion and founded on the determinants of health, takes a uniquely Canadian approach to the health of Canadians.

In the first section, the emphasis is on primary health care principles; action strategies for the promotion of health and prevention of illness and injury; culture; public health science; informatics; and emerging threats to the health of Canadians. This section sets the stage for the process that follows, and for the wonderful stories that are told of working in and with communities across the country. These are wonderful illustrations of how evidence informs practice and policy.

How can communities be involved in their health? What leverage can be created when communities work with health professionals to improve their health? Citizens working together have the capacity to change society for the betterment of all. Health at the community and national levels creates the foundation for growth and prosperity in all of Canada.

It is through citizens living in strong, vital communities across Canada that the health of all Canadians will improve. While the Canadian Health Care system is an important safety net, it is through upstream intervention and a focus on all the determinants of health that the health status of Canadians will make the greatest gains.

Knowledge and experience of communities and the ways of working with citizens in the community setting is fundamental for researchers, practitioners, educators, and policy makers who are involved in health and health care. *Canadian Community as Partner: Theory & Multidisciplinary Practice* brings together the knowledge of leading experts in community health from across Canada.

Sheilah Sommer
President, Canadian Public Health Association
November 30, 2006

Preface

Since the first edition of *Canadian Community as Partner: Theory & Practice* was published, I have had the pleasure of meeting many practitioners and students who have used it to learn and to inform their practice. I also discovered that community groups have used the book to guide their own projects. This has been most exciting for me! The book was originally written to provide a "made-in-Canada" resource for exactly these purposes: education, practice, and community development.

Canada continues to be a leader on the international stage in public health and health promotion, thanks in large part to the leadership exhibited by the Canadian Public Health Association, the Canadian Consortium of Health Promotion Research, and others. However, we have not often recognised the importance of the grassroots approach to community practice; in this book we tell the stories of community projects that use the community as partner process and principles of primary health care.

The first edition began in 2000 when I met Bets Anderson at a conference in Boston, then invited Judith McFarlane to Calgary, and began a lasting collegial publishing partnership. This second edition began immediately after the printing stopped on the first one, as stories started coming in from the field. I am indebted not only to the original authors but to the people of Canada whose stories we share in this edition.

The book is organised in three sections; a *theoretical* section that sets the stage for how and why we work as partners with the communities we serve; a *process* section that details the activities of the community process in action; and a third section of *stories* that tell the tales of working in and with communities from sea to sea to sea.

PART I: THEORETICAL FOUNDATIONS

In this section of *Canadian Community as Partner*, the reader is invited to appreciate the fundamental principles of community practice. It uses the Ottawa Charter (1986) as its primary framework, incorporating the determinants of health, epidemiologic principles, the appreciation of culture and informatics, and a discussion of the challenges to health that Canadians face now and in the near future. Fundamental to community practice is the interdisciplinary nature of teamwork; hence, there are no references to the professions that comprise the community health workforce.

PART II: THE PROCESS OF COMMUNITY AS PARTNER

This section begins with the model that guides the process of working in and with communities. In subsequent chapters, each step of the process is detailed with specific examples. All of the steps emphasize the importance of social justice, equity, and public participation, and the determinants of health.

PART III: COMMUNITY AS PARTNER IN PRACTICE: CASE STORIES

The eight chapters in this section tell the stories of field-based practitioners of population health promotion from several disciplinary viewpoints. All action strategies of the Charter are illustrated, along with stories that touch many populations across the country. The projects presented took place in several different settings, illustrating how practitioners partner across sectors. Regardless of the geography, these stories will resonate, and as the community as partner process is used in future, we will hear (in time for the next edition) more success stories from every province and territory of Canada.

Ardene Robinson Vollman, PhD, RN

Acknowledgments

Without the efforts of Judith McFarlane and Elizabeth (Bets) Anderson over two decades and five editions of their original book, *Community as Partner*, this Canadian edition would never have been written.

Without the support of my family, I might not have embarked on the publishing journey that brings me to the second edition. My husband, Ken, has been a tireless cheerleader; my two sons, Mike and Rob, and Mike's wonderful wife Joanna, have been very gracious when writing kept me busy. My late mother, Lillian Robinson, my sister, Jacquie Simpson, and my friend Candy Jordan have believed in me throughout this process and have encouraged me in so many ways.

My students in Nursing and in Community Health Sciences have kept my feet firmly on the ground; they make me very proud as I watch them venture into community practice and make a difference in their worlds.

To my colleagues—especially Drs. Fran Racher, Wilfreda "Billie" Thurston, Lynn Meadows, Jennifer Hatfield, Tom Noseworthy, and Professor Roxie Thompson Isherwood—thank you. To Corey Wolfe of Lippincott Williams & Wilkins—my appreciation for your ongoing support. To the contributors to this edition—my heartfelt gratitude for your efforts to make this book a success.

To the readers—this is for you. Enjoy.

Contents

PART I
Theoretical Foundations 1

1 Population Health Promotion: Essentials and Essence of Practice 2
Ardene Robinson Vollman
INTRODUCTION 2
FOUNDATIONS OF COMMUNITY PRACTICE 4
A FRAMEWORK FOR HEALTH PROMOTION IN CANADA 7
GLOBAL CONFERENCES ON HEALTH PROMOTION 11
POPULATION HEALTH 14
POPULATION HEALTH PROMOTION 20
POPULATION HEALTH APPROACH 22
IMPLICATIONS OF POPULATION HEALTH PROMOTION FOR "COMMUNITY AS PARTNER" 23
SUMMARY 23

2 Ethics for Community Practice 26
Frances E. Racher
INTRODUCTION 26
KEY CONCEPTS IN ETHICAL PRACTICE 27
ETHICAL DIVERSITY UNDERPINS COMMUNITY PRACTICE 28
ETHICAL THEORIES 28
ETHICAL FOUNDATIONS OF PUBLIC HEALTH AND COMMUNITY PRACTICE 39
ADVANCES IN ETHICS FOR COMMUNITY PRACTICE 42
ETHICAL CHALLENGES IN COMMUNITY PRACTICE 44
SUMMARY 45

3 Epidemiology, Demography, and Community Health 48
Dana S. Edge
INTRODUCTION 48
DEMOGRAPHY AND EPIDEMIOLOGY 49
CONTEMPORARY COMMUNITY HEALTH PRACTICE 50
EPIDEMIOLOGIC APPROACHES TO COMMUNITY HEALTH RESEARCH 50
LEVELS OF PREVENTION IN COMMUNITY PRACTICE 55
DESCRIPTIVE MEASURES OF HEALTH 56
ANALYTIC MEASURES OF HEALTH 62
SOURCES OF COMMUNITY HEALTH DATA 68
SCREENING FOR HEALTH CONDITIONS 70
DECISION MAKING IN SCREENING: PRACTICAL AND ETHICAL CONSIDERATIONS 72
OUTBREAK MANAGEMENT 73
SUMMARY 74

4 Creating Supportive Environments for Health: Social Network Analysis 77
Malcolm Shookner, Catherine M. Scott, and Ardene Robinson Vollman
INTRODUCTION 78
SUNDSVALL CONFERENCE AND STATEMENT 78
THE PHYSICAL ENVIRONMENT AND HUMAN HEALTH 80
ACTION PROCESS FOR CREATING SUPPORTIVE ENVIRONMENTS FOR HEALTH 83

ECOLOGICAL PERSPECTIVE: OVERLAPPING ENVIRONMENTAL INFLUENCES ON HEALTH 85
ENVIRONMENTS AND SETTINGS 86
SOCIAL CAPITAL AND SOCIAL NETWORKS 87
SUMMARY 91
ACKNOWLEDGMENTS 92

 5   Developing Personal Skills: Empowerment   94
Lewis Williams
INTRODUCTION 95
PERSONAL EMPOWERMENT IN CONTEXT 97
HEALTH AND EMPOWERMENT 99
LITERACY AND HEALTH FOR ALL 100
POWER-CULTURE, EMPOWERMENT, AND HEALTH 102
THE EMPOWERMENT TERRAIN 106
A CRITICAL POSTMODERN APPROACH TO EMPOWERMENT 108
A HEALTH PROMOTION EXAMPLE 108
SUMMARY 110

 6   Strengthening Community Action: Public Participation and Partnerships for Health   113
Catherine M. Scott and Gail L. MacKean
INTRODUCTION 114
COMMUNITY DEVELOPMENT 114
BUILDING COMMUNITY CAPACITY 115
METHODS OF COMMUNITY DEVELOPMENT 116
THE COMMUNITY DEVELOPMENT PROCESS 117
PUBLIC PARTICIPATION IN HEALTH 118
COLLABORATION AND PARTNERSHIPS 123
A PARTNERSHIP FRAMEWORK 127
PARTNERSHIP CONFIGURATION 129
PARTNERSHIP ORGANIZATION 131
A PROCESS MODEL OF PARTNERSHIP DEVELOPMENT 131
APPLICATION OF THE TOOLS—KEY CONSIDERATIONS 133
SUMMARY 135

 7   Building Healthy Public Policy   138
Wilfreda E. Thurston
INTRODUCTION 138
WHAT IS PUBLIC POLICY? 139
HOW IS PUBLIC POLICY DEVELOPED? 139
POLICY COMMUNITIES, NETWORKS, AND PARTNERSHIPS 143
PARTNERSHIPS 145
SUMMARY 145

 8   Reorienting Health Services   148
Laurie Fownes and Ardene Robinson Vollman
INTRODUCTION 149
PRIMARY HEALTH CARE 149
TOWARD AN INTEGRATED MODEL OF HEALTH 151
THE SETTINGS APPROACH TO HEALTH 154
CAPACITY BUILDING AND THE REORIENTATION OF HEALTH SERVICES 158
HEALTH SECTOR REFORM 159
SUMMARY 160

9 Honouring Culture and Diversity in Community Practice   164
Frances E. Racher and Robert C. Annis
INTRODUCTION 164
THE CULTURAL LANDSCAPE OF CANADA 165
KEY CONCEPTS RELATED TO CULTURE AND ETHNICITY 171
MULTICULTURALISM IN CANADA 172
THE CANADIAN MOSAIC AND THE AMERICAN MELTING POT 175
BARRIERS TO MULTICULTURALISM 177
FACILITATORS OF MULTICULTURALISM 180
COMMUNITY PRACTICE IN MULTICULTURAL ENVIRONMENTS 181
SUMMARY 187

10 Community Health Informatics   190
Tracy Halbert
INTRODUCTION 190
COMMUNITY-BASED HEALTH INFORMATICS 191
HEALTH STATUS: HEALTH DETERMINANTS, SERVICES, AND CHOICES 193
COMMUNITY HEALTH POLICY DEVELOPMENT 193
HEALTH INFORMATICS METHODS AND REQUIREMENTS 194
SUMMARY 201

11 Emerging Threats to Community Health   204
Monique Stewart
INTRODUCTION 204
IDENTIFICATION OF EMERGING PUBLIC HEALTH ISSUES 205
INFLUENZA PANDEMIC 206
ENVIRONMENTAL HEALTH 207
INFECTIOUS DISEASES 208
CHRONIC DISEASES 210
MENTAL HEALTH 211
SUMMARY 213

PART II
The Process of Community as Partner 217

12 A Model to Guide Practice   218
Ardene Robinson Vollman
INTRODUCTION 218
MODELS 219
ASSESSMENT 230
ANALYSIS, DIAGNOSIS, AND PLANNING 232
INTERVENTION 232
EVALUATION 234
PARTNERSHIP PLANNING AND TEAMWORK 235
SUMMARY 236

13 Community Assessment   238
Ardene Robinson Vollman
INTRODUCTION 238
THE COMMUNITY ASSESSMENT TEAM 239

GETTING TO KNOW THE COMMUNITY 241
PLANNING THE ASSESSMENT 243
METHODS OF DATA COLLECTION 245
ELEMENTS OF A COMMUNITY ASSESSMENT 253
SUBSYSTEMS 259
SUMMARY 276

14   Community Analysis and Diagnosis   280
Ardene Robinson Vollman
INTRODUCTION 280
COMMUNITY ANALYSIS 281
SAMPLE COMMUNITY ANALYSIS 283
EVALUATION 303
SUMMARY 304

15   Planning a Community Health Program   306
Ardene Robinson Vollman
INTRODUCTION 306
PLANNING IN PARTNERSHIP WITH THE COMMUNITY 307
PRIORITIZING COMMUNITY DIAGNOSES 310
PLANNED CHANGE 311
DEVELOPING A PROGRAM LOGIC MODEL 317
SUMMARY 325

16   Implementing a Community Health Program   327
Ardene Robinson Vollman
INTRODUCTION 327
PROMOTING COMMUNITY OWNERSHIP 328
IMPLEMENTING A UNIFIED PROGRAM 330
SETTING COMMUNITY AND POPULATION HEALTH GOALS 330
COMMUNITY HEALTH FOCUS 331
COMMUNITY INTERVENTIONS 335
EVALUATION 342
SUMMARY 344

17   Evaluating a Community Health Program   346
Marcia Hills and Simon Carroll
INTRODUCTION 347
EVALUATION PRINCIPLES 349
THE EVALUATION PROCESS 350
COMPONENTS OF EVALUATION 352
EVALUATION STRATEGIES 354
SELECTED METHODS OF DATA COLLECTION 354
SUMMARY 366

PART III
Community as Partner in Practice *371*

18   Community Profile: Exemplar Health District   373
Ardene Robinson Vollman
INTRODUCTION 373

DEMOGRAPHIC DATA 374
HEALTH DETERMINANTS 377
HEALTH STATUS 384
OBSERVATIONS AND RECOMMENDATIONS 392
REGIONAL HEALTH INDICATORS 394
SUMMARY 394

19 Assessing the Health of Communities in Northern Canada   397
Gwen K. Healey and Frances E. Racher
INTRODUCTION 397
INUIT WOMEN'S HEALTH 398
PROMOTING YOUTH PARTICIPATION IN COMMUNITY DEVELOPMENT THROUGH PHOTOVOICE 403
SUMMARY 412

20 Promoting the Health of Pregnant Women   414
Truc Huynh, Dorothy Nicolaou, and Aliyah Mawji
INTRODUCTION 414
EMPOWERING IMMIGRANT WOMEN IN CANADA 415
THE SILK ROAD: HEALTH PROMOTION IN NORTHERN PAKISTAN 422
SUMMARY 430

21 Promoting the Health of Schoolchildren   432
Jenean Johnson, Heather McElroy, and Candace Lind
INTRODUCTION 432
ORAL HEALTH PROGRAMMING—GETTING TO THE EVIDENCE 433
PROMOTING SCHOOL HEALTH THROUGH A PARTNERSHIP MODEL 440
SUMMARY 446
ACKNOWLEDGMENTS 446

22 Youth Engagement in Health Promotion   449
Michelle Sullivan, Nancy Sullivan, Donna Hardy-Cox, Annette Johns, Sharon M. Yanicki, and Karoline Philipp
INTRODUCTION 450
WAY OUT THERE: YOUTH ENGAGEMENT IN SOCIAL POLICY ACTION PLANNING 450
COMMUNITY PARTNERSHIPS FOR POSTSECONDARY TOBACCO REDUCTION 459
SUMMARY 468

23 Workplace Health Promotion   470
Roxanne Felix, Donna Pierrynowski Gallant, and Mary Ann Murray
INTRODUCTION 470
WORKPLACE HEALTH PROMOTION IN A MUNICIPAL GOVERNMENT SETTING 471
RESPONSIVE WORKPLACE STRATEGIES FOR PANDEMIC INFLUENZA 479
SUMMARY 487

24 Promoting the Health of Vulnerable Populations   493
Jim Frankish, Catherine M. Scott, and Wilfreda E. Thurston
INTRODUCTION 493
WORKING WITH VULNERABLE POPULATIONS IN URBAN SETTINGS 494
WOMEN'S PERSPECTIVES ON POVERTY: PHOTOVOICE AS A TOOL FOR SOCIAL CHANGE 501
SUMMARY 506
ACKNOWLEDGMENTS 506

25 Using Technology to Promote the Health of Homebound Seniors   508
Antonia Arnaert
INTRODUCTION 508

BACKGROUND 509
TELESENIOR: A TELE-HOMECARE PROJECT 510
EVALUATION 514
LESSONS LEARNED 516
SUMMARY 517
ACKNOWLEDGMENTS 517

Appendix A: A Model Assessment Guide for Nursing in industry   521

Appendix B: Assessment of an industry   527

Index   535

Part 1

Theoretical Foundations

Chapter 1
Population Health Promotion: Essentials and Essence of Practice / 2

Chapter 2
Ethics for Community Practice / 26

Chapter 3
Epidemiology, Demography, and Community Health / 48

Chapter 4
Creating Supportive Environments for Health: Social Network Analysis / 77

Chapter 5
Developing Personal Skills: Empowerment / 94

Chapter 6
Strengthening Community Action: Public Participation and Partnerships for Health / 113

Chapter 7
Building Healthy Public Policy / 138

Chapter 8
Reorienting Health Services / 148

Chapter 9
Honouring Culture and Diversity in Community Practice / 164

Chapter 10
Community Health Informatics / 190

Chapter 11
Emerging Threats to Community Health / 204

Population Health Promotion: Essentials and Essence of Practice

ARDENE ROBINSON VOLLMAN

Chapter Outline

Introduction
Foundations of Community Practice
A Framework for Health Promotion in
   Canada
Global Conferences on Health Promotion
Population Health

Population Health Promotion
Population Health Approach
Implications of Population Health
   Promotion for "Community as
   Partner"
Summary

Learning Objectives

After studying this chapter, you should be able to:

❖ Describe the philosophical foundations of population health promotion

❖ List the five principles and eight essentials of primary health care

❖ Outline the challenges, mechanisms, and strategies of the Canadian framework
   for health promotion

❖ Detail the prerequisites for health and the action strategies for health promotion as described in the Ottawa Charter for Health Promotion

❖ List the factors that determine health

❖ Understand the evolution of population health promotion

Introduction

In the 20th century, many gains in health status among the people of
the developed world were achieved. Much was accomplished through four means:
(1) advances in knowledge about the causes of disease, (2) development of new
technologies and pharmaceuticals to treat and cure many diseases, (3) creation of

vaccines and environmental solutions to prevent disease transmission and acquisition, and (4) innovations in surveillance techniques to measure health status. However, it has become increasingly accepted that health is more than the absence of disease—it is a broad manifestation of wellness of body, mind, and environment and is viewed as an essential resource for everyday living. In this chapter, the history and the evolution of thought around the concept of health as it relates to individuals, families, groups, and communities is chronicled. Many of the principles and concepts presented in this chapter are discussed more fully in other parts of the book.

In this text, the generic term "health worker" or "health team" is used to connote the multidisciplinary and intersectoral approach that underlies successful community practice. Although initially designed for nurses, this book is intended to be useful to community social workers, nutritionists, health educators, community medicine physicians, pharmacists, and health promoters. It also recognizes that health teams should have members of the public involved in all levels of activities to ensure that the foundational principles of community practice are implemented.

As you will see as you progress through this book and learn the processes of community assessment, planning, and evaluation, it will become evident that no single person or agency is capable of addressing the many and complex health problems of communities and populations. Because health is determined by a complex mix of factors, maintaining and creating health requires ongoing action from multiple partners whose mandates support similar goals. Hence, community health workers rely on cooperation with other workers, collaboration among agencies involved in similar work, and partnerships with people, communities, public and private sectors, and business to effect change that has a positive impact on the health of people.

Partnerships may be formed across *sectors* (i.e., broad fields of activity, such as education, health, justice, etc.), and at different *levels*. Levels may be defined by geography, by scope of mandate (e.g., municipal, provincial), or by vertical level within organizations (e.g., senior management, front-line). Action is more effective when it includes vertical as well as horizontal partnerships and collaboration. Horizontal links are created when partnerships are formed at the same level. For instance, to deal with an outbreak of infection in a day care centre, the health district's environmental health officer and community nurse, the school board's preschool education specialist, and the social worker from children's services may be involved in the follow-up action. To illustrate vertical collaboration, to set health policy regarding tobacco, a health region will work with the federal health department, the provincial health ministry, and the municipality, all of whom have different jurisdictions in policy development and enforcement. Horizontally, each partner may also need to work with justice counterparts (e.g., Royal Canadian Mounted Police, provincial police, local by-law enforcement) and other departments to effect change in tobacco policy.

Key to all community practice is the principle of "doing with," not "to" or "for," the people served. This theme is pervasive in all the documents that form the foundation of community practice. The title of this book is *Community as Partner*, meaning that community workers partner not only with professional colleagues to serve the people in communities but also with members of those communities and groups. In the following section, how this principle became the key theme in community practice will be described.

FOUNDATIONS OF COMMUNITY PRACTICE

Whatever discipline in which community workers are trained, several documents published in the last quarter of the 20th century have been instrumental in the development of guiding principles of ethical community practice. Many of the seminal documents that form this foundation have originated in Canada.

The Lalonde Report

The publication of the report *New Perspectives on the Health of Canadians* in 1974 under the auspices of the then minister of National Health and Welfare, the Honourable Marc Lalonde, heralded a change in the focus of health on disease to a focus on health (Lalonde, 1974). The Lalonde Report, as it has become known, argues that health is not achievable from health care services alone, but from the interaction of health services with human biology, lifestyle, and the environment in which we live. This report suggested that health is tied to overall conditions of living, particularly the environment and the behaviours chosen by people. Lalonde's approach was directed primarily toward the individual and toward individuals taking responsibility for their health. Proponents of the approach tended to focus on behaviours, and when illness or injury resulted, people felt "blamed" for not carrying out the recommended health behaviours, or not doing them "enough." Interventions focused on telling people what the healthy behaviour was, but did not address the social conditions that militated against its adoption. For instance, mothers were taught to follow Canada's Food Guide, but for women living in poverty, the means to purchase wholesome food were not accessible. People wishing to bike to work or school, as exhorted by *ParticipAction* advocates, took their lives in their hands as they competed with large vehicles for road space. This emphasis on lifestyle captured the attention of governments, and the social-environmental elements were consequently downplayed in health policy and funding until the next decade when it became evident that the health education and social marketing approach alone was not adequate to create the reduction in health expenditures envisioned by politicians and health planners who initially embraced this new perspective.

Although the Lalonde Report had obvious limitations, it did stimulate thought in a new direction and led to other important outcomes, not the least of which was the attention sparked across sectors such as economics, education, social welfare, and justice regarding the environmental imperatives of creating healthy people in healthy nations. As a result, the Lalonde Report received international attention, and in response to the growing concern about the disparities in health status between developed and undeveloped countries and between people with many resources and those with few, the World Health Organization (WHO) convened a meeting of member countries.

Declaration of Alma-Ata

The WHO member states met in Alma-Ata, Kazakhstan, in September 1978 to develop an action plan to achieve the goal of "Health for All by Year 2000," proposed as the vision by the 30th World Health Assembly (held in 1977). From this conference came the *Declaration of Alma-Ata* (WHO, 1978) on primary health care, viewed as the bridge between the Lalonde perspective and the influence of postmodern thinkers such as Marxists and other critical social activists who critiqued social structures to better understand and transform the dominant social order. As historical, cultural, and gendered social constructions were questioned, new ways of working with people emerged so that the people themselves (not the politicians or experts) could shape the world in which they live.

The Declaration of Alma-Ata (Box 1-1) became the philosophy of community action for health. Its emphasis on social justice, equity, public participation, appropriate technology, and intersectoral collaboration focused action on the needs of the population and the root causes of ill health, challenging the system to move from the traditional biomedical model (disease) to a framework that promoted health. Influenced by the work of Freire (1970) and others, the Declaration of Alma-Ata called for health providers to work *with* people to assist them in making decisions about their health and how to meet health challenges in ways that are affordable, acceptable, and sustainable in the long term. The Declaration also explicitly

---

BOX 1-1

The Declaration of Alma-Ata: Primary Health Care

Primary health care is essential health care based on practical, scientifically sound, and socially acceptable methods and technology made universally accessible to individuals and families in the community through their full participation and at a cost that the community and country can afford to maintain at every stage of their development in the spirit of self-reliance and self-determination. It forms an integral part both of the country's health system, of which it is the central function and main focus, and of the overall social and economic development of the community. It is the first level of contact of individuals, the family, and community with the national health system bringing health care as close as possible to where people live and work and constitutes the first element of a continuing health care process. (Article VI)

stated the elements of a health system that were essential to the achievement of health for all:

◆ Education about the prevailing health problems and their prevention and control
◆ Safe food supply and adequate nutrition
◆ Adequate supply of safe water and basic sanitation
◆ Maternal and child care, including family planning
◆ Immunization against basic infectious diseases
◆ Prevention and control of locally endemic diseases
◆ Appropriate treatment of common diseases and injuries
◆ Essential drugs

People who are homeless are one of the most vulnerable population groups in society, exposed to multiple hazards in a nonsupportive environment, diminishing their ability to stay healthy or to take the necessary steps to seek the services they need to become healthy. In many instances, homeless people fear and distrust formal health and social services and, as a result, make contact only when their situations are most dire and their health and social conditions have deteriorated extensively. Services that might be available to this population through the combined efforts of outreach teams, soup kitchens, shelters, and churches using a primary health care framework are illustrated in Table 1-1.

Other services that may be provided include postal facilities, distribution of welfare cheques, legal assistance, job skills education, work placement services, "inn from the cold" shelter in winter, bottled water in the heat of summer, transportation vouchers, and assisted housing. In every community that faces the challenge of homelessness, formal and informal agencies work with tireless volunteers to deliver these services in ways that respect the principles of Alma-Ata by:

◆ Ensuring that health and health services are geographically, financially, and culturally within reach of people living in poverty, ethnic and cultural minorities, rural residents, stigmatized populations, men and women across the life span
◆ Facilitating public participation and empowerment through citizen involvement in service planning, provision, and evaluation
◆ Creating conditions that support intersectoral and interdisciplinary collaborations and private–public–charity partnerships
◆ Adapting technology to the community and population's social, economic, and cultural needs and to its high-risk groups in ways that are sustainable in the long term
◆ Focusing on health promotion and disease and injury prevention within the context of the lives of the people served

Primary health care is more than the first point of contact with the health system. It implies the application of the primary health care philosophy that ensures public participation at all levels of the system, social justice and equity, and a system that balances prevention and promotion with the demands for care, cure, and rehabilitation. Primary health care also extends beyond the health system to the other societal systems that create conditions where health, not disease and injury,

TABLE 1-1
Essentials of Primary Health Care With an Application to Community Practice

ESSENTIALS OF PRIMARY HEALTH CARE	SERVICES OFFERED TO HOMELESS PEOPLE
Education about the prevailing health problems and their prevention and control	Education and counselling for alcohol and drug addictions; needle exchanges and safe havens for injecting drug users; safer sex education; violence prevention
Safe food supply and adequate nutrition	Meals; food bank; collective kitchen
Adequate supply of safe water and basic sanitation	Clothing; laundry and shower facilities and supplies (e.g., soap, shampoo, feminine hygiene products)
Maternal and child care, including family planning	Free male and female condoms; bad date reports for sex trade workers; prenatal care; parenting classes; preschool; respite care for parents (e.g., Calgary Children's Cottage)
Immunization against basic infectious diseases	Hepatitis B vaccination; childhood vaccines; influenza and pneumococcal vaccine
Prevention and control of locally endemic diseases	Directly observed tuberculosis medications; methadone clinics
Appropriate treatment of common diseases and injuries	Wound and foot care; dental care; mental illness treatment; infections; frostbite; fractures; general health conditions
Essential drugs	HIV medications; prenatal vitamins; lice treatments; antibiotics for communicable diseases

can flourish. It can exist not only in community practice but also in other aspects of human services when applied as a pervasive philosophy rather than just as a set of activities. We can see primary health care in action in participatory research, in emancipatory political action, in empowerment education in schools, and in other social movements where social justice, equity, and participation are valued.

A FRAMEWORK FOR HEALTH PROMOTION IN CANADA

In recognition of the social aspects of health promotion and as a signator of the Declaration of Alma-Ata, the Canadian government in 1986 published the discussion paper *A Framework for Health Promotion* (coined "the Epp Framework" for the Honourable Jake Epp, National Minister of Health and Welfare; Epp, 1986) in preparation for the WHO First International Health Promotion Conference in Ottawa held in that same year (Fig. 1-1).

The times during which the Epp Framework was developed were characterized by rapid and irreversible social change due to shifting family structures, an aging population, and wider participation in the workforce by women. These conditions exacerbate certain health problems, create pressure for new kinds of social support,

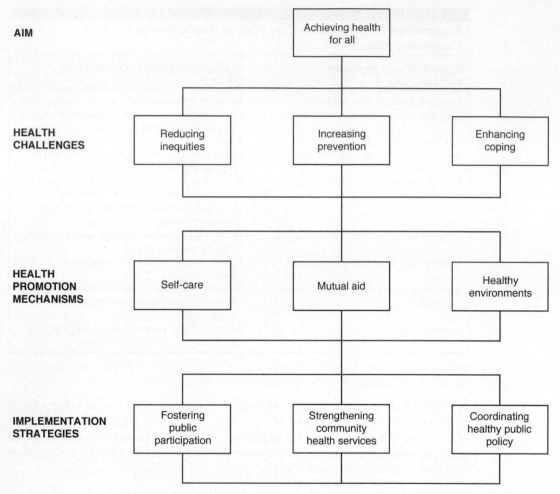

AIM

Achieving health
for all

HEALTH
CHALLENGES

Reducing
inequities

Increasing
prevention

Enhancing
coping

HEALTH
PROMOTION
MECHANISMS

Self-care

Mutual aid

Healthy
environments

IMPLEMENTATION
STRATEGIES

Fostering
public
participation

Strengthening
community
health services

Coordinating
healthy public
policy

FIGURE 1-1   ◆   A Framework for Health Promotion in Canada.

and force community workers to seek new approaches to deal effectively with the impact of these social forces on the future health of Canadians.

The framework defines health as a part of everyday living, an essential dimension of the quality of our lives. In this context, quality of life "implies the opportunities to make choices and gain satisfaction from living." Health is a state that individuals and communities alike strive to achieve, maintain, or regain and is influenced by circumstances, beliefs, culture, and socioeconomic and physical environments. This document reaffirmed the WHO definition of health promotion as "the process of enabling people to increase control over, and to improve, their health."

The **aim** of health promotion is the achievement of health for all. Although the prospects for health of Canadians have improved over recent decades, three major issues remain that are not being adequately addressed by current health policies and practices:

◆ Disadvantaged groups have significantly lower life expectancy, poorer health, and a higher prevalence of disability than the average Canadian.
◆ Various forms of preventable diseases and injuries continue to undermine the health and quality of life of many Canadians.
◆ Many thousands of Canadians suffer from chronic disease, disability, or various forms of emotional stress and lack adequate community support to help them cope and live meaningful, productive, and dignified lives (p. 1).

To achieve the goal of "health for all," ways must be found to overcome three *challenges*: reduce inequities in health status between Canadians with low and high incomes; increase the prevention effort and find new and more effective means to prevent injuries, illness, chronic conditions, and disabilities; and find ways to enhance people's ability to manage and cope with chronic conditions, disabilities, and mental health problems.

In the latter part of the 20th century, chronic conditions and mental health problems replaced communicable diseases as the predominant health problems among Canadians in all age groups. People with disabilities and mental health problems need skills and community support to lead stable and quality lives. Family members, especially women, care for others on a regular basis and also need support. Home support services, home nursing, and respite care services can enhance the coping capacity of both those with disabilities and their care providers.

Three *mechanisms* intrinsic to health promotion are self-care, or the decisions and actions individuals take in the interest of their own health; mutual aid, or the actions people take to help each other; and healthy environments, or the creation of conditions and surroundings conducive to health.

Self-care refers to the decisions made and the behaviours practised by an individual specifically for the preservation of health; encouraging self-care means encouraging healthy choices. An older person using a walking stick when sidewalks are icy, a teenager choosing a fruit for a snack, people engaging in physical activity, choosing not to smoke—these are all examples of self-care. Beliefs, access to appropriate information, and being in surroundings that are supportive are factors that play important roles in making healthy choices.

Mutual aid refers to people's efforts to work together to deal with concerns; it implies people helping each other; supporting each other emotionally; and sharing ideas, information, and experiences. Frequently referred to as social support, mutual aid may arise in the context of the family, the community, a voluntary organization, a self-help group, informal networks, or a special interest association.

Strong evidence indicates that people who have social support are healthier than those who do not; social support enables people to live interdependently within a *healthy environment* while still retaining their independence. A parent with a special-needs child, an older person recovering from a stroke, an adolescent using drugs—these are people who not only need professional services but also need the understanding and the sense of belonging that comes with being in a socially, physically, and economically supportive environment built in a manner that supports interaction and community integration to preserve and enhance health where we live, worship, work, play, and learn. From this perspective, the environment is all encompassing; it includes the buildings in our community, the air we breathe, and the jobs we do. It is also the education, transportation, justice, social services, political, and health systems.

The three leading *strategies* by which we can act in response to the challenges are fostering public participation, strengthening community services, and coordinating healthy public policy. These strategies, in addition to the mechanisms, are mutually reinforcing; one strategy or mechanism on its own will not create significant outcomes.

Public participation is essential to the achievement of health for all Canadians. Encouraging public participation means helping people take part in decisions that influence or control factors that affect health. People (citizens, residents, schools, workplaces, communities) must be equipped and enabled to act, to channel their energy, skills, and creativity to build community capacity and enhance social capital. (Refer to Chapter 6 for more information.)

Community services play a critical role in preserving health, particularly if they are expressly oriented toward promoting health and preventing disease/injury. A health promotion and disease/injury prevention orientation means that community services will need to focus more on dealing with the major health challenges we have identified. Greater emphasis will need to be placed on providing services to groups that are disadvantaged, communities will need to become more involved in planning services, and links between communities and their services and institutions will need to be strengthened. In these ways, community health services will assume a key role in fostering self-care, mutual aid, and the creation of healthy environments.

Public policy has considerable potential to influence people's everyday lives; it has the power to provide people with opportunities for health or to deny them such opportunities. All policies, and hence all sectors, have a bearing on health. What we seek is *healthy public policy*. All policies that have direct or indirect bearing on the health of Canadians need to be coordinated. The list is long and includes the broad determinants of health (discussed in greater detail later in this chapter), and income security, employment, education, housing, economy, agriculture, transportation, justice, and technology. It is not an easy undertaking to coordinate policies among various sectors, all of which obviously have their own priorities, because health is not necessarily a priority for other sectors. Conflicting interests may exist between and among sectors. Take, for example, tobacco. Health promoters are proponents of a smoke-free environment, but some Canadian farmers cultivate this product for their livelihood. Therefore, changes in tobacco policy have broad implications for the economy as well as health. For public policies to be healthy, they must respond to the health needs of people and their communities; this is so whether they are developed in government offices, legislatures, board rooms, church halls, union meetings, schools, workplaces, or seniors' recreation centres.

GLOBAL CONFERENCES ON HEALTH PROMOTION

In 1986, the WHO convened the First International Conference on Health Promotion, which resulted in the publication of the *Ottawa Charter for Health Promotion*, jointly with the Canadian Public Health Association and Health and Welfare Canada (WHO, 1986). The Ottawa Charter explicitly identified the *prerequisites for health* as peace, shelter, education, food, income, a stable ecosystem, sustainable resources, and social justice and equity. The health promotion processes of enabling, advocating, and mediating were identified. *Advocacy* aims to create the socioenvironmental conditions necessary for health. *Enabling* aims to ensure equal opportunities for achieving health and reducing inequities in health status. *Mediation* between different interests is required to ensure the collaboration needed among disciplines, agencies, and sectors to coordinate action and policy efforts. In the Charter, five *strategies* for health promotion were identified: building healthy public policy, creating supportive environments, strengthening community action, developing personal skills, and reorienting health services (Fig. 1-2). This landmark document built on the Declaration of Alma-Ata and Canadian leadership and is considered to be the formal beginning of what is referred to as "the new public health movement." It was hailed as a signal for change in direction and policy for the reorientation of the health system.

Five International Health Promotion Conferences have followed since 1986: in Adelaide, Australia; Sundsvall, Sweden; Jakarta, Indonesia; Mexico City, Mexico; and Bangkok, Thailand. At each conference, participants reaffirmed commitment to the Ottawa Charter and extended the discourse by focusing research and discussion on a single Ottawa Charter strategy and making recommendations for action.

In Adelaide, Australia (WHO, 1988), participants called on those who make public policy to examine and be responsive to the health impacts of their policies. Pleas were made for industrialized nations to provide assistance to underdeveloped nations to reduce health disparities. Four priority areas for action were identified: support for the health of women; elimination of hunger and malnutrition; reduction of tobacco growing and alcohol production; and the creation of more supportive environments by aligning with the peace, environmental, and health movements.

The Third International Conference was held in Sundsvall, Sweden, in 1991 (WHO, 1991). Here, the theme was on supportive environments for health, and the Conference highlighted four aspects of supportive environments: (1) the social dimension, which includes the ways in which norms, customs, and social processes affect health, (2) the political dimension, which requires governments to guarantee democratic participation in decision making and the decentralization of responsibilities and

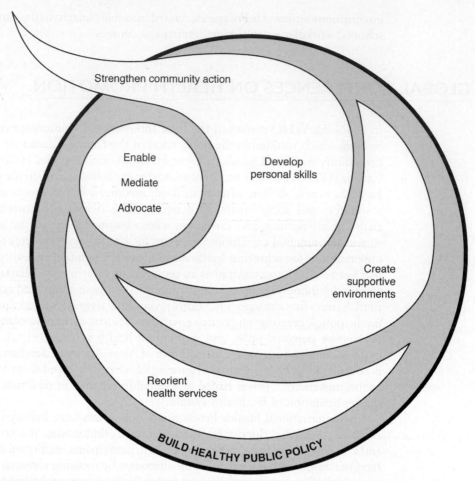

FIGURE 1-2 ◆ Ottawa Charter for Health Promotion. (Note: for an explanation of the logo, see http://www.who.int/healthpromotion/conferences/previous/ottawa/en/index4.html)

resources, (3) the economic dimension, which requires a rechannelling of resources for the achievement of "Health for All" and sustainable development, including safe and reliable technology, and (4) the need to recognize and use women's skills and knowledge in all sectors to develop a more positive infrastructure for supportive environments. Conference recommendations for action were to strengthen advocacy through community action, particularly through groups organized by women; enable communities and individuals to take control of their health and environment through education and empowerment; build alliances to strengthen cooperation between health and environment campaigns; and mediate between conflicting interests in society to ensure equitable access to a supportive environment for health.

Six years later, at the Fourth International Conference in Jakarta, Indonesia (the first to be held in a developing country), the *Jakarta Declaration on Leading Health Promotion into the 21st Century* (WHO, 1997) expanded the conditions (prerequisites) for health to include also social security, social relations, empowerment of women, sustainable resource use, and respect for human rights. "Above all, poverty is the greatest threat to health." The statement noted the need for comprehensive approaches that work on several levels, within various settings, and effective partnerships among all levels of government, nongovernmental organizations (NGOs), and private and public sectors. Five priorities were set: (1) promote social responsibility for health, (2) increase investments for health development, (3) consolidate and expand partnerships for health, (4) increase community capacity and empower the individual, and (5) secure an infrastructure for health promotion.

In 1999, the Fifth Global Health Promotion Conference was held in Mexico City, Mexico (WHO, 1999); the theme was on bridging the equity gap and recommended strengthening the "art and science" (evidence base) of health promotion and strengthening political skills and actions for health promotion to ensure healthy public policy. Processes suggested to achieve the recommendations were solidarity among practitioners and activists through networks, alliances, and partnerships; mobilization of resources; development of community capacity; development of human resources; and the creation of networks and associations of practitioners for mutual support and personal development.

Most recently, a sixth global conference was health in Bangkok, Thailand, in 2005, resulting in an affirmation of the Ottawa Charter and extending it to the globalized world (WHO, 2005). The Bangkok Charter provides new direction to health promotion by calling for policy coherence, investment and partnering among governments, international organizations, and civil society and the private sector to create a worldwide collaboration to fulfil the promise of the Ottawa Charter and deliver the strategies that will ensure health for all peoples. The challenges faced in achieving the aim of health promotion means addressing the changing global health context, including harnessing the effects of the double burden of communicable and chronic diseases, widening inequities, rapid urbanization, and the degradation of environments, all of which contribute to increasing the gaps in health status and causing significant health inequalities between nations of the world. As Professor Sir Michael Marmot (2005), Chair of the WHO Commission on the Social Determinants of Health, stated: "It is not inevitable that there should be a spread of life expectancy of 48 years among countries and 20 years or more within countries. A burgeoning volume of research identifies social factors at the root of much of these inequalities in health." The Bangkok Charter (WHO, 2005) calls for all sectors and settings to advocate for health based on human rights and solidarity; invest in sustainable policies, actions, and infrastructure to address the determinants of health; build capacity for policy development, leadership, health promotion practice, knowledge transfer, research, and health literacy; regulate and legislate to ensure a high level of protection from harm and enable equal opportunity for health and well-being for all people; and partner and build alliances with public, private, nongovernmental, and international organizations and civil society to create sustainable actions. It recommends four key commitments:

◆ Make the promotion of health central to the global development agenda.
◆ Make the promotion of health a core responsibility for all governments.
◆ Make the promotion of health a key focus of communities and civil society.
◆ Make the promotion of health a requirement for good corporate practice.

In 2007, the International Union for Health Promotion and Education (IUHPE) will hold its 19th World Conference, "Health Promotion Comes of Age: Research, Policy & Practice for the 21st Century," in Vancouver, British Columbia, further advancing the health promotion agenda in Canada and around the globe.

POPULATION HEALTH

Canadian influence on global health promotion is strong on the international scene; Canadian researchers, policymakers, educators, and practitioners have contributed significantly to each of the WHO conferences. For instance, the Healthy Cities movement began in Canada and has become a dominant force in European countries. Health promotion research, supported by Health Canada through the formation of five funded Canadian Centres for Health Promotion in 1995, has had international impact. Much of the work of these centres has been presented at WHO global conferences. However, on the home front, leadership in health promotion has been challenged by traditional biomedical and economic rationalist approaches to policy, care, and research that pervade the Canadian health context. The influence of biostatisticians, epidemiologists, and social demographers is evident by the attraction of policymakers to the population health perspective. Leadership for health promotion at Health Canada has been dispersed, a quarterly journal on the field has been cancelled, funding for the five centres has not been sustained, and none of the 13 Canadian Institutes for Health Research (CIHR) has been dedicated to health promotion research. Instead, the term "population health" has become preeminent (Box 1-2).

CIHR's 13 institutes are Aboriginal Peoples' Health; Aging; Cancer Research; Circulatory and Respiratory Health; Gender and Health; Genetics; Health Services and Policy Research; Human Development, Child and Youth Health; Infection and Immunity; Musculoskeletal Health and Arthritis; Neurosciences, Mental Health and Addiction; Nutrition, Metabolism and Diabetes; and Population and Public Health.

Population health is the term used to describe an approach that is founded on epidemiologic principles, statistical measures, and economic conservatism. Population health provides the data that underscore the importance of factors other than the health care system in determining or influencing the health of large groups (populations). Population health, like health promotion, focuses on the larger scope than the individual. Unlike health promotion, however, it is not rooted in empowerment,

> **BOX 1-2**
>
> **Definition of Terms**
>
> ---
>
> **Primary health care:** first described in the Declaration of Alma-Ata (WHO, 1978), primary health care refers to the five principles on which action on "health for all" must be based: equitable access to health and health services, public participation, appropriate technology, intersectoral collaboration, and reorientation of the health system to promotion of health and prevention of disease and injury. The Declaration further details eight essentials—services that nations must have in place to create positive conditions for health.
>
>   **Critical social action theory:** attempts to describe and explain oppressive social conditions that limit people from reaching their full potential. In relation to health, its ultimate goal is to liberate (emancipate) people from health-damaging environmental conditions (Stevens & Hall, 1992). This approach involves exposing inequities, empowering citizen engagement, improving health literacy, and creating change.
>
>   **Health promotion:** the process of enabling people to exercise control over those factors and conditions that influence their health. Health promotion is viewed as a collective, rather than individual, activity and has five key strategies: develop personal skills, create supportive environments, strengthen community action, build healthy public policy, and reorient health services.
>
>   **Population health:** the health of a population as measured by health status indicators and as influenced by social, economic, and physical environments; personal health practices; individual capacity and coping skills; human biology; early childhood development; and health services.
>
>   **Population health promotion:** integration of population health concepts with the principles that guide action on health promotion in efforts to maximize the likelihood of reinforcing and maintaining synergistic effects in health programming.
>
>   **Population health approach:** a strategic administrative focus on the complex interrelated conditions and factors that influence population health, which uses information regarding patterns and trends in health status indicators to create healthy public policy and respond to the needs of Canadians through targeted intervention programs.

community development, qualitative research, social justice, or political advocacy. It purports to be more objective in its stance, citing facts and suggesting causal pathways, without necessarily recommending action. Once the four health fields were articulated in the Lalonde Report (1974), population health scientists stepped up study on the impacts of lifestyle and the environment on health status. This activity led to the identification of a broader range of health determinants, the specification of targets for health promotion, and the description of settings where health promotion can occur.

Although a certain tension exists because of some philosophical differences (Coburn & Poland, 1995), the two perspectives are complementary. Health promoters appreciate the legitimacy that population health scientists have given to their long-standing concern about the impact of social forces on health (Labonté,

1995). Population health scientists are now accepting findings from qualitative research and experiential/traditional knowledge as legitimate evidence.

Determinants of Health

Central to population health science was the question: "Why are some people healthy and others are not?" (Evans, Barer, & Marmor, 1994). Because health and social services are provincial matters, several provinces commissioned studies to address this concern, leading to the publication of reports that suggested that the impacts of health care services on the health of citizens were far less than expected and that lifestyles and the social, economic, and physical environments had a potentially larger impact on health status. As technologies improved and extensive databases were created and used to correlate various factors, national population health surveys were carried out, and the scientific community began to create models that suggested causal pathways for health. Canadian Institute for Advanced Research (CIAR) scientists Evans and Stoddard (1990) chronicled the evolution of a model that illustrates feedback loops for human well-being and economic costs (Fig. 1-3).

This model uses the absence of disease as the definition of health because it is more easily operationalized than definitions proposed by health promotion proponents. As well, deaths (and to some extent illness and injury) can be counted, so "absence or presence of disease" became an index to measure health status. In its

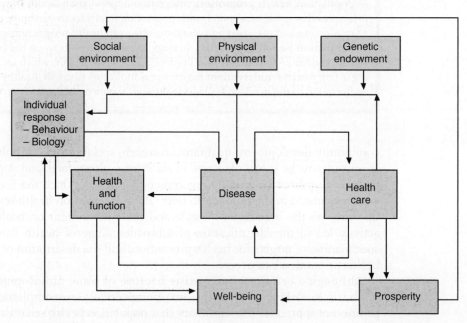

FIGURE 1-3   ◆   Feedback loop for human well-being and economic costs.

initial conceptualization, the authors described people getting sick or injured from unspecified reasons and presenting themselves to the health care system, where the diseases or injuries are diagnosed, treatment needs are defined, and the system responds. The level of response is determined by the access to care and technology, and its provision in turn reduces the level of disease/injury and the person returns to health. However, as technology advanced and health care costs rose in response to demands, evidence was growing that interventions and structural changes outside the health system were needed to effect further improvements in the health status of the population.

The four-field framework described by Lalonde was incorporated into the CIAR model, so instead of the "unspecified factors" that contributed to illness and injury, human biology, lifestyle, and environment were added to the mix. However, in the years subsequent to the publication of the Lalonde Report, lifestyle choices were increasingly seen to be influenced by social and physical environmental factors, and it was found that underlying conditions influence susceptibility to a whole range of diseases as well as personal sense of well-being and productivity. This complex interaction of factors has provided the foundation for a vast array of research on human behaviour, biologic responses to social and physical environments, and the effects of economic trade-offs on health and well-being. Research has shown that living and working conditions, such as housing, income, social support, work stress, and education, make a difference in the number and quality of years lived (Frank, 1995).

To further describe the evidence being generated by population health scientists, the Federal/Provincial/Territorial Advisory Committee on Population Health (ACPH) published in 1994 its discussion document *Strategies for Population Health: Investing in the Health of Canadians*. The Canadian Health Network and others have extended the list of health determinants, which now comprises 12 determinants, and researchers are continuing to refine our understanding and will perhaps expand the list further in years to come. The current accepted list of determinants, along with their descriptions, are found in Table 1-2.

Target Populations

By incorporating the determinants, health services and health promotion activities have become targeted to specific groups within the population that had "needs" or deficits that could be addressed to improve health status. This approach rested on the foundation of risk factor assessment; that is, if people will reduce or eliminate risk-taking behaviours, and if risky environments could be fixed, then population health would improve. Therefore, individuals, groups, or aggregates of individuals, families, communities, and society itself became targets for action and intervention.

Many programs were directed toward individuals and aggregates—developing personal skills for healthy behaviours through health education and social marketing. Because, for instance, adolescent pregnancy is viewed as detrimental to health of women and their infants, campaigns to strengthen families, enhance the availability

TABLE 1-2
Determinants of Health

Income and social status	Health status improves at each step up the income and social hierarchy. Higher income levels affect living conditions such as safe housing and the ability to buy sufficient and healthy food.
Social support networks	Support from families, friends, and communities is associated with better health. The health effect of the support of family and friends who provide a caring and supportive relationship may be as important as risk factors such as smoking, physical activity, obesity, and high blood pressure.
Education	Health status improves with level of education. Education increases opportunities for income and job security and gives people a sense of control over their lives—key factors that influence health.
Employment and working conditions	Unemployment, underemployment, and stressful work are associated with poorer health. Those with more control over their work and fewer stress-related demands on the job are healthier.
Social environments	The values and norms of a society affect the health and well-being of individuals and populations. Social stability, recognition of diversity, safety, good relationships, and cohesive communities provide a supportive society, which reduces or removes many risks to good health.
Physical environments	Physical factors in the natural environment (e.g., air and water quality) are key influences on health. Factors in the human-built environment, such as housing, workplace safety, and community and road design are also important influences.
Personal health practices and coping skills	Social environments that enable and support healthy choices and lifestyles, as well as people's knowledge, behaviours, and coping skills for dealing with life in healthy ways, are key influences on health.
Healthy child development	The effect of prenatal and early childhood experiences on subsequent health, well-being, coping skills, and competence is very powerful. For example, a low weight at birth links with health and social problems throughout life.
Culture	Culture comes from both personal history and wider situational, social, political, geographic, and economic factors. Multicultural health issues demonstrate how necessary it is to consider the interrelationships of physical, mental, spiritual, social, and economic well-being.
Gender	Gender refers to the many different roles, personality traits, attitudes, behaviours, values, relative powers, and influences that society assigns to the two sexes. Each sex has specific health issues or may be affected in different ways by the same issues.
Biology and genetic endowment	Physical characteristics we inherit play a part in deciding how long we live, how healthy we will be, and how likely we are to get certain illnesses.
Health services	It benefits people's health when they have access to services that prevent disease as well as maintain and promote health.

From www.canadian-health-network.ca and http://www.phac-aspc.gc.ca/ph-sp/phdd/determinants/index.html#determinants also, Frankish, C. J., Moulton, G. E., Quantz, D., Carson, A. J., Casebeer, A. L., Eyles, J. D., et al. (2007). Addressing the non-medical determinants of health: A survey of Canada's health regions. *Canadian Journal of Public Health, 98*(1), 41–47.

of birth control, delay the onset of sexual activity, and promote abstinence were mounted across the nation. Motor vehicle mortality was addressed through programs aimed primarily at young men who drive while under the influence of alcohol and programs that exhorted people to use seatbelts in vehicles. The "BreakFree" campaign for youth tobacco reduction is an example of how program planners further categorized the target population through demographics. Youth were surveyed and then described in terms of subpopulations of youth, and messages were targeted accordingly, on the assumption that rural and urban youth, athletes, and honours students would respond to different marketing strategies to reduce tobacco use.

Other programs were directed to creating more supportive family environments for health; for instance, children of families living in poverty were provided educational opportunities in such programs as Head Start that prepared them for school entry, Nobody's Perfect that enhanced parenting skills, and Brighter Futures that supported early childhood development through family nutrition and prenatal support.

At the same time as Canadians' attitudes toward health and wellness were changing, social conventions were being altered so that behaviours such as tobacco use, substance use, domestic violence, and drinking and driving have become increasingly socially unacceptable. In addition, the move toward self-determination through public participation in policy decision making has become an imperative rather than a luxury. Canadians now expect to be consulted on matters that relate to health, and health is defined more broadly than the absence of disease.

Settings

Not only have the targets for health interventions expanded from the individual level but also settings for health service provision and health promotion expanded from health settings (e.g., hospitals, clinics, etc.) to settings where people live, work, worship, play, and go to school. The WHO Healthy Cities, Comprehensive School Health, and Healthy Workplace movements were attempts to develop strong communities and build social capacity and human capital that would enhance and strengthen the ability of communities, schools, and workplaces to influence the health and well-being of their residents, students and teachers, and employees.

The environment or context provided by various settings also contributes to health. As settings began to change and adapt in response to the needs and preferences of society, so, too, did environmental change affect people. That people behave or respond differently in different situations, contexts, and settings has led program planners to view the environment as a predisposing, enabling, and reinforcing factor for individual and collective behaviour (Green, Poland, & Rootman, 2000). Green and Kreuter (1991) state that the effectiveness of a health strategy depends on its fit with the target population, the health issue involved, and the environment in which it is applied. Using the setting as a focus fosters outcomes that are adaptable and sensitive to particular traditions, cultures, and circumstances. A multilevel, multicultural, multisectoral intervention runs the risk of being expensive and perhaps essentially meaningless, as well as not evaluable, because of the breadth of its target, lack of focus, and inability to specify indicators for assessing effectiveness. Hence, we are seeing the implementation of healthy workplace projects, comprehensive school health programs, and parish health initiatives as means of influencing the health of Canadians.

POPULATION HEALTH PROMOTION

In response to the growing debate and tension among health promotion practitioners and population health scientists, Hamilton and Bhatti (1996), instead of entering the debate, offered for discussion a model they termed *Population Health Promotion* (Fig. 1-4). This model has been adapted over time to embrace levels of action, determinants of health, action strategies, and the foundations for practice in health promotion (Flynn, 1999).

In this model, the central concepts and action strategies of the Ottawa Charter for Health Promotion, 12 determinants of health, and targets and/or settings are integrated with evidence-based decision making to ensure that policies and programs focus on the right issues, take effective action, and produce sound results.

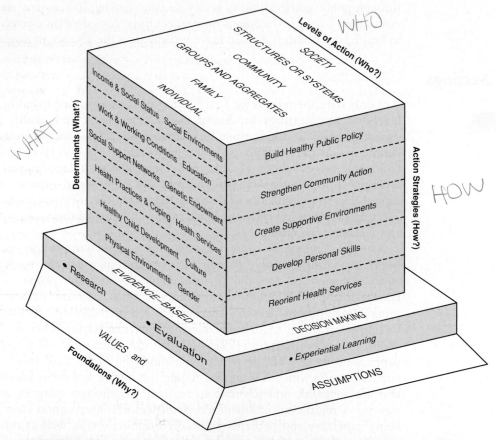

FIGURE 1-4 ◆ Population health promotion model. (Redrawn by Flynn [1999] from Hamilton, N. & Bhatti, T. [1996]. *Population health promotion: An integrated model of population health and health promotion*. Ottawa: Health Canada.)

Evidence is derived from three principal sources: research, experience, and evaluation studies. The model is based on the following underlying assumptions and values:

◆ Policy and program decision makers agree that comprehensive action needs to be taken on all the determinants of health using the knowledge gained from research and practice.

◆ It is the role of health organizations to analyze the full range of possibilities for action, to act on those determinants that are within their jurisdiction, and to influence other sectors to ensure their policies and programs have a positive impact on health. This can best be achieved by facilitating collaboration among stakeholders regarding the most appropriate activities to be undertaken by each.

◆ Multiple points of entry to planning and implementation are essential; however, there is a need for overall coordination of activity.

◆ Health problems may affect certain groups more than others. However, the solution to these problems involves changing social values and structures. It is the responsibility of the society as a whole to take care of all its members.

◆ The health of individuals and groups is a combined result of their own health practices and the impact of the physical and social environments in which they live, learn, work, pray, and play. There is an interaction among people and their surroundings. Settings, consisting of places and things, have a physical and psychological impact on people's health.

◆ To enjoy optimal health, people need opportunities to meet their physical, mental, social, and spiritual needs. This is possible in an environment that is based on the principles of social justice and equity and where relationships are built on mutual respect and caring, rather than on power and status.

◆ Health care, health protection, and disease prevention initiatives complement health promotion. Comprehensive approaches will include a strategic mix of the different possibilities for action. Meaningful participation of people in the development and operationalization of policies and programs is essential for them to influence the decisions that affect their health. (Hamilton & Bhatti, 1996, p. 3)

Hamilton and Bhatti (1996) make the distinction between risk factors and risk conditions. *Risk factors* are elements, often behaviour patterns, that tend to dispose people to poorer health and are modifiable through strategies that create individual behaviour change. *Risk conditions*, on the other hand, are general circumstances over which people have little or no control that are known to affect health status. Risk conditions are usually a result of public policy and are modified through collective action and social reform.

The population health promotion model allows for the integration of new knowledge from research, experience, and evaluation. It offers an analytic tool to assess situations that put people at risk, to assess populations at risk, and to move away from a victim-blaming approach to a more comprehensive determination of factors that contribute to ill health and injury.

POPULATION HEALTH APPROACH

Health Canada and the Public Health Agency of Canada have adopted the *population health approach* by which action is focused toward improved health outcomes, a sustainable and integrated health system, increased national growth and productivity, and strengthened social cohesion. The key elements of this approach are:

◆ Address the determinants of health, recognizing that they are complex and interrelated.
◆ Focus on the health of populations.
◆ Invest upstream.
◆ Base decisions on evidence.
◆ Apply multiple strategies to act on the determinants of health.
◆ Collaborate across levels and sectors.
◆ Use mechanisms to engage citizens.
◆ Increase accountability for health outcomes.

More detail on this approach is available from the Health Canada website (**http://www.phac-aspc.gc.ca/ph-sp/phdd/**). In this chapter, the current understanding of the *determinants of health* has been presented; our knowledge will continue to further develop, evolve, and be refined as interventions are implemented and success chronicled. *Investing upstream* means directing attention at the root causes of illness and injury, rather than at the symptoms that are evident. In this way, interventions can be placed earlier in the causal stream and provide greater gains in population health. Traditional and new sources of qualitative and quantitative research and evaluation *evidence* are used to set priorities and identify best practices for influencing health; this is called evidence-based decision making. A *variety of strategies* applied in a variety of settings are required to create joint action among health and other sectors to effectively influence the factors and improve the health of Canadians. *Collaboration* and horizontal management strategies will require agreement on common goals, coordinated planning, development of related policies, and implementation of integrated programs and services. To do this means that citizens need to be engaged in all aspects of health and social service priority setting, the determination of appropriate interventions, and the review of outcomes. (Chapter 6 discusses *public participation* in detail.) Accountability requires that process, impact, and outcome evaluations be undertaken to assess changes in health status and that the results of evaluations be reported widely not only to the scientific community but also to the public.

In summary, this approach has been articulated by the government of Canada as a unifying force for the entire spectrum of health system interventions—from prevention, promotion, and protection to diagnosis, treatment, care, and rehabilitation—that integrates and balances actions among them. As an approach, population health targets factors that influence the health of Canadians across the life span, identifies variations in patterns of health, and uses the resulting knowledge to plan and implement interventions and policies to improve the nation's health status. Even though health and social services are funded by the provinces and territories, Health Canada and the Public Health Agency of Canada exercise strong leadership roles in setting direction and standards in efforts to improve Canadians' health.

IMPLICATIONS OF POPULATION HEALTH PROMOTION FOR "COMMUNITY AS PARTNER"

In 1986, the WHO took the lead in providing the scope, definition, and a framework for action to create "Health for All by Year 2000" as mandated by the Declaration of Alma-Ata (WHO, 1978). The Ottawa Charter serves to this day as the foundation of health promotion, and as action has taken place, the evidence generated by evaluation and research has expanded. Health Canada has sponsored several population health surveys, created the Canadian Institutes for Health Research (CIHR) and the Canadian Institute of Health Information (CIHI) to gather and report evidence, and has realigned the organization to support and promote a population health approach. Health promotion is a key means of taking action on population health. Consequently, this book is written to be consistent both with the population health approach and the fundamental principles of health promotion. In Chapter 2, the ethics of community practice are discussed. Chapter 3 presents the basics of epidemiology as the foundation of understanding patterns of health in populations. The five strategies of the Ottawa Charter are presented in Chapters 4 through 8. Part 1 ends with chapters discussing culture and diversity, health informatics, and emerging threats to community health. In Part 2, the process of working with community is detailed, and in Part 3, case stories are presented that offer examples of successful population health promotion interventions in a variety of settings with a range of target groups.

SUMMARY

In this chapter, the history and development of the modern approach to health is chronicled. The Lalonde Report (1974) signalled a paradigm shift in how health was viewed, and the Declaration of Alma-Ata (WHO, 1978) provided the foundational philosophy by which to attain the goal of "health for all." Five subsequent International Health Promotion Conferences extended the understanding of the processes (advocacy, enabling, and mediating) and five action strategies for practice. The Canadian Institute of Advanced Research in population health furthered the understanding of the determinants of health, creating conditions for the formation of a population health promotion model (Hamilton & Bhatti, 1996). The policy stance now taken by Health Canada and the Public Health Agency of Canada is based on its population health approach to policy and programming.

Thus, the stage is set for readers to further investigate key concepts and develop a process for partnering with communities to enhance health and well-being.

References

Coburn, D., & Poland, B. (1995). The CIAR vision of the determinants of health: A critique. *Canadian Journal of Public Health, 87*(5), 308–310.

Epp, J. (1986). Achieving health for all: A framework for health promotion. Ottawa: National Health and Welfare.

Evans, R., Barer, M., & Marmor, T. (Eds.). (1994). Why are some people healthy and others not? New York: Aldine.

Evans, R., & Stoddard, G. (1990). Producing health, consuming health care. *Social Science and Medicine, 31*(12), 1347–1363.

Federal/Provincial/Territorial Advisory Committee on Population Health (1994). *Strategies for population health: Investing in the health of Canadians.* Ottawa: Health Canada.

Flynn, L. (1999). *An adaptation of the Hamilton and Bhatti (1996) Population Health Promotion Model.* Manitoba and Saskatchewan Region: Health Canada.

Frank, J. (1995). Why "population health"? *Canadian Journal of Public Health, 86*(3), 162–164.

Frankish, C. J., Moulton, G. E., Quantz, D., Carson, A. J., Casebeer, A. L., Eyles, J. D., et al. (2007). Addressing the non-medical determinants of health: A survey of Canada's health regions. *Canadian Journal of Public Health, 98*(1), 41–47.

Freire, P. (1970). *Pedagogy of the oppressed.* New York: Continuum.

Green, L. W., & Kreuter, M. W. (1991). *Health promotion planning: An educational and environmental approach.* Mountain View, CA: Mayfield.

Green, L. W., Poland, B., & Rootman, I. (2000). The settings approach to health promotion. In B. Poland, L. W. Green, & I. Rootman (Eds.), *Settings for health promotion.* Thousand Oaks, CA: Sage.

Hamilton, N., & Bhatti, T. (1996). *Population health promotion: An integrated model of population health and health promotion.* Ottawa: Health Canada.

Labonte, R. (1995). Population health and health promotion: What do they have to say to each other? *Canadian Journal of Public Health, 86*(3), 165–168.

Lalonde, M. (1974). *New perspectives on the health of Canadians.* Ottawa: National Health and Welfare.

Marmot, M. (2005). New Bangkok charter for health promotion adopted to address rapidly changing global health issues; WHO press release: August 11, 2005. Retrieved June 2, 2007 from **http://www.who.int/mediacentre/news/releases/2005/pr34/en**

Stevens, P. E., & Hall, J. M. (1992). Applying critical theories to nursing in communities. *Public Health Nursing, 9*(1), 2–9.

World Health Organization. (1978). *declaration of Alma-Ata on primary health care.* Geneva, Switzerland: Author.

World Health Organization. (1986). *Ottawa charter for health promotion.* Geneva, Switzerland: Author.

World Health Organization. (1988). *Adelaide recommendations.* Geneva, Switzerland: Author.

World Health Organization. (1991). *Sundsvall statement on supportive environments for health.* Geneva, Switzerland: Author.

World Health Organization. (1997). *Jakarta declaration on leading health promotion into the 21st century.* Geneva, Switzerland: Author.

World Health Organization. (1999). *Health promotion: Bridging the equity gap.* Geneva, Switzerland: Author.

World Health Organization. (2005). *Bangkok Charter for health promotion in a globalized world.* Geneva, Switzerland: Author.

Internet Resources _____

www.who.int/healthpromotion/conferences/previous/adelaide/en/
Adelaide Recommendations

http://www.who.int/healthpromotion/conferences/6gchp/bangkok_charter/en/
Bangkok Charter

www.canadian-health-network.ca
Canadian Health Network

www.who.int/hpr/NPH/docs/declaration_almaata.pdf
Declaration of Alma-Ata

http://www.iuhpeconference.org/
IUHPE Conference Canada 2007

http://www.who.int/healthpromotion/conferences/previous/jakarta/en/
Jakarta Declaration

http://www.who.int/healthpromotion/conferences/previous/mexico/en/
Mexico Conference Report

www.who.int/healthpromotion/conferences/previous/ottawa/en/
Ottawa Charter

http://www.phac-aspc.gc.ca/ph-sp/phdd
Population Health Approach

www.who.int/healthpromotion/conferences/previous/sundsvall/en/
Sundsvall Statement

2

Ethics for Community Practice

FRANCES E. RACHER

Chapter Outline

Introduction
Key Concepts in Ethical Practice
Ethical Diversity Underpins Community
    Practice
Ethical Theories
Ethical Foundations of Public Health and
    Community Practice

Advances in Ethics for Community
    Practice
Ethical Challenges in Community
    Practice
Summary

Learning Objectives

After studying this chapter, you should be able to:

❖ Define the key concepts in ethical practice

❖ Outline the differences between ethical pluralism and ethical relativism

❖ Discuss the ethical theories of rule ethics, virtue ethics, and feminist ethics

❖ Delineate the ethical principles of rule ethics and their application to practice

❖ Describe the ethical foundations of public health and community practice

❖ Identify ethical challenges in community practice and apply ethical principles, foundations, and strategies for their resolution

Introduction

*T*raditionally, health care and human services ethics have focused on the individual client. Defining the community as client or partner, however, requires a different ethical approach, an approach focused on the aggregate, community, or societal level. In this chapter, the evolution of rule ethics, virtue ethics, and feminist ethics will move the community practitioner from considerations of the traditional ethical principles to consider also the ethical foundations of public health and community practice. Challenges in ethical practice are identified, and the discussion of ethical principles and foundations prepares the practitioner for application of ethical theory to practice. Practitioners are encouraged to consider relationships, environments, and dialogues with and among health professionals and the communities in which they work. Together, answers can be sought to ethical dilemmas. Through discussion and action based on respect for all people and their inclusion, diversity, participation, and empowerment, solutions can be achieved. Advocacy is required to reach the goals of social justice and healthy interdependence among peoples and their communities.

KEY CONCEPTS IN ETHICAL PRACTICE

Ethics is the philosophical study of morality, the discipline that deals with the rightness or wrongness of actions. Ethics is the systematic examination and critical reflection on living morally, designed to illuminate behaviour that should be taken in consideration of ordinary actions, judgments, and justifications (Beauchamp & Childress, 2001). The terms *ethics*, from ancient Greek roots, and *morality*, from Latin origin will be used interchangeably.

Practical ethics involve the use of ethical theory and methods of analysis to examine moral problems, practices, and policies. *Professional ethics* emphasize the primacy of relationships in light of practitioner obligations to those served (Storch, 2004). *Bioethics*, a relatively new field of inquiry first coined in the early 1970s, is the systematic study of the moral dimensions of the life sciences and health care, employing a variety of ethical methodologies in an interdisciplinary setting (Johnstone, 2004).

Values are attitudes or beliefs about the importance of a goal, object, principle, or behaviour (Canadian Nurses Association, 2002). Values are ideals that have importance or significance to individuals, groups, communities, or societies. For example, the *Canadian Charter of Rights and Freedoms* documents the societal values of individual freedom, health, fairness, honesty, and integrity (Department of Justice, 1982). *Principles* are fundamental guiding standards for action, the precursors for more specific rules of conduct (Volbrecht, 2002). *Ethical principles* are general standards of conduct derived from moral theory, used to guide moral behaviour and support the uptake of consistent moral perspectives and positions (Keatings & Smith, 2000). Ethical principles are stated in many professional codes of ethics. Examples of ethical principles are beneficence and autonomy. *Virtues* are defining traits, strengths of character, and standards for noble conduct that predispose the possessor to consistent excellence of intent and human performance. Virtue denotes the quality or practice of moral excellence (Johnstone, 2004). Compassion, respectfulness, and trustworthiness are commonly identified virtues.

ETHICAL DIVERSITY UNDERPINS COMMUNITY PRACTICE

Diversity or pluralism of moral values and beliefs is characteristic of multicultural countries such as Canada. *Ethical pluralism* or *moral diversity* maintains the position that culturally diverse societies display multiple moral standards that may lead to conflicting moral realities. However, divergence in values and differences in moral standards that exist across cultural boundaries are valued and considered to be resources that have historically led to the evolution of moral thinking (Volbrecht, 2002).

Ethical pluralism rejects the perspective of *ethical relativism*, the position that moral judgments can be viewed as right or wrong relative to the norms or standard patterns of behaviour of a particular culture or society. Different societies have different cultural norms and thus different moral codes (Card, 2004). Consider Critical Thinking Exercise 2-1.

Ethical relativism does not provide direction in situations when cultures conflict, neither is guidance afforded when individuals belong to multiple cultures with differing perspectives. For example, an individual may belong to various groups that may include ethnic, religious, professional, and organizational cultures.

Ethical pluralism emphasizes understanding difference rather than striving for uniformity to ensure that moral systems are truly responsive to the lived realities and experiences of all human beings, not just the select few who hold positions of power (Johnstone, 2004). Moral diversity ensures that no one point of view dominates. Diversity of values and beliefs is crucial to morality's survival, as it prompts critical reflection, inviting revision and creative refinement.

ETHICAL THEORIES

Health care professionals and community members regularly make ethical decisions. These ethical decisions and the moral actions of individuals, organizations,

CRITICAL THINKING EXERCISE 2-1
Ethical Relativism and Ethical Pluralism

Ethical relativism may allow for polygamy, honour killings, infanticide, or euthanasia as cultural or religious norms in particular countries or situations. Can you identify other cultural or religious customs or norms that may be acceptable in some countries and not others? What are some cultural or religious customs that come into conflict in our Canadian society as we strive to achieve ethical pluralism? What strategies are used to address these ethical conflicts? To support ethical pluralism?

and communities are influenced by ethical theory. Three ethical theories, including rule ethics, virtue ethics, and feminist ethics, are of primary concern in community health.

Rule Ethics or Ethical Principlism

Two systems, teleology and deontology form the foundation of rule ethics. *Teleology* (Greek for "logic of ends") or consequentialism is concerned about ends, goals, purposes, and outcomes. Rightness is viewed in terms of good produced as consequences of action. *Deontology* (Greek for "what is due" or duty) is the theory of rights and duties based on unconditional respect for persons. Deontology requires doing right, regardless of consequences (Tschudin, 2003).

HISTORICAL EVOLUTION OF RULE ETHICS

Rule ethics were developed in the 18th and 19th centuries during the Enlightenment period, an intellectual movement that celebrated the power and value of individual human reason. Until this time, early virtue ethics were predominant and emphasized the importance of a good upbringing, education, and mentors in the development of character and moral judgment. Virtue ethics smacked of social privilege and advantages available only to upper class. During the Enlightenment era, individuals claimed the right to think for themselves, work for themselves, and govern themselves (Volbrecht, 2002). Moral authority no longer resided with kings, feudal lords, and bishops. Individuals assumed the power to rationally discover universal truths and moral judgment-applied rules or principles (Table 2-1).

TWO SCHOOLS OF RULE ETHICS

The goal of rule ethics is to delineate moral duties and obligations within a manageable set of rules. Utilitarianism and Kantianism are the most influential theories of rule ethics in contemporary moral philosophy and current health care ethics. Although significant differences exist between Utilitarianism and Kantianism, both theories are seen to have contributed to the development of a set of ethical principles or moral rules (Johnstone, 2004; Volbrecht, 2002).

Utilitarianism, the most popular form of teleology or consequentialism, is a moral perspective based on the goal of achieving the greatest good for the greatest number of people. Weighing consequences, benefits, or detriments that result from one's actions is instrumental in determining moral conduct and course of action. Utilitarianism is not concerned directly with a person's intentions but only with the outcome of the action. The end can justify the means; a moral outcome can justify unethical actions (Card, 2004).

By comparison, *Kantianism*, a form of deontology, is an ethical perspective based on respect for persons and action based on moral duty or good will. Morality is ensured by following the rules and acting from good intentions. The consequences of the actions are not of fundamental concern. Unconditional respect for persons

TABLE 2-1		
Historical Development of Rule Ethics		
ERA OF EARLY VIRTUE ETHICS	**ENLIGHTENMENT ERA CHANGE**	**EVOLUTION TO RULE ETHICS**
• Good upbringing, good education, and mentors lead to development of moral judgment and character • Social privilege and advantage available only to upper classes	• Authority related to accidents of birth, inheritance of wealth, or social position rejected • Power and value of individual human reason celebrated	• Rational analysis and logical deduction of conclusions from universal principles emphasized • All declared equal in virtue of capacity to reason, to deliberate, to choose
• Religious and intellectual authority within the church	• Individuals claimed right to think for themselves • Modern science evolves	• Individual reason is arbiter of truth • Empirical and quantitative evidence emphasized
• Political authority vested in the monarchy	• Individuals claimed right to govern themselves • Rise of nation states and republican governments	• Individual effort / integrity valued over social status • Individual represented in process of governing
• Economic authority lay with feudal lords	• Individuals claimed right to work for themselves • Collapse of feudalism	• Individual effort / ingenuity valued over social position • Rise of capitalism
• Moral authority vested in kings, feudal lords, and bishops	• All moral agents began on an equal footing with regard to moral judgment	• Moral authority in power of individuals to rationally discover universal truths • Moral judgment based on a set of rules
Adapted from Volbrecht, R. (2002). *Nursing ethics: Communities in dialogue.* Upper Saddle River, NJ: Prentice Hall.		

may require moral action to be taken regardless of the outcome or consequence (Card, 2004).

ETHICAL PRINCIPLES FOR PRACTICE

An ethical principle is a standard for moral behaviour, derived from moral theory—an essential norm in a system of thought used to form the basis of moral reasoning in that system. *Principlism* is a view that a set of principles can be developed from multiple ethical theories to be used in concrete applications. Ethical principlism reasons that ethical decision making and problem-solving are best undertaken by application of sound moral principles (Johnstone, 2004). The search for these principles consumed bioethicists in the later portion of the 20th century, resulting in the seminal work *Principles of Biomedical Ethics* by Beauchamp and Childress (1979), who documented four key ethical principles—autonomy, beneficence, nonmaleficence, and justice. The strength of these four principles is in their compatibility with both teleological and deontological theories.

An ethical principle is considered to be *prima facie* or relative to another principle that may have equal weight or priority in a particular situation. Some individuals may consider some principles to be *a priori*—that is, a priority, more important, or binding. The four ethical principles of autonomy, beneficence, nonmaleficence, and justice are considered to be *prima facie*. Beauchamp (2003) continues to demonstrate the relevance of these principles:

> *I believe that method in ethics begins with moral convictions that inspire the highest confidence and that appear to have the lowest level of bias. They serve as first principles and conditions of more specific moral conceptions. I take these principles to be universally valid norms that warrant us in making intercultural and cross-cultural judgments about moral depravity, morally misguided beliefs, savage cruelty, and other moral failures (p. 269).*

In recent literature, fidelity and veracity have been included (Aiken, 2004; Purtilo, 2005; Scoville Baker, 2004) in addition to a principle that some have called respect for persons (Scoville Baker) and others have called sanctity of life (Keatings & Smith, 2000). These seven ethical principles form the basis of rule ethics currently applied in community practice.

The principle of *autonomy* is focused on the right of self-determination that grants importance to independence and individual freedom. People should be free to make choices and entitled to act on their decisions, provided that their actions do not violate or impinge on the moral interests of others (Johnstone, 2004). In health care, autonomy involves respect for clients' rights to make decisions about and for themselves and their care. Informed consent is based on the principle of autonomy and a person's right to information required to make informed decisions about one's health care. Health care providers act to support the autonomy of clients and provide information to them on which to base their decisions.

Limitations can be placed on autonomy in situations where individual choices interfere with the rights or well-being of others. As is often the case in community practice, personal choice or autonomy may be restricted by concern for the well-being of the community. For example, clients generally have the autonomous right to refuse treatment. However, if a contagious disease that has implications for the community or society, such as tuberculosis, is diagnosed, clients can be required to take prescribed medication and may be isolated or quarantined for a time to prevent the spread of the infectious disease to others.

Beneficence is an age old requirement of the *Hippocratic Oath* for health professionals to "do good." The expectation is for health care providers to act for the benefit of others; to be knowledgeable and technically competent; and to ensure that their provision of care does good and benefits clients and their well-being. Beneficence requires potential benefits to individuals and society be maximized and potential harms minimized, while promotion of the common good and protection of individuals are considered (Vollman, 2004).

The principles of beneficence and autonomy may be at odds in community practice. For example, a community health initiative such as immunization, undertaken on a community-wide basis, may conflict with the autonomy of people whose religious beliefs do not support this practice. Community-wide initiatives often will not be viewed as beneficial to all sectors of the community (Scoville Baker, 2004) or by all sectors of the community.

Nonmaleficence, the partner of beneficence, also comes from the *Hippocratic Oath*. Nonmaleficence requires that harmful acts not be committed—*Primum non nocere*—first, do no harm. By extension, the principle of nonmaleficence requires that health care professionals protect from harm those who cannot protect themselves—those who are children, those who may live in poverty, those with disability, or those on the margin of society.

The principle of nonmaleficence is distinctly different from the principle of beneficence as demonstrated by Beauchamp and Childress (2001), and obligations to nonmaleficence may override obligations to beneficence. For example, allocation of resources to the benefit of one group is not morally defensible if the action takes resources from meeting more basic needs of others for necessities such as food and shelter. In such situations, doing no harm to one group takes precedence over doing good for another group. The practice of community health requires advocacy for the benefit, well-being, and protection from harm for all people in general and for populations and groups who are vulnerable in particular.

Community conflict arises when the benefits identified as the priority for one group conflict with harm identified as the priority for another group. For example, a group of rural residents may support the development of intensive livestock operations to provide anticipated employment and economic benefit to their community, while other community groups may be more concerned about the anticipated negative environmental impact in their community.

The principle of *justice* is based on obligations of fairness, regarding treatment of individuals and groups within society; the distribution of potential benefits and potential burdens (distributive justice); and the ways that those who have been unfairly burdened or harmed are compensated (compensatory justice). Philosophical discussions of justice consider *procedural* and *substantive* rules of justice. Procedural rules focus on the process of distribution noted in maxims such as "first come, first served" and "'due process." Rules of justice are based on perceptions of fairness, with maxims such as "to each according to need." Distributive justice or the distribution of benefits (education) and burdens (taxes) may be viewed from the perspectives of communitarianism, egalitarianism, libertarianism, or utilitarianism.

Community practice is traditionally based on utilitarianism, adheres to the axiom "the greatest good for the greatest number," and supports the position that maximizing benefits to socially disadvantaged groups ultimately benefits society as a whole. Community practitioners advocate for distribution of health promotion and chronic disease prevention resources in ways that are fair and equitable to benefit the most people. Community health providers also focus on the needs of vulnerable populations and advocate for the distribution of resources to compensate for the shortfalls or build individual capacity to address the difficulties that members of these groups may be experiencing. At times, these two perspectives come into conflict, creating ethical dilemmas for community practitioners and communities.

Respect for persons is based on the belief that human beings have worth and moral dignity. Persons are worthy moral agents and should be treated as ends in themselves, not merely as means to ends. Respect for persons is the foundation of all other principles and for some is subsumed, along with fidelity and veracity under the principle of autonomy (Johnstone, 2004). Persons who are respected and have moral dignity can rightfully determine their own destiny, make choices, and take action. Respect for persons ensures their right to privacy and confidentiality. Sometimes in public health, the individual right to privacy is usurped by the public benefit of disclosure. For example, regulations were changed to allow the use of large health databases for epidemiological research to benefit society, without the informed consent of those people whose information was held in the database (Bayer & Fairchild, 2004).

The principle of the *sanctity of life* is directly related to the respect for persons and may conflict with the principle of autonomy. For example, when persons with terminal illnesses are living in extreme pain, they may consider assisted suicide to be the preferred option. In Canada, the right for an individual to choose assisted suicide does not carry more weight than the societal belief in the sanctity of life. The principle of autonomy is superseded by the value of sanctity of life based on the principle of respect for persons (Keatings & Smith, 2000).

In community health promotion and community development, the respect for persons is extended to respect for their experience as knowledge and their abilities and capacities as community members to contribute to decision making and planning at the community level. Respect for persons applies to all persons and supports the inclusion and participation of all community members in community endeavours.

The principle of *fidelity* is about faithfulness and focuses on maintaining loyalty, keeping promises, and being faithful in relationships. Being faithful entails meeting the client's reasonable expectations of the health care provider, including basic respect, competency, honesty, promise-keeping, and adherence to policies and laws (Purtilo, 2005). Whether working with individuals or communities, health professionals must be careful in making promises and steadfast in keeping them. Commitments may be as simple as attending meetings or as extensive as delivering survey findings back to community leaders.

The principle of *veracity*, the duty to tell the truth and be honest, is derived from respect for persons and their autonomy. As this principle is specific in directing behaviour, some consider it to be a second-level principle to guide behaviour and support the intent to be benevolent or to maintain fidelity in relationships with clients (Purtilo, 2005). Kant gave veracity a central role and considered truthfulness to be an absolute duty to be upheld without exception.

Veracity is essential in building and maintaining trust in relationships with individuals, groups, and communities. Health care providers working in and with communities must be truthful and transparent in the work they undertake and the relationships they establish. Health professionals have a responsibility to be clear and truthful about who they are, what roles they play, and what they bring to the community. Health practitioners, as community advocates, should help to ensure that research undertaken in or with the community also meets the burden of veracity and that researchers are truthful in disclosing what they can and cannot contribute to the community as well as how they may and may not benefit the community.

CRITIQUE OF RULE ETHICS

The application of ethical principles and the theoretical limitations of the principles have raised concerns about the effectiveness of rule ethics. Problems commonly associated with the application of rule ethics include (1) deciding correctly which principles apply in a given situation, (2) interpreting correctly the imperatives or required actions of the principles in a given situation, (3) deciding correctly the relative weights of given principles, (4) balancing the demands of different principles in situations where equally weighted demands might conflict, (5) deciding whether ethical principles apply at all, and (6) resolving disagreements in prioritizing ethical principles in a given situation (Johnstone, 2004).

Broader theoretical limitations of the principles themselves are identified by Rodney, Burgess, McPherson, and Brown (2004), who argued that (1) a lack of consensus exists concerning the nature of fundamental ethical principles, (2) ethical principles are not easily prioritized or applied to concrete moral situations, (3) reliance on ethical principles may lead to the exclusion of other variables known to influence ethical practice, (4) ethical principles do not reflect the breadth and diversity of concepts available in the general ethics literature, and (5) rule ethics fosters a prescriptive formal approach by which principles are applied in a process-dominated manner.

Critics argue that rule ethics neglect or exclude important aspects of the moral experience of health care professionals, including moral judgments, the significance of emotions and experience, and the relational nature of professional practice (Volbrecht, 2002). Moral sensitivity and responsiveness to one's relational responsibilities does not lend itself to rule-making. The capacity to make contextual moral judgments and discern morally appropriate responses exceeds the will to take the right action and the analytic skills to apply rules to situations.

Rule ethics is criticized for reflecting typically masculine characteristics of autonomy, rationality, and independence of the moral subject, in contrast to an ethic of care that reflects more typically feminine characteristics of responsiveness to relational responsibilities, emotional connectedness, and contextuality (Volbrecht, 2002). The principle-based approach is also criticized for being culturally specific and inattentive to a multicultural society; weak in insisting on action related to issues such as access to health care or the creation of choices for vulnerable groups; and missing the subtle pervasive power dynamics that infuse individual, family, and community relationships within current hierarchies (Rodney et al., 2004).

Emerging ethical theory emphasizes the importance of community as the context where values and virtues are collectively shaped and practical moral reasoning is exercised (Volbrecht, 2002). Community and relationships are central themes in virtue ethics and feminist ethics.

Virtue Ethics or Moral Virtues

While rule ethics is action based, virtue ethics is agent based. Instead of duties and obligations, virtue ethics focuses on characteristics of the moral agent. Ancient Greeks, including Aristotle, initially conceived of ethics in this manner. Early virtue ethics, however, fell out of favour during the Enlightenment era (Table 2-1), as the valued human characteristics became the purview of birthright and social station. With the dissatisfaction of rule ethics, the value of virtue ethics has been revisited in the development of many codes of ethics.

CRITERIA OF VIRTUE ETHICS

The main criteria of virtue ethics involve the type of person one should strive to be and the sort of life one ought to live. Virtue ethics involves the integration of seeing, feeling, and acting. Virtue connotes the moral excellence of intent and behaviour. Goodness is prior to rightness, and various virtues, such as loyalty, courage, and honesty, are necessary for good actions (Tschudin, 2003). An action is deemed morally acceptable if an ideally virtuous agent would perform the same action under the same circumstances. Virtues are good, independent of any desire or ethical situation; every action depends on the person. Telling the truth is essential, not because of the importance of autonomy or informed consent but because it is required to achieve the virtue of truthfulness and to demonstrate integrity. Tschudin argues that the practice of self-awareness is vital in considering conflicting personal, professional, and social dimensions, because self-awareness and personal integrity keep a person sane in situations that require the consideration of multiple factors and options. Since individuals live in communities that significantly affect their character development and persons can be nurtured or marred accordingly, virtue ethics asserts that people are not only responsible for developing good character as individuals but also have responsibilities for the kind of communities they collectively develop (Volbrecht, 2002).

APPLICATION OF VIRTUE ETHICS

Volbrecht (2002) identifies compassion, fidelity to trust, moral courage, justice, mediation, self-confidence, resilience, practical reasoning, and integrity as nursing virtues. These virtues are offered not as an exhaustive list but as fodder for discussion and further development. Professional codes of ethics often identify values and virtues that are considered essential for ethical practice. Values and virtues overlap when the ideals of importance are defining traits or standards for noble conduct. For example, some values articulated in the *Code of Ethics for Registered Nurses* (Canadian Nurses Association, 2002) such as dignity, confidentiality, fairness, and accountability could also be defined as virtues of importance to the profession of nursing and applicable to all health care professions.

Caring is often considered to be a virtue. Tschudin (2003) discussed eight major ingredients for caring in general and five Cs of caring particular to nursing and health care professionals. The eight major ingredients included knowledge, alternating rhythms (between past and present, between attention to detail and to the whole), patience, honesty, trust, humility, hope, and courage. In health care, the term *alternating rhythms* is consistent with the concept of critical reflection, considering the context. The five Cs of caring include compassion, competence, confidence, conscience, and commitment. In both cases, the characteristics of caring could be defined as virtues for public health or community practice.

CRITIQUE OF VIRTUE ETHICS

The major criticism of virtue ethics is that virtues are not always compatible, and no process is offered to resolve this type of conflict (Glannon, 2005). For example, disclosure of negative information may trigger negative consequences, and the virtue of compassion comes into conflict with the virtue of honesty. In a community setting, compassion for members of a vulnerable group may come in conflict with courage required to address the broader community.

Some argue that virtue ethics entails (1) a justification of circularity whereby the virtuous person does what is good, and what is good is what the virtuous person does; (2) the inability to explain its force or power as a moral guide in the absence of obligations, maxims, or principles; and (3) unrealistic and unattainable expectations imposed on people to be excellent (Johnstone, 2004). Proponents respond by questioning the need to justify virtuous actions, rejecting the expectation that virtue ethics can be reduced to a set of ethical rules, and spurning the belief that expecting moral excellence is an unrealistic prospect. Virtue ethics contributes much to moral reasoning, to a comprehensive moral philosophy, and to ethical health care practice.

Feminist Ethics

Feminist ethics is viewed by some as an extension of virtue ethics, as it emphasizes an ethics of care that involves human connectedness and the importance of interpersonal relationships (Glannon, 2005). Feminist ethics strives to address the imbalance of power between men and women and places them on equal footing. Feminist ethics draws attention to the distinguishing characteristics of relationships and the power within those relationships at individual, group, community, and societal levels. Based on the core ideal of achieving social justice, feminist ethics extends the principle of justice and the notion of distributive justice to consider social structures and contexts. Feminist ethics is committed to the constructive process of designing alternative ways to restructure relationships, social practices, and institutions, with the ultimate goal of social transformation that will empower all people to live freer and fuller lives (Volbrecht, 2002).

HISTORIC EVOLUTION OF FEMINIST ETHICS

While philosophers such as Aristotle and Kant supported the belief in women's infe-riority to men, which they explained in terms of women's allegedly defective capac-ity to reason, others including Plato and Mill, now viewed as early pioneers in fem-inist ethics, opposed women's subordination and the historically dominant belief in women's inherent inferiority (Jaggar, 1991). During the 18th and 19th centuries, some writers formulated positions on women's morality that viewed men and women as distinct but equal in moral virtues, others declared moral virtue as gender neutral, and still others recognized women's morality as distinct and either superior or potentially superior to that of men (Volbrecht, 2002). The first wave of feminism used arguments from these positions to advocate for voting rights for women.

Resurgence of feminist ethics in the 1960s coincided with feminist activism, as grassroots activists were joined by academic feminists, and debate on practical issues of contemporary social life such as abortion, equality of opportunity, and domestic labour churned (Jaggar, 1991). By the late 1970s, feminists were ques-tioning the ability of traditional ethical theories to address "women's issues"; oth-ers were recognizing the difficulties associated with using traditional ethical theo-ries to address issues in a complex, multicultural world; and still others were identifying the contributions that feminist ethics could make to address these con-cerns and other ethical issues.

In the early 1980s, feminist ethics was dedicated to rethinking the deepest issues in ethical theory, in light of a moral sensibility perceived as distinctively feminine (Jaggar, 1991). The work of Carol Gilligan (1982) revolutionized discussions in moral theory and feminism, as she argued that women speak with a different voice than men and espoused a feminine ethic of care that considers responsibility to care and relationships between people as opposed to a masculine ethic of justice that considers ethical principles, conflicting duties, and consequences.

APPLICATION OF FEMINIST ETHICS

The traditional framework for ethical practice involves (1) identification of the issue, (2) analysis of the context of the situation, (3) exploration of potential options, (4) application of ethical decision making process and criteria, (5) imple-mentation of the plan, and (6) evaluation of the outcome and the process. Vol-brecht (2002) suggested a feminist ethics decision making process that extends the traditional framework, to include five specific actions at step four of the traditional process. To apply feminist ethics in decision making, Volbrecht recommends the following:

◆ Identifying social practices that underlie and contribute to the ethical problem or situation
◆ Examining and evaluating ways that these social practices may contribute to the oppression of the social group involved, by considering imbalances of power and the related social construction of reality

♦ Considering ways that a relational account of justice reveals the harm done to the oppressed group
♦ Considering unique insights that those people who have been marginalized by social practices can provide to guide relational, societal, and institutional restructuring
♦ Designing new ways to restructure or resist oppressive practices

Feminist ethics and its application strive to strengthen connectedness and relationships, eliminate oppression, balance power, and achieve social justice. Inclusion, participation, empowerment, social justice, advocacy, and the interdependence of these concepts are key considerations of feminist ethics from the individual to the societal level. These concepts may be also considered as foundational principles for public health and community practice. As such, they will be discussed in more detail later in this chapter.

CRITIQUE OF FEMINIST ETHICS

The primary criticism of feminist ethics comes from those who believe in the application of ethical principles in a rational manner, without complication of emotions or concern for relationships. Proponents of feminist ethics cover a continuum from recognizing this approach as a complement that extends rule ethics and virtue ethics, to advocating for the application of feminist ethics in completely new and evolving ways. Feminist ethics and its application at the broader community level continue to be advanced. The evolution from rule ethics to virtue ethics to feminist ethics and their differentiations are reviewed in Table 2-2. To understand the contributions of each theory to practice, consider Critical Thinking Exercise 2-2.

CRITICAL THINKING EXERCISE 2-2
Rule Ethics, Virtue Ethics, and Feminist Ethics
Consider that your community is struggling with a decision about where to build a centre for vocational rehabilitation for people living with developmental challenges. Two neighbourhoods are being considered, but in each case, the residents are worried about the potential decrease in property values and are organizing to prohibit building in their neighbourhood. Compare and contrast how decisions would be made using rule ethics, virtue ethics, and feminist ethics, each in isolation of the other theories. What could each theory offer to a process and an outcome, if all three theories were considered concurrently for their potential contributions?

TABLE 2-2
Distinguishing Moral Perspectives

RULE ETHICS	VIRTUE ETHICS	FEMINIST ETHICS
Masculine perspective is conceived as foundational.	Masculine and feminine human virtues form the basis.	Feminine perspective is seen as foundational.
Humans are viewed as separate individuals.	Humans are viewed by their moral characteristics.	Humans are viewed in terms of their relationships.
Duties, obligations, and outcomes determine morality.	Traits and characteristics of virtuous people determine morality.	Responsibilities to care determine morality.
Focus is on independence, autonomy, and rationality.	Focus is on character, virtues, and good judgment; integrates reason and emotion.	Focus is on connection, sharing, and community.
Conflict is resolved through the application of ethical principles.	Virtuous persons resolve conflict using good judgment in relation to the context of the situation.	Conflict is resolved in ways that preserve and strengthen connections and relationships.
Moral decision making involves the logical application of universal rules.	People apply human virtues to make good judgments while considering the situation.	Moral decision making is attentive to the context of relationships.
Ethical principles give direction to care delivery.	Care providers demonstrate the virtues of caring in their practice.	Ethics of care guide relationships and health care practice.
What actions are right and wrong? What moral rules or ethical principles should be developed, and how should they be applied?	What traits and characteristics are virtues? What kind of person should one be? What kind of community do we want to be?	How can oppressive practices be eliminated? How can relationships, social practices, and institutions be restructured to empower men and women?

ETHICAL FOUNDATIONS OF PUBLIC HEALTH AND COMMUNITY PRACTICE

Seven concepts are foundational in public health and community practice, including inclusion, diversity, participation, empowerment, social justice, advocacy, and interdependence. Of particular importance are the interrelationships of and among these concepts that weave a strong web on which to base community practice.

Inclusion

Inclusion or the act of being included means being accepted and able to participate fully within the family, the community, and the society in which one lives (Guildford, 2000). People who are excluded, whether because of poverty, ill-health, gender, race, or lack of education, do not have the opportunity for full participation in the social and economic benefits of the community or the society. *An Inclusion Lens* offers tools for analyzing practices, programs, policies, and legislation to determine their ability to promote the social and economic inclusion of individuals, families, and communities (Shookner, 2002). Values that underpin this work are social justice and diversity. Ultimately, the goal is to provide a new way to encourage change that will transform organizations, communities, and society as a whole.

Diversity

Diversity is the condition of being diverse, differing from one another, composed of distinct or unlike elements or qualities. Earlier in the chapter, diversity has been discussed in relation to moral diversity and ethical pluralism. The value of diversity among people is key in ethical pluralism and required for the evolution of moral thought. Valuing diversity requires "recognition and respect for the diversity of cultures, races, ethnicity, languages, religions, abilities, age and sexual orientation; valuing all contributions of both men and women to the social, economic, and cultural vitality of society" (Shookner, 2002, p. 2).

Participation

Engaging people in determining the ways a society guides its actions, makes decisions on public policy, and delivers programs and services is called public participation, or citizen engagement. The desired outcome of participation in decision making is greater social cohesion as evidenced by the creation of shared values, the reduction of health and wealth disparities, and the building of community spirit and capacity for action (Vollman, 2004).

Increasingly, community and public health agencies are generating opportunities to involve citizens in processes of service planning and program evaluation. Public involvement strategies must be designed and planned in collaboration with stakeholders to facilitate informed and meaningful public participation. Discussion of public participation is found in Chapter 6.

Empowerment

Empowerment is both a process and an outcome (Vollman, 2004). As a process, empowerment is the development of knowledge and skills that increase one's mastery over decisions that affect one's life. As an outcome, empowerment is the achievement of mastery. To gain mastery or be empowered, people must be able to predict, control, and participate in their environments. At the community or population level, empowerment has been described as community competence. Community empowerment is exhibited as residents actively participate and promote inclusion, communicate with respect and in ways that accommodate and manage conflict, demonstrate commitment to collectively determined goals, foster and share leadership and decision making, create supportive environments, strive for social justice, and nurture intercommunity relationships. Effective community practitioners engage with communities and act as resources to them as they strive to achieve the many aspects of community empowerment.

Social Justice

Social justice is ideologically neutral and open to people of all political and religious affiliations, all socioeconomic brackets, all cultures and ethnic groups, both sexes, and all ages (Vollman, 2004). The field of activity may be literary, scientific, religious, political, economic, cultural, or athletic, across the spectrum of human social activities. The virtue of social justice allows for people of good will to reach different, even opposing, practical judgments about the material content of the common good (ends) and ways to get there (means). Social justice is based on the application of equity, rights, access, and participation.

Social justice counters oppression and powerlessness. The role of community workers is to support inclusion and empowerment of people living on the margins of society so they may freely participate on footings of respect. Empowerment is the guarantor of equity and justice, and freedom is the result—freedom to fully participate in public decisions (Vollman, 2004).

Advocacy

Advocacy can be defined as the act of disseminating information to influence opinion, conduct, public policy, or legislation. It is the pursuit of influencing outcomes, including public policy and resource allocation decisions within political, economic, and social systems and institutions, which directly affect people's lives. Advocacy consists of organized efforts and actions to highlight critical issues that have been ignored and submerged, to influence public attitudes, and to enact and implement laws and public policies so that visions of a just, decent society become reality. The goal of advocacy is to promote social justice and equity. Human rights—political, economic, and social—are the overarching framework for this vision (Vollman, 2004). Community workers, as advocates, represent the interests of the people in the community, intervene to investigate problems and resolve conflicts, assist in capacity building within the community to advocate on its own behalf, review and comment on public policy, and disseminate information to the community and across communities.

Interdependence

Another key concept in public health and community practice is the recognition of the interdependence of the people, an interdependence that is the essence of community (American Public Health Association, 2002). Public health strives for the health of entire communities and recognizes that the health of individuals is tied to the life of the community. Interdependence relates to the interdependence of and among human beings and also the interdependence of people with the world in which they live—their social, economic, and physical environments.

ADVANCES IN ETHICS FOR COMMUNITY PRACTICE

Early bioethics focused on the health of the individual and individual autonomy, not population health (Callahan & Jennings, 2002). However, population health and public health have come to the foreground as a result of the reminders posed by acquired immune deficiency syndrome (AIDS) and severe acute respiratory syndrome (SARS) that infectious disease has not been conquered. Efforts of public health management of infectious diseases has raised ethical questions related to the principle of autonomy and individual choice, which is often found in conflict with the collective good in public or population health. Ethical issues related to the determinants of health and access to employment, education, health services, and healthy environments have added to the ethical challenges presented by population health. Public health issues related to epidemiological research and the use of large population databases without expressed consent of members of the population, surveillance related to AIDS, confinement related to SARS, and restrictions related to tobacco consumption have generated ethical issues calling for the birth of public health ethics (Bayer & Fairchild, 2004).

A Public Health Code of Ethics

As a result, the American Public Health Association (APHA) (2002) has developed the *Public Health Code of Ethics*. In sharp contrast to medical ethics, public health is concerned more with populations than with individuals and more with prevention than with cure (Thomas, Sage, Dillenberg, & Guillory, 2002). The code states key principles for the ethical practice of public health. Public health is understood as "what we in society, do collectively to assure the conditions for people to be healthy" (American Public Health Association, 2002, p. 1). The code highlights the ethical principles that follow from the distinctive characteristics of public health. A key belief that underlies several of the principles is the interdependence of the people, which is the essence of community. Table 2-3 contains the 12 *Principles of the Ethical Practice of Public Health*.

The APHA is based on many of the ethical foundations discussed earlier in the chapter. Public health and this code give priority to the common good over the individual, prevention (and some might argue care) over cure, public participation, advocacy, empowerment, social justice, and evidence-based decision making. The code recommends providing information and obtaining community consent for decisions on policies and programs, acting in a timely manner, applying varied approaches in respect of diversity, and respecting and enhancing social and physical environments. Public health institutions are expected to strive to protect confidentiality of information, ensure professional competence of their employees, and engage in collaborations and affiliations that build public trust and organizational effectiveness. Although challenges will occur as conflicts arise in the application of the 12 principles, and the setting of priorities among them

---

TABLE 2-3

Principles of Ethical Practice in Public Health

1. Public health should address principally the fundamental causes of disease and requirements for health, aiming to prevent adverse health outcomes.
2. Public health should achieve community health in a way that respects the rights of individuals in the community.
3. Public health policies, programs, and priorities should be developed and evaluated through processes that ensure an opportunity for input from community members.
4. Public health should advocate and work for the empowerment of disenfranchised community members, aiming to ensure that the basic resources and conditions necessary for health are available to all.
5. Public health should seek the information needed to implement effective policies and programs that protect and promote health.
6. Public health institutions should provide communities with the information they have that is needed for decisions on policies or programs and should obtain the community's consent for their implementation.
7. Public health institutions should act in a timely manner on the information they have within the resources and the mandate given to them by the public.
8. Public health programs and policies should incorporate a variety of approaches that anticipate and respect diverse values, beliefs, and cultures in the community.
9. Public health programs and policies should be implemented in a manner that most enhances the physical and social environment.
10. Public health institutions should protect the confidentiality of information that can bring harm to an individual or community if made public. Exceptions must be justified on the basis of the high likelihood of significant harm to the individual or others.
11. Public health institutions should ensure the professional competence of their employees.
12. Public health institutions and their employees should engage in collaborations and affiliations in ways that build the public's trust and the institution's effectiveness.

Public Health Leadership Society (2002). *Principles of the Ethical Practice of Public Health*. New Orleans, LA: Author.

---

dependent on circumstance, they are an effort at documentation of explicit guidelines for public health practice. Beyond the principles, the code also includes statements of values and beliefs underlying the code and notes related to the individual principles.

A Health Promotion Code of Ethics?

As a result of the publication of the APHA code of ethics, the question has been raised about the need for a code of ethics for health promotion (Sindall, 2002). Although health promotion has had little to say about its moral foundations, the *Ottawa Charter for Health Promotion* (as discussed in the previous chapter) can be considered as a statement of values and moral commitment. Sindall challenges the field of health promotion and its practitioners to effectively establish the moral credibility of health promotion through (1) conferences and other forums for discussion of health promotion, bioethics, human rights, and social philosophy; (2) papers on ethical topics in health promotion journals and on the ethics of health promotion in journals of other disciplines; (3) incorporation of ethics courses into the health promotion curriculum; and (4) consideration of the value of developing a code of ethics.

Unquestionably, responsibilities for moral thought, discussion, and action regarding public health and health promotion lay with health care professionals. However, the ethical foundations of community practice require the inclusion, diversity, empowerment, and participation of communities and their members in this work. Social justice, advocacy, and interdependence must underpin the process.

Ethics as Communal Dialogue

Ethics or morality exists on individual, group, community, and societal levels. Ethics, as communal dialogue, is a dynamic, ongoing conversation among members of a community about values and principles needed to make society and people's lives as civilized and fruitful as possible (Volbrecht, 2002). Ethics is a process of reflecting consciously on moral beliefs and consists of an ongoing dialogue about community values and community actions that should be taken in light of those values. Ethical pluralism promotes ongoing dialogue among community members facilitating the development and identification of a community's shared moral understandings and expectations of its members and the community as a whole (Volbrecht, 2002).

ETHICAL CHALLENGES IN COMMUNITY PRACTICE

A variety of ethical challenges that exist within public health and community practice have been discussed throughout this chapter. An exhaustive list is neither reasonable nor possible. However, the chapter will conclude with a brief summary of some of the general challenges in community practice that continue to keep practitioners, communities, and society as a whole "ethically engaged." Refer to Box 2-1 for a list of ethical challenges. Consider Critical Thinking Exercise 2-3.

CRITICAL THINKING EXERCISE 2-3
Identifying and Managing Ethical Dilemmas in Community Practice
Consider Critical Thinking Exercise 2-2. What might your role be as a community practitioner? What action might you take? How might social justice be achieved?

BOX 2-1

Ethical Challenges in Community Practice

- The conflict continues between respecting individual autonomy and benefiting or protecting the collective or the community.
- Protecting individual right to privacy and informed consent may conflict with sharing individual information for the benefit of the health of the public.
- The goals of social justice and empowerment can be very difficult to achieve, and many barriers may need to be identified and addressed in community practice.
- Facilitating and ensuring inclusion and diversity in community participation though challenging is fundamental to effective community practice.
- Fostering and maintaining effective and caring relationships with the various professionals, clients, organizations, and communities with whom one engages requires commitment and consistent effort.
- Appropriate boundaries in community work with individuals, groups, and communities, though often difficult to establish and maintain, are essential to effective community practice.
- Working with multiple partnerships offers challenges in supporting and ensuring processes through which all groups are respected, involved, contributing as able, included in decision making, and benefiting equitably.
- Issues of social justice and conflict arise in striving to support the autonomy and rights of the community while facilitating the empowerment and rights of a group within the community who may have been marginalized and are experiencing vulnerability.
- Values, roles, and responsibilities within one's profession, organization of employment, and community of practice may come into conflict.
- Protection of clients, co-workers, and others, including one's self, requires considerations of autonomy, informed consent, advocacy for marginalized groups, and risk management in daily practice.
- Advocacy has the potential to generate conflict, and community practitioners are challenged to build and apply skills in mediation, negotiation, and conflict resolution.
- Community practitioners are expected to prevent or disclose conflicts of interest; be transparent in their intentions; and act with honesty, truthfulness, loyalty, and integrity.

SUMMARY

The application of rule ethics, virtue ethics, and feminist ethics offers ways to address ethical dilemmas and resolve ethical conflict. Feminist ethics have made way for the revolutionary inclusion of responsiveness to relational responsibilities, emotional connectedness, and contextuality in discussions of ethical practice. Inclusion, diversity, participation, empowerment, social justice, advocacy, and interdependence and their interrelationships create a foundation to effectively underpin and support ethical community practice. The genesis of a public health code of ethics, conversations about ethics in health promotion, and identification of ethical challenges in community practice extend the dialogue. The interdependence, relationships, and collaboration among health care professionals and members of the organizations, communities, and societies in which they practice will facilitate the further development of moral thought and continue the evolution of ethical theory to underpin ethical community practice.

References

Aiken, T. (2004). *Legal, ethical and political issues in nursing* (2nd ed.). Philadelphia: FA Davis Co.

American Public Health Association. (2002). *Public Health Code of Ethics*. Washington, DC: Author. Retrieved June 15, 2007, from **http://www.apha.org/programs/education/progeduethicalguidelines.htm.**

Bayer, R., & Fairchild, A. (2004). The genesis of public health ethics. *Bioethics, 18*(6), 473–492.

Beauchamp, T., & Childress, J. (1979). *Principles of biomedical ethics*. New York: Oxford University Press.

Beauchamp, T., & Childress, J. (2001). *Principles of biomedical ethics* (5th ed.). New York: Oxford University Press.

Beauchamp, T. (2003). Methods and principles in biomedical ethics. *Journal of Medical Ethics, 29,* 269–274.

Callahan, D., & Jennings, B. (2002). Ethics and public health: Forging a strong relationship. *American Journal of Public Health, 92*(2), 169–176.

Canadian Nurses Association. (2002). *Code of ethics for registered nurses*. Ottawa: Author.

Card, R. (2004). *Critically thinking about medical ethics*. Upper Saddle River, NJ: Pearson Prentice Hall.

Department of Justice. (1982). *Canadian Charter of Rights and Freedoms*. Ottawa: Author. Retrieved March 13, 2006, from **http://laws.justice.gc.ca/en/charter/index.html**.

Gilligan, C. (1982). *In a different voice*. Cambridge: Harvard University Press.

Glannon, W. (2005). *Biomedical ethics*. New York: Oxford University Press.

Guildford, J. (2000). *Making the case for social and economic inclusion*. Halifax: Atlantic Region, Health Canada.

Jaggar, A. (1991). Feminist ethics: Projects, problems, and prospects. In C. Card (Ed.), *Feminist ethics*. Lawrence, KS: University Press of Kansas.

Johnstone, M. (2004). *Bioethics: A nursing perspective* (4th ed.). Sydney: Churchill Livingstone.

Keatings, M., & Smith, O. (2000). *Ethical and legal issues in Canadian nursing* (2nd ed.). Toronto: WB Saunders.

Public Health Leadership Society (2002). *Principles of the Ethical Practice of Public Health*. New Orleans, LA: Author.

Purtilo, R. (2005). *Ethical dimensions in the health professions* (4th ed.). Philadelphia: Elsevier Saunders.

Rodney, P., Burgess, M., McPherson, G., & Brown, H. (2004). Our theoretical landscape: A brief history of health care ethics. In J. Storch, P. Rodney, & R. Starzomski (Eds.), *Toward a moral horizon: Nursing ethics for leadership and practice* (pp. 56–76). Toronto: Pearson Prentice Hall.

Scoville Baker, S. (2004). Ethical quandaries in community health nursing. In E. Anderson & J. McFarlane (Eds.), *Community as partner: Theory and practice in nursing* (4th ed., pp. 83–113). Philadelphia: Lippincott Williams & Wilkins.

Shookner, M. (2002). *An inclusion lens: Workbook for looking at social and economic exclusion and inclusion*. Halifax, NS: Health Canada, Population and Public Health Branch.

Sindall, C. (2002). Does health promotion need a code of ethics? *Health Promotion International*, *17*(3), 201–203.

Storch, J. (2004). Nursing ethics: A developing moral terrain. In J. Storch, P. Rodney, & R. Starzomski (Eds.), *Toward a moral horizon: Nursing ethics for leadership and practice* (pp. 1–16). Toronto: Pearson Prentice Hall.

Thomas, J., Sage, M., Dillenberg, J., & Guillory, V. (2002). A code of ethics for public health. *American Journal of Public Health*, *92*(7), 1057–1059.

Tschudin, V. (2003). *Ethics in nursing: The caring relationship*. Edinburgh: Butterworth Heinemann.

Volbrecht, R. (2002). *Nursing ethics: Communities in dialogue*. Upper Saddle River, NJ: Prentice Hall.

Vollman, A. (2004). Ethics and advocacy in community practice. In A. Vollman, E. Anderson, & J. McFarlane (Eds.), *Canadian Community as Partner* (pp. 106–123). Philadelphia: Lippincott Williams & Wilkins.

Internet Resources

http://www.apha.org/
American Public Health Association

http://www.ccepa.ca/index.html
Canadian Centre for Ethics in Public Affairs

http://laws.justice.gc.ca/en/charter/index.html
Canadian Charter of Rights and Freedoms

http://www.cna-nurses.ca/CNA/practice/ethics/code/default_e.aspx
Canadian Nurses Association—Code of Ethics

http://www.nursingethics.ca/
Nursing Ethics Resources

http://www.phen.ab.ca/index.asp
Provincial Health Ethics Network of Alberta

http://www.publichealthlaw.net/Reader/toc.htm
Public Health Law and Ethics: A Reader

http://www.apha.org/NR/rdonlyres/1CED3CEA-287E-4185-9CBD-BD405FC60856/0/ethicsbrochure.pdf
Public Health Leadership Society—Principles of the Ethical Practice of Public Health

3

Epidemiology, Demography, and Community Health

DANA S. EDGE

Chapter Outline

Introduction
Demography and Epidemiology
Contemporary Community Health Practice
Epidemiologic Approaches to Community
   Health Research
Levels of Prevention in Community Practice
Descriptive Measures of Health

Analytic Measures of Health
Sources of Community Health Data
Screening for Health Conditions
Decision Making in Screening:
     Practical and Ethical Considerations
Outbreak Management
Summary

Learning Objectives

To assess community health needs and to plan, implement, and evaluate programs to meet those needs, the community health professional must understand basic concepts in epidemiology and demography.

After studying this chapter, you should be able to:

❖ Interpret and use basic epidemiologic, demographic, and statistical measures of community health

❖ Apply principles of epidemiology and demography to your community practice

Introduction

Demography and epidemiology are sciences used for studying populations and population health. To promote, maintain, and restore the health of populations, the community health professional integrates and applies concepts from these fields. In this chapter, we explore the meaning and usefulness of these concepts.

When program planners partner with communities, they contribute their expertise supported by the relevant science; in other words, they come armed with the statistics and models that explain health and disease patterns in community health. This information might include the current health status of the population according to a number of accepted indicators, allowing local data to be compared with data from other jurisdictions regionally, nationally, and internationally. By being able to see trends and patterns, strengths and risk factors can be identified, and working together, residents and community workers can develop plans and set priorities to address concerns and build on community assets. Epidemiologic and sociodemographic data have traditionally formed the scientific foundation of population health practice so that comparative and comprehensive evidence is available to inform decision making. Regardless of what epidemiologic and demographic information reveals, *how* decision making unfolds at the community level is essential to population health practice. Principles of primary health care—in particular, public participation and intersectoral collaboration—must be honoured at the local level if efforts to improve the health of Canadians are to be affordable and sustainable over time. Therefore, being able to communicate effectively to a variety of stakeholders with standard measures of health and wellness is critical to the community health worker.

DEMOGRAPHY AND EPIDEMIOLOGY

Demography (literally, "writing about the people," from the Greek *demos* [people] and *graphos* [writing]) is the science of human populations and is concerned with population size, density, characteristics, and change. Examples of demographic research are descriptions and comparisons of populations according to such characteristics as age; ethnicity; sex; socioeconomic status; geographic distribution; and patterns of birth, death, marriage, and divorce. Demographic studies often have health implications that may or may not be addressed by the investigators. The census of the Canadian population is an example of a comprehensive descriptive demographic study that is conducted every 5 years.

Epidemiology ("the study of what is upon the people," from the Greek *logos* [study], *demos* [people], and *epi* [upon]) is the science of population health and is characterized by the study of the distribution and the determinants of health-related states (Last, 2001). Epidemiology overlaps with demography. Epidemiologic studies may take on the intrigue of detective stories as investigators track the factors associated with illness and death. In fact, a number of works concerning epidemiologic studies have become popular classics (e.g., *The Andromeda Strain* [Crichton, 1969]; *The Hot Zone* [Preston, 1994], *Outbreak* [Petersen, 1995]; and *Miss Evers' Boys* [Feldshuh, 1997]).

Epidemics, defined as outbreaks of illnesses greater than expected levels in a population, were a major focus of early epidemiological work. In 1854, Dr. John Snow, a British anaesthesiologist, and William Farr, a statistician, conducted what is now considered to be a classic epidemiologic study; their collaboration capitalized on a naturally occurring phenomenon during a cholera epidemic in the SoHo district of London (Morabia, 2004). At that time, the mode of transmission of cholera was unknown, although Snow suspected it was spread through contaminated water. In the area of London most affected, households randomly received their water supply from either the Lambeth Company or the Southwark & Vauxhall Company. Early in the outbreak, Snow went door-to-door to determine the name of the household water supplier. By mapping the cholera outbreak cases, using group comparisons, and applying epidemiologic principles, Snow and Farr determined that death rates from cholera were eight to nine times greater in households served by the Southwark & Vauxhall Company. The water supplied by Southwark & Vauxhall came from portions of the Thames River into which London sewage was discharged. Thus, this early epidemiologic work established the waterborne mode of transmission of cholera (Snow, 1936). Near the end of the epidemic, to make a political statement and prevent further transmission of cholera, Dr. Snow removed the handle of the Broad Street pump, eliminating the source of the cholera outbreak.

CONTEMPORARY COMMUNITY HEALTH PRACTICE

Today, advanced epidemiologic and demographic research methods are used not only to study outbreaks such as *Escherichia coli* food poisoning and severe acute respiratory syndrome (SARS) but also to investigate environmental conditions, lifestyles, health promotion strategies, and other factors that influence health. This chapter provides an introduction to epidemiologic and demographic concepts that are useful for community practice. Additional reading and in-depth discussion can be found in numerous textbooks (e.g., Fletcher & Fletcher, 2005; Gordis, 2004; Lilienfeld & Stolley, 1994; Rothman, 2002; Timmreck, 1998).

EPIDEMIOLOGIC APPROACHES TO COMMUNITY HEALTH RESEARCH

In studying the determinants of population health, investigators are guided by epidemiologic models. This section describes three models and explains how each might guide the approach to the same problem.

The problem to be considered is an increase in the infant mortality rate (IMR) in a hypothetical community. The IMR is a particularly important health index that should be understood even by health professionals whose main concern is not maternal or child health. Because infant mortality is influenced by a variety of biologic and environmental factors affecting infants and mothers, the IMR is both a direct measure of infant health and an indirect measure of community health as a whole. Infant mortality rates, as well as the mortality of children under the age of five years, are used as basic indicators of a nation's health status by the World Health Organization (WHO, 2005).

The Epidemiologic Triad

The epidemiologic triad or agent–host–environment model is a traditional view of health and disease, developed when epidemiology was concerned chiefly with communicable disease. As you will see, however, the model is applicable to other conditions as well. In the model, the *agent* is an organism capable of causing disease. The *host* is the population at risk for developing the disease. The *environment* is a combination of physical, biologic, economic, and social factors that surround and influence both the agent and the host. According to this model, by examining the characteristics of, changes in, and interactions among the agent, host, and environment, health (and illness) can be more holistically understood.

Figure 3-1 shows the triad in its normal state of equilibrium. Equilibrium does not signify optimum health but simply the usual pattern of illness and health in a population. Any change in one of the sides (agent, host, or environment) will result in disequilibrium—in other words, a change in the usual pattern.

How would this model guide the investigation of an increased IMR? To understand this, let us consider the three facets of the model.

AGENT

At first glance, it might be concluded that any investigation should focus on types of infections as agents that cause infant deaths. However, major causes of infant mortality in Canada and the United States include prematurity, low birth weight, birth injuries, congenital malformations, sudden infant death syndrome (SIDS), injuries, and homicides. Therefore, the investigation will try to determine whether

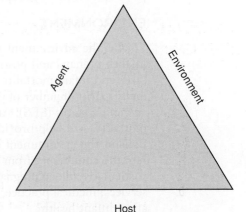

FIGURE 3-1 ◆ The epidemiologic triangle is the traditional view, showing health and disease as a composite state of three variables.

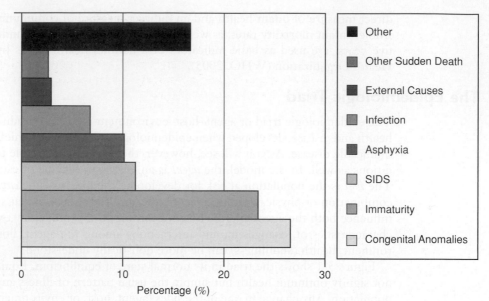

FIGURE 3-2 ◆   Leading causes of infant mortality, Canada.

there has been a change in any of these other agents. Figure 3-2 illustrates the leading causes (agent) of infant mortality in Canada during 1999 (Health Canada, 2003).

HOST

Investigators also will want to know the characteristics of the host—in this case, the infant population. This involves examining infant birth and death patterns in terms of age, ethnicity, sex, and birth weight. These characteristics have been shown to be important risk factors for infant mortality. By studying these factors, it may be possible to identify groups of infants who are at particularly increased risk of dying.

ENVIRONMENT

Finally, the environment must be assessed. The mother is a significant part of an infant's prenatal and postnatal environment. Therefore, investigators will analyze birth and infant mortality patterns according to factors such as maternal age, ethnicity, parity (number of previous live births), prenatal care, education, and socioeconomic status (SES). Analysis of these factors, which are also related to infant mortality, will help provide further identification of at-risk groups. Other conditions in the environment also need to be considered. For instance, has migration into the community from other areas increased? Has adult morbidity or mortality, particularly among pregnant women, increased? Have there been changes in health services, medical practice, policies, personnel, funding, or other factors that could affect infant health?

The analysis of these three areas—the agent, host, and environment—should provide information regarding groups at risk for increased infant mortality and may point the way toward a program aimed at reducing that risk. Thus, the epidemiologic triad, although it was designed with a communicable disease orientation, can provide a useful guide for studying the multifaceted problem of infant mortality as well as other health problems.

The Person–Place–Time Model

An approach similar to the epidemiologic triangle is one that guides the investigators to consider the health problem in terms of person, place, and time (Fletcher & Fletcher, 2005; Timmreck, 1998). The investigators examine characteristics of the persons affected (the host in the triangle model), the place (environment) or location, and the time period involved (which could relate to the agent, host, or environment). In studying infant mortality according to the person–place–time model, infant and maternal factors are considered traits of "person." Aspects of "place" are such factors as whether the community is rural or urban, affluent or poor. Aspects of "time" might include seasonal variation, age-specific patterns, or trends in mortality.

The Web of Causation

The web of causation (MacMahon & Trichopoulos, 1996) views a health condition not as the result of individual factors but of complex interactions among multiple factors. One factor may lead to others, which, in turn, lead to others, all of which may interact with one another to produce the health condition. Factors can be at the *macro* (multisystem, societal) level, *meso* (familial, local) level, or *micro* (individual) level.

Central to this model is the concept of synergism, wherein the whole is more than the sum of its separate parts. For example, the effects of a *Shigella* infection on an infant, combined with the effects of poverty, youth, and low educational level of the mother, are more deleterious to infant health than the sum of the effects of the individual risk factors.

Use of the web of causation may result in a more expansive study of infant mortality than one guided by other models. Ideally, investigators using this model first identify all factors related to infant mortality. Next, secondary components that are related to each of the initial factors are identified. These two comprehensive steps provide the outline for the web of causation for infant mortality. Finally, investigators examine the relationships among all the identified components of the web and attempt to determine the most feasible point of intervention to improve infant mortality in the community. Figure 3-3 depicts a web of causation for infant mortality. Other webs are proposed in literature related to specific issues (e.g., myocardial infarction, lead poisoning, adolescent pregnancy, addiction).

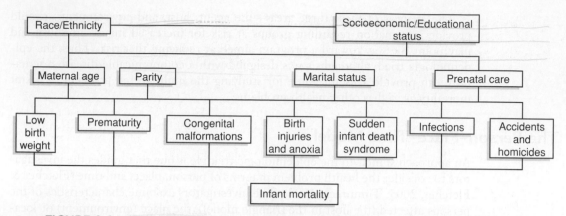

FIGURE 3-3 ◆ A web of causation for infant mortality based on information available from birth and death certificates.

This multifaceted approach addresses the concept of causation in a manner consistent with current knowledge of human health. However, it may be overwhelming to carry out in everyday practice, and some would argue that the concept oversimplifies the complexity of disease causation (MacMahon & Trichopoulos, 1996). Regardless, using a web of causation model can serve as a starting point to examine a facet of the web, acknowledging that other relationships exist. Thorough examination of one portion of the web may provide sufficient information for initiation of useful actions to improve community health.

The Haddon Matrix: Application of the Epidemiologic Triad

In the field of injury control, Haddon developed a matrix in the early 1970s to guide the development of public health strategies to prevent automobile crashes (Haddon, 1999; Runyan, 1998; Runyan, 2003). Using the epidemiologic triad of host–agent–environment (columns) and the concepts of pre-event, event, and post-event as prevention time points (rows), a matrix is formed and potential risk and protective factors can be filled in (Fig. 3-4). Interestingly, the Haddon Matrix has resurfaced in the literature as a conceptual model that is applicable for more than injury prevention and has been suggested for disaster planning and SARS preparedness (Barnett et al., 2005).

In this section, we showed how three models each provide a slightly different approach to a community issue and how the Haddon Matrix can be used to identify preventive approaches. Community issues can be related to "problems" or "wellness," and in future chapters, you will see how the models can apply to both situations. As you continue to study community health, you will find other models that can guide your practice and investigation. There is no one "correct" model; as you gain experience, you will be able to choose or adapt those that are most appropriate for your work.

| Phase | Influencing Factors | | | |
	Host	Agent / Vehicle	Physical Environment	Social Environment
Pre-event	Fatigue Substance use Uncorrected vision Distraction Cell phone use Seat-belt use	Poor maintenance of vehicle Bald tires Excessive speed	Poor visibility from weather Slick roads Inadequate street lighting Poor road signage Nighttime	Culture that discourages seat-belt use Inadequate enforcement of speed limit laws Poor public investment in road maintenance or snow clearing
Event	Driver's body impacted by vehicle Driver's pre-existing physical condition & health	Impact of vehicle with roadside object (e.g. guardrail) or another vehicle Vehicle size, airbags, suspension, and crash rating	Local environment (e.g. ambient temperature ground condition) Distance to hospital(s) with trauma centres Time of day for discovery	Ambulance service Good samaritan laws
Post-event	Driver's ability to recover Medical and nursing care received post-injury Prevention of complications Psychological impact	Severity of physical injuries Severity of psychological impact	Availability of rehabilitation facility	Workplace benefits Extra health insurance coverage Family and social support

FIGURE 3-4   ◆   Use of Haddon Matrix.

LEVELS OF PREVENTION IN COMMUNITY PRACTICE

The concept of prevention is a key component of modern community health. In popular terminology, prevention means intervening before an event occurs. In community health, three levels of prevention are practised: primary, secondary, and tertiary.

Primary prevention involves true avoidance of an illness or adverse health condition through health promotion activities and protective actions. Primary prevention encompasses a vast array of intervention strategies, including nutrition, hygiene, sanitation, immunization, environmental protection, health education, and housing, to name but a few. Research into the causes of health problems provides the basis for primary prevention. For example, just as Snow's 1854 investigation of cholera paved the way for provision of clean water to the residents of London, modern research into motor vehicle injuries has led to the use of seat belts and air bags.

Secondary prevention is the early detection and treatment of adverse conditions. Secondary prevention may result in the cure of illnesses that would be incurable at later stages, the prevention of complications and disability, and confinement of the spread of communicable diseases. An important component of secondary prevention is screening, the examination of asymptomatic people for disorders such as tuberculosis, diabetes, hypertension, and the Papanicolaou (Pap) smear, a commonly used screening test for the detection of cervical cancer. By 2006, to prevent motor vehicle injuries in populations at the highest risk, all provinces with the exception of Saskatchewan instituted graduated licences for new drivers. Reductions in collisions within this high-risk group have already been documented; in British Columbia, collisions by new drivers decreased by 16% during the first three years following the introduction of graduated licensing (ICBC, 2006).

Tertiary prevention is used after diseases or events have already resulted in damage to individuals. The purpose of tertiary prevention is to limit disability and to rehabilitate or restore the affected people to their maximum possible capacities. Examples of tertiary prevention include provision of "meals on wheels" for the homebound, physical therapy services for stroke victims, and mental health counselling for rape victims. With respect to motor vehicles, the adaptation of vehicles for paraplegic individuals and those with prosthetic lower limbs is an example of tertiary prevention.

To plan appropriate methods of primary, secondary, and tertiary prevention, the community health professional must first assess the health of the community (Sahai et al., 2005). The following section covers some basic measures used in community health assessment.

DESCRIPTIVE MEASURES OF HEALTH

Demographic Measures

Certain human characteristics, or demographics, may be associated with wellness or illness. Age, sex, ethnicity, income, and educational level are important demographics that may affect health outcomes. For example, men are more likely than women to die from certain heart diseases (Statistics Canada, 2006a), First Nations peoples are three to five times more likely to have diabetes than other Canadians (Health Canada, 2002), and adolescent women are more likely than adult women to have low-birth-weight infants (Health Canada, 2003). To plan interventions for population health, the community health worker must be familiar with the demographic characteristics of the community and with the health problems associated with those characteristics.

Morbidity and Mortality

Although epidemiology encompasses wellness as well as illness, wellness is difficult to measure. Therefore, many measures of "health" are expressed in terms of *morbidity* (illness) and *mortality* (death). Most Canadian indices of health are published by Health Canada and listed on the Public Health Agency of Canada website and include reports on communicable diseases and chronic diseases as well as other important topics and links to other relevant sites. An excellent source of U.S. morbidity and mortality data is *Morbidity and Mortality Weekly Report* from the Centers for Disease Control and Prevention (CDC).

Incidence

The *incidence* of a disease or health condition refers to the number of individuals in a population who develop the condition during a specified period of time (normally, a calendar year). The calculation of incidence, therefore, generally requires that a population be followed over a period of time in what is called a prospective (forward-looking) study.

Prevalence

The *prevalence* of a disease or condition refers to the total number of individuals in the population who have the condition at a particular time. Thus, prevalence may be calculated in a "one-shot" cross-sectional ("slice of time") or retrospective (backward-looking) study.

Interpretation of Incidence and Prevalence

Measures of incidence and prevalence provide different information and have different implications. For example, an increase in the prevalence of cancer means that there are more persons with cancer in the population. This may be because there are more new cases (in other words, increased incidence) or because persons with cancer are living longer. In either case, the community may need to direct resources toward cancer. However, if knowledge of incidence is lacking, it will be difficult to decide whether to target the resources toward primary prevention of cancer or toward secondary prevention (diagnosis and treatment) and tertiary prevention (rehabilitation) services.

Rates

Incidence and prevalence usually are expressed as mathematical measures called rates. Because epidemiology is the study of population health, these measures must relate the occurrence of a health condition to the population base. Rates do exactly this. They express a mathematical relationship in which the numerator is the number of persons experiencing the condition and the denominator is the population at risk, or the total number of persons who have the possibility of experiencing the condition.

Rates must not be confused with other proportions that do not use the population at risk as the denominator. For example, the death rate from cancer is not the same as the proportion of deaths from cancer. In each, the numerator is the number of deaths from cancer. However, the denominators differ. In the death rate, the denominator includes all persons at risk of dying from cancer. Therefore, the cancer death rate is an expression of the risk of dying from cancer. In the proportion of deaths, also called proportionate mortality, the denominator is the total number of deaths from all causes. Therefore, the proportionate cancer mortality simply describes the proportion of deaths attributable to cancer.

CALCULATION OF RATES

Rates are calculated in this general format:

$$\text{Rate} = \frac{\text{number of people experiencing condition}}{\text{population at risk for experiencing condition}} \times K$$

K is a constant (usually 1,000, 10,000, or 100,000) that allows the ratio, which may be a very small number, to be expressed in a meaningful way. Let us apply this formula to the calculation of the IMR, which estimates an infant's risk of dying during the first year of life.

EXAMPLE OF A RATE: THE INFANT MORTALITY RATE

The IMR usually is calculated on a calendar-year basis: the number of infant deaths (deaths before the age of 1 year) in 1 year is divided by the number of live births (infants born alive) during that year. The numerator represents the number of infants experiencing the "condition" of dying in the first year of life, and the denominator represents the population of infants at risk for dying in the year.

In 2003, there was an average of 5.3 infant deaths for every 1,000 live births in Canada. In Alberta in 2004, there were 40,779 live births and 258 infant deaths reported. To compare the infant mortality rate with the Canadian average, we calculate a rate. Applying the formula for a rate, we divide 258 by 40,779 and find that 0.0063 of an infant died during the first year of life. Because it is difficult to relate to 0.0063 of an infant, we multiply by a constant (K), in this case 1,000, and find that 6.3 infants per 1,000 live births died during the first year of life; that is, the IMR was 6.3 infant deaths per 1,000 live births in that year. In comparison to the most recent national data available, we can say that Alberta has a higher IMR than the national average. How does this compare with other provinces and territories?

By comparing rates rather than raw numbers, we can then rank parts of the country by IMR to determine areas of greatest need for intervention. In 2003, New Brunswick had the lowest infant mortality rate at 4.1 infant deaths per 1,000 live births, whereas Nunavut had the highest rate at 19.8 per 1,000 (Statistics Canada, 2006b). Regional variations also occur within provinces. For example, in Alberta for the same time period, the mortality rate was significantly higher in the Chinook, David Thompson, Aspen, and Northern Lights health regions than the provincial average (Child Health Surveillance Project Data Group, 2005). Each of these areas has very different actual numbers of births, but by comparing rates,

TABLE 3-1

Infant Mortality (rate per 1,000 live births) in Canada, 1993–2003*

YEAR	INFANT MORTALITY RATE
1993	6.3
1994	6.3
1995	6.1
1996	5.6
1997	5.5
1998	5.3
1999	5.3
2000	5.3
2001	5.2
2002	5.4
2003	5.3

*Includes stillbirths of unknown gestational period. Newfoundland, New Brunswick, and Québec do not report fetal death of less than 500 g.

health program planners are able to determine where need is greatest for programming to improve birth outcomes.

Additionally, trends can become apparent by tracking rates longitudinally over time. In Table 3-1, we can see that the trend in the national IMR decreased for the first 5 years and has stabilized over the 10-year period.

INTERPRETATION OF RATES

Rates enable researchers and practitioners to compare different populations in terms of health problems or conditions. To assess whether the population in a specific community is at greater or lesser risk for the problems or conditions, the rates for the community should be compared with rates from similar communities, from the province or territory, or from Canada as a whole.

In almost all countries, IMRs have declined dramatically over the last century with improvements in sanitation, nutrition, infant feeding, and maternal and child health care, although the decline has been slower in recent years (Kramer et al., 2005). Nevertheless, disparities in the risk of infant mortality remain, including in Canada (Luo et al., 2004; Martens & Derksen, 2002; Rockwell, 2001). Estimates of preventable infant mortality enable us to better understand the nature of the disparities between population subgroups and the factors that may be responsible and help to direct interventions toward areas where improvement is possible.

Some caution must be taken in interpreting rates. Like most statistical measures, rates are less reliable when based on small numbers. This must be kept in mind when assessing relatively infrequent events or conditions or communities with small populations.

Many rates are based on data from a calendar year, which may also present some difficulties. When calculating an IMR for a particular year, such as 2003, be aware

---

BOX 3-1

Causes of Infant Mortality

- Late fetal, neonatal, and postneonatal deaths among babies weighing less than 1,500 g may be largely attributable to factors affecting maternal health. Late fetal deaths among babies weighing ≥1,500 g may result from suboptimal maternal care. For example, regions characterized by relatively high rates of late fetal death among babies with normal birth weight may benefit from better access to caesarean delivery.
- Suboptimal newborn care or lack of access to neonatal intensive care is likely to contribute to early neonatal (0–6 days of age) deaths among babies with birth weight ≥1,500 g and late neonatal deaths among babies with intermediate birth weight, between 1,500 and 2,499 g.
- Infant deaths during the late neonatal (7–27 days) period for birth weight ≥2,500 g and postneonatal (28–364 days) deaths for birth weight ≥1,500 g may be largely attributable to factors in the infant environment (e.g., access to immunization, injury prevention, and control).

From Health Canada Perinatal Health Indicators: **http://www.phac-aspc.gc.ca/rhs-ssg/phic-ispc/index.html** and Canadian Perinatal Health Report 2003 **http://www.phac-aspc.gc.ca/publict/cphr-rspc03/index.html.**

---

that some of the infants who die during the 2003 calendar year were actually born in 2002 and thus were not part of the 2003 population at risk (denominator), and some of the infants who were born in 2002 might die in 2003 (numerator) and not be reflected in the 2002 IMR. Also, populations may increase or decrease during a calendar year. In such cases, the midyear population estimate (June 30) is generally used because the population at risk cannot be determined exactly. A study that follows a cohort, or specified group, prospectively can help overcome the limitations of the conventionally calculated calendar-year rate.

Box 3-1 presents more information regarding causes of infant death.

COMMONLY USED RATES

Table 3-2 summarizes a number of important rates. Note that the measures of natality and mortality are, in essence, measures of incidence of the conditions of "being born" and "dying." Note also the various ways in which the denominator, or population at risk, is determined in different rates.

CRUDE, SPECIFIC, AND ADJUSTED RATES

Rates that are computed for a population as a whole are called *crude rates*. Subgroups of a population may have differences that are not revealed by the crude rates. Rates that are calculated for subgroups are referred to as *specific rates*. Specific rates help identify groups at increased risk within the population and also facilitate

TABLE 3-2
Commonly Used Rates

Measures of Natality

$$\text{Crude birth rate} = \frac{\text{Number of live births during time interval}}{\text{Estimated midinterval population}} \times 1{,}000$$

$$\text{Fertility rate} = \frac{\text{Number of live births during time interval}}{\text{Number of women aged 15-44 at midinterval}} \times 1{,}000$$

Measures of Morbidity and Mortality

$$\text{Incidence rate} = \frac{\text{Number of new cases specified health conditions during the time interval}}{\text{Estimated midinterval population at risk}} \times 1{,}000$$

$$\text{Prevalence rate} = \frac{\text{Number of current cases of specified health condition at a given point in time}}{\text{Estimated population at risk at same point in time}} \times 1{,}000$$

$$\text{Crude death rate} = \frac{\text{Number of deaths during time interval}}{\text{Estimated midinterval population}} \times 1{,}000$$

$$\text{Specific death rate} = \frac{\text{Number of deaths in a subgroup during time interval}}{\text{Estimated midinterval population of subgroup}} \times 1{,}000$$

$$\text{Cause-specific death rate} = \frac{\text{Number of deaths from specified cause during time interval}}{\text{Estimated midinterval population}} \times 1{,}000$$

$$\text{Infant mortality rate} = \frac{\text{Number of deaths of infants aged } <1 \text{ year during time interval}}{\text{Total live births during time interval}} \times 1{,}000$$

$$\text{Neonatal mortality rate} = \frac{\text{Number of deaths of infants aged } <28 \text{ days during time interval}}{\text{Total live births during time interval}} \times 1{,}000$$

$$\text{Postneonatal mortality rate} = \frac{\text{Number of deaths of infants aged } \geq 28 \text{ days but } <1 \text{ year during time interval}}{\text{Total live births during time interval}} \times 1{,}000$$

comparisons between populations that have different demographic compositions. Most frequently, specific rates are computed according to demographic factors such as age, ethnicity, or sex.

In comparing populations with different distributions of a factor that is known to affect the health condition being studied, the use of *adjusted rates* may be advisable. An adjusted rate is a summary measure that statistically removes the effect of the difference in the distributions of that characteristic. In essence, adjustment produces an estimate of what the crude rate would be if the populations were identical in respect to the factor for which adjustment is made. A rate can be adjusted for age, ethnicity, sex, or any factor or combination of factors suspected of affecting the rate. Adjusted rates are helpful in making community comparisons, but they are hypothetical as the numerical value of an adjusted rate depends on the standard population used in the standardization calculations (Gordis, 2004). Therefore, adjusted rates must be interpreted with care.

ANALYTIC MEASURES OF HEALTH

As you have learned, rates are used to describe and compare the risks of dying, becoming ill, or developing other health conditions. It is also desirable to determine if health conditions are associated with, or related to, other factors. The related factors may point the way to preventive actions (e.g., the linking of air pollution to health problems has led to environmental controls). To investigate potential relationships between health conditions and other factors, analytic measures of community health are required. In this section, three analytic measures are discussed: relative risk, odds ratio, and attributable risk.

Relative Risk

To determine if a relationship or association exists between a health condition and a suspected factor, it is necessary to compare the risk of developing the health condition for the population exposed to the factor with the risk for the population not exposed to the factor. The *relative risk* (RR) *ratio* does exactly this by expressing the ratio of the incidence rate of those exposed and those not exposed to the suspected factor:

$$RR = \frac{\text{incidence rate among those exposed}}{\text{incidence rate among those not exposed}}$$

The RR tells us whether the rate in the exposed population is higher than the rate in the nonexposed population and, if so, how many times higher it is. A high RR in the exposed population suggests that the factor is a *risk factor* in the development of the health condition.

Internal and External Risk Factors

The concept of RR is understood readily when one group of people clearly is exposed and another is not exposed to an external agent such as a virus, cigarette smoke, or an industrial pollutant. However, it may be confusing to see RRs applied to internal factors such as age, race, or sex. Nevertheless, as can be seen in the next example, persons are also "exposed" to intrinsic factors that may carry as much risk as extrinsic ones.

EXAMPLE OF RELATIVE RATE: DIABETES

Type 2 diabetes mellitus is complicated by conditions such as ischemic heart disease, peripheral vascular disease, cerebral vascular disease, retinopathy, renal vascular disease, and peripheral neuropathy. Complications of diabetes lead to a poorer quality of life and premature death.

There is general agreement that type 2 diabetes has a genetic basis but that environmental factors, the most important of which is obesity, are also involved in the disease onset. It appears that nongenetic factors may be subject to intervention, and studies of controlling obesity are needed, especially by diet and exercise. Participation in a community-based exercise program can successfully facilitate weight loss in a group of individuals with type 2 diabetes. Participation decreases fasting blood glucose values and decreases the need for insulin or oral hypoglycaemic agents, or both.

DIABETES AND THE FIRST NATIONS

Health Canada (2002) reports that, according to the 1996–1997 National Population Health Survey (NPHS), 3.2% of the Canadian population aged 12 and over has a diagnosis of diabetes. However, among Aboriginal people aged 12 and over living on reserves rather than in towns or cities off the reserve to which they belong, the rate was 8.5%. With this information, we can calculate a relative risk. Among on-reserve Aboriginals (those "exposed" to the intrinsic condition of being First Nations people living on a reserve), the rate was 8.5/100, and among non-Aboriginals living off reserves in Canada (those "not exposed" to the condition), the rate was 3.2/100. Thus, the RR of diabetes for Aboriginal people living on reserves compared with Canadians in general can be calculated as follows:

$$RR = \frac{8.5 \text{ per } 100}{3.2 \text{ per } 100} = 2.67$$

In other words, the risk of diabetes is almost three times greater for on-reserve Aboriginals than for Canadians in general. Clearly, First Nations ancestry is a risk factor. The risk factor itself cannot be altered, but the information provided by this analysis can be used to plan protective services for the population at greatest risk (e.g., Canadian Diabetes Strategy–Aboriginal Initiative).

We must be cautious in making generalizations, however, because further analysis indicates that diabetes rates differ across the country. The prevalence in the Cree-Ojibwa living in North West Ontario and North East Manitoba has been reported as 46/1000 (RR = 1.43), whereas among the Dene Tlicho in the Northwest Territories, nearly 10% of adults were found to be hyperglycaemic (RR = 3.12) (Young, 1988). On the Kahnawake reservation near Montreal, 12% of Mohawks aged 45 to 65 were known diabetics compared with 3.2% of Canadians in the same age group (RR = 3.8) (Macauley, Montour, & Adelson, 1988). Rates rise in people over age 65, regardless of ethnicity, with 23% of Aboriginal seniors compared with 10.4% of senior Canadians diagnosed with diabetes (Health Canada, 2001).

Odds Ratio

Calculation of the RR is straightforward when incidence rates are available. Unfortunately, not all studies can be carried out prospectively as is required for the computation of incidence rates. In a retrospective study, the RR must be approximated by the *odds ratio* (OR).

TABLE 3-3			
Cross Tabulation for Calculation of Odds Ratio			
	HEALTH CONDITION		
	Present	Absent	Total
Exposed to factor	a	b	$a + b$
Not exposed to factor	c	d	$c + d$
TOTAL	$a + c$	$b + d$	$a + b + c + d$

As shown in Table 3-3, the OR is a simple mathematical ratio of the odds in favour of having a specific health condition when the suspected factor is present and the odds in favour of having the condition when the factor is absent. The odds of having the condition when the suspected factor is present is represented by a divided by b in the table (a/b). The chance of having the condition when the factor is absent is represented by c divided by d (c/d). The odds ratio is thus:

$$\frac{a/b}{c/d} = \frac{ad}{bc}$$

An example may help. When toxic shock syndrome (TSS), a severe illness involving high fever, vomiting, diarrhea, rash, and hypotension or shock, was first reported in the early 1980s, it was neither practical nor ethical to consider cases only on a prospective basis. Therefore, existing cases were compared retrospectively with controls. Early studies noted an association between TSS and tampon use and suggested that users of a specific brand of superabsorbent tampon might be at especially high risk. To clarify the issue, researchers analyzed data from TSS cases and controls, all of which used tampons. Let's use the TSS data in Table 3-4 to calculate the OR for users of the specific brand of tampon.

$$OR = \frac{ad}{bc} = \frac{30(84)}{30(12)} = 7$$

Users of the specific brand were seven times more likely to develop TSS than were users of other brands. Based on this and other studies, the brand was voluntarily withdrawn from the market.

Relative Rate and Odds Ratio: Caution in Interpretation

A word of caution: Regard a high OR or RR with appropriate concern, but do not allow the finding to obscure the potential involvement of other factors. Refer to Table 3-4 again and note that 12 persons in the sample had TSS although they did not use the specific brand of tampon. In other words, this product was not the sole cause of TSS. Subsequent research showed that certain superabsorbent materials in

TABLE 3-4			
Toxic Shock Syndrome Cases Among 156 Tampon Users			
	TOXIC SHOCK SYNDROME		
BRAND OF TAMPON USED	Present	Absent	Total
Suspected brand	30	30	60
Other brands	12	84	96
TOTAL	42	114	156

Data from Centers for Disease Control and Prevention. (1980, September 19). Follow up on toxic shock syndrome. *Morbidity and Mortality Weekly Report, 29,* 441–445.

tampons or certain aspects of tampon use foster growth of *Staphylococcus aureus*, the probable causal organism in TSS (CDC, 1981, 1983; Davis et al., 1980).

In addition to assessing the strength of the association based on either the OR or RR, the confidence interval (CI) surrounding the estimate must be evaluated. Since RR and OR are ratios, an estimate of 1.0 indicates that there is no difference between the variables being compared. Therefore, if the confidence interval includes the integer "1," then the estimate is considered statistically "nonsignificant" (e.g., OR =1.8, 95% CI = 0.6–2.3).

Attributable Risk and Attributable Risk Percent

Another measure of risk is *attributable risk* (AR), or the difference between the incidence rates for those exposed and those not exposed to the risk factor. This measure estimates the excess risk attributable to the factor being studied. It shows the potential reduction in the overall incidence rate if the factor could be eliminated.

AR = incidence rate in exposed group *minus* incidence rate in nonexposed group. AR usually is further quantified into attributable risk percent:

$$\frac{\text{attributable risk}}{\text{incidence rate in exposed group}} \times 100$$

This provides an estimate of the percentage of occurrences of the health condition that could be prevented if the risk factor were eliminated. For example, studies of the relationship between physical inactivity and mortality from coronary heart disease (CHD) showed that the percent of AR associated with physical inactivity was 35% (CDC, 1993). Thus, improved physical activity has the potential to greatly reduce CHD mortality.

Cause and Association

Ultimately, community health professionals hope to determine causes of health conditions so that steps can be taken to improve health. In view of the complexity of the human body and human behaviour, establishing causality is difficult. Therefore, investigations of population health generally examine relationships or *associations* between variables. The variables are the characteristics or phenomena (such as age, occupation, or physical exercise) and the health conditions (such as heart disease) being studied.

VARIABLES AND CONSTANTS

An important requirement in any study is that the factors studied must have the potential to vary from person to person. If a factor cannot vary, it is not a variable but a constant. It is impossible to establish an association between a constant and a variable because the constant, by definition, cannot change when the variable changes. Thus, a study that looks only at men cannot establish an association between sex and, for example, heart disease; the study has made sex a constant. A study that looks only at persons with heart disease cannot establish an association between heart disease and any other variable; heart disease has become a constant in the study.

CONTROL OR COMPARISON GROUPS

To ensure that associations between variables can be examined, *control groups* or *comparison groups* may be needed. A study of heart disease might compare persons with the disease with a control group of persons without the disease. An investigation of a new treatment would study persons who receive the treatment and a control group of persons who do not receive the treatment.

INDEPENDENT AND DEPENDENT VARIABLES

Frequently, variables are referred to as *dependent* or *independent*. The dependent variable is the outcome or result that the investigator is studying. It is a characteristic that conceivably could be altered (e.g., health status, knowledge, or behaviour). The independent variable is the presumed "cause" of or contributor to variation in the dependent variable. For example, in the heart disease study cited earlier (CDC, 1993), physical inactivity, the independent variable, is seen to contribute to heart disease, the dependent variable. An independent variable may be a naturally occurring event or phenomenon such as level of usual physical activity, exposure to ultraviolet radiation, or type of employment, or it might be a planned intervention such as an exercise regimen, a medical treatment, or an educational program. An independent variable might also be an intrinsic quality such as age, ethnicity, or sex. Note that these intrinsic qualities, although they cannot vary within an individual, can vary from person to person; thus, they can be studied as independent variables.

CONFOUNDING VARIABLES

When an association is identified between variables, it is tempting—but incorrect—to assume that one variable causes the other. If, for example, a study found that communities with lower salaries for public health workers had higher crime rates, we could not conclude that low public health salaries led to high crime rates. Common sense suggests that economic conditions might influence both salaries and crime; that is, economic conditions intervene in the study and confound the results. Any factor that is associated with both the independent (exposure) and dependent (disease) variables is considered a confounding variable.

CRITERIA FOR DETERMINING CAUSATION

If an association is found between variables, it means that variables tend to occur or change together, but it does not prove that one variable causes the other. Because of the possibility of confounded results, guidelines for determining causation have been identified. An association must be evaluated against these criteria; the more criteria that are met, the more likely it is that the association is causal. However, an association may meet all the criteria for causation and later be shown to be spurious because of factors that were not known at the time the study was done. For this reason, investigators must interpret their results with great caution; rarely can results be shown to be causal. Nine widely used guidelines for evaluating causation, first established by Bradford Hill in 1965, are listed below (Gordis, 2004). Of these, time sequence, strength of association, and consistency with existing knowledge are argued to be the most critical (MacMahon & Trichopoulos, 1996).

1. The association is strong. The strength of the relationship may be evaluated statistically by a variety of measures. For example, the higher the RR or OR with a narrow CI, the stronger the association.
2. Consistency with other knowledge. An association that contradicts current scientific views must be evaluated very carefully. However, associations may be inconsistent with current knowledge simply because current knowledge is not as advanced as a new discovery.
3. The association is temporally correct. The hypothesized cause of the health condition must occur before the onset of the condition.
4. Dose–response relationship. A strong argument can be made for a causal relationship if the risk of disease or condition increases with increased exposure. However, absence of a dose–response relationship does not necessarily rule out a causal relationship.
5. Consideration of other alternative explanations. Not all potential intervening variables can be explored, of course, but alternate explanation for the association, including the possibility of confounding, must be examined carefully before considering an association to be causal.
6. The association is biologically plausible. Consistency with existing biologic knowledge is sought; however, there have been instances where the epidemiologic identification of a syndrome or disease has preceded the biological understanding of a disease (e.g., HIV/AIDS).
7. Replication of findings. The same association must be found repeatedly in other studies, in other settings, and with other methods.

8. Cessation of exposure. If a causal exposure or factor for a condition is removed, it is expected that the incidence of the disease would also decrease. While this is normally the case, there are instances where the pathologic progression of a disease is irreversible by the time the exposure is removed, and the occurrence of the condition may not fall accordingly.
9. The association is specific. The hypothesized cause should be associated with relatively few health conditions. For example, speaking English may be associated with many health conditions, but it is a cause for none. This criterion must be tempered by the knowledge that certain factors or behaviours, such as cigarette smoking, have been shown to have multiple effects.

The usefulness of information to a community depends on its accuracy, completeness, and reliability. If data are to provide a realistic profile of a community, identify issues placing people at risk, and assess areas of strength on which to build programs, then planners must have confidence in the information they gather and in the interpretations made by residents and community workers. Hence, data must be from credible sources, collected by ethical and valid methods, appropriate to the issues involved, and detailed enough to allow quality interventions to be developed. In the next section, common sources of data are identified and, when combined with assessment strategies presented in Chapter 13, can form a solid foundation for community action.

SOURCES OF COMMUNITY HEALTH DATA

To be an effective community health professional, you will also need to interpret and use data from various sources. In this section, we present the use of several important sources of data.

Census

The census is the most comprehensive source of population data for Canada. Every 5 years, under the Statistics Act, the government of Canada enumerates the population and surveys it for basic demographics such as age, sex, marital status, and mother tongue as well as numerous other factors such as employment, ethnicity, housing, income, migration, and education.

Canada's first census was in 1666, when Jean Talon counted the 3,215 inhabitants of the Colony of New France, noting their age, sex, marital status, and occupation. Approximately 98 colonial and regional censuses took place between then and Canada's first official census in 1871. The Census Act (1870) required that enumeration of the population take place every 10 years, providing the cornerstone for representative government. Since 1951, Canada has conducted a census every 5 years. Up to and including the 1966 census, all data collection was conducted by interview; in 1971, self-enumeration began. Refinements have been made to methods of data collection as technology has advanced; questions have changed as information needs have developed with changing populations, immigration, wars, and social trends. (Statistics Canada, 2006c)

The 2006 Census took place May 1–16; approximately 32.5 million people were to be "counted in" during the census. At the same time that households received a Census of Population questionnaire, farm operations received a Census of Agriculture form. An adult in each household is required to complete the questionnaire and return it to Statistics Canada or complete the form on-line. The short form of the questionnaire, containing eight questions, was sent to 80% of all households, and the long form of the questionnaire went to one in five households and contained the original 8, plus 53 additional questions. In remote areas such as Baffin Island, a census enumerator conducts household interviews.

Census reports are available in public libraries; in municipal, provincial, and federal government offices; and on the Internet. Although census data are comprehensive, bias does occur. For example, people may answer personal questions dishonestly. Perhaps more significant, the census is believed to under-represent low-income residents, residents of First Nations reserves, and transients. These people are more difficult to locate and enumerate and tend to be less likely to respond to census surveys. However, efforts are made to capture information on as many people as possible; forms are available in more than 50 languages, in braille, and in large print. Forms are also available in electronic formats, and a census representative is available to collect the data in person if necessary. People are required by law to complete census forms every 5 years, and there are penalties for those who refuse or who do not tell the truth. Additional information on the Canadian census can be found at **http://www12.statcan.ca/english/census01/home/Index.cfm**.

Vital Statistics

Vital statistics are the data on legally registered events (such as births, deaths, marriages, and divorces) collected on an ongoing basis by government agencies. Provincial health departments usually publish vital statistics annually. Health Canada also gathers data from the provinces and publishes annual volumes as well as periodic reports on specific topics. Vital statistics for provinces and territories can be found online.

Beginning researchers tend to consider vital statistics "hallowed" because they are, after all, legal data. However, legality does not guarantee validity. For example, the manner in which cause of death is recorded on death certificates is inconsistent. The numbers of unmarried but cohabiting couples—and the occasional news reports of newly discovered bigamists—also demonstrate that marriage and divorce records are also not completely valid measures of reality. Despite their limitations, vital statistics are often the best available data, and much useful information can be gained from them.

Notifiable Disease Reports

The Public Health Agency of Canada (PHAC) reports data collected by provincial and local health departments on legally reportable diseases and also periodically requests voluntary reporting of non-notifiable health conditions of special interest. Canada Communicable Disease Report (CCDR), other reports on chronic diseases, and reports on special topics are available from the PHAC.

Even legally mandated disease reports may not be representative of all cases of the disease. Thus, they may not provide valid description of a disease as it exists in the community. In practice, health care providers may fail to report diseases that should be reported; for instance, chickenpox (varicella) is consistently underreported.

Medical and Hospital Records

Medical and hospital records are used extensively in community health research. These records, however, do not provide a completely representative or valid picture of community health. In the first place, not all persons with health problems receive medical attention, so medical records are obviously biased. Second, medical documentation is not always complete. Finally, hospitalized patients are also more likely to have another illness along with the one being studied. This phenomenon, called Berkson's bias, creates the likelihood of finding a false association between the two illnesses (Last, 2001).

Social Welfare Reports

Statistics Canada as well as Human Resources and Social Development Canada (HRSDC) publish regular reports on current issues about the social situation experienced by Canadians. A survey of the websites of these organizations can offer the community professional insight into social conditions such as homelessness, poverty, education, and the economy. Other national Internet sites offer opinion and analysis of social and economic conditions. There are also regional "think tanks" that offer comment on issues specific to people in groups of provinces.

Various national and provincial professional associations also offer publications on issues relevant to their disciplines. As with any site, you must be cautious in interpreting the opinions and analysis because they will come from a particular perspective and are trying to make an argument that supports their specific viewpoint. Seeking information from several sites will provide the community health professional with a broad perspective on issues.

SCREENING FOR HEALTH CONDITIONS

Thus far, we have focused on methods for studying community health problems and assessing health risks for populations. In this section, we discuss screening, a method of secondary prevention. Screening is an effort to detect unrecognized or preclinical illness among individuals. Screening tests are not intended to be diagnostic. Their purpose is to rapidly and economically identify persons who have a high probability of having (or developing) a particular illness so that they can be referred for definitive diagnosis and treatment.

Considerations in Deciding to Screen

Screening goes further than identifying groups at risk for illness; it identifies individuals who may actually have an illness. Screening carries an ethical commitment to continue working with these individuals and provide them access to diagnostic and treatment services. In general, screening should be conducted only if:

◆ Early diagnosis and treatment can favourably alter the course of the illness
◆ Definitive diagnosis and treatment facilities are available, either through the screening agency or through referral
◆ A group being screened is at risk for the illness (in other words, the group is likely to have a high prevalence of the illness)
◆ Screening procedures are reliable and valid

Ideally, a screening test should be simple to perform, cause minimal distress to patients, and be low cost. Acceptability by the public and clinicians is also crucial for the adoption and implementation of any screening test (Fletcher & Fletcher, 2005).

Screening Test Reliability and Validity

Reliability refers to the consistency or repeatability of test results; *validity* refers to the ability of the test to measure what it is supposed to measure. A few considerations specific to screening tests are discussed below.

SCREENING TEST RELIABILITY

A reliable screening test yields the same result even when administered by different screeners. Training for all screening personnel in use of the test is essential. Lack of reliability may suggest that the screeners are administering the test in an inconsistent manner or that a chemical reagent is unstable.

SCREENING TEST VALIDITY: SENSITIVITY AND SPECIFICITY

To be valid, a screening test must distinguish correctly between those individuals who have the condition and those who do not. This is measured by the test's sensitivity and specificity, as shown in Table 3-5.

Sensitivity is the ability to correctly identify individuals who have the disease—that is, to identify a true positive. A test with high sensitivity will have few false negatives.

Specificity is the ability to correctly identify individuals who do not have the disease or to call a true negative "negative." A test with high specificity has few false positives.

TABLE 3-5
Sensitivity and Specificity of a Screening Test

	REALITY	
SCREENING TEST RESULTS	Diseased	Not Diseased
Positive	True positive	False positive
Negative	False negative	True negative
TOTAL	Total diseased	Total not diseased

$$\text{Sensitivity (true-positive rate)} = \frac{\text{True positives}}{\text{Total diseased}}$$

$$\text{Specificity (true-negative rate)} = \frac{\text{True negatives}}{\text{Total not diseased}}$$

$$\text{False-negative rate} = \frac{\text{False negatives}}{\text{Total diseased}} \quad or \quad 1 - \text{Sensitivity}$$

$$\text{False-positive rate} = \frac{\text{False positives}}{\text{Total not diseased}} \quad or \quad 1 - \text{Sensitivity}$$

RELATIONSHIP BETWEEN SENSITIVITY AND SPECIFICITY

Ideally, a screening test's sensitivity and specificity should be 100%; in practice, however, screening tests vary in this regard. As shown in Table 3-5, sensitivity, or the true-positive rate, is the complement of the false-negative rate, and specificity, or the true-negative rate, is the complement of the false-positive rate. Thus, as sensitivity increases, specificity decreases, and vice versa. Therefore, decisions regarding screening test validity may require uncomfortable compromises, as you will see from the following examples.

DECISION MAKING IN SCREENING: PRACTICAL AND ETHICAL CONSIDERATIONS

Suppose you are screening for a deadly disease that is curable only if detected early, and you have a choice between a test with high sensitivity and low specificity or one with high specificity and low sensitivity. To save the most lives, you need high sensitivity; that is, a low rate of false negatives (people who *have* the disease but are not detected by the screening test). However, if you select the test with high sensitivity, its low specificity means that you will have a high number of people who do *not* have the disease but whom the test identifies as having it (false positives). Using such a test will alarm many people needlessly and will cause unnecessary expenses by over-referring them for nonexistent disease. Which test would you choose?

Now, suppose you are screening for the same disease, but the diagnostic and treatment facilities in the community are already overloaded, and further budget cuts are projected. To minimize unnecessary referrals of false positives, you would want the test with high specificity. However, because of the low sensitivity of this test, you will have to weigh the benefits of a low false-positive rate against the ethics of a high false-negative rate. Is it justifiable to lull the undetected diseased persons into a false—and potentially fatal—sense of security? Which test would you choose now?

Decisions regarding screening involve seeking the most favourable balance of sensitivity and specificity. Sometimes, sensitivity and specificity can be improved by adjusting the screening process (e.g., adding another test or changing the level at which the test is considered positive). At other times, evaluating sensitivity and specificity may result in a decision not to conduct a screening program because the economic costs of over-referral or the ethical considerations of under-referral outweigh the usefulness of screening. An understanding of the principles discussed in this section will help you make informed decisions regarding community screening.

OUTBREAK MANAGEMENT

The emergence of newly identified infectious diseases in the past 20 years (e.g. HIV, Ebola virus, SARS, etc.) highlights the importance of preparedness of the public health system as well as an organized, logical approach to the investigation of outbreaks. Critical with any report of an outbreak is early verification of the diagnosis, plus the establishment of an epidemic (Mausner & Kramer, 1985; Timmreck, 1998). Key to diagnosis verification is ascertaining what constitutes a "case" and that laboratory and clinical assessments are accurate; simultaneously, potential missing cases are searched for. If previous records exist about the prevalence of a disease, it is important to compare the current findings with historical data. Once the existence of an epidemic has been established, identification of "when" (time), "where" (place), and "who" (person) occurs. Plotting the occurrences on a map and the cases on a time line assists in describing the nature of the epidemic. Determination as to whether the epidemic has a common source versus whether it is propagated aids in identifying potential control measures. Finally, it is important to analyse the findings and develop and test hypotheses. Appropriate public health agencies are notified once an epidemic is verified and it has been determined who is at risk. This is not always easily accomplished, particularly when dealing with a new condition or disease not previously known.

A case in point was the 2003 SARS outbreak in Toronto, Ontario, as there was no diagnostic test, no treatment, and very little information on the characteristics of the viral agent (Basrur, Yaffe, & Henry, 2004). The SARS outbreak was unique in that it was propagated within hospitals and to households that had contact with patients (Svobada et al., 2004; Varia et al., 2003). A total of 224 SARS cases were documented among Toronto residents, and of 23,300 people identified as contacts, 13,374 were placed in quarantine (Basrur, Yaffe, & Henry, 2004). The strain on the public health system was enormous, particularly given the clinical uncertainty of the disease (Affonso, Andrews, & Jeffs, 2004). The need for comprehensive disease control strategies with strong communication linkages between health agencies was one of the most salient lessons learned from the experience. The Canadian Notifiable Diseases On-line can be accessed at **http://dsol-smed.phac-aspc.gc.ca/dsol-smed/ndis/index_e.html**.

SUMMARY

In this chapter, you have been introduced to demography, the broad science of populations, and epidemiology, the specific science of population health. Examples have been offered as to how these two sciences can be used to accurately assess a community's health status in order to appropriately intervene as a community health professional. Answers to many health questions can be obtained by examining existing data and by remaining inquisitive. Our practice is better informed through applying demographic and epidemiologic principles to community problems.

References

Affonso, D. D., Andrews, G. J., & Jeffs, L. (2004). The urban geography of SARS: Paradoxes and dilemmas in Toronto's health care. *Journal of Advanced Nursing, 45*(6), 568–578.

Barnett, D. J., Balicer, R. D., Blodgett, D., Fews, A. L., Parker, C. L., & Links, J. M. (2005). The application of the Haddon Matrix to public health readiness and response planning. *Environmental Health Perspectives, 113*(5), 561–566.

Basrur, S., Yaffe, B., & Henry, B. (2004). SARS: A local public health perspective. *Canadian Journal of Public Health, 95*(1), 22–24.

Centers for Disease Control and Prevention. (1981, June 30). Toxic shock syndrome—United States, 1970–1980. *Morbidity and Mortality Weekly Report, 30*, 25–33.

Centers for Disease Control and Prevention. (1983, August 5). Update: Toxic shock syndrome—United States. *Morbidity and Mortality Weekly Report, 32*, 398–400.

Centers for Disease Control and Prevention. (1993, September 10). Public health focus: Physical activity and the prevention of coronary heart disease. *Morbidity and Mortality Weekly Report, 42*, 398–400.

Child Health Surveillance Project Data Group. (2005). *Alberta Child Health Surveillance Report 2005*. Edmonton, AB: Alberta Health and Wellness.

Crichton, M. (1969). *The Andromeda strain*. New York: Alfred A. Knopf.

Davis, J. P., Chesney, P. J., Ward, P. J., LaVenture, M., & the Investigation and Laboratory Team. (1980). Toxic shock syndrome: Epidemiologic features, recurrence, risk factors, and prevention. *New England Journal of Medicine, 303*, 1429–1435.

Feldshuh, D. (1997). *Miss Evers' boys*. New York: Home Box Office Production with Anasazi Productions.

Fletcher, R. W., & Fletcher, S. W. (2005). *Clinical epidemiology: The essentials* (4th ed.). Philadelphia: Lippincott Williams & Wilkins.

Gordis, L. (2004). *Epidemiology* (3rd ed.). Philadelphia: Elsevier Saunders.

Haddon, W. Jr. (1999). The changing approach to the epidemiology, prevention and amelioration of trauma: The transition to etiologically rather than descriptively based. *Injury Prevention, 5*, 231–236.

Health Canada. (2001). *Diabetes among Aboriginal people in Canada: The evidence*. Ottawa: Aboriginal Diabetes Initiative.

Health Canada. (2002). *Diabetes in Canada* (2nd ed.). Ottawa: Centre for Chronic Disease Prevention and Control, Population and Public Health Branch, Health Canada.

Health Canada. (2003). *Canadian perinatal health report 2003*. Ottawa: Minister of Public Works and Government Services Canada.

ICBC. (2006). Insurance Corporation of British Columbia: Driver Licensing. Retrieved July 28, 2006, from **http://www.icbc.com/licensing.**

Kramer, M. S., Barros, F. C., Demissie, K., Liu, S., Kiely, J., & Joseph, K. S. (2005). Does reducing infant mortality depend on preventing low birthweight? An analysis of temporal trends in the Americas. *Paediatric and Perinatal Epidemiology, 19*(6), 445–451.

Last, J. M. (Ed.). (2001). *A dictionary of epidemiology* (4th ed.). Toronto: Oxford University Press.

Lilienfeld, D. E., & Stolley, P. D. (1994). *Foundations of epidemiology* (3rd ed.). New York: Oxford University Press.

Luo, Z-C., Kierans, W. J., Wilkins, R., Liston, R. M., Uh, S-H., & Kramer, M. S. (2004). Infant mortality among First Nations versus non-First Nations in British Columbia: Temporal trends in rural versus urban areas, 1981-2000. *International Journal of Epidemiology, 33*(6), 1252–1259.

Macauley, A. C., Montour, L. T., & Adelson, N. (1988). Prevalence of diabetic and atherosclerotic complications among Mohawk Indians of Kahnawake, PQ. *Canadian Medical Association Journal, 139*, 221–224.

MacMahon, B., & Trichopoulos, D. (1996). *Epidemiology: Principles and methods* (2nd ed.). Boston: Little, Brown.

Martens, P. J., & Derksen, S. (2002). A matter of life and death for Manitoba's children: An overview of birth rates and mortality rates. *Canadian Journal of Public Health, 93*[Suppl 2], S21–S26.

Mausner, J. S., & Kramer, S. (1985). Epidemiology—An introductory text (2nd ed.). Philadelphia: WB Saunders.

Morabia, A. (2004). *A history of epidemiologic methods and concepts*. Boston: Birkhäuser Verlag.

Petersen, W. (1995). *Outbreak*. Los Angeles, CA: Warner Brothers Entertainment.

Preston, P. (1994). *The hot zone*. New York: Random House.

Rockwell, F. S. (2001). Infant mortality among status Indians on Vancouver Island, British Columbia: Evidence of variability within the Status Indian population. *Canadian Journal of Pubic Health, 92*(6), 453–456.

Rothman, K. J. (2002). *Epidemiology: An introduction*. Toronto: Oxford University Press.

Runyan, C. W. (1998). Using the Haddon matrix: Introducing the third dimension. *Injury Prevention, 4*, 302–307.

Runyan, C. W. (2003). Introduction: Back to the future—Revisiting Hadon's conceptualization of injury epidemiology and prevention. *Epidemiologic Reviews, 25*, 60–64.

Sahai, V. S., Ward, M. S., Zmijowskyj, T., & Rowe, B. H. (2005). Quantifying the iceberg effect for injury: Using comprehensive community health data. *Canadian Journal of Public Health, 96*(5), 328–332.

Snow, J. (1936). Snow on cholera, being a reprint of two papers by John Snow, M.D., together with a biographical memoir by B. W. Richardson, M.D., and an introduction by Wade Hampton Frost, M.D. New York: Commonwealth Fund.

Svobada, T., Henry, B., Shulman, L., Kennedy, E., Rea, E., Ng, W., et al. (2004). Public health measures to control the spread of the severe acute respiratory syndrome during the outbreak in Toronto. *New England Journal of Medicine, 350*, 2352–2361.

Statistics Canada. (2006a). Selected leading causes of death, by sex, 1997. Retrieved July 24, 2006, from **http://www40.statcan.ca/l01/cst01/health36.htm.**

Statistics Canada. (2006b). Infant mortality rates, by province and territory. Retrieved July 24, 2006, from **http://www40.statcan.ca/l01/cst01/health21a.htm.**

Statistics Canada. (2006c). History of the Census of Canada. Retrieved July 24, 2006, from **http://www12.statcan.ca/english/census01/Info/history.cfm**.

Timmreck, T. C. (1998). *An introduction to epidemiology* (2nd ed.). Boston: Jones & Bartlett.

Varia, M., Wilson, S., Sarwal, S., McGeer, A., Gournis, E., Galanis, E., et al. (2003). Investigation of a nosocomial outbreak of severe acute respiratory syndrome (SARS) in Toronto, Canada. *Canadian Medical Association Journal, 169*(4), 285–292.

WHO. (2005). Child and adolescent health and development. Progress Report 2004-2005. Geneva: World Health Organization. Available at http://www.who.int/child-adolescent-health/New_Publications/overview/ISBN_92_4159422_5.pdf.

Young, T. K. (1988). *Health care and cultural change: The Indian experience in the central subarctic*. Toronto: University of Toronto Press.

Internet Resources

http://www.phac-aspc.gc.ca/publicat/ccdr-rmtc/index.html
Canada Communicable Disease Report (CCDR)

http://www.phac-aspc.gc.ca/publications_e.html
Public Health Agency of Canada

http://www.phac-aspc.gc.ca/id-mi/index.html
PHAC reports on communicable diseases

http://www.phac-aspc.gc.ca/cd-mc/index.html
PHAC reports on chronic diseases

http://www.cdc.gov/mmwr/
Centers for Disease Control and Prevention, Morbidity and Mortality Weekly Report

http://www.phac-aspc.gc.ca/publicat/dic-dac2/english/01cover_e.html
Health Canada report, Diabetes in Canada (2nd ed.)

http://www.hc-sc.gc.ca/fnih-spni/pubs/diabete/2001_evidence_faits/index_e.html
Health Canada report Diabetes among Aboriginal People in Canada: The Evidence

http://www.hrsdc.gc.ca/en/gateways/nav/left_nav/publications.shtml
HRSDC publications

http://www.hrsdc.gc.ca/en/cs/sp/sdc/pkrf/publications/research/2002–000662/page00.shtml
HRSDC publication Low Income in Canada: 2000–2002, Using the Market Basket Measure

http://www.socialpolicy.ca/cush/index.htm
Canada's Social History

http://www.conferenceboard.ca
Conference Board of Canada

http://www.ciar.ca
The Canadian Institute of Advanced Research

http://www.fraserinstitute.ca
The Fraser Institute

http://www.ualberta.ca/PARKLAND
The Parkland Institute

http://www.cwf.ca
Canada West Foundation

http://www.phac-aspc.gc.ca/publicat/cphr-rspc03/index.html
PHAC reports on perinatal health (including IMR)

Creating Supportive Environments for Health: Social Network Analysis

MALCOLM SHOOKNER
CATHERINE M. SCOTT
ARDENE ROBINSON VOLLMAN

Our societies are complex and interrelated. Health cannot be separated from other goals. The inextricable links between people and their environment constitutes the basis for a socio-ecological approach to health. The overall guiding principle for the world, nations, regions and communities alike, is the need to encourage reciprocal maintenance— to take care of each other, our communities and our natural environment. The conservation of natural resources throughout the world should be emphasized as a global responsibility.

Changing patterns of life, work and leisure have a significant impact on health. Work and leisure should be a source of health for people. The way society organizes work should help create a healthy society. Health promotion generates living and working conditions that are safe, stimulating, satisfying and enjoyable.

Systematic assessment of the health impact of a rapidly changing environment—particularly in areas of technology, work, energy production and urbanization—is essential and must be followed by action to ensure positive benefit to the health of the public. The protection of the natural and built environments and the conservation of natural resources must be addressed in any health promotion strategy. OTTAWA CHARTER (1986)

Chapter Outline

Introduction
Sundsvall Conference and Statement
The Physical Environment and Human
  Health
Action Process for Creating Supportive
  Environments for Health

Ecological Perspective: Overlapping
  Environmental Influences on
  Health
Environments and Settings
Social Capital and Social Networks
Summary

Learning Objectives

After studying this chapter, you should be able to:

❖ Describe the links between creating supportive communities, an ecological perspective, social capital, and social networks

❖ Discuss the role of environments in health

❖ Discuss the rationale for a settings approach to health interventions

❖ Describe strategies for creating supportive environments

Introduction

O n a day-to-day basis, people are influenced by, and influence, environments within which they live, learn, work, play, and pray. The population health promotion model introduced in Chapter 1 is based on an ecological perspective that acknowledges health as a product of interdependence between people and ecosystems. Based on this point of view, individuals are not solely responsible for their actions; environments influence the way people view the world and the choices they make.

Following the 1986 Global Health Promotion Conference held in Ottawa (World Health Organization, 1986), the Canadian effort to understand the relationship between health and the environment was extended when a commission recommended actions for Canada to move toward healthier environments for its citizens. Five components for action were identified: ending prejudice and oppression; creating a new vision of environmental choice; fostering technology for assessing our environment; accommodating diversity through participation; and becoming world experts in intersectoral action in the design of healthy environments (Small, 1990). Four strategies for action arise from a commitment to make healthy environments available to all Canadians: political vision and leadership in all five action components listed above; scientific and social research and industrial incentive to produce materials that are cleaner, less risky, and less damaging; public education about environmental effects on health; and legislative review and re-examination of policies to ensure that individuals control their environments.

SUNDSVALL CONFERENCE AND STATEMENT

At the Third International Conference on Health Promotion that focused on Supportive Environments for Health, in Sundsvall, Sweden, in June 1991, participants from 81 countries issued a call to people in all parts of the world to actively engage

BOX 4-1

Dimensions of a Supportive Environment for Health

1. The *social* dimension, including ways in which norms, customs, and social processes affect health
2. The *political* dimension, including democratization, decentralization of power and resources, and commitment to human rights and social justice
3. The *economic* dimension, including sustainable development and reliable and safe technology
4. A positive *infrastructure*, which includes and values women's skills and knowledge

World Health Organization. (1991). Sundsvall Statement on Supportive Environments for Health. Third International Conference on Health Promotion, Sundsvall, Sweden, June 9–15, 1991. Retrieved June 4, 2007 from **http://www.who.int/hpr/NPH/docs/sundsvall_statement.pdf.**

in making environments more supportive to health: "The way forward lies in making the environment—the physical environment, the social and economic environment, and the political environment—supportive to health rather than damaging to it" (World Health Organization, 1991) (Box 4-1).

A supportive environment is of paramount importance for health; environment and health are interdependent and inseparable. Participants noted the significant health inequalities as reflected in the widening gap in health status both within nations and between rich and poor countries; millions of people live in extreme poverty and deprivation in an increasingly degraded environment; an alarming number of people suffer from the tragic consequences of armed conflicts; and rapid population growth is a major threat to sustainable development forcing people to survive without clean water and adequate food, shelter, or sanitation. Thus, action to create supportive environments must be coordinated at local, regional, national, and global levels to achieve solutions that are truly sustainable.

The Sundsvall Statement suggests that interventions to achieve health for all must reflect two basic principles: equity and public action. *Equity* is the priority in creating supportive environments for health. Any action and resource allocation should be based on clear priorities and a commitment to those marginalized by poverty, gender, race, or disability. *Public action* must recognize the interdependence of all living beings and manage all natural resources effectively, taking into account the needs of future generations and recognizing the importance of involving indigenous peoples in sustainable development activities.

There were four key action strategies identified at Sundsvall to create supportive environments at community level: *strengthen advocacy* through community action, particularly through groups organized by women; *enable communities* and individuals to take control over their health and environment through education and empowerment; *build alliances* for health and supportive environments in order to strengthen the cooperation between health and environmental campaigns and strategies; and *mediate* between conflicting interests in society in order to ensure equitable access to supportive environments and health.

THE PHYSICAL ENVIRONMENT AND HUMAN HEALTH

In this section, the mechanisms by which contaminants enter human populations are presented. Airborne contaminants and other environmental toxins (e.g., tobacco smoke) affect people exposed to them. Some hazards can seem innocuous, but people are becoming increasingly sensitive to commonly occurring environmental conditions. Perfume is such an instance; hence, we are seeing more "scent-free" buildings, conferences, and meetings as people become aware of these situations. Following are summaries from the report "Health and the Environment—Partners for Life" (Health Canada, 1997).

The Natural Environment

Over past decades, the environment has been used as a convenient biological, radioactive, physical, and chemical waste disposal site. In some parts of Canada, the results of this environmental abuse have caused many Canadians, particularly those populations that live near manufacturing and processing plants, or in remote areas, to have detectable levels of contaminants (e.g., mercury and lead) in their blood, hair, and body tissues. In the 1970s, leaded gasoline was phased out, resulting in the dramatic decline of air lead contamination to trace levels. However, contaminants of both natural and human origin that are still found in the air, water, food, and soil have many adverse effects on human health (e.g., cancer, birth defects, respiratory diseases, and gastrointestinal illness).

Air Quality

Air is the mixture of gases that surrounds the planet and makes up the atmosphere; it consists of 21% oxygen and 78% nitrogen by volume, plus traces of other gases and water vapour. However, its composition may vary from one location to another and between indoors and outdoors because of contamination with particulate matter or other gases. These airborne contaminants pose health risks either directly through inhalation or indirectly through their effects on the environment (e.g., pollution of the water supply or contamination of foods). When inhaled and depending on its physical properties, amount, the rate and depth of breathing, and the health of those exposed, air pollution can cause a variety of health effects.

Asthma, a respiratory disease, affects more than one million Canadians and is chronic among children and the leading cause for school absence. It can be triggered by a variety of airborne contaminants (e.g., dust, pollen, pets, scents, and tobacco smoke) and often leads to hospitalization.

Natural sources of outdoor contaminants include smoke from forest fires, wind-blown dust particles from soil and volcanoes, fungi, bacteria, plants, and animals. Pollutants are also released from motor vehicles, industrial processes, burning fuels, and the like. The level of contamination in outdoor air is influenced by population density, degree of industrialization, local pollution emission standards, season, climate, and daily weather conditions. Air pollutants may originate from local sources or from remote locations, travelling thousands of kilometres from one part of the world to another through the phenomenon called "long-range atmospheric transport."

Canadians spend nearly 90% of their time indoors. Outside air quality can affect the quality of indoor air, but pollutants can also arise from poor ventilation that allows contaminants from building materials, furnishings, heating, cooking, consumer products (e.g., tobacco, perfumes), and the soil to build up indoors. This often results in "sick buildings."

Ultraviolet (UV) radiation is one of the main causes of skin cancer in Canada. While some exposure to UV radiation is beneficial (because it helps produce vitamin D, although dietary sources are also available), UV rays pose a health hazard to anyone who is exposed for long periods of time. In 1995, more than 55,000 Canadians developed various forms of skin cancer, and the incidence for malignant melanoma has substantially increased in recent years. The increased incidence of skin cancer is attributed in part to sun tanning, but scientists are also concerned about the depletion of the earth's ozone layer, which acts to prevent UV radiation from penetrating the atmosphere.

Water Quality

Canada contains 15% of the earth's fresh water supply, but 60% of Canada's supply exists far from the heavily populated areas where it is needed for human use. The proportion that is accessible, although generally of high quality, often contains small amounts of environmental contaminants. Compared with other transmission media, such as food and air, drinking water is a minor source of most pollutants—although it is the principal source of exposure to some micro-organisms and to water disinfection by-products.

About 87% of Canadians receive municipal tap water that is treated. Chlorine is a simple, effective, yet relatively inexpensive agent for destroying harmful micro-organisms in tap water. With a few exceptions, the most serious contamination problems involve tap water from untreated sources, such as private wells. Recent outbreaks of water-borne disease have affected thousands of people and have been responsible for several deaths.

Water fluoridation helps to prevent tooth decay in children without endangering their health. However, even at optimal levels in some children, fluoride may cause dental fluorosis, a generally mild condition involving tooth discoloration. Despite claims to the contrary, there is no evidence that fluoridated water causes heart disease, cancer, thyroid problems, birth defects, miscarriages, or hearing or vision problems.

About 100,000 home water treatment devices are sold annually in Canada. When not used properly, some devices can become health hazards. Studies have shown that levels of bacteria present in water that has passed through an improperly maintained home filtration device may be up to 2000 times higher than levels in unfiltered water.

Chemical and Biological Hazards

Canadians are exposed to environmental contaminants primarily through food despite strict control by federal and provincial legislation and by voluntary actions taken by food producers, processors, and packagers. Contaminants can enter the food supply via a number of different routes and from different sources. Contamination may occur at the site of production, in the processing plant, at the distribution centre, in the retail outlet, in the refrigerator at home, or even on the kitchen counter. Exposure to food-borne contaminants is affected by many factors: food availability, the preparation method, the amount and type eaten, age, occupation, sex, health status, culture, religion, socioeconomic factors, geography, and the nature of the contaminant. People who have high intakes of wild game, birds, fish, and shellfish are exposed to higher levels of contamination because certain organic pesticides that are no longer registered in Canada may persist in soil or enter the environment through long-range atmospheric transport from countries where they are still in use. Some groups are more susceptible than the general population to the effects of food-borne contaminants (e.g., unborn fetuses, breast-fed infants, the elderly, and people with weakened immune systems). However, proper food handling and cooking practices could prevent most adverse incidents.

The Built Environment

We are as much a part of our fabricated or built environment as we are part of our natural environment. The built environment encompasses all of the buildings, spaces, and products that are created or significantly modified by humans. It includes our homes, schools, workplaces, parks, business areas, and roads. It extends overhead in the form of electric transmission lines, underground in the form of waste disposal sites and subway trains, and across the country in the form of highways. The way communities are planned and built, including such aspects as the availability of affordable housing, public transportation and bicycle paths, and the design of public spaces, can also affect health. For example, people are more likely to exercise when recreation and sport facilities are located near their homes. Commuting can have a negative impact on the psychological state of commuters and the quality of social life. Available parks and green spaces provide opportunities for reducing stress and meeting spiritual needs. Urban planners must keep in mind the needs of people with limited mobility, the proximity of required services to sustain a community (e.g., schools, community centres, shopping), the negative effects of overcrowding, and the need for safety and security.

Risk Assessment

The assessment and management of environmental risks (whether they result from personal choice or substances, processes, or products in the environment) involves a process that identifies the specific hazards, estimates the associated level of risk, develops and analyzes potential options for managing that risk, selects and implements a risk management activity, and monitors and evaluates the impact of the strategy chosen.

How people judge risks, that is, *risk perception*, affects how they act and the decisions they make about avoidance, control, or protection. Risk perception is affected by many factors (e.g., age, sex, education, region of the country, values, and previous exposure) and changes over time as new information becomes available. *Risk communication* must take these factors into account. Risk communication involves the exchange of information about the existence, nature, form, severity, or acceptability of health or environmental risks (Health Canada, 1997). Some examples of risk communication include the provision of information to the public to assist people with making decisions (e.g., food product labels), alerting the public to a significant risk (e.g., weather alerts, smog warnings), calming concerns (e.g., severe acute respiratory syndrome transmission), and putting certain public concerns in perspective.

ACTION PROCESS FOR CREATING SUPPORTIVE ENVIRONMENTS FOR HEALTH

A planning approach called the Action Process for Creating Supportive Environment for Health Action Plan (APCSEH), adapted from MacArthur (2002), suggests following concrete steps that begin with the preparatory stages of gaining commitment, forming partnerships, and creating the processes of working together; followed by assessment, analysis, public participation, and priority setting; and completed by the planning approval, launch, and evaluation stages (Fig. 4-1).

Several other strategies draw from community theory and practice for the creation of supportive environments. Shapiro and Cartwright (1994) describe a recent innovative Australian pilot project that addresses health advancement in elderly populations. The strategies used for this project can serve as a template for strategies to be used in the creation of supportive environments elsewhere:

♦ Develop structures that bring people together
♦ Organize activities that would provide people with the skills to conduct their own ongoing health education and promotion within the community
♦ Facilitate nongovernmental organizations (NGOs) and private businesses to become involved with the people in the community
♦ Establish activities that would encourage professionals to become equal partners with the people in the community and to share health information and resources

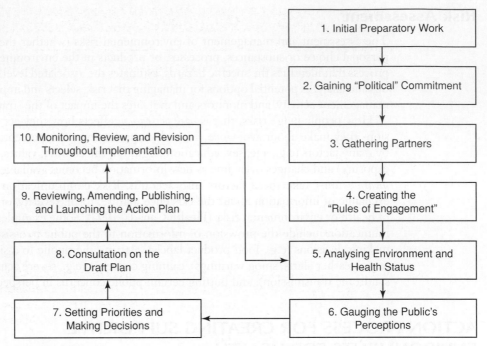

FIGURE 4-1 ◆ Action Process for Creating Supportive Environments for Health.

◆ Develop structures that would enable the community to identify its needs and initiate action to meet those needs
◆ Involve public participation in priority setting and planning
◆ Set up structures to enhance future involvement of community people

Once the community context is favourable to intervention, community developers can then engage the group in identifying risk groups, organising interventions, and mobilizing resources for ongoing action.

As models of health promotion have evolved over the past three decades, the targets for health interventions have shifted from a preoccupation with individual-level behaviour change to an ecological approach that considers interactions among the target population, the health issue involved, and environmental influences. Many initiatives focus on creating supportive environments through particular settings (e.g., work, school, home, etc.) as a starting point to address the determinants of health (e.g., World Health Organization Healthy Cities, Comprehensive School Health, Healthy Workplace).

Environments may predispose, enable, and reinforce individual and collective behaviour; they may also limit choices and behaviours (Green & Kreuter, 1999). Many groups of Canadians are exposed to unhealthy environments. Devaluing or undervaluing groups of people (e.g., people who are homeless, women, immigrants, elderly, gays and lesbians, Aboriginals, and people who have disabilities) and

---

BOX 4-2

Definition of Terms

Ecological perspective: Focuses on the interactions between humans and their environment.

Environment: Surrounds individuals wherever they go and whatever they do; is composed of physical, political, economic, sociocultural, and biological components.

Setting: Establishes boundaries within which health promotion interventions take place (e.g., work, school, home settings); defines the population involved in an intervention and the location of the intervention (Poland et al., 2000).

Social capital: The networks of social relations that may provide individuals and groups with access to resources and supports (PRI, 2005).

Social networks: A basic component of social structure derived from patterns of relations between individuals (or organizations or countries).

---

environmental issues (e.g., climate change, pollution, affordable housing, workplace determinants, urban development) has generated tremendous disparities across the economic, sociocultural, and physical components of the environment with which people interact, and yet, ensuring that all citizens have access to supportive environments benefits society as a whole.

In the next part of this chapter, we will explore how local communities can take action to influence the environments that impact their lives. We describe in the ecological perspective, using it as a starting point for describing overlapping environmental influences on health. We then briefly distinguish environments from settings, the latter being the focus of many health promotion interventions. The ecological perspective reflects complex interactions among determinants of health and as such implies that strategies for creating supportive environments adopt an interdisciplinary, multisectoral approach. We lay the foundation for later chapters by highlighting the role of social capital in population health promotion (Box 4-2).

ECOLOGICAL PERSPECTIVE: OVERLAPPING ENVIRONMENTAL INFLUENCES ON HEALTH

The field of social ecology focuses on relationships between human populations and their environments. The word *environment* means different things to different people. For some, it is limited to a discussion of physical components of an environment—air, water, and soil quality. While threats to the physical components of an environment can have direct and immediate impacts on health, our discussion of human environments is somewhat broader. Using an ecological perspective means that we include the physical components as well as political, economic, sociocultural, and biological environmental influences in our discussion (Fig. 4-2). By adopting this

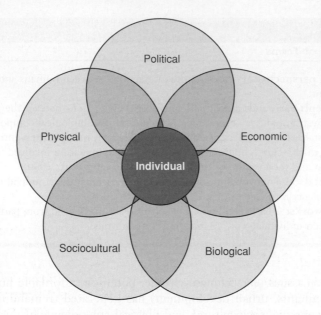

FIGURE 4-2 ◆ An ecological model of the influences on human environments.

perspective, the proponents of population health promotion explicitly focus interventions toward *populations and their environments*. While such a broad perspective does more accurately reflect the influences on human health, it also complicates things. If health is determined by the complex interplay between people and the environment that surrounds them, then population health interventions must take this complexity into account, thus requiring cross-disciplinary and cross-sectoral collaboration to create supportive environments.

ENVIRONMENTS AND SETTINGS

The broad definition of *environments* is helpful for thinking about the complex influences on human health, but it is not as helpful for thinking about how to implement strategies that focus on creating supportive environments. It is perhaps more helpful to think in terms of specific settings in which people interact (e.g., workplaces, schools, communities) and to look at the environmental influences within that setting in order to develop strategies that are feasible, focused, evaluable, and effective. The Jakarta Declaration on Leading Health Promotion into the 21st Century (World Health Organization, 1997) states that "*settings for health* offer practical opportunities for the implementation of comprehensive strategies" (p. 2).

A more focused settings-based approach means that interventions can be tailored to the characteristics of the setting. Environments that are created within a setting can predispose, enable, and reinforce individual and collective behaviour (Poland et al., 2000). For example, the sociocultural and political environmental influences in a particular setting may either enable people to interact with one another, to share resources and ideas, or they may constrain such behaviour; people behave differently in different settings. The success of health strategies therefore depends on their fit with (1) the people who are involved, (2) the health issue being addressed, and (3) the environmental characteristics of the setting (Green & Kreuter, 1999). Fownes and Vollman discuss settings more fully in Chapter 8.

SOCIAL CAPITAL AND SOCIAL NETWORKS

The term *social capital* has come into increasing prominence over the past 20 years. The origins of social capital can be traced back to the nineteenth century classics of sociology (Woolcock, 1998). As with many terms that rise to prominence, there are differing opinions about its meaning and its implications for the design of health interventions. The definition that we use comes from a social capital project commissioned by the Government of Canada between 2003 and 2005 that uses social networks as its central component: "*Social capital refers to the networks of social relations that may provide individuals and groups with access to resources and supports*" (PRI, 2005). Social capital definitions differ from other *capital* definitions because they relate to the quality and quantity of social processes and what flows from the links, rather than the common measures of individual well-being and success (e.g., income levels). For example, human capital is about *what* you know, and social capital is concerned with *whom* you know.

Two forms of the concept of social capital are bonding and bridging. *Bonding* social capital relates to the value assigned to social networks that are quite dense, where most members have close connections with one another (e.g., close-knit families, workplace teams, professional groups). *Bridging* social capital is the value generated from social networks that cut across groups, creating connections that have the potential to bring in resources that a group does not currently have or to share information between groups. While bonding social capital is frequently described in terms of its negative potential (i.e., for excluding others or creating an insular environment), the appropriate balance of these two forms of social capital is dependent on the setting or context.

Creating supportive environments is about building social capital (as well as other forms of capital, such as economic and cultural). Tapping into and possibly strengthening social networks has the potential to facilitate the achievement of common goals. Social networks have the potential to bring many benefits (e.g., goods and services, connections to jobs and funding sources, emotional support) and to enable or constrain behaviours (e.g., family and friends may influence choices related to diet and exercise); they also have the potential to exclude people and break apart communities. There is much debate about the potential for using social capital to create more supportive environments; some people argue that it may be possible to facilitate the development of bridging social capital but not bonding. Whatever strategies are used, it is important to remember that the value of different forms of social capital is dependent on the context (Putnam, 2001; Woolcock, 2001).

The following case study provides an example of an initiative that was designed to create supportive environments. We encourage you to think about the following questions as you read:

◆ What environmental components (physical, political, economic, sociocultural, and biological) influenced the evolution of the project?
◆ Were there clear settings within which the strategies evolved? How did this influence the project?
◆ What role did social networks play in the development and implementation of the strategies?
◆ What types of social capital were evident? How did these influence the development of the project?

Community-Based Management of Marine Infrastructure in Coastal Communities

CONTEXT

As communities face increasing levels of social and economic volatility, as they are in Atlantic Canada, they have to adapt or become "resilient." A resilient community is "one that takes intentional action to enhance the personal and collective capacity of its citizens and institutions to respond to and influence the course of social and economic change" (Colussi et al., 2000). The Rural Communities Impacting Policy (RCIP) Project was a partnership between the Coastal Communities Network (CCN) and the Atlantic Health Promotion Research Centre (AHPRC) at Dalhousie University in Nova Scotia. Over 5 years (2001–2006), the RCIP Project carried out a number of activities to help rural communities use social science research to develop and influence policies that affect the health and sustainability of their communities. The RCIP Project used this definition:

> A "healthy community" is one where people, organizations and local institutions work together to improve the social, economic and environmental conditions that make people healthy—the determinants of health. (RCIP, 2006)

The RCIP Policy Work Group, chaired by a community resident and CCN Board member, brought community, academic, and government participants together on a regular basis over the 5-year term of the RCIP Project. This group focused on policy change by identifying the issues to be addressed at the Rural Policy Forum, assigning student interns to community research projects, monitoring and supporting the community research projects, receiving and reviewing the research findings, and promoting the policy change strategies that were being pursued as a result of the research.

THE ISSUE

Many coastal communities in Nova Scotia are facing the daunting challenge of maintaining and managing their wharves. The current system of Harbour Authorities was created by Small Craft Harbours (SCH) and the Department of Fisheries and Oceans (DFO) to give communities more control over their wharves. Unfortunately, this system often does not effectively address the needs of these communities, and many feel that they are worse off now than they were before Harbour Authorities were introduced. Furthermore, DFO has divested many wharves in Nova Scotia, leaving some communities with full responsibility for a wharf if they wish to maintain a viable fishing livelihood. These divested wharves are as important as those that DFO continues to support; this is particularly true in the Bay of Fundy, where high tides and unpredictable weather often require fishermen to head to shore away from their home port (RCIP Rural Policy Forum, 2004).

In January 2004, the CCN released a report that generated compelling evidence of the importance of wharves and harbours as essential to the economic, social, and cultural viability of coastal communities in Nova Scotia noting that, "*the overall social and economic well being of the province is immensely affected by developments in the coastal zone*" (CCN, 2004). Wharves are "sustaining structures" for coastal communities and for the province as a whole. As a result of this research, the issue of harbour management was identified by the RCIP Policy Work Group for inclusion in the Rural Policy Forum organized by the RCIP Project.

Ideas for wharf management solutions involving communities working together have been discussed for many years in many different forums. In February 2004, at the RCIP Rural Policy Forum, ideas for action began to form. A group consisting of fishermen, community organizations, funders, and policy makers recognized the need for improved wharf management and agreed that collaborative management could be the solution. A pilot project was proposed in the harbours along the Upper Bay of Fundy, along the Kings County shore. The Upper Bay of Fundy Marine Resource Centre (MRC) agreed to be the focal point for getting people to work together, a base of operations to connect disparate groups, and a common and neutral ground for working together on wharves in new, collaborative ways. The MRC would pull together all the harbour management groups in the area and work to assist them in making decisions about appropriate courses of action. A student intern from the RCIP Project, with community sponsorship from MRC, would conduct research to support the pilot project. The RCIP Policy Work Group would have a link to this project through a representative from one of the harbour authorities on the MRC. A policy change strategy was identified—that the DFO change its policy about dealing with harbour management groups individually.

UPPER BAY OF FUNDY WHARF PILOT PROJECT

In April 2004, the Upper Bay of Fundy Wharf Pilot Project was formed to create an alternative community-based system for managing and maintaining wharves in Kings County. Representatives from Delhaven Harbour Authority, Harbourville

Restoration Society, Scots Bay Harbour Authority, and Harbour Authority of Halls Harbour agreed to pursue the pilot project, supported by the MRC. During the summer of 2004, the RCIP intern researched best practices in harbour management and documented the process of collaboration among the local harbour management groups (De Sousa, 2004).

The report proposed that collaborative, community-based resource management be pursued as a strategy to manage sustainably the physical environment, both natural and built (wharves and harbours) marine infrastructure that contributes to the economic and social development of coastal communities. In so doing, these communities would be taking action on the determinants of health that affect their livelihoods and sustainability—physical and social environments around the wharves, adequate income from the fisheries to sustain families and the community, and safe working conditions for fishermen and others using the wharves.

Further support for the innovation in community-based management of wharves and harbours was included in the 2005 Rural Policy Forum agenda. The focus of the workshop was on *Kings Harbours: A Community Network* as they moved toward incorporation and forming their board of directors. Two years after the initial meetings through RCIP, *Kings Harbours: A Community Network* continues to move ahead with its mission:

> . . . to preserve, protect and promote the traditional Nova Scotian values of community identity, independence, self-reliance and self sufficiency through the restoration, development and continuous maintenance of the wharves and harbours of Kings County for the benefit of all. (RCIP Rural Policy Forum, 2005)

The group hopes to receive funding from a variety of government sources in 2006 that will allow them to hire staff and begin activities that will raise their profile and create more public awareness of the challenges facing wharves and harbours and the integral role they play in coastal communities and the greater community of Kings County.

POLICY CHANGE STRATEGY

Communities learning to work together to manage their resources and influence government policies to support them are part of a long-term strategy needed for the survival and sustainability of coastal and rural communities in Nova Scotia.

Since people in communities were taking the leadership role in this pilot project, the role of Small Craft Harbours, DFO, and other funders had to be redefined. The Harbour Authorities system created by DFO was an attempt at co-management between communities and government. Although the responsibilities were given to the community, control remained with the government (RCIP Rural Policy Forum, 2004).

DFO has shown interest in and support of Kings Harbours by sponsoring a few local meetings. The Harbour Authority Advisory Council (HAAC) of DFO was a subject of discussion in the 2005 Rural Policy Forum, to ensure that community needs are being met. DFO is now cooperating with harbour management groups acting collaboratively by sitting down together with them to find solutions to wharf maintenance, repair, and financing. This is an example of building healthier public policy for coastal communities.

KEYS TO SUCCESS

Upon reflection around the RCIP Policy Work Group table, the keys to the success of this project are:

- ◆ Community leaders in each of the four harbour management groups who had a common vision and took risks to work together to achieve it, rather than compete for scarce resources
- ◆ Participatory model of research in which community partners identified the research to be done and a policy change strategy to pursue
- ◆ RCIP Partners, the CNN and the AHPRC, creating a supportive environment at the provincial level among community, government, and academic participants to be receptive to and promote policy change
- ◆ CCN providing ongoing support and encouragement to local leaders and groups to participate and play leading roles to develop the research and policy change agendas
- ◆ AHPRC ensuring that quality research was being conducted
- ◆ Rural Policy Forum bringing together community, university, and government participants to focus on the issue of wharf and harbour management and identify solutions

This case study demonstrates that communities can have a positive impact on the conditions that affect their health and sustainability. They can find their own solutions to problems that they face with support from government and academic partners. Community, government, and academic partners can create an "enabling environment" by working collaboratively toward a common goal—the health and sustainability of rural communities in Nova Scotia. Policies that affect communities can be changed to make them healthier.

SUMMARY

Creating supportive environments for health is a complex undertaking. Some of the lessons learned in the cases described in this chapter are summarized in Table 4-1.

Recognizing that individuals are surrounded by overlapping environmental influences is fundamental to the ecological perspective underpinning population health promotion. Developing strategies that address only physical environmental influences without considering social, political, or economic contexts will be of limited value when attempting to address health issues. Social networks connect people, groups, and communities and as such are important social structures through which community development can take place. The resources and supports generated

TABLE 4-1	
Lessons Learned	
PROJECT PHASE	**DESCRIPTION AND KEY CONSIDERATIONS**
Development of vision for project	A small group coming together based on a perceived need
Identification of other potential participants	Making sure that all who should be at the table are there
Understanding the context	Taking stock of the overlapping environmental influences and identifying appropriate settings
Developing the ground rules (structures and processes for project management)	Communication, decision making, dealing with conflict, dealing with power
Obtaining commitment to proceed	Explicit commitment from each participant to work within the ground rules
Implementation	Being prepared to change direction based on life circumstances, changing membership, new opportunities, etc.
Maintenance and sustainability	Paying ongoing attention to the needs of participants
Winding down	Recognizing when the time has come to move on

through social networks can help to build social capital, creating environments that foster the potential of all citizens.

At this point in time, this type of work is not "how we do business" in health systems. It requires time and commitment on the part of all involved, resources that are frequently in short supply. But that is not to say that we should avoid advocating for supportive environments at home, work, and play for ourselves and for others. Creative approaches are needed to ensure that every Canadian has access to resources and supports to control his or her life. The challenge, according to Michael Woolcock (1998):

> . . . is to identify the mechanisms that will create, nurture, and sustain the types and combinations of social relationships conducive to building dynamic participatory societies, sustainable equitable economies and accountable developmental states. (p. 186)

ACKNOWLEDGMENTS

The Kings Harbours Community Network developed as part of a larger, 5-year project Rural Communities Impacting Policy, co-sponsored by the Coastal Communities Network and the Atlantic Health Promotion Research Centre at Dalhousie University. I would like to thank the people who had the vision to create the Kings Harbours Project—Ishbel Munro (Coastal Communities Network), Holly MacDonald (Harbourville Restoration Society), and Glen Travis (Upper Bay of Fundy Marine Resource Centre). I would also like to thank the RCIP student intern who conducted the participatory research that provided documentation for this case study, Erica de Sousa. —*MS*

I would like to thank Anne Hofmeyer for her feedback regarding the section on social capital —*CS*

References

Coastal Communities Network (CCN). (2004). *Between the land and the sea: The social and economic impact of wharves and harbours on coastal communities.* New Glasgow, NS. Available at **http://www.coastalcommunities.ns.ca/publications.php**.

Colussi, M., Lewis, M., Lockhart, S., Perry, S., Rowcliffe, P., & McNair, D. (2000). *The community resilience manual.* Making Waves. Vol. 10, No. 4. Vancouver: Centre for Community Enterprise. Available at **http:// www.cedworks.com/communityresilience01.html**.

De Sousa, E. (2004). *Sustaining structures: Exploring the collaborative management of wharves in Kings County.* Rural Communities Impacting Policy Project. Halifax: Coastal Communities Network & Atlantic Health Promotion Research Centre, Dalhousie University. Available at **http://www.ruralnovascotia.ca/internreports.asp**.

Green, L. W., & Kreuter, M. W. (1999). *Health promotion: An educational and ecological approach* (3rd ed.). Mountain View, CA: Mayfield Publishing Company.

Health Canada. (1997). *Health and the Environment—Partners for Life.* (Cat. H49-112/1997E, ISBN 00662-26149-6). Ottawa: Public Works and Government Services Canada.

MacArthur, I. D. (2002). *Local environmental health planning: Guidance for local and national authorities.* WHO Regional Publications, European Series, No. 95. Copenhagen, Denmark: World Health Organization Regional Office for Europe.

Poland, B. D., Green, L. W., & Rootman I. (Eds.). (2000). *Settings for health promotion: Linking theory and practice.* Thousand Oaks, CA: Sage Publications.

PRI. (2005). *Social capital as a public policy tool: Project report.* Ottawa, ON: Policy Research Initiative for the Government of Canada.

Putnam, R. D. (2001). *Bowling alone: The collapse and revival of American community.* First Touchstone Edition. New York: Simon & Schuster.

Rural Communities Impacting Policy Project (RCIP). (2006). Healthy and sustainable rural communities. RCIP Health and Sustainability Backgrounder. Available at **http://www.ruralnovascotia.ca/backgrounder.asp**.

RCIP Rural Policy Forum. (2004). Wharves and Harbours background paper and workshop notes, February 27. Available at **http://www.ruralnovascotia.ca/policyforum.asp**.

RCIP Rural Policy Forum (2005). Rural Policy Forum Report. Available at **http://www.ruralnovascotia.ca/policyforum2005.asp**.

Shapiro, M., & Cartwright, C. (1994). Community development in primary health care. *Community Development Journal, 29*(3), 222–231.

Small, B. (1990). Healthy environments for Canadians: Making the vision a reality. AEHA Quarterly, Winter. Retrieved June 4, 2007 from **https://www.environmentalhealth.ca/w90vision.html**.

World Health Organization. (1986). Ottawa charter for health promotion. Geneva, Switzerland: Author. Retrieved June 4, 2007 from **http://www.who.int/hpr/NPH/docs/ottawa_charter_hp.pdf**.

World Health Organization. (1991). Sundsvall Statement on Supportive Environments for Health. Third International Conference on Health Promotion, Sundsvall, Sweden, June 9–15, 1991. Retrieved June 4, 2007 from **http://www.who.int/hpr/NPH/docs/sundsvall_statement.pdf**.

World Health Organization. (1997). *Jakarta Declaration on Leading Health Promotion into the 21st Century.* Geneva, Switzerland: Author.

Woolcock, M. (1998). Social capital and economic development: Towards a theoretical synthesis and policy framework. *Theory and Society, 27*(2), 151–208.

Woolcock, M. (2001). The place of social capital in understanding social and economic outcomes. *Canadian Journal of Policy Research, 2,* 11–17.

5

Developing Personal Skills: Empowerment

LEWIS WILLIAMS

*H*ealth promotion supports personal and social development through providing informa-tion, education for health, and enhancing life skills. By so doing, it increases the options available to people to exercise more control over their own health and over their environments, and to make choices conducive to health.

Enabling people to learn, throughout life, to prepare themselves for all of its stages and to cope with chronic illness and injuries is essential. This has to be facilitated in school, home, work and community settings. Action is required through educational, profes-sional, commercial and voluntary bodies, and within the institutions themselves.
OTTAWA CHARTER (1986)

Chapter Outline

Introduction
Personal Empowerment in Context
Health and Empowerment
Literacy and Health for All
Power-Culture, Empowerment,
   and Health

The Empowerment Terrain
A Critical Postmodern Approach
   to Empowerment
A Health Promotion Example
Summary

Learning Objectives

After studying this chapter, you should be able to:

❖ Understand how the development of personal skills as an effective means of enabling people to increase control over and improve their health is closely related to and contingent on collective and sociopolitical forms of empowerment

❖ Understand how health and empowerment are culturally contingent constructs

❖ Understand how empowerment is mediated by cultural-power dynamics and the relevance of critical and postmodern theories in explaining these processes

Introduction

The development of personal skills* as a means to achieving Health for All is one of five action areas of the Ottawa Charter for Health Promotion (WHO, 1986). At the heart of this action is the notion of individual empowerment—the development of personal capacities and the mobilization of these toward health promoting behaviours and increased control over health. However, in the 20 years since the Ottawa Charter came into being, much and little has changed. Many people throughout Canada and other parts of the world still struggle for the basic prerequisites for health—peace, shelter, education, food, and income—and at a larger level, organizations concerned with the governance and regulation of the societies within which we live continue to fall short of providing the conditions conducive to a stable and sustainable ecosystem, social justice, and equity among people. The Charter represented a huge leap forward in approaches to health, at least in Western biomedically driven health system contexts, in that it clearly went beyond the lifestyles approach to health to make the links to the influence of ecological factors. However, it was drafted when health promotion theory was even less developed than it is today and was implicitly Western in its conceptualization of how Health for All might be actualized. Since that time, significant shifts have occurred in terms of the contextual factors that shape individual empowerment, understandings of what individual empowerment means, and how it is actualized.

Contextual factors shaping individual empowerment have become increasingly influenced by various forms of globalization, including sociohistoric processes of colonization. Contemporary globalization describes an accelerated constellation of processes by which nations, businesses, and people are becoming more interconnected and interdependent. Two forms of globalization are relevant here. Economic globalization refers to the increasing flow of capital, labour, and goods across national boundaries. At local levels, it is characterized by flatter tax rates, decreased state regulation and levels of assistance to those in need, and the concentration of wealth and employment opportunities in urban centres. Cultural globalization refers to the globalization of perception and consciousness, the transmission of cultural symbols and systems (including knowledge systems), and the actual movement of people across and within national borders. Both processes are closely linked, as the ability to produce and disseminate culture on a large scale is closely tied to economic power. The globalization of economy and culture are quite relevant to individual empowerment because they influence the ways people think, how they see and feel about

---

*Personal skills are hereafter referred to as personal capacities. Personal capacities refer to the broad array of attributes that can be ascribed to the individual—for example, self-identity, knowledge, life skills, literacy, biological characteristics, and the like.

themselves (self-identity) and others, and more generally shape the power relations within which opportunities for individual empowerment are embedded.

Both forms of globalization continue to contribute to the increased wealth, power, and health inequities between people. For example, the National Council of Welfare's (2006) report on welfare incomes in Canada for 2005 paints a dismal picture of income inequalities—a picture that is becoming worse every decade. When adjusted for inflation, many welfare incomes were lower in 2005 than they were in 1986. Paradoxically, paralleling these developments has been increased attention to health determinants and population health promotion based approaches to well-being by health care systems and governments in Canada (Hamilton & Bhatti, 1996; Health Canada, 2005). In particular, literacy and culture, both of which are fundamentally shaped by global phenomena, are increasingly recognized as shaping access to other health determinants such as income and social status, housing, health care, employment and working conditions, and personal health practices and coping skills (Ronsman & Rootman, 2004).

Meanings of individual empowerment on the whole have been shaped within neo-colonial contexts that privilege Western identities, biomedically oriented beliefs, and knowledge systems over others, including those of indigenous peoples throughout the world and Canada. On the whole, such meanings have tended to view the individual as being a discrete entity—part of but separate from the environment. While to some extent individual empowerment occurs within the social context, the development of personal skills and capacities (often used as a proxy for individual empowerment, as in the Ottawa Charter) is often conveyed as occurring within the individual. Indigenous conceptualizations of individual empowerment on the other hand are more anchored to ideas of having a secure cultural identity and are more relational with respect to extended family, land, and metaphysical realities. Individual empowerment continues to serve as an important public health construct and tool. However, the evolution of this construct has continued to develop largely according to Western cultural norms and worldviews and warrants some cultural critique.

Actualizing individual empowerment and the understanding of how and why this occurs, as with health promotion, generally remains a much undertheorized area. Some of the most significant Western-based theoretical work rightfully makes the interconnections between individuals and social structures. For example, empowerment has been conceived as a multilevelled construct involving intrapersonal, interpersonal, and sociopolitical elements (Wallerstein, 1992) and as a process progressing along a dynamic continuum of action from individual and small group development to community organization, partnerships, and advocacy/political action (Rissel, 1994). In this sense, individual empowerment is contingent on collective empowerment and the creation of supportive environments, and the latter two are equally contingent on individual empowerment. However, on the whole, empowerment theory has generally stopped short of theorizing the forms of power inherent in these processes. Neither has it given much consideration to the identity and cultural power relations that mediate these processes. Both issues have gained increasing relevance in globalized societies that continue to be shaped by capitalist, neo-colonial relations.

In this chapter, you are encouraged to think critically about the concept of individual empowerment and its application within public health through (1) making linkages between individual, collective, and sociopolitical forms of empowerment; (2) critiquing and extending meanings of well-being and individual empowerment to include those of indigenous peoples and other groups; (3) demonstrating the relevance of cultural-power dynamics to empowerment processes, both as they mediate the access of different groups to environmental capacities and as they influence people's experiences of power and powerlessness; and (4) proposing the empowerment terrain and critical postmodern theory as ways of usefully conceptualizing the intricacies of empowerment.

PERSONAL EMPOWERMENT IN CONTEXT

Within public health contexts, individual empowerment is often taken to mean the development of personal skills via activities aimed at health education, life-skills enhancement, and personal and social development. Often, the underlying rationale and intent of these activities within public health programs is that they will reduce risk behaviours for specific diseases. For example, since diet, physical activity, stress management, and tobacco smoking remain the most important proximal causes of chronic disease, interventions have most often focused on the individual determinants of behaviour change. While person-based approaches have much to offer, rates of recidivism from individualized behaviour change interventions can be very high as individuals slip back into their normal (less healthy) behaviour patterns in environments that are not conducive to healthy personal practices. Evidence abounds that the translation of an individual's knowledge and skills into health promoting behaviours and practices are undoubtedly strongly influenced by socioecological influences such as income, housing quality, location, and social capital (Heyman et al., 2006; Raphael, 2004). For example, even if we know the power of regular physical activity with respect to physical and mental health benefits, formidable barriers may reside in our work, family, neighbourhood, and cultural circumstances. The temptation to use comfort measures such as food, alcohol, or tobacco may be hard to resist if people lack social sources of that comfort; people who feel depressed, socially isolated, or trapped may sense a lack of personal control over their circumstances and might therefore find it difficult to make (and follow through) on healthy choices.

Obviously, in itself, personal empowerment (i.e., the development and mobilization of personal capacities by individuals) is not enough to achieve healthier communities. Sustained changes in health promoting behaviours require the transformation of risk environments to those that support healthy behaviours. While earlier research tended to emphasize empowerment as an individual construct and emphasized its psychological components, later definitions begin to emphasize its group and sociopolitical elements. Wallerstein (1992) describes empowerment as "a social action process that promotes participation of people, organizations and communities towards the goals of increased individual and community control, political efficacy, improved quality of life and social justice."

Rissel (1994) similarly makes the connections between the intrapersonal aspects of empowerment, such as self-esteem and self-efficacy; mediating structures that promote collective participation, such as group consciousness-raising activities; and macro factors, which refer to social and political activities. This conceptualization potentially makes the link among the five action strategies of the Ottawa Charter and clearly articulates the need to address risk environments as well as risk behaviours. As will become evident through the application of the power-culture lens to empowerment and health later in this chapter, the development of personal skills and their successful mobilization toward increased control over health is inseparable from other forms of empowerment. The idea of empowerment as process and its incorporation of Rissel's concepts of psychological empowerment and community empowerment are represented in Figure 5-1.

Sen (2000) describes empowerment as the ability of individuals and communities to live lives that they have reason to value. Individual empowerment is linked to collective forms of empowerment and includes the development of personal skills and capacities that allow a satisfying and healthy life: positive self-identity, cultural connectedness, sense of belonging, critical thinking, knowledge acquisition, and the general ability to negotiate one's environment. Both individual and collective forms of empowerment require health contexts to be aligned—that is, health-related systems and policy organizations are in accord with community needs and realities.

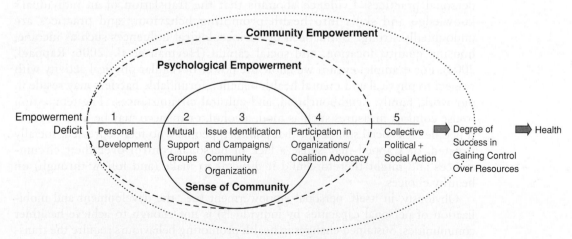

FIGURE 5-1 ◆ Community empowerment components and process.

Expanding Sen's idea, empowerment is further defined as:

> . . . *a process of enabling individuals and communities to express consciously constructed (cultural) identities and aspirations through access to capacities such as land, language, housing, economic resources and decision making institutions in ways that are mutually empowering. (Williams, 2005)*

This definition of empowerment recognizes that health, as self-defined by communities, and empowerment, as the means to health, are both culturally contingent. The definition also recognizes the importance of countering the influence of culturally dominant discourses and practices over groups at the margins and therefore includes the concept of authentic expression through consciously constructed identities. Authentic expression refers to chosen forms of expression that are self-defined as being congruent with people's sense of self and identity. The definition recognizes that the material expression of a community's aspirations, worldviews, and cultural systems must be sufficiently supported by access to economic resources, social structures, and decision making institutions (environmental supports). Where life circumstances do not support the expression of people's identities and cultural systems, the development and mobilization of personal and community capacities (empowerment processes—in particular, those that concern literacy as an active and multiple phenomena) and alignment of health systems and policy organizations with community needs and realities (the development of healthy public policies and sociopolitical transformation) are a key means through which desired changes may be made.

The interrelationships among social identities, cultural systems, and empowerment processes, as reflected in this latter definition and more recent work (Williams, Labonté, & O'Brien, 2003) is of increasing relevance to achieving the World Health Organization (WHO) goal of Health for All. While the need for empowerment initiatives to deal comprehensively with community differences is acknowledged, various aspects of identity and culture are often compartmentalized, as are discussions regarding the impact of ethnic cultures on development, or literature drawing the connections between gender identities and women's health. Furthermore, the limited understanding of how social identities and cultural systems mediate empowerment processes has tended to be confined to either individual or community levels of empowerment. As you proceed through this chapter, however, it will become more apparent how and why this area is increasingly relevant. Health disparities are greater for groups at the economic and cultural margins of our societies.

HEALTH AND EMPOWERMENT

Health in itself is culturally constructed, contingent on worldview. Worldviews are embedded in deeply held values and cultural beliefs, influencing how we experience our world and explain these experiences. They incorporate our perceptions about the nature of life, how human beings interact with each other, and the natural world. Indigenous approaches to health are distinct from Western constructions (which currently predominate in health-related discourses and public policies) in that they place emphasis on wholeness, connection, balance, harmony, and growth. For First Nations peoples, for example:

> The development of the individual is interwoven with the well-being of the community and of the nation. Moreover, an individual's identity, status and place in the world are tied not only to the [extended] family, but also to one's ancestors and community. This leads to a way of viewing mental health [individual empowerment] that is very different from Western models that focus on individuation, independence and self-reliance. (Aboriginal Healing Foundation, 2006, p. 24).

Such approaches have been developed to specifically advance the health status of indigenous peoples in response to a dominant paradigm that compartmentalizes and individualizes health. These models are holistic and culturally connected; that is, they contextualize mental well-being within culturally specific frameworks and are about empowerment or self-determination in a broader sense. They also make the connections between health status and access to determinants of health. While Western conceptualizations of empowerment are now rightfully making the connections between individual and collective forms of empowerment—that is, individual empowerment cannot occur without collective empowerment and changes to environmental conditions—these remain distinct from indigenous approaches. For indigenous peoples, empowerment is generally much more a collective phenomenon within which the individual is metaphysically indistinct from his or her extended family, ancestors, land, and historical tribal context.

Cultural identity and worldview and the means to express these are then central to how health is conceptualized and empowerment is realized. Chandler and Lalonde (1998) illustrate this in the Canadian context in their research on cultural continuity and suicide rates in First Nations communities in British Columbia. Their results demonstrate a compelling inverse relationship among community control (e.g., over education, health, justice, and cultural facilities), self-government factors, and youth suicide in First Nations communities. They report, for example, striking suicide rates of 120 per 1,000 youth in communities that do not govern themselves, compared with 20 per 1,000 youth in communities with self-government. It may be, for indigenous peoples at least, that development of personal skills and capacities, including a secure sense of cultural identity and the means to express these—empowerment in its fullest sense—is actually a project of decolonization, including claiming back indigenous meanings of health and empowerment.

LITERACY AND HEALTH FOR ALL

There are many forms of literacy, such as conversation, reading and writing, linguistic, cultural, spiritual, and technological. Literacy may be regarded as a tool or the means by which people negotiate their environments in order to achieve full health and human potential.

Literacy is central to the development of personal capacities and empowerment and is an important determinant of health. Low literacy affects health directly in that people without functional reading ability tend to make ineffective use of the health care system, manage chronic diseases poorly, experience difficulty using medication, and exercise fewer safety precautions in the workplace. Low literacy also has indirect effects on health related to difficulty obtaining and retaining employment, low income, low self-esteem, social isolation, and the abuse of alcohol and tobacco. Indeed, the impact of these indirect effects may have a more pervasive influence on health than the direct effects (Hauser & Edwards, 2006; Ronsman & Rootman, 2004). Furthermore, Ronsman and Rootman (2004) suggest that literacy is clearly linked to or associated with other determinants of health, such as income and social status, culture, gender, quality of living and working conditions, personal health practices and coping skills, and healthy child development. "These other determinants moreover, directly affect the quality of housing, food security and to some extent healthcare services. Undoubtedly, health has a strong impact on literacy, just as literacy impacts on health" (Ronsman & Rootman, 2004, p. 159). See Figure 5-2.

Canada has significant problems with low levels of literacy. The International Adult Literacy and Life Skills Survey (IALLSS), carried out by Statistics Canada in cooperation with the Organization for Economic Co-operation and Development (OECD), provides a comprehensive picture of literacy in Canada and compares Canada's literacy rates with six other OECD countries. Forty-eight percent of the adult population—some 12 million Canadians—performed below a level of literacy that is considered desirable for coping with the demands of our knowledge and information based society (Hauser & Edwards, 2006). Literacy as practised

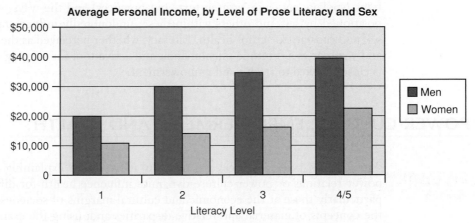

FIGURE 5-2 ◆ Personal income, prose literacy, and sex.

and measured in Canada is profoundly influenced by culture and language. Aboriginal, Francophone, and immigrant peoples have lower literacy scores relative to the rest of the population. Literacy studies have drawn attention to the importance of first language acquisition to literacy, and Aboriginal practitioners have found Native language studies to be an important precursor or complement to literacy studies in English or French. Social exclusion is thought to be a primary barrier to well-being and learning. Conceivably, when one feels more grounded in one's own culture, language, and traditions, literacy will improve (Ronsman & Rootman, 2004).

Approaches to defining and measuring literacy are based on worldview. To date, Western conceptualizations that primarily assess literacy through prose and document literacy, numeracy, and problem solving have predominated in Canada. Non-Western peoples have considerably different conceptualizations. The rainbow approach to literacy proposes that there are several forms of Aboriginal literacy, each of which can be characterized by a colour. For example, red is mother tongue literacy, while green is English and/or French literacy; yellow is the literacy of symbolism and blue the literacy of technology; indigo is spiritual literacy, and violet is holistic literacy—an appreciation of the interconnections between mind, body, spirit, and family for a healthy life. "When viewed in these terms literacy is not [just] a skill to be learned but an approach to life that includes healthy relationships, healthy nutrition, language instruction, ceremonial practices and family literacy" (Hauser & Edwards, 2006, p. 25). Being literate is about visioning a future in which an Aboriginal way of being will continue to thrive (Antone, Gamlin, & Provost-Turchetti, 2003).

Literacy is increasingly thought of as an active phenomenon deeply linked to personal and cultural identity and self-determination. Freire (1970) helped to transform literacy from a received ability to read and write to an individual's capacity to put those skills to work in shaping the course of his or her own life. Literacy is strongly linked to the ability to think critically about discourses and belief systems (spoken language, written text, and practices) and the ways in which one is positioned by self and others within these, undoubtedly influencing our sense of self and capacity to act for health. Literacy, whether perceived as the ability to read and write or as a multiple phenomenon and active tool for shaping one's own life, is closely linked to health and empowerment.

POWER-CULTURE, EMPOWERMENT, AND HEALTH

This section takes a critical postmodern approach to explaining how cultural-power relations or power-culture dynamics influence health for different groups, particularly those at the economic and cultural margins of societies. It introduces the concepts of material and relative disparities and, using the example of mental

> ## BOX 5-1
> ### Definition of Power-Culture
>
> *Power-culture* refers to the interplay of dynamics of power and culture that are operative in any one context and influence all stages of self-determination or empowerment, including the development and mobilization of personal skills. Different levels of power, such as individual, group, or institutional, are brought into dynamic interaction with different cultural systems (such as ethnicity, gender, sexual identity, or class), resulting in various forms of empowerment relations (Williams, 2001; Williams & Labonté, in press).

well-being, demonstrates how dynamics of power and culture structure environments, placing these groups at increased risk of health disparities relative to economically and culturally powerful groups (Box 5-1).

There is now overwhelming evidence that for individuals, higher socioeconomic position is associated with better health; however, debate continues regarding the extent to which income inequalities within societies are a predictor of health (Heyman et al., 2006). Nevertheless, there is sufficient evidence that both material and relative deprivation have significant implications for health and empowerment. *Material deprivation* refers to lack of access to environmental capacities conducive to health, including the alignment of communities' realities and cultural values with the rules, norms, and conventions on which institutions and public policies are based. *Relative deprivation*, or relative access to environmental capacities, is significant with respect to both health and empowerment in two ways. Firstly, inequalities in incomes are important in that by virtue of having 'less', some sectors of the population are excluded socially and materially from the life of society. This creates inequities in communities' capacities for meaningful participation, a key element of individual and collective forms of empowerment. Secondly, relative inequalities have been shown to impact on health through psychosocial pathways such as stress, self-esteem, and associated feelings of powerlessness (Brunner, 1997, & Wilkinson, 1999a, as cited in Williams, 2001).

Using the lens of power-culture provides another way of thinking how material and relative deprivation structure health (and empowerment). Different levels of power (individual, group, and institutional) are brought into dynamic interaction with different cultural systems (such as ethnicity, gender, class, sexuality), differentially shaping health contexts and opportunities for empowerment. The effects of material and relative disadvantage on the health of groups at the economic and cultural margins and the ways in which power-culture dynamics shape these are particularly evident with respect to the mental well-being.

Among those displaying symptoms of poorer mental health relative to other populations are Aboriginal and migrant peoples, rural communities, youth, low-income groups, GLBT (gay/lesbian/bisexual/transgendered people), people with disabilities, and elders. Such experiences of mental health are also gendered, strongly influenced by social power, roles, and identity (Williams, 2005). Overall, mental health status of indigenous peoples is significantly worse than that of nonindigenous peoples by almost every measure—suicide rates for Aboriginal youth in Canada, for example, are roughly five to six times higher than for non-Aboriginal youth (Health Canada 2006; Kirmayer, Simpson, & Cargo, 2003). Research largely demonstrates that the mental health of migrants, particularly those with low income and education, tends to erode over time in response to pressures of racism, poverty, and social exclusion and to lesser degrees the vulnerability of migrants to stress by the disruption of social and cultural networks. Members of sexual minority groups also bear excessive burdens of mental disease; for example, lesbians have rates of depression, anxiety disorders, and suicidal ideation that are two to three times higher than women in the general population (McNair, 2003). The experiences of these groups are by no means homogeneous, as members occupy a range of social, economic, and cultural locations. For example, the experience of immigrant people will vary, contingent on ethnic, class, and gender identities; associated social statuses; and access to social and structural forms of power. However, research also reveals clear patterns across groups even when other factors are controlled.

Access to environmental supports (structural forms of power) for mental wellbeing is clearly mediated by sociocultural identities and statuses with groups at the economic and cultural margins having consistently less access than others. Many examples across these groups in Canada are evident—relative to national averages, Aboriginal peoples live in substandard housing conditions (Table 5-1), immigrants (particularly recent immigrants) have lower rates of labour force participation, and women and people with disabilities have lower income levels (Williams, 2005).

TABLE 5-1	
Housing Disparities in Aboriginal Homes in Canada	
HOUSING DESCRIPTION	**ABORIGINAL COMPARED TO NON-ABORIGINAL HOMES**
In need of major repairs	Twice as many
No piped water supply	Ninety times as many
No bathroom facilities	Five times as many
Number of persons per dwelling	Thirty percent higher
Owner-occupied dwellings	Thirty-four percent fewer owners
No flush toilet	Ten times as many

Adapted from Adelson, N. (2005). The embodiment of inequity. Health disparities in Aboriginal Canada. *Canadian Journal of Public Health, 96*(S2), S45–S61.

Experiences of relative deprivation have significant implications for health, including the ways in which marginalized groups are discriminated against or negatively positioned with respect to self-identity by members of dominant groups. The media is a powerful influence on the positions accorded these groups: media reports influence public opinion and public policy development and the ways that people treat each other. The ability to produce and disseminate culture on a large scale is closely tied to economic or material forms of power. Members of economically and culturally dominant groups (e.g., Caucasian, male, middle class) tend to control major sources of media and therefore hold the power to construct beliefs about groups, particularly those who do not have access to these forms of power.

Take Note

Examine a local or national newspaper for examples of the ways in which people and newspaper media depict Aboriginal people, women, people with disabilities, people living in poverty, and members of GLBT communities.

The effects of relative deprivation in terms of these forms of discriminatory positions and signifying practices are enormous. Studies have found racism to be a determinant of mental well-being, either through institutionalized forms or via the disempowering ways in which individuals and groups are positioned by more economically and culturally dominant groups. For example, the Fourth National Survey of Ethnic Minorities (UK) finds an association between interpersonal racism and mental illness. Those who had experienced racial attacks are three times more likely to suffer from depression and five times more likely to suffer from psychosis (Williams, Neighbors, & Jackson, 2003) and a comprehensive review of U.S. literature found that 92% of studies reported a positive association between psychological distress and the experience of racism (McKenzie, 2004). Homosexual and bisexual men and women have been found to be consistently discriminated against across a number of categories. For example, they are more likely to be fired from a job, denied a promotion, forced out of the neighbourhood by neighbours, and given inferior medical care than their heterosexual counterparts.

Same-sex-attracted young people have higher rates of homelessness and cannot necessarily rely on support and protection of their families of origin. This group is more likely to engage in self-endangering behaviours, such as abusing alcohol and other drugs, vomiting or taking laxatives to lose weight, and thinking about planning and attempting suicide (Fisher & Ackman, 2002). Clearly, risk behaviours and their health outcomes occur within the context of risk environments. Such environments are shaped by differential access of groups to material and structural health capacities (i.e., the extent to which social structures reflect their identities, cultural norms, and practices). The meanings people attribute to their experiences and the subsequent modes of subjectivity they adopt are key to personal identity, empowerment, and health. People are either "active subjects who take up positions from which (they) can exercise power within a particular social practice or (they) are subjected to the definition of others" (Jordan & Weedon, 1995). However, the extent to which people can adopt new beliefs and practices is circumscribed by social power relations. Put another way, how people feel about themselves, their life chances, and their perceived and real ability to make changes is clearly linked to health outcomes. The development of personal capacities (skills) and their mobilization is closely related to self and cultural identity and their ability to think critically. Further, access to mediating structures such as networks and institutions that reflect one's aspirations, cultural identity, and day-to-day realities depends on having personal capacity.

THE EMPOWERMENT TERRAIN

The empowerment terrain provides a useful means of conceptualizing the interrelationships between social identities, cultural systems, and empowerment processes. Developed by Williams (2001, 2005), the *empowerment terrain* refers to the landscape of elements that exist both within and outside of individuals whose dynamic interaction constitute an individual's or community's capacity to exercise control over health and well-being. The *internal empowerment terrain* refers to the more subjective or psychological elements of empowerment—consciousness, identity, and culture. Consciousness includes knowledge, skills, ability to think critically, and intuition (Spretnak, 1991). Identity includes one's sense of self, belonging, and self-esteem. Culture refers to "a signifying system [either through language, the way we dress, what and how we eat, and how we socialize etc.] through which necessarily [among other things] a social order is communicated, reproduced, experienced and explored" (Jordan & Weedon, 1995, p. 8). The internal empowerment terrain is conceptualized as the individual capacities or the internal world that people carry from one locale to another. The ways in which these elements combine begins to structure the internal empowerment terrain and thus empowerment capacities of the individual.

The *external empowerment terrain* refers to the more outwardly orientated, material elements and relational aspects of empowerment. These are physical and other economic resources (e.g., housing and income), social structures, discourses, community social networks, and community cohesiveness and strategic partnerships to which one may have access. Globalization (including sociohistoric and contemporary processes of colonization) is also considered to be an important element that currently characterizes the external empowerment terrain and that has very real material effects on the lives of people. The combinations of these elements structure the external empowerment terrain. Empowerment is

TABLE 5-2	
Key Elements of Internal and External Empowerment Terrains	
INTERNAL EMPOWERMENT TERRAIN	**EXTERNAL EMPOWERMENT TERRAIN**
Consciousness • Knowledge, critical thinking, spontaneity, and intuition	Colonization Economic globalization • Global movement of capital and goods
Identity • Sense of self and herstory/history • Self-esteem, sense of belonging	Cultural globalisation • The globalisation of culture via migration, electronic, and print media
Culture • Internalised systems of meaning • Worldviews and symbols shared by a collective	Economic and other physical resources • Housing, access to health care, and the like
	Dominant social structures (rules, norms, conventions) and institutions (democracy, neoliberalism, religion, professions) that transmit cultural systems
	Social and interorganizational networks

constrained or enabled by the elements that constitute both internal and external empowerment terrains (Table 5-2).

Neither the external nor the internal empowerment terrains exist independently of one another. Both are mediated by the other and are constituted by the flow of actions between actors. For example, discourses are articulated within print media and policies and also are internalized by people. Positions and self-identity are reconstituted via the mediating influences of internal empowerment terrain elements (e.g., consciousness, self-esteem, knowledge) on the external elements and vice versa. Some empowerment capacities appear to be more clearly located either within the internal or external empowerment terrain; for instance, access to public health services that are institutionally supportive of one's culture (external) or a strong sense of culture and identity (internal). However, an interdependent relationship exists between the two. A strong sense of identity assists one in accessing culturally appropriate health services and, in turn, is nurtured by those same social structures. Some empowerment capabilities even more clearly span both people's internal and external worlds, such as an alliance with another group, which may be both formalized (institutional aspects) and also have subjective elements (the felt relationship as in a sense of connection/belonging).

The empowerment capacity of individuals and communities to act and make changes of their choice is undermined by deprivations within any of the empowerment terrain elements. For example, unemployment undermines empowerment capacity through loss of income, self-reliance, self-confidence, and psychological and physical health. Sen (2000) refers to this process as *capability deprivation*. Such deprivations in empowerment capacities are often linked to health determinants such as income or housing conditions, to inequities within populations of wealth and power, and to health itself.

A CRITICAL POSTMODERN APPROACH TO EMPOWERMENT

According to postmodern philosophers, reality is socially and culturally constructed, and pluralism is a fact of life. Critical postmodernists are concerned with power, oppression, and inequality. In this section, empowerment is discussed using these postmodern principles. Theoretically, this conceptualization of empowerment rests on postmodern thought wherein the ensuing power-culture dynamics are unstable and shifting, contingent on the relative natures of empowerment elements operative within particular locales. It also bases its account of empowerment relations on conceptualizations of power that suggest power is dispersed throughout the social system (empowerment terrain), is fluid and unpredictable (particularly at micro, interpersonal, community levels), yet also more deterministic in nature at macro levels (Williams, 2001).

Power-culture dynamics are constituted by various elements of the internal and external empowerment terrains that are operative within any context. These empowerment terrains will be contingent on who is present (and the internal empowerment terrains they bring with them) and the context (external empowerment terrain). Thus, power-culture dynamics and ensuing relations of empowerment will vary from situation to situation. At community levels, for instance, power-culture dynamics will be influenced by the differential access of individuals and communities to structural power, whereas at the macro, institutional level, the relationship becomes more deterministic. Large amounts of structural power are leveraged through the institutionalization of discourses and practices that reproduce particular cultural systems, representing the interests of those communities (Box 5-2).

A HEALTH PROMOTION EXAMPLE

The mobilization of identities and cultural systems as capacities for individual and community empowerment within health-related initiatives is increasingly apparent within Canada and throughout other parts of the world.

For example, First Nations communities in Canada are increasingly asserting their rights to combine traditional, locally based approaches with Western models. Such projects often require activities that (1) articulate and build awareness among community members about local, traditional approaches; (2) strengthen connections

BOX 5-2
Example of Power-Culture Dynamics

A group of Métis women confront a Caucasian male employed by a government-housing agency about his refusal to allocate their friend a subsidized rental unit. The employee of the government-housing agency has institutional power and knowledge of the Western-based cultural norms of the organization's procedures.

The collective power of several Métis women is likely to produce a different set of empowerment relations (power with) than if there were just one woman. If the Métis women have good self-esteem, are educated, and have knowledge of European bureaucratic structures (power within), the power-culture dynamics and ensuing empowerment relations will alter again.

If they take their case to the media and receive sympathetic treatment, then they will have been able to access the institutional power of the media. However, their treatment by the media will probably be contingent upon (a) who is reporting the story, (b) which discourses influence the way the story is told, and (c) how the Métis women are positioned as subjects.

The power-culture relations fluctuate from situation to situation, although consistently influenced by dominant social structures and cultural systems.

to mediating structures such as health advocacy groups; and (3) advocate for public policy development to enable programs that better reflect community-defined and culturally-based approaches to healing.

One such participatory action research project currently occurring in Saskatchewan is with a Cree First Nation of approximately 2,200 members, about 1,500 of whom live on-reserve; many of the remainder live locally in surrounding areas. On-reserve members receive a variety of federally and provincially funded mental health promotion related services as well as nonfunded services. Funded services largely correspond to Western health models, while unfunded services (provided by elders and other band members) tend to be based more on Cree concepts and traditions. The Health Centre director estimates that some 38 practitioners provide mental health–related services; however, only two of these, a mental health therapist and a Fetal Alcohol Spectrum Disorder therapist, are hired specifically for this purpose. Policies and programs intended to address mental health issues with on-reserve people have also attempted to incorporate prevention and promotion strategies alongside treatment approaches. However, the vast majority of on-reserve health services remain largely entrenched in treatment frameworks that address underlying determinants of well-being.

This project seeks to explore Saskatchewan Cree concepts of mental health and how they may be incorporated and used to provide more effective approaches to mental well-being. Focus groups are currently being held with on-reserve elders and youth to determine locally and culturally based perspectives of what supports well-being. These are being followed by interviews with health practitioners and managers to determine how these community-based perspectives match current practice and programming. The project will have an advocacy component to incorporate Cree cultural perspectives into policy and programs.

These processes are not dissimilar to Torre's (as cited in Rissel, 1994) description of empowerment as process. However, what is different is that such initiatives actively work with cultural identities and systems (at individual, community, and organizational capacities) to address systematic cultural-power inequities. Power-culture becomes an important tool for analyzing and taking action to address such inequities.

SUMMARY

The development of personal capacities skills as a means of achieving Health for All is closely connected to collective and sociopolitical forms of empowerment as health promoting environments enable the translation of personal skills and knowledge into health promoting behaviours. While efforts have been directed into theorizing empowerment as a process and conceptualizing its measurement, little attention has been given to the ways in which empowerment processes are influenced by cultural identities, social status, and other forms of power. Empowerment (the development and mobilization of personal and community capacities) is closely connected to identity, culture, and literacy. It can be conceptualized as the expression of aspirations, personal identity, and culture through the development of personal capacities and skills and access to material capacities or environmental supports such as land, language, economic resources, and the like.

Health and empowerment mean different things to different groups. Health is a culturally contingent construct, as is empowerment. Literacy is a key health determinant and a marker variable for other health determinants such as income, housing, and occupation. It is closely connected to the development of personal skills and capacities (including positive self-identity and critical thinking), cultural identity, and empowerment. Literacy in a broad sense, that is, multiple literacies, may be thought of as the means by which we negotiate our environments in the pursuit of health and human potential.

Power-culture is a potentially useful framework for thinking about and analyzing how the dynamics produced between different forms of power and cultural systems influence access to material capacities, experiences of power (and powerlessness), and health outcomes. Developing personal skills is not just a matter of increasing capacities such as knowledge, life skills, and reading and writing but ultimately is closely linked to self-identities, beliefs, and worldviews of individuals and communities in ways that enable the diverse development and expression of human potential.

The Ottawa Charter remains an important blueprint toward achieving health for all. The legacies of colonization and current processes of Western Capitalist expansion that paradoxically make our societies more culturally heterogeneous but continue to perpetuate disparities in economic and cultural power between groups mean that addressing cultural-power inequities must be a key part of health promotion. Beginning points for this are (a) thinking more critically about the ways in which the development of personal skills and capacities are intricately linked to cultural identity, worldview, and social institutions and (b) building these considerations into health promotion initiatives.

References

Aboriginal Healing Foundation. (2006). *Final report of the Aboriginal Healing Foundation: Vol. III. Promising healing practices in Aboriginal communities.* Ottawa: Author.

Antone, E., Gamlin, P., & Provost-Turchetti, L. (2003). *Literacy and learning: Acknowledging Aboriginal holistic approaches to learning in relation to Best Practices Literacy Training Programs.* Toronto: Ontario Institute for Studies in Education, University of Toronto.

Chandler, M., & Lalonde, C. (1998). Cultural continuity as a hedge against suicide in Canada's First Nations. *Transcultural Psychiatry, 35,* 191–219.

Fisher, B., & Akman, J. (2002). Normal development in sexual minority youth. In Jones, B. & Hill, M. (Eds.), *Review of Psychiatry: Vol. 21. Mental health issues in lesbian, gay, bisexual, and transgender communities* (pp. 1–13). Arlington, VA: American Psychiatric Press.

Freire, P. (1970). *Pedagogy of the oppressed.* New York: Continuum.

Hamilton, N., & Bhatti, T. (1996). *Population health promotion: An integrated model of population health and health promotion.* Ottawa: Health Canada.

Hauser, J., & Edwards, P. (2006). *Literacy, health literacy and health: A literature review.* Prepared for the Canadian Public Health Association Expert Panel on Health Literacy.

Health Canada. (2005). *The integrated pan-Canadian healthy living strategy.* Ottawa: Author.

Health Canada. (2006). *The human face of mental health and mental illness in Canada.* Ottawa: Author.

Heyman, J., Hertzman, C., Barer, M., & Evans, R. (2006). *Healthier societies: From analysis to action.* Oxford: Oxford University Press.

Jordan, G., & Weedon, C. (1995). *Cultural politics: Class, race, gender and the postmodern world.* Oxford: Blackwell Publishers.

Kirmayer, L., Simpson, C., & Cargo, M. (2003). Healing traditions: Culture, community and mental health promotion with Canadian Aboriginal peoples. *Australian Psychiatry, 11*(S1), S15–S23.

McKenzie, K. (2004). Tackling the root cause. *Mental Health Today,* Nov., 30–32.

McNair, R. (2003). Lesbian health inequalities: A cultural minority issue for health professionals. *Medical Journal of Australia, 178,* 643–645.

National Council of Welfare. (2006). *Welfare incomes 2005.* Ottawa: Government of Canada.

Raphael, D. (2004). *Social determinants of health: Canadian perspectives.* Toronto: Canadian Scholars' Press Inc.

Rissel, C. (1994). Empowerment: The holy grail of health promotion? *Health Promotion International, 9*(1), 39–47.

Ronsman, B., & Rootman, I. (2004). Literacy: One of the most important determinants of health today. In Raphael, D. (Ed.), *Social determinants of health: Canadian perspectives* (pp. 155–170). Toronto: Canadian Scholars' Press Inc.

Sen, A. (2000). *Development as freedom.* New York: Alfred A. Knopf.

Spretnak, C. (1991). *States of grace: The recovery of meaning in the postmodern age.* San Francisco: HarperCollins Publishers.

Wallerstein, N. (1992). Powerlessness, empowerment and health: Implications for health promotion programmes. *American Journal of Health Promotion, 6*(3), 197–205.

Williams, D., Neighbors, H., & Jackson, J. (2003). Racial/ethnic discrimination and health: Findings from community studies. *American Journal of Public Health, 93*(2), 200–208.

Williams, L. (2001). *Identity, power and culture: Frameworks for self-determination of communities at the margins.* Unpublished doctoral dissertation, Massey University, Auckland.

Williams, L. (2005). Taking a population health approach to mental well-being: Identity, power and culture. Opening Keynote, 2005 Summer School, *Taking a population health approach to mental well-being: Identity, power and culture.* Saskatoon: Prairie Region Health Promotion Research Centre.

Williams, L., & Labonté, R. (in press). Empowerment for migrant communities: Paradoxes for practitioners. *Critical Public Health.*

Williams, L., Labonté, R., & O'Brien, M. (2003). Empowering social action through narratives of culture and identity. *Health Promotion International, 18*(3), 33–40.

World Health Organization. (1986). *Ottawa charter for health promotion.* Ottawa: Author.

6

Strengthening Community Action: Public Participation and Partnerships for Health

CATHERINE M. SCOTT

GAIL L. MacKEAN

*H*ealth promotion works through concrete and effective community action in setting priorities, making decisions, planning strategies and implementing them to achieve better health. At the heart of this process is the empowerment of communities—their ownership and control of their own endeavours and destinies.

Community development draws on existing human and material resources in the community to enhance self-help and social support, and to develop flexible systems for strengthening public participation in and direction of health matters. This requires full and continuous access to information, learning opportunities for health, as well as funding support.
OTTAWA CHARTER (1986)

Chapter Outline

Introduction
Community Development
Building Community Capacity
Methods of Community Development
The Community Development Process
Public Participation in Health
Collaboration and Partnerships
A Partnership Framework

Partnership Configuration
Partnership Organization
A Process Model of Partnership
    Development
Application of the Tools—
    Key Considerations
Summary

Learning Objectives

After studying this chapter, you should be able to:

❖ Describe the links between strengthening community action, community development, public participation, collaboration, and partnerships

❖ Describe elements of community development methods and processes

❖ Discuss the role of public participation in health

❖ Understand the roles of partnerships in population health promotion

❖ Describe common characteristics of collaboration and partnerships

Introduction

Over the past several decades, population health interventions have met with varying levels of success. Increasingly, health professionals, researchers, policy makers, and the public have acknowledged that meaningful participation of stakeholders in conceptualizing, developing, and implementing health interventions is vital to the success of such initiatives. Over the past two decades, population health promotion policies and programs have placed high priority on active public participation in activities that effect health. This is evident in the Population Health Promotion (PHP) model. Comprehensive action strategies to improve health are embedded within the model; Strengthening Community Action (SCA) is one of its cornerstones, specifically addressing the need for public engagement in health.

SCA combines community development processes with the goal of stimulating social action for health. Engaging public participation in a social change agenda, however, raises a host of questions. For example:

◆ How is *community* defined and by whom?

◆ Whose agenda(s) is (are) being addressed?

◆ In what areas can public participation have meaningful impact (i.e., rather than being token involvement)?

◆ How do individuals, communities, and organizations work with health systems to meaningfully address joint goals?

In this chapter, we begin to address these questions. We start with an overview of theory that informs the process of community development. We then discuss how the public can participate in individual level care, health systems decision making, and population health promotion with particular focus on the development of interdisciplinary and intersectoral partnerships to address health. We argue that developing in-depth understanding of community development processes, public participation, and collaboration is fundamental to strengthening community action and ultimately to achieving population health goals.

COMMUNITY DEVELOPMENT

When people think about *community*, they may be thinking in terms of geographic or demographic boundaries. While such definitions may be useful in some circumstances, they can be of limited value when it comes to community organizing. People often attach themselves to, and are active in, communities that stretch beyond their place of residence (e.g., school and work communities). Thinking of communities as collectives of people who share common values and concerns provides a broader definition that more accurately reflects the way that people think about and organize their social relationships.

Community development can be defined as "a process of social change, which brings community members together, in an equitable fashion, to work cooperatively to identify community strengths and needs, and to address common issues that affect their health" (Denetto & Wiebe, 1999). It involves building of collective commitment, resources, and skills that can be deployed for purposive community change, building on community strengths to address community needs. It means that members of a community work together to develop their capacity and competencies, identify and meet their needs, and participate more fully in society. Community development is therefore concerned with people working together to create opportunities for learning through experience and collective effort to influence decisions that affect them. Thus, individual involvement and collective activity go hand-in-hand; the aim is for people in a community to join together with others to address community needs in such a way that all who take part, professionals and nonprofessionals alike, develop their own potential as members of society (Box 6-1).

BUILDING COMMUNITY CAPACITY

What does it mean to develop community capacity? It means members of a community developing a positive difference in their capacity and skills because they actively participate in activities directed toward meeting their needs in some way.

BOX 6-1
Developing Communities: Where Do We Start?

Start where people are, because it reflects a respect for the rights of individuals and communities to affirm their own values and ways of living. Secondly, one should recognize and build on community strengths instead of only assessing the community needs. Thirdly, while we need to work closely with communities, to respect their capacities and rights to self-determination, we must at the same time strive to live up to our own ethical standards and those of our profession in not letting blind faith in the community prevent us from seeing and acting on the paramount need for social justice. Fourth, high level community participation must be fostered. Fifth, one should not forget sense of humour in their work. Sixth, the role of political analysis and activism in health education must be recognized. Health problems and their solutions need to be re-framed in terms of their political, economic, and social contexts. Think globally, act locally, foster individual and community empowerment, and finally, work for social justice. (Minkler, 1994)

Not every activity that benefits a community can be seen as promoting community capacity building as described. Kretzmann and McKnight (1993) describe community development as "building community from the inside out." They suggest that people external to the community of interest (e.g., urban planners and professionals from public, private, and nonprofit organizations) traditionally view communities as entities with deficits or problems to be addressed, usually through the provision of services. Thus, community residents begin to view themselves as victims who need the services of outside agencies to survive. The pervasive nature of this deficiency model has a devastating effect on a community and its residents. Residents become demoralized and disempowered, mutual support and community problem-solving abilities weaken, and hope for improvement disappears as funding for services is ever dependent on problems being worse than last year or more intractable than the problems of other communities, or funding will disappear. A cycle of dependence is the result, and community leadership is undermined.

An alternative is to focus not on problems associated with a deficiency model but to take a capacity building approach. Evidence indicates that when local community members are committed to investing in citizens and their community, they can successfully develop and mobilize their assets, capacities, and abilities to construct a new social reality—one that is based on opportunity, competence, and empowerment. This community development approach focuses on community assets, not deficiencies.

METHODS OF COMMUNITY DEVELOPMENT

Although there are no prescribed methods to community development because each community will have unique challenges and assets, several social and environmental conditions can facilitate the process:

◆ Trust and the presence of community bonds
◆ Effective and inclusive communication methods
◆ Presence of responsive organizations and community facilities
◆ Adequate and appropriate levels and mix of skills across the community
◆ Preparedness to engage with government and external stakeholders
◆ Shared commitment and entrepreneurial spirit
◆ Resilience and flexibility to deal with conflict and change
◆ The ability to sustain its commitments, networks, and outcomes

External champions in the form of local politicians or professional service providers (e.g., health care providers and community workers) are helpful to the community development process, but such supporters must take care to allow community control over directions, agendas, and processes and not highjack the process for their professional purposes. This is particularly the case when undertaking community-based research (Box 6-2).

> ### BOX 6-2
> #### Community-Based Research and Participatory Action Research
>
> Savan & Sider (2003) describe community-based research (CBR) as a range of participatory research approaches that includes action research, participatory action research (PAR), and collaborative inquiry. CBR:
>
> - Is a collaborative project between different constituencies (i.e., most often academic researchers, community agency representatives, people who have experienced the issue of focus)
> - Values different sources of knowledge, promotes different methods of discovery, and assumes that multiple methods of dissemination will be required
> - Goals are social action and social change for the purpose of social justice
>
> (Strand, 2002, as cited in Stoecker, 2002).

THE COMMUNITY DEVELOPMENT PROCESS

Often, there is an external catalyst that brings people together against a common "foe." In some instances, it has been reactions against crime (e.g., gangs, prostitution, violence); in others, it has been a result of externally imposed decisions (e.g., urban renewal, school closings, hospital relocations) or a common issue facing many residents (e.g., poverty, AIDS, homelessness). Whatever the impetus, people come together to take action. It is in these initial gatherings that community development begins, gains momentum, creates leaders, and focuses efforts. There are several steps in the community development process (Table 6-1).

The community development process involves commitment, resources, and skills. Each community has its unique starting point. For instance, some communities know exactly what they want but either do not know how to get there or need support. Other communities rarely get decisions made because of deep-rooted conflicts or historical divisions among groups of people who stubbornly refuse to cooperate. Some communities have experienced too much change too quickly, and old-timers and newcomers have not yet formed a common bond. Other communities have given up trying to do anything because too many people have moved away and the energy of those remaining has been sapped, resulting in general apathy. Whatever the starting point, and no matter what the community is facing, certain time-tested principles must be kept in mind:

- Have patience: Community development takes time.
- Be flexible: There will be ups and downs.
- Be resilient: Adversity builds character.
- Encourage others: Many hands make light work.
- Be organized: You will be ready when opportunity knocks.
- Embrace challenge: Opportunities are often found in threats.

TABLE 6-1	
Steps in the Community Development Process	
Defining the issue	Articulate the issue; what is known about it, and who is affected.
Initiating the process	Research the veracity of the issue and perspectives, identify the full range of stakeholders, and gather people together to create commitment for action.
Planning community conversations	Invite all stakeholders to participate; develop both informal and formal processes of consultation that allow all viewpoints to be properly aired.
Talking, discovering, and connecting	Prepare handouts that outline the issue and why you are gathering information and mobilizing the community; connect with key people and community members; share information and garner support.
Creating an asset map	Develop lists as you talk to people and initiate relationships, communicate regularly and widely; attract resources.
Mobilizing the community	Bring people together in central locations to discuss options, share experiences, create a common vision, and plan activities.
Taking action	Involve and educate community members, help to shape opinion; and galvanize commitment.
Planning and implementing	Have a vision in mind of what must change so community-driven initiatives improve the situation, organize people and work, and sustain efforts.

◆ Build networks: Champions are sometimes located in strange places.
◆ Communicate, communicate, and communicate!

America Speaks (1996) has distilled criteria that characterize communities that successfully sustain citizen engagement (Box 6-3).

As health professionals, and as health organizations, are there strategies in addition to community development that we can use to engage individuals, groups, and communities in decisions that affect their health and their health care? What kinds of health and health care decision making can the public be effectively involved in and how? Can the public engage in health services planning and development decisions? Can patients and families participate more actively in decisions around their own health and health care? In this next section, we address some of these questions by providing an overview of what is known about public participation in health.

PUBLIC PARTICIPATION IN HEALTH[1]

History

Over the past two decades, there has been increasing attention paid to involving the public in decisions that affect their health and their health care. A number of social trends have influenced this movement; these trends include increasing distrust in authority, access to information, and an emphasis in the health sector on health

---

[1]The content of the "Public Participation in Health" section of this chapter was developed in 2006 in collaboration with the Strengthening Community Action and Public Participation Committee, Healthy Living Department, Calgary Health Region.

BOX 6-3

Nine Criteria for Sustaining Citizen Engagement

1. Political, civic, and corporate leadership have vision and understand the importance of listening to all voices in the community.
2. Community activists have vision, are self-initiating, and focus on the common good.
3. Institutional and grassroots leaders recognize that the changes necessary are systemic, and both individuals and institutions carry responsibility for making the necessary changes.
4. Media outlets—print, television, radio, and the Internet—have embraced civic/public journalism values and commit resources to building community.
5. Sufficient technology infrastructure is in place to support community-wide and region-wide dialogue and deliberation processes.
6. Community projects flow across political jurisdictions and reflect a natural ecological and economic region.
7. There is an existing infrastructure of citizen involvement so that people who participate in the project have opportunity to stay involved for the long term.
8. Resources are committed to capacity building for people at all economic levels in the community, reflecting the skill sets needed for leadership in the next century.
9. There is an established and expressed public trust, respect, and compassion among the people engaged in the civic life of the community.

America Speaks. (1996). How sustainable is your community citizen involvement? Retrieved March 4, 2006 from **www.americaspeaks.org/library/sustainable_cmty.pdf.**

promotion and population health. Public participation is central to the World Health Organization's (WHO) definition of health *promotion*, which is "the process of enabling people to increase control over and to improve their health" (WHO, 1986). Fostering public participation is one of three strategies for enabling people to have more influence in areas that affect their health, outlined in the 1986 federal document, Achieving Health for All: A Framework for Health Promotion (Health and Welfare Canada, 1986).

Range of Activities

The public as individuals, groups of people, organizations, and entire communities are participating in a variety of activities that ultimately have an impact on their health. This participation encompasses an extensive range of activities in a variety of contexts. For example:

◆ Individual patients and their families participating in decisions, with frontline health care providers, about their own health and health care
◆ Groups participating at an operational level in planning particular health care services (e.g., new parents participating in the development of pre- and postnatal

services; children and families participating in the planning and design of a children's hospital)

◆ Citizens participating in the establishment of governance-level policies and priorities for a Health Region (e.g., provincial governments have devolved authority for health services planning and delivery to regional health boards that are comprised of local citizens; community health councils, advisory to regional health boards, provide opportunities for additional public input into governance-level policies and priorities)

◆ Communities participating in decision making on issues that impact the broader determinants of health (e.g., building of safe playgrounds, development of community gardens, creation of bicycle paths)

Three Lenses

Public participation in health theory and practice has evolved concurrently in three areas, all influenced by common societal trends but with different foci. Health and health care is viewed through a somewhat distinct lens in each of these areas, with each of these areas having its own body of literature and unique language:

◆ The population health promotion lens
◆ The health systems decision making lens
◆ The individual patient/client care lens

This trifocal lens is illustrated in Figure 6-1. These are not three distinct lenses; rather, they blur into each other. This is illustrated by having dotted lines separating the lenses. Also, no one of these lenses is more important than the other. Rather, the area of focus or lens changes, depending on the context of the public participation processes. This is illustrated by having the central portion of the trifocal lens shift, as each of these lenses is described.

Common values and principles underpin all three lenses, and together they encompass multiple ways that the public can participate in health. Providing opportunities for public participation, as viewed through any of these three lenses, builds public capacity to participate generally, regardless of the lens through which participation is being viewed. The centrality of information in public participation

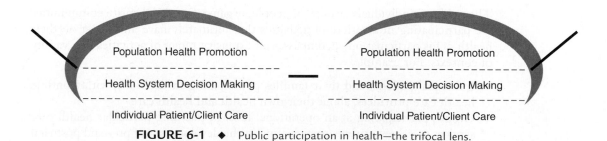

FIGURE 6-1   ◆   Public participation in health—the trifocal lens.

FIGURE 6-2 ◆ The population health
promotion lens.

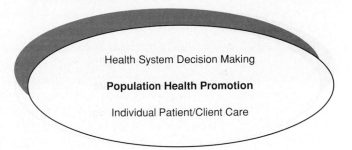

processes (Abelson et al., 2004) is an important consideration here. Members of the public gain health-related knowledge through participating in their own health care and in planning for health care and other services as stakeholders and/or citizens. They also gain confidence in the importance of their experience-based knowledge and in their ability to give voice to their experiences in a way that positively contributes to health planning and decision making processes. In short, the more ways that members of the public can participate in health-related planning and decision making, the more their capacity to participate grows.

Through the population health promotion lens (Fig. 6-2), public participation is viewed as central to SCA. Community participation is aimed at addressing the broad determinants of health, inclusive of but going far beyond those addressed by the health care system. The underlying rationale for SCA is that involving communities in their health has benefits for the health of the population.

Through the health system decision making lens (Fig. 6-3), public participation is viewed as a mechanism for incorporating public values and perspectives into various levels of health services decision making. The emphasis here is on developing health policies and making health services decisions that are in the public interest. Members of the public (citizens and/or stakeholders) are invited to participate in some type of public consultation process that is sponsored by the health services organization. These consultation processes can be one-time events (e.g., town-hall meetings, day-long deliberative process) or ongoing initiatives (e.g., issue-specific task forces, standing advisory councils). Although public views and perspectives are listened to and considered through these consultation processes, the ultimate

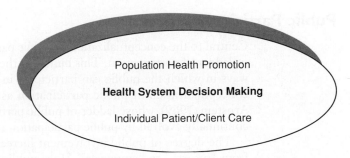

FIGURE 6-3 ◆ The health system
decision making lens.

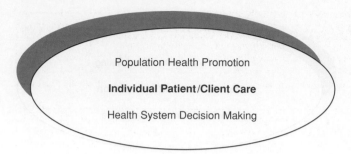

FIGURE 6-4 ◆ The individual patient/client care lens.

accountability for any policies developed and decisions made remains with the sponsoring organization. The health care management and health policy body of literature explores and explains public participation from this perspective.

Through the individual patient/client care lens (Fig. 6-4), public participation is viewed as patient (and family) involvement in decisions about their own health and health care. This lens extends a health promotion perspective to the individual patient care level by advocating for enabling patients (and their families) to assume more control over their own health and health care. This kind of patient (and family) participation is described in the literature on patient–health care provider relationships and patient and family-centered care. At this level, there is evidence that involving individuals in their own health, and the health of family members, benefits the health of the individual (and their family) (American Academy of Pediatrics, 2003; MacKean, Thurston, & Scott, 2005). In practice, these three public participation lenses are not mutually exclusive, but the ways in which they are integrated is rarely explicitly described and explained.

Benefits

A number of benefits from public participation have been described in the respective bodies of literature related to each of these lenses. Broadly described, these include improved decision making, increased public capacity to participate in decisions that affect health, health care and related services that are more responsive to the public's needs, and ultimately improved individual and population health.

Public Participation Spectrum

Central to the conceptualization of public participation is the concept of a spectrum or ladder of participation. This builds on the understanding that there is a range of ways in which the public can participate in decisions that can affect health. This conceptualization of public participation as a spectrum is generally attributed to Arnstein (1969), whose ladder of public participation has been widely adopted and continually evolved by public participation researchers and practitioners.

The degree of public involvement increases as one moves across the spectrum from "inform" to "empower." More public involvement is not necessarily better

Increasing Public Involvement →

	Inform	Input	Engage	Collaborate	Empower
Description	Information out—Information goes from a health organization to the public	Information in—input comes from the public to a health organization	A health organization and the public talk and understand each other	A health organization and the public work together over a period of time	A health organization works with the public to build capacity
Purpose	Creating awareness, public education	Getting citizen and/or stakeholder input, advice, and feedback	In-depth exploration of views, perspectives, and interests, with emphasis on listening and achieving mutual understanding	To make decisions and/or develop policy on an issue	To enable the public to make decisions and take action in areas that affect health
Public participation scenarios	A social marketing campaign is used to increase public awareness about active living strategies	A broad community survey is used to obtain public input on playground safety	A structured public consultation day is held to explore a geographic community's perspectives on the determinants of health	A health organization works collaboratively with community partners on issues (e.g., comprehensive school health, smoke-free municipalities)	Communities make decisions in areas that impact health through community development and social action

FIGURE 6-5 ◆ Public participation spectrum. (Adapted from Smith, B.L. [September, 2003]. Public policy and public participation: Engaging citizens and community in the development of public policy. Prepared for: Population and Public Health Branch, Atlantic Regional Office, Health Canada. Retrieved June 7, 2007 from http://www.phacaspc.gc.ca/canada/regions/atlantic/Publications/Public_policy/index.html.; International Association of Public Practitioners [2003]. Public Participation Spectrum. Retrieved June 7, 2007 from http://www.iap2.org/displaycommon.cfm?an=5.)

than less public involvement; rather, it depends on the context of the public participation. This spectrum is illustrated in Figure 6-5.

COLLABORATION AND PARTNERSHIPS

Addressing complex health and social issues requires that people work together to explore their differing perspectives and develop strategies to move forward. Increasingly, public health professionals are encouraged to work in collaboration and develop partnerships with the public in order to more effectively address health and health service issues (Raphael, 2004; Scott & Thurston, 2004). As is illustrated in the public participation spectrum (Fig. 6-5), collaboration and partnerships are strategies that involve high levels of public participation. In this section, we provide an overview of the concepts of collaboration and partnerships and introduce strategies for more effectively engaging the public in decisions related to population health promotion, health systems decision making, and individual care.

> **BOX 6-4**
>
> **Collaborative Processes**
>
> Barbara Gray defines *collaboration* as "a process in which those parties with a stake in the problem actively seek a mutually determined solution" (Gray, 1989, p. xviii). Collaboration may be motivated by a desire to advance a shared vision or a need to resolve conflict. The expected outcome of collaboration may be the exchange of information or the development of a joint agreement (Gray, 1996). Participating organizations form a new structure to address the mission. Such relationships involve detailed planning and communication as well as the pooling of resources.

Terminology and Meaning

Collaboration and partnerships are terms that are frequently used synonymously. Although they are closely linked, they have distinct meanings.

Collaboration is an umbrella term often used for a range of strategies for building relationships to address health and social issues (Box 6-4). Gray (1989, 1999) makes clear distinctions between collaboration, coordination, and cooperation when she suggests that cooperation and coordination "often occur as part of the process of collaboration" (p. 15). Coordination and cooperation are informal interactions that lay the foundation for the development of more formal relationships. Similarly, Winer and Ray (1994) suggest that all three of these concepts exist along a continuum of increasing intensity with cooperation at one end, coordination in the middle, and collaboration representing the more intense end of the relationship scale.

Partnerships are a type of collaboration. *Partnerships* occur when the purpose of collaboration is to advance a shared vision of a need and the expected outcome is to develop and implement a joint agreement to address the problem and bring the vision into reality. As a result, referent organizations (i.e., managing bodies such as committees) are usually created to address agreements (Alberta Public Health Association, 2000) (Box 6-5). Some commonly identified characteristics of partnerships include:

◆ Shared authority, responsibility, and management
◆ Shared liability, risk-taking, accountability, and rewards
◆ Detailed communication strategies

> **BOX 6-5**
>
> **What Is a Referent Organization?**
>
> A referent organization is formed as a result of a collaborative effort. The functions of this organization include regulation of relationships and activities, appreciation of emergent trends and issues, and infrastructure support (Gray, 1989).

> **BOX 6-6**
> **Framework and Models**
>
> **Framework:** "Descriptive categories are placed within a broad structure of both explicit and assumed propositions . . . its propositions summarize and propose explanations for vast amount of data. It is not a theory, however, because the propositions are not systematically derived in a deductive fashion" (Denzin, 1970).
> **Models:** Symbolic representation of the concepts that make up a theory; may draw on a number of theories or empirical findings to further understanding of a problem in a specific context (Polit & Hungler, 1995).

- Joint investment of resources (time, work, funding, material, expertise, information) and reputation
- The development of a new structure (i.e., referent organization)
- Explicit awareness of the influence of power differences—often assumed to be equal but rarely so

Over the past 10 years, there has been an explosion of literature on the topic of collaboration and partnerships. Partnership theory derives from many different theoretical perspectives and practice situations; correspondingly, a number of frameworks and models have developed (Box 6-6). By their very nature, frameworks and models leave out much of the detail of the theories they represent and frequently do not make explicit links to theories from which they are derived. Application of such tools therefore involves acknowledging the contexts within which they were developed and determining whether they are relevant (or irrelevant) for the context within which they are being applied. Models and frameworks must be applied with a measure of flexibility that accounts for contextual realities.

When they are compared, it is evident that partnership and collaborative models share a number of components (Huxham & Vangen, 2005; Scott & Thurston, 2004):

- The context within which they are developed (also described as the environment, extra-local relations, and external factors)
- Common interest (vision or domain)
- Characteristics of the members or partners (culture, structures, resources, representation, reputation)
- Characteristics of the partnership (principles, common purpose, vision, culture, structures, processes, representation, reputation, resources, outcomes)
- Communication (open, frequent, formal and informal, shared language, respectful)

Collaboration is not a static process; it is generally described as flexible and iterative, having characteristics in common with the community development process. Development of partnerships usually commences with a few potential partners exploring issues of common interest, articulating a common vision, and

> **BOX 6-7**
>
> **Collaborative Advantage and Inertia**
>
> **Collaborative advantage:** something is achieved that could not have been achieved by any one individual, group, or organization working alone (Huxham & Vangen, 2005).
>
> **Collaborative inertia:** a situation that arises when the apparent rate of work output from a collaboration is slowed considerably compared to what a casual observer might expect to be able to achieve (Huxham, 1996, p. 4).

developing a preliminary strategy before approaching other potential partners. Before commitment to proceed is achieved, many relationship-building activities are required. Achieving "collaborative advantage" and moving through "collaborative inertia" (Huxham & Vangen, 2005) is dependent on remaining responsive to changes (Box 6-7). Changes in membership and context require ongoing negotiation of purpose, strategies to build and maintain trust among members, accepting accountability, attention to the role of power, identifying resources, developing and adapting action plans, agreeing on communication strategies, and adopting a broad understanding of leadership (Huxham & Vangen, 2005) (Box 6-8). Many process descriptions emphasize the importance of evaluation strategies throughout (Scott & Thurston, 1997). Resources that were frequently discussed in relation to the process of moving the partnership forward are people, time, and commitment.

In the following sections, we describe a partnership framework and partnership models that reflect collaborative characteristics. The tools that we use were originally developed based on a qualitative study conducted in 1993, which focused on the development of partnerships among community agencies working with vulnerable groups (Scott-Taplin, 1993). Since that time, the framework has been applied in a variety of health and social settings and has been demonstrated to have continued relevance.

> **BOX 6-8**
>
> **What Does Leadership Mean?**
>
> In collaborative contexts, leadership is NOT about a single formal leader influencing members to achieve goals. Three leadership media—structures, processes, and participants—influence whether or not collaborative advantage is achieved. Leadership is about balancing the facilitative roles (i.e., embracing, empowering, involving, mobilizing the structures, processes, and participants) with directive roles (i.e., manipulating the collaborative agenda and playing politics) (Huxham & Vangen, 2005).

A PARTNERSHIP FRAMEWORK

The partnership framework (Table 6-2) described in this chapter is comprised of five categories: extra-local relations, domain, partner characteristics, partnership characteristics, and communication.

Extra-Local Relations

Extra-local relations are described as the external influences on the partnership, including the social context and the political and economic systems within which the partnership is based. All programs are situated within social contexts. Although extra-local relations may not play a predominant role in a partnership, they must always be considered. In this framework, extra-local relations that may influence the partnership are distinguished by whether they exert influence on administrative level or at the service provision activities. Organizations, communities, and individuals not directly involved in the partnership are potential sources of extra-local influence.

Domain

The domain is the area of interest that is the focus of partnership activities (e.g., HIV/AIDS prevention). Partners may come to a partnership representing interests in several different domains; however, at the partnership level, these differing interests are focused in an attempt to address one particular domain. If the existence of the domain is recognized and supported by all players (i.e., funders, the community, potential partners, and program personnel), partnership initiatives are more likely to succeed.

Partner Characteristics

Partner characteristics are those factors that distinguish the partners. Each partner will bring distinctive characteristics to the partnership that will directly and indirectly influence its development. These characteristics include:

◆ The structure and processes of the partner agency
◆ The resources that the partner and the partner representative are able to contribute to the partnership initiative
◆ Representation of the target group in the partner agency
◆ The reputation of the partner, of the personnel working for the partner, and of the group(s) served by the partner agency

The importance of formal representation of the target group in partner agencies is something that needs to be discussed when developing the partnership. The characteristics of this representation will vary from partner to partner. For example, agencies might involve the target group at the board or management committee level, whereas other agencies might seek feedback through more indirect means

TABLE 6-2
Partnership Framework

CATEGORIES	Properties	Dimensions		
		PARTNERSHIPS		
Extra-local factors	Administrative	Organizational		
	Service provision	Individual		
		Community		
Domain	Recognition	Funders		
	Support	Community		
		Vulnerable group		
		Partners		
		Personnel		
Partnership characteristics	Groundwork	Research	Activities	
	Organizational structure	Administrative		
		Operational		
	Resources	Funding	Space	
		Personnel	Time	
		Material		
	Representation	Areas	Characteristics	
	Reputation	Positive	Negative	
Partner characteristics	Organizational structure	Administrative		
		Operational		
	Resources	Commitment	Funding	
		Knowledge	Time	
		Skills		
	Representation	Areas	Characteristics	
	Reputation	Partners		
		Personnel		
		Vulnerable group		
Communication	Type	Formal	Informal	
	Area	Service recipient		
		Personnel		
		Partnership		
		Partner		
		Community		
Operations	Type	Administrative		
		Service provision		
	Area	Service recipient		
		Personnel		
		Partnership		
		Partner		
		Community		

Adapted from Scott-Taplin, C. M. (1993). *The development of partnerships among community agencies working with vulnerable groups* (p. 107). Calgary: University of Calgary.

(e.g., surveys, public forum). It is important that partners accept the legitimacy of a range of representation strategies.

Partnership Characteristics

Each partnership initiative is unique. This uniqueness is a function of the way in which a partnership is established and the individuals and organizations that participate in its development. The characteristics that distinguish a partnership include:

♦ The groundwork completed before the initiation of the partnership
♦ The structure and processes of the partnership
♦ The resources available to the initiative
♦ The representation of the target group within the partnership
♦ The reputation of the partnership

Partnerships that are effective are those that develop strategies to break down professional territorial barriers. These strategies include the implementation of communication mechanisms and professional development opportunities that encourage collaboration (Scott & Thurston, 1997).

Communication

Communication affects all of the categories previously discussed. Recognition of formal and informal types of communication is vital to the success of a partnership. The type of communication that occurs between partners will directly or indirectly affect the partnership. There is a need for both formal and informal communication strategies. It is suggested that ongoing evaluation of communication strategies will facilitate the determination of strategies that are appropriate for the partnership at a given time (Scott-Taplin, 1993).

PARTNERSHIP CONFIGURATION

The configuration of categories, properties, and dimensions must be unique to the specific requirements of the partnership. It is recommended that all categories and their associated properties and dimensions be appraised and adapted to meet the specific needs of individual partnership initiatives.

Categories within the framework must never be considered in isolation. Each category interacts with each of the other categories. Changes in one area may directly, or indirectly, influence changes in all other categories. Just as the cogs within a toy must all work together to propel the toy, within this framework, all of the categories and their properties and dimensions must be considered and configured to advance the partnership toward a common vision.

The configuration will vary from partnership to partnership with some categories taking precedence in some partnerships and other categories taking precedence in

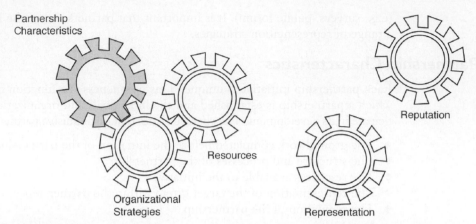

FIGURE 6-6 ◆ Failure to include essential elements in the partnership. In this example, the partnership has failed to address the issue of representation of the partners. As a result, the partnership is not as successful as it otherwise would have been. (Redrawn from Scott-Taplin, C. M. [1993]. *The development of partnerships among community agencies working with vulnerable groups.* Unpublished master's thesis, University of Calgary, Calgary, AB.)

others. Failure to assess each of the elements in the framework to determine its appropriateness for a specific partnership model may result in some essential elements being neglected (Fig. 6-6), some nonessential elements being implemented (Fig. 6-7), or some essential elements being implemented improperly (Fig. 6-8). In any of these situations, the result may be that increased work will be required to ensure the success of the partnership or the partnership may fail to achieve the vision.

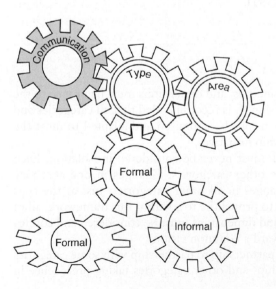

FIGURE 6-7 ◆ Inclusion of nonessential elements in the partnership. In this example, some unnecessary formal communication strategies have been implemented. As a result, effective communication is essentially blocked. (Redrawn from Scott-Taplin, C. M. [1993]. *The development of partnerships among agencies working with vulnerable groups.* Unpublished master's thesis, University of Calgary, Calgary, AB.)

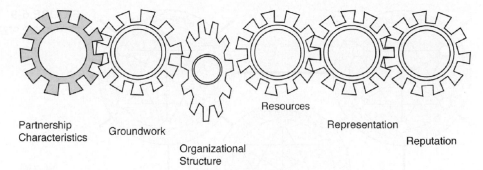

FIGURE 6-8 ◆ Improper configuration of elements in the partnership model. In this example, the organizational structure that has been selected does not meet the needs of all of the partners. As a result, more work is required to advance the vision of the partnership. (Redrawn from Scott-Taplin, C. M. [1993]. *The development of partnerships among community agencies working with vulnerable groups.* Unpublished master's thesis, University of Calgary, Calgary, AB.)

PARTNERSHIP ORGANIZATION

The model of partnership organization (Fig. 6-9) extends the description of partnerships. This model portrays the categories of the partnership framework enmeshed in the partnership culture. All of the categories are displayed in a relationship of mutual dependency. The linkages (direct and indirect) between each of the categories within the model will vary from partnership to partnership.

It is important to note that although the characteristics of the partners are part of the partnership culture, the organizational culture of individual partners may overlap with, or be distinct from, the partnership culture. The similarity between the partnership culture and the culture of the individual partners should be carefully considered when forming a partnership. If the partnership and partners' cultures are in conflict, decisions will have to be made about whether the partnership is appropriate for some partners or whether the inclusion of those partners is important enough to warrant extra resources being devoted to support their participation. For example, some additional strategies may be required to make successful a partnership between a government organization that is based on hierarchical structures and a nonprofit organization based on feminist principles of equity and consensus decision making. It is also important to recognize that partners may develop relationships with one another that are external to the partnership. Consideration should be given to how such external relationships may influence the partnership.

A PROCESS MODEL OF PARTNERSHIP DEVELOPMENT

It is one thing to recognize that specific elements in the partnership framework are essential or nonessential for the development of a partnership; it is quite another to

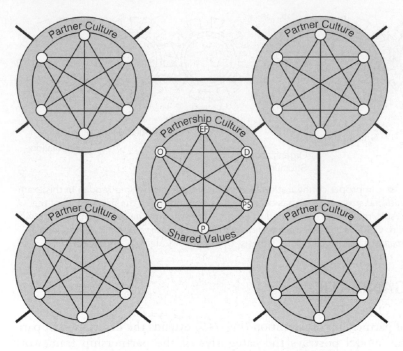

FIGURE 6-9 ◆ A model of partnership organization.

EF– Extra-local relations   P– Partner Characteristics
D – Domain   C– Communications
PS– Partnership Characteristics   O– Operations

determine when to implement each of these elements. The process model describes some phases of partnership development (Fig. 6-10).

As described earlier, development of a partnership is an iterative process. Although elements of the process are arranged around a circle, after the partnership has been initiated, the order in which these activities occur will vary from one partnership initiative to the next. As the partnership evolves, some elements of the process may need to be revisited.

The process begins with the awareness of a need. It is important to discuss the formation of the partnership with potential partners early in the process. This informal group will formulate a vision for the collaborative initiative. When the vision has been formulated, this group will be able to:

◆ Identify potential actions that will support attaining the vision
◆ Identify extra-local relations that may affect the partnership
◆ Identify essential partnership characteristics
◆ Identify other potential partners
◆ Contact the partners that are so identified
◆ Identify communication strategies

The next stage of the process involves going to the identified partner agencies to discuss their potential commitment to the project. Before proceeding,

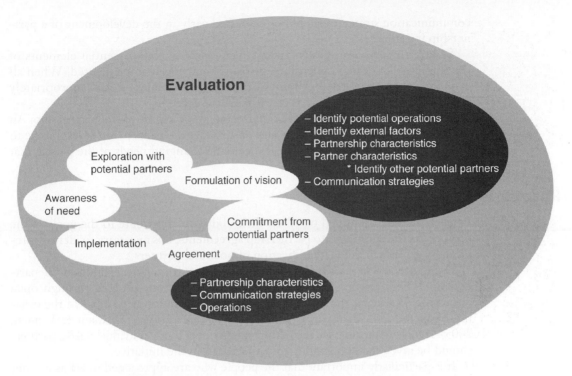

Evaluation

- Identify potential operations
- Identify external factors
- Partnership characteristics
- Partner characteristics
  * Identify other potential partners
- Communication strategies

Exploration with potential partners

Formulation of vision

Awareness of need

Commitment from potential partners

Implementation

Agreement

- Partnership characteristics
- Communication strategies
- Operations

FIGURE 6-10 ◆ A process model for partnership development.

it is recommended that potential partners achieve agreement on issues relating to partnership characteristics and communication strategies. Once these factors have been established, the partnership initiative can be implemented. Evaluation procedures are an integral part of the entire development process.

APPLICATION OF THE TOOLS—KEY CONSIDERATIONS

Complex interactions within and among categories imply that there is no single right way to develop and structure a partnership initiative (Scott & Thurston, 1997). The proposed framework and models must only be used to guide such initiatives. This being said, the framework suggests some actions that may encourage the success of these ventures.

Prior to developing a relationship of the intensity and formality of a partnership, some coordinating activities are necessary. The completion of groundwork prior to the establishment of a partnership may facilitate the identification of the elements of the framework that are required for a specific partnership. Issues relating to extra-local relations, domain, partnership characteristics, partner characteristics, and communication strategies should be discussed early in the development of a partnership initiative.

Failure to complete these activities may result in some essential elements of the framework not being identified or being improperly implemented. When all elements of the partnership framework have been reviewed and appropriately implemented, the partnership is more likely to succeed.

An evaluative component should permeate every aspect of the partnership. An overall commitment to evaluation may ensure that the partnership is responsive to the external environment and that it meets the changing needs of the people that it serves.

Partner Identification

Partners may be identified based on their ability to contribute to the goals of the project. Before entering into partnership agreements, it is necessary to identify preliminary criteria to guide identification of potential partners.

Each potential partner will seek specific benefits from participation in the partnership. These reasons for participation should be acknowledged through open discussion. Balancing the overall aims of the collaboration with those of the organizations and individual participants is an ongoing process (Huxham & Vangen, 2005). If it is not possible for the partnership to meet these individual needs, partners should be given the opportunity to withdraw from the initiative.

It is particularly important that the people who are approached to act as partner representatives be committed to the issue that will be addressed by the partnership. It is essential to develop strategies to maintain a high level of commitment and trust as experienced partner representatives leave and as new partner representatives join the partnership.

In the current economic climate, there is increasing pressure on partnership initiatives to achieve the objectives that they identify. Care should be taken to select partner representatives who will provide different skills required for advancing the partnership. An additional factor to consider when identifying potential partners is the impact of differences between the organizational culture of the partnership and the organizational culture of potential partners. The more divergent the organizational cultures, the more resources will be required to advance the partnership.

Partnership Characteristics and Communication Strategies

It is not possible to overemphasize the importance of clearly describing the reason for the partnership. It is essential to develop agreement on definitions regarding the vision, goals, and objectives of the partnership. All of the partner representatives must be talking the same language when they come to the partnership table. Agreement on these and other partnership characteristics and communication strategies should be in place before a partnership is formally established. Some more successful partnerships have implemented a formal time for discussing partnership issues during each partnership meeting.

Guiding Principles

The results of research regarding the development of partnerships have emphasized the need for partners to agree on the basic guiding principles for the partnership. Although specific principles that are adopted by a partnership will vary, the following general principles have been identified as being valuable for creating sustainable partnerships (Himmelman, 1996; Labonte, 1993; Scott & Thurston, 1997; Winer & Ray, 1994):

◆ Membership is not assumed. Partners will agree to the mission, goals, objectives, activities, and guiding principles that have been established for the partnership.

◆ All partners and partner representatives are recognized for their unique and essential contributions to the partnership.

◆ All partners agree to share the risks, responsibilities, and rewards associated with the partnership.

◆ All partners agree to how power is distributed and used within the partnership. Power is shared but may not be equally distributed among the partners.

◆ All partners recognize the need for the partnership to enhance the capacity of individual partners while working to achieve a common purpose.

◆ The structure of the partnership will remain flexible to accommodate changing needs.

◆ Administration of partnership contracts will be assigned to members as appropriate.

◆ All communication (formal and informal) and activities undertaken on behalf of the partnership or relating to the partnership will embody the principles of social justice and equity.

SUMMARY

In this chapter, we have described links between strengthening community action, community development, public participation, collaboration, and partnerships. We have argued that developing in-depth understanding of community development processes, public participation, and collaboration is fundamental to strengthening community action and ultimately to achieving population health goals. The positive effects of healthy communities become evident as citizens participate in making choices and decisions that affect the quality of community life.

References

Abelson, J., Forest, P. G., Eyles, J., Casebeer, A., MacKean, G. (2004). Will it make a difference if I show up and share? A citizens' perspective on improving public involvement processes for health system decision making. *Journal of Health Sciences and Policy Research*, 9(4), 205–212.

Alberta Public Health Association. (2000). Partnership guidelines. Retrieved June 4, 2007 from **http://www.cms.apha.ab.ca/files/partnership.pdf.**

American Academy of Pediatrics, Institute for Family Centered Care. (2003). Policy statement: Family-centered care and the pediatrician's role. *Pediatrics, 112*(3), 137–142.

America Speaks. (1996). How sustainable is your community citizen involvement? Retrieved March 4, 2006, from **www.americaspeaks.org/library/sustainable_cmty.pdf**.

Arnstein, S. R. (1969). A ladder of participation. *American Institute of Planners Journal, 35*, 216–224.

Denzin, N. K. (1970). *The research act: A theoretical introduction to sociological methods*. Chicago: Aldine Publishing.

Denetto, S., & Wiebe, V. (1999). Role of community facilitator. Unpublished document. Winnepeg, Canada: Winnipeg Regional Health Authority.

Gray, B. (1989). *Collaborating—Finding common ground for multiparty problems*. San Francisco: Jossey-Bass.

Gray, B. (1996). Cross-sectoral partners: Collaborative alliances among business, government and communities. In C. Huxham (Ed.), *Creating collaborative advantage* (pp. 57–79). Thousand Oaks, CA: Sage Publications.

Gray, B. (1999). The evolution of collaborative research in the last decade: Toward a dynamic theory. In S. Schruijer (Ed.), *Multi-organizational partnerships and cooperative strategy* (pp. 9–16). Tilburg: Dutch University Press.

Health and Welfare Canada. (1986). *Achieving health for all: A framework for health promotion*. Ottawa: Minister of Supply and Services.

Himmelman, A. T. (1996). On the theory and practice of transformational collaboration: From social service to social justice. In C. Huxham (Ed.), *Creating collaborative advantage* (pp. 19–43). Thousand Oaks, CA: Sage Publications.

Huxham, C. (Ed.). (1996). *Creating collaborative advantage*. Thousand Oaks, CA: Sage Publications.

Huxham, C., & Vangen, S. (2005). *Managing to collaborate: The theory and practice of collaborative advantage*. London, UK: Routledge, Taylor and Francis Group.

Kretzmann, P., & McKnight, J. (1993). Building communities from the inside out: A path toward finding and mobilizing a community's assets. Evanston, IL: Institute for Policy Research.

Labonte, R. (1993). Community development and partnerships. *Canadian Journal of Public Health, 84*, 237–240.

MacKean, G. L., Thurston, W. E., & Scott, C. M. (2005). Bridging the divide between families and health professionals' perspectives on family centered care. *Health Expectations, 8*, 74–85.

Minkler, M. (1994). Challenges for health promotion in the 1990s: Social inequities, empowerment, negative consequences, and the common good. *American Journal of Health Promotion, 8*(6), 403–413.

Polit, D. F., & Hungler, B. P. (1995). *Nursing research, principles and methods*. (5th ed.) Philadelphia: Lippincott.

Raphael, D. (2004). *Social determinants of health: Canadian perspectives*. Toronto, ON: Canadian Scholars' Press.

Savan, B., & Sider, D. (2003). Contrasting approaches to community-based research and a case study of community sustainability in Toronto, Canada. *Local Environment 8*(3), 303–316.

Scott, C. M., & Thurston W. E. (1997). A framework for the development of community health agency partnerships. *Canadian Journal of Public Health, 88*, 416–420.

Scott, C.M., & Thurston, W. E. (2004). The influence of social context on partnerships in Canadian health systems. *Gender, Work and Organization, 11*(5), 481–505.

Scott-Taplin, C. M. (1993). *The development of partnerships among community agencies working with vulnerable groups*. Unpublished master's thesis, University of Calgary, Calgary, AB.

Stoecker, R. (2002). Practices and challenges of community-based research. *Journal of Public Affairs Supplement, 1*(6), 219–239.

Winer, M., & Ray, K. (1994). *Collaboration handbook: Creating, sustaining, and enjoying the journey.* St. Paul, MN: Amherst H. Wilder Foundation.

World Health Organization. (1986). Ottawa Charter for Health Promotion. Geneva, Switzerland: Author.

7

Building Healthy Public Policy

WILFREDA E. THURSTON

*H*ealth promotion goes beyond health care. It puts health on the agenda of policy makers in all sectors and at all levels, directing them to be aware of the health consequences of their decisions and to accept their responsibilities for health.

*Health promotion policy combines diverse but complementary approaches including legis-
lation, fiscal measures, taxation and organizational change. It is coordinated action that
leads to health, income and social policies that foster greater equity. Joint action contributes
to ensuring safer and healthier goods and services, healthier public services, and cleaner,
more enjoyable environments.*

*Health promotion policy requires the identification of obstacles to the adoption of healthy
public policies in non-health sectors, and ways of removing them. The aim must be to make
the healthier choice the easier choice for policy makers as well.* OTTAWA CHARTER (1986)

Chapter Outline

Introduction   Policy Communities, Networks, and Partnerships
What Is Public Policy?   Partnerships
How Is Public Policy Developed?   Summary

Learning Objectives

After studying this chapter, you should be able to:

❖ Describe policy making processes

❖ Discuss the role of communities in policy development

❖ Acknowledge the need for critical social analysis throughout the policy cycle

Introduction

*H*ealthy public policies are those that influence the health of
populations; they are described as "ecological in perspective, multisectoral in scope
and participatory in strategy" (Milio, cited in Pederson et al., 1988, p. iii). This

chapter discusses the processes by which healthy public policy is developed so as to provide population health practitioners with a broad view into how they might influence public policies. Public participation is touched on but is explored more thoroughly in Chapter 6. In this chapter, we present a framework for understanding the development of public policy. We argue that the processes of policy development and evaluation should include economic analysis and must also address disparities so that reduction of health inequities is an intended outcome of public policies.

WHAT IS PUBLIC POLICY?

Public policy as defined by Pal (2001) is "a course of action or inaction chosen by public authorities to address a given problem or interrelated set of problems" (p. 2). Once a problem or issue has been given public attention, inaction or failure to formulate a response is a deliberate policy decision. "We have no position" is a policy statement. Public policies deal with public problems, not with the operations and structures through which the policies (or lack of policy) will be implemented. Public policies act as a set of guidelines or as a framework for action. Once a problem has been identified, governments have three general categories of policy instruments: do nothing; act indirectly (e.g., educate, provide funds); or act directly through state agencies, corporations, or in partnership with private or nonprofit organizations (Pal, 2001).

Public policy in a democracy is made by elected officials (Pal, 2001). Thus, it is distinguished from the organizational policies made by administrators, managers, or frontline staff within public organizations. Public policy is also separate from corporate policy or policies made by nongovernmental organizations. That does not mean that there is no interaction among these various locations of policy.

HOW IS PUBLIC POLICY DEVELOPED?

Howlett and Ramesh (1995) present five aspects of a policy cycle:

◆ Agenda setting
◆ Policy formulation
◆ Decision making
◆ Policy implementation
◆ Policy evaluation

Figure 7-1 is a representation of how the processes work together. These processes are not considered to be linear because there may be several iterations for each before a public policy is stated. This should be contrasted with what Pal

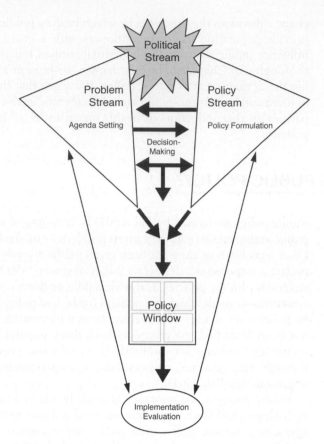

FIGURE 7-1 ◆ A nonlinear, nonrational policy process.

(2001) identified as the more commonly promoted rational decision making model that assumes a linear process, where problems and the solutions are broken into discrete parts, would result in a more efficient and predictable government. We argue that linear models are incompatible with much of healthy public policy because analysis inevitably reveals the complexity and nonlinear nature of most problems and their solutions (Miller et al., 1998). Healthy Cities (HC) projects as described by the World Health Organization (WHO) are examples of ecological, multisectoral, and participatory healthy public policy initiatives. HC initiatives focus on the setting where people live and work (e.g., home, school, work, community) to support the development of policies that address broad determinants of health (e.g., income and social status, social support networks, education, working conditions, social environments, physical environments, gender, culture). Knowledge of public policy processes and theory provides a foundation for such population health initiatives.

Agenda Setting

Agenda setting is the process through which problems come to the attention of elected officials or policy makers. This is the problem recognition stage. The problem stream is the process whereby a problem or lack of an ideal state becomes perceived as a problem that public bodies should address. Decision makers receive feedback from both external and internal sources (Howlett & Ramesh, 1995). The strength of the policy network (discussed later in this chapter) clearly affects this feedback process. Pal (2001) emphasizes the difference between problem recognition and problem definition. The way a problem is defined shapes the options available.

Gender-based analysis (GBA), defined as identifying how problems are different for women and men and girls and boys or how policies and programs impact the sexes differently, has been argued to be essential in good policy development (Vlassoff & Moreno, 2002). GBA is one means to ensure that policies create equity rather than perpetuating inequalities (Spitzer, 2005). It is supported by Canadian federal policy (Women's Health Bureau, 2003) as well as the WHO and Pan-American Health Organization (PAHO); however, GBA is not yet common practice. Analyzing data that has been segregated by sex is only a minimum for GBA.

Many of the public health problems that face practitioners in the new millennium (e.g., HIV/AIDS, poverty and chronic disease, violent injury) are complex, and public health practitioners cannot be sure of the effects of interventions. Koppenjan and Klijn (2004) have described these as "wicked societal problems" (p. 6), which reminds us that the task of creating healthy public policy is not simple (Box 7-1).

Policy Formulation

The policy stream is the process whereby experts and analysts pose solutions to the problem and is consistent with the stage of policy formulation. When solutions

---

BOX 7-1

Tobacco Policies: Gender and Diversity?

On a population level, public health policy has been successful in reducing smoking rates. A group of researchers examined the evidence for tobacco policies published between 1990 and 2004. Articles were analyzed for evidence of gender-based analysis and diversity analysis. They identified that studies often do not collect or report the data needed to do these assessments; therefore, it is difficult to plan policies that positively impact groups such as girls or Aboriginal people.

From Greaves, L., Johnson, J., Bottorff, J., Kirkland, S., Jategaonkar, N., McGowan, M., et al. (2006). What are the effects of tobacco policies on vulnerable populations? A better practices review. *Canadian Journal of Public Health, 97,* 310–315.

become joined to problems, argued Kingdon (cited in Howlett & Ramesh, 1995), and a favourable political stream exists, a policy window opens. The political stream refers to social and political context. The policy window refers to a favourable opening for a public policy. Even if the work of the problem and policy streams goes well, if the political stream is not favourable—for instance, if any public policy is going to attract vociferous opposition—then the policy window may never open. For example, when the issue of domestic violence was first raised in the House of Commons in 1982, some members made jokes and laughed. In general, the public was outraged by the response of some of their elected officials. Public pressure widely reported in the media prompted a House of Commons report on domestic violence from the Standing Committee on Health.

The latter example also highlights the influential role of the media (Phillips & Orsini, 2002) in both reflecting and shaping the political stream. Pal (2001) writes about "ideas in good currency," ideas that "sound right to most people" (p. 121). Similarly, Engberg-Pedersen and Webster (2002) talk about a political space for the poor where public policies can be generated. An important aspect of political space is the range of ideas that are circulating in the political stream. As Koppenjan and Klijn (2004) point out, some actors in the policy game have more power than others to hinder or realize the agenda setting and the identification of potential solutions. Understandings of power and how it circulates may therefore be important in analyzing a policy network. Gerrard, Thurston, Scott, and Meadows (2005), for instance, describe how some policies have eroded the capacity of rural women to participate in policy development and monitoring.

Decision Making

In the decision making stage, policy makers select from among policy options developed in the formulation stage. Even at this stage, the policy making process may cease when options that satisfy competing agendas (agendas other than solving that particular societal problem) or that are low cost and low risk are not evident. Alternatively, politicians may float a policy idea to gauge public reaction. Sufficient negative reaction may mean that the policy never sees implementation.

Economic analysis can be useful in choosing a public policy alternative. Farrier and Weber (1998) emphasized that "cost is a half-word" (p. 135) when assessing public health policies. Estimating both the costs and benefits, and if possible the direct and indirect costs and benefits, of a policy can form an important aspect of rationales for policies along with statistical, moral, and ethical arguments.

Many public policies have been developed in Canada and other countries since the House of Commons report mentioned previously, yet the reported rates of domestic violence remain as high as in 1982. It is hoped that evaluation of programs and policies assists policy advocates in policy formation and modification.

Policy Implementation and Evaluation

Policy implementation is the process by which governments put solutions or policies into effect. Policy evaluation includes processes by which results of policies are monitored. Evaluation can lead back to a fuller understanding of either the problem or potential solutions. There are several possible explanations for why domestic violence rates have not been reduced; for example, women may be more likely to report than in the past and they may report earlier, record-keeping may have improved so that more cases enter public statistics, or the policies enacted may not be addressing the causes of domestic violence. Evaluations can help to assess whether social change has occurred and how it occurred (Thurston & Potvin, 2003).

Health economics aims to join both costs and outcomes in evaluation of health policies and in so doing makes the assumptions and values of the decision makers clear. This approach to health economics will therefore encourage understanding of the agenda setting, policy formulation, and decision making phases of healthy public policy. Few economic evaluations have been completed in health promotion overall (Rush, Shiell, & Hawe, 2004); in fact, in their study of economic evaluations conducted between 1990 and 2001, Rush, Shiell and Hawe (2004) did not find any that addressed projects aimed at building healthy public policy. This is an increasingly important aspect of policy evaluation.

POLICY COMMUNITIES, NETWORKS, AND PARTNERSHIPS

People who are concerned about a particular policy issue are considered by Howlett and Ramesh (1995) to form a policy community (Fig. 7-2). These people

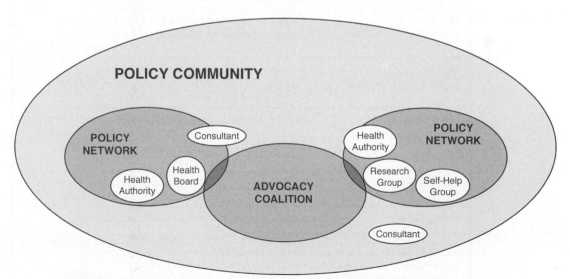

FIGURE 7-2 ◆ Policy subsystems: Policy communities, networks, and advocacy coalitions.

may include members of the general public, representatives of organizations, government employees, and elected or appointed officials. They further distinguish the actors in the policy cycle. "Policies are made by policy subsystems consisting of actors dealing with a public problem. . . . Policy subsystems are forums where actors discuss policy issues and persuade and bargain in pursuit of their interests" (Howlett & Ramesh, 1995, p. 51). Some members of the policy community interact on a regular basis, and these form a policy network. Advocacy coalitions form yet another subset of the policy community and comprise "actors from a variety of public and private institutions at all levels of government who share a basic set of beliefs (policy goals plus causal and other perceptions) and who seek to manipulate the rules, budgets and personnel of governmental institutions in order to achieve these goals over time" (Howlett & Ramesh, 1995, p. 126). Doern and Phidd (1992) suggest "Bureaucracy is also a system of delegation that immediately creates an impetus for 'bottom-up' policy initiatives emanating from departments that possess their own agendas reinforced and challenged by their policy communities" (p. 154). Actors in the policy subsystem vary in knowledge and expertise and in ultimate goals. The arrows in Box 7-2 point to the importance of a varied membership in a policy network and the role of advocacy coalitions and the broader policy community. The problem and policy streams rely on experts and analysts examining problems and proposing solutions, but these people need accurate information to do their jobs well.

BOX 7–2

Levels of Public Participation with a Regional Health Authority (RHA)

Level	Objective
Information Publics ◄——— RHA	Publics are informed about the issue and process, misconceptions are clarified, communication of decisions made.
Input Publics ———► RHA	Publics' perceptions, opinions, and advice are sought and may be used in decision making. Decision making is retained by the RHA.
Consultation Publics ◄——► RHA	Publics' informed perceptions, opinions, and advice are sought and may be used in decision making regarding the issue. Consultation is an interactive exchange. Decision making is retained by the RHA.
Partnership Publics ◄——► RHA	Publics participate in a partnership process. Decision-making is joint between the RHA and the public.
Delegation RHA ———► Publics	Decision making is delegated to the publics.

Two assumptions are relevant to the level provided below:
1. The publics are informed about the issue and process at each level.
2. Regardless of the level selected, the RHA is accountable for the decisions and outcomes.

Howlett and Ramesh (1995) suggest that dense policy networks, where both the government and society are strong and close partnerships between the two are possible, result in more "cohesive and long-term policies" (p. 65). Networks where the government and society are both weak will produce "ineffective and short-sighted policies" (p. 65). Doern and Phidd (1992) go further in saying that the absence of a network "may make coherent policy impossible" (p. 77). This would suggest that strengthening policy networks might be necessary in some instances. Further, it is important to keep in mind that other advocacy coalitions can create competition for the time and attention of the policy makers.

We would argue that discussion and analysis of power and equity must be a central focus of the purpose of interorganizational arrangements or that participation is more likely to be about social control than social change (Cooke & Kothari, 2001). It is the critical analysis that distinguishes social justice participation from social control participation. One of the unintended consequences of ignoring power and equity is that participation of social elites can be strengthened at the expense of redistribution of power (Hildyard et al., 2001). The interactions among citizens, social movements, the political representation system, and government apparatus create opportunities for participation (Briskin, 1999).

Healthy public policy strengthens communities, and a policy process built on participation strengthens the ability of communities to develop the ways and means to address its issues, to nurture the talent and leadership that enhance the quality of community life, to tackle problems that threaten the community, and to take advantage of opportunities that can help create conditions for people to mutually support and care for each other. In this section, we review how individual citizens and communities develop this capacity and what it contributes to health and quality of life.

PARTNERSHIPS

Interdependence among sectors that influence the health of populations has made intersectoral action critical to addressing the wicked problems of pubic health. In Canada, emphasis has been placed on the need for intersectoral action to effectively address the broad determinants of health (Evans et al., 1994). Strengthening the impact of intersectoral policy requires detailed knowledge of collaborative planning and evaluation strategies. Scott and MacKean (Chapter 6) present an overview of collaboration literature and describe a partnership framework and process model that has been used effectively for planning and evaluation.

SUMMARY

"Public policy is a highly complex matter, consisting of a series of decisions, involving a large number of actors operating within the confines of an amorphous, yet inescapable, institutional set-up, and employing a variety of instruments. Its complexity poses grave difficulties for those seeking a comprehensive understanding of the subject" (Howlett & Ramesh, 1995, p. 198).

A brief introduction to the literature on public policy was presented with the intent of emphasizing the complexities of policy processes. Policy that is designed to effectively address population health must do so with a critical social lens to scrutinize all elements of the policy cycle from construction of the problem to evaluation of the solutions. We have also linked the purposes, processes, and outcomes of developing strong communities and strengthening social action to the policy development process. The positive effects of healthy communities become evident as citizens participate in making choices and decisions that affect the quality of community life.

References

Briskin, L. (1999). Mapping women's organizing in Sweden and Canada: Some thematic considerations. In L. Briskin & M. Eliasson (Eds.), *Women's organizing and public policy in Canada and Sweden* (pp. 3–47). Montreal: McGill-Queen's University Press.

Cooke, B., & Kothari, U. (2001). The case for participation as tyranny. In B. Cooke & U. Kothari (Eds.), *Participation: The new tyranny?* (pp. 1–15). London: Zed Books.

Doern, G. B., & Phidd, R. W. (1992). *Canadian public policy: Ideas, structure, process.* (2nd ed.). Toronto: Nelson.

Engberg-Pedersen, L., & Webster, N. (2002). Introduction to political space. In N. Webster & L. Engberg-Pedersen (Eds.), *In the name of the poor: Contesting political space for poverty reduction* (pp. 1–29). London: Zed Books.

Evans, R. G., Barer, M. L., & Marmor, T. R. (1994). *Why are some people healthy and others not? The determinants of health populations.* Hawthorne, NY: Aldine de Gruyter.

Farrier, M., & Weber, M. L. (1998). A model for the assessment of cost in workplace health promotion: Cost is a half word. In W. E. Thurston, J. D. Sieppert, & V. J. Wiebe (Eds.), *Doing health promotion research: The science of action* (pp. 135–160). Calgary, AB: University of Calgary Health Promotion Research Group.

Gerrard, N., Thurston, W. E., Scott, C. M., & Meadows, L. M. (2005). Silencing women in Canada: The effects of the erosion of support programs for farm women. *Canadian Women's Studies, 24,* 59–66.

Hildyard, N., Hegde, P. H., Wolvekamp, P., & Reddy, S. R. (2001). Pluralism, participation and power: Joint forest management in India. In B. Cooke & U. Kothari (Eds.), *Participation: The new tyranny?* (pp. 56–71). London: Zed Books.

Howlett, M., & Ramesh, M. (1995). *Studying public policy: Policy cycles and policy subsystems.* Toronto: Oxford University Press.

Koppenjan, J., & Klijn, E-H. (2004). *Managing uncertainties in networks.* London: Routledge.

Miller, W. L., Crabtree, B. F., McDaniel, R., & Stange, K. C. (1998). Understanding change in primary care practice using complexity theory. *Journal of Family Practice, 46,* 369–376.

Pal, L. A. (2001). *Beyond policy analysis: Public issue management in turbulent times.* (2nd ed.). Scarborough, ON: Nelson Thomson Learning.

Pederson, A. P., Edwards, R. K., Marshall, V. W., Allison, K. R., & Kelner, M. (1988). *Coordinating healthy public policy: An analytic literature review and bibliography.* Ottawa: Minister of National Health and Welfare.

Phillips, S. D., & Orsini, M. (2002). Mapping the links: Citizen involvement in policy processes (CPRN Discussion Paper No. F/21). Ottawa: Canadian Policy Research Networks.

Rush, B., Shiell, A., & Hawe, P. (2004). A census of economic evaluations in health promotion. *Health Education Research, 19,* 707–719.

Spitzer, D. (2005). Engendering health disparities. *Canadian Journal of Public Health, 96,* S78–S96.

Thurston, W. E., & Potvin, L. (2003). Evaluability assessment: A tool for incorporating evaluation in social change programs. *Evaluation, 9,* 453–469.

Vlassoff, C., & Moreno, C. G. (2002). Placing gender at the centre of health programming: Challenges and limitations. *Social Science and Medicine, 54,* 1713–1723.

Women's Health Bureau. (2003). *Exploring concepts of gender and health.* Ottawa: Health Canada.

Internet Resources

http://www.calgaryhealthregion.ca/hecomm/pubpolicy/pubpolicy.htm
Alberta

http://www.healthservices.gov.bc.ca/prevent/
http://www.firstcallbc.org/childyouth/poverty.htm
British Columbia

http://www.uregina.ca/sipp/
Saskatchewan

http://www.fcpp.org/main/about.php
Manitoba

http://www.ccnpps.ca/2/Home.htm
Quebec

http://www.opc.on.ca./english/policy/index.htm
Ontario

http://www.nscommunitylinks.ca/publications/actionplan.doc
Nova Scotia

http://www.infonet.st-johns.nf.ca/nhhp/docs/policy.html
Newfoundland

http://www.policyalternatives.ca/
http://www.napo-onap.ca/en/index.php
http://www.povnet.org/
National

http://www.swc-cfc.gc.ca/pubs/gbaguide/gbaguide_e.html
http://www.cwhn.ca/network-reseau/2-4/genderlens.html
http://www.hc-sc.gc.ca/hl-vs/pubs/women-femmes/gender-sexes_e.html
http://www.uwinnipeg.ca/admin/vh_external/pwhce/pdf/sightingGba.pdf
Gender-Based Analysis

http://www.cpalanka.org/profile.html
http://www.centerwomenpolicy.org/
http://www.iwpr.org/index.cfm
International

Reorienting Health Services

LAURIE FOWNES

ARDENE ROBINSON VOLLMAN

T he responsibility for health promotion in health services is shared among individuals, community groups, health professionals, health service institutions and governments. They must work together towards a health care system that contributes to the pursuit of health.

The role of the health sector must move increasingly in a health promotion direction, beyond its responsibility for providing clinical and curative services. Health services need to embrace an expanded mandate that is sensitive and respects cultural needs. This mandate should support the needs of individuals and communities for a healthier life, and open channels between the health sector and broader social, political, economic and physical environmental components.

Reorienting health services also requires stronger attention to health research as well as changes in professional education and training. This must lead to a change of attitude and organization of health services [that] refocuses on the total needs of the individual as a whole person. OTTAWA CHARTER (1986)

Chapter Outline

Introduction

Primary Health Care

Toward an Integrated Model of Health

The Settings Approach to Health

Capacity Building and the Reorientation of Health Services

Health Sector Reform

Summary

Learning Objectives

After studying this chapter, you should be able to:

❖ List the principles of primary health care and discuss how they influence health reform

❖ Understand the role of health promotion and prevention approaches in the traditional biomedical model and in a reformed system

❖ Discuss the healthy settings approach and the healthy communities movements

❖ Identify the role of capacity building strategies in the reorientation of health services
❖ Reflect on what an integrated model of health would contribute to the health system

Introduction

*D*espite efforts in recent decades to reform the Canadian health care delivery system so that it reflects changing understandings of health, challenges have emerged that have limited the success of innovative and timely reforms. As a result, a reorientation of health services has been an ongoing and critical debate within the sector. This chapter focuses on the fifth action strategy for health promotion, *reorienting health services* (World Health Organization [WHO], 1986). Health systems are defined "as comprising all the organizations, institutions and resources that are devoted to producing health actions" (WHO, 2000, p. xi). The reorientation of health services in Canada includes a call for action by provincial governments that are charged with delivering health services, the federal government that governs national health policy, social and economic sectors, nongovernmental and voluntary organizations, local authorities, industry, and the media.

We begin with a focus on primary health care (PHC), then overview some shifts that have occurred within the Canadian health system, including a transition away from the traditional biomedical model toward models aimed at health promotion and disease prevention. This is followed by a review of the settings approach to health promotion with emphasis on the health promoting hospital, school health, and healthy community movements. We conclude with an exploration of an integrated model of health.

PRIMARY HEALTH CARE

The 1974 Lalonde Report paved the way for recommendations on strengthening the PHC system in Canada and around the globe. The International Conference on Primary Health Care, held at Alma-Ata in 1978, catalyzed action on reorienting the health care delivery systems to address the health inequalities between people in developed countries and those living in developing nations. Developed countries also used the Declaration of Alma-Ata (WHO, 1978) to examine their internal contexts and assess the inequalities in access to health that existed among their own citizens. The stated goal was to achieve Health for All by the year 2000; regrettably, that goal was not achieved. PHC is a philosophy as much as a framework and refers to five principles on which action for Health for All must be based: equitable access to health and health services; public participation; appropriate technology;

intersectoral collaboration; and the reorientation of the health system to promotion of health and prevention of disease and injury. In recent years, these principles have been reframed to include "universal access and coverage on the basis of need; health equity as part of development oriented to social justice; community participation in defining and implementing health agendas; and intersectoral approaches to health" (WHO, 2003a, p. 103). These principles reflect the complex health issues that communities encounter and the need to address health inequities (WHO, 2003a).

At the systems level, there has been a shift toward a more encompassing perspective (WHO, 2003a). Using the PHC philosophy, an integrated health systems approach links acute and chronic health care needs and recognizes the importance of both preventive and curative health systems (WHO, 2003a). WHO (2003a) identified some of the benefits of using an integrated model, including a "demonstrated reduction in health care costs, lower use of health care services, and improved health status" (p. 108).

One of the defining characteristics of PHC is the relationship between patient care and public health care (WHO, 2003a). In the late 1990s, WHO developed a health systems performance assessment framework as an analytic tool to assess the effect of PHC concerns for equity and actual population health outcomes (WHO, 2003a). Understanding of health service and system requirements has shifted over time, as there have been changes in different levels of health systems. For example, there have been shifts in demographic and epidemiological situations fuelled by factors such as disease, poverty, and income inequality (WHO, 2003a). Health system capabilities have also shifted, including technology, structures, and functions (WHO, 2003a). These shifts have also influenced the context of policy-making and health care delivery, responsibilities of governments, and required a process of redefining health sector objectives (WHO, 2003a). Important factors that influence the process of addressing these shifts includes "chronic underfunding of publicly financed health services . . . [and] processes of decentralization and health sector reform [which] have had mixed effects on health care system performance" (WHO, 2003a, p. 107).

The Declaration of Alma-Ata states that PHC, based on population health principles, advocates a basic level of health services as essential to the health of populations (WHO, 2003a). Initially conceived as both a health development strategy and a level of health service (Kekki, 2003; WHO, 1978), the basic principles and values of PHC promote access to health (not health care itself) based on equity, social justice and participation, to create services that are affordable, accessible, practical, scientifically sound, and socially acceptable (Kekki, 2003; WHO, 1978). Eight essential services were named in the Declaration as components of PHC, suggesting that if these services were provided in an organized fashion, the population would have a good chance for health. If people were educated concerning prevailing health problems, they would learn and implement methods of preventing and controlling them. A secure food supply promotes proper nutrition, and an adequate supply of safe water and basic sanitation prevents debilitating gastrointestinal diseases that cause premature death. Maternal and child health care, including family planning, would foster reproductive rights and reduce infant mortality. Immunization against the major infectious diseases, particularly for children, would reduce mortality from these causes and give children a better chance to live to adulthood. If locally endemic diseases could be prevented and controlled, if appropriate treatment of common diseases and injuries were available, and if essential drugs were provided at reasonable cost, then people would have access to health. With health, the populace could be more productive, bringing prosperity to the nation (WHO, 1978).

The Declaration of Alma-Ata was created to mobilize political will and to set into motion a process of national health reforms (Pan American Health Organization [PAHO] & WHO, 2003). Since that time, WHO recognizes that numerous changes have occurred globally. For example, there have been "dramatic changes in the pattern of disease, in demographic profiles, and in socioeconomic environment which present new challenges to PHC" (WHO, 2003b, p. 8). These shifts have included changes in government roles and responsibilities, program delivery, and policy development and implementation. The role of nongovernmental organizations has shifted so that they are now included as important stakeholders in health and health care (WHO, 2003b).

WHO (2003b) identified four strategic imperatives for integrating PHC into their corporate strategies, including to reduce excess mortality among marginalized populations, to reduce leading risk factors to health, to develop sustainable health systems, and to develop enabling policy and institutional environment. For the first strategy, interventions should "directly impact on the major causes of mortality, morbidity and disability" (WHO, 2003b, p. 6) among marginalized populations. To address the second strategy, health promotion and prevention approaches should address known risk factors. For the third, financially sustainable approaches that are supported by leaders and populations should be sought. Finally, to integrate the fourth strategy, PHC policy "must be integrated with other policy domains, and play its part in the pursuit of wider social, economic, environmental and development policy" (WHO, 2003b, p. 7).

TOWARD AN INTEGRATED MODEL OF HEALTH

How we understand health has been largely influenced by the different health models through which we have viewed health systems. The biomedical model dominated the health sector and narrowly defined health as the absence of disease. WHO provided a broader definition of health as the state of complete physical, mental, and social well-being and not merely the absence of disease and infirmity. The Lalonde Report (1974) expanded our understanding even further by acknowledging that lifestyle factors influence health. These definitions fuelled the debate about what health entailed and led to a re-examination about the way in which we define, measure, and understand health. Labonté (1995) reviewed the historical approaches to health and acknowledged that the notions of health, illness, and disease may overlap. Labonté (1995) described three main approaches to defining health, including medical (absence of disease), behavioural (lifestyle factors), and socioenvironmental. The evolving definitions of health allowed us an opportunity to reflect on the importance of having an emerging understanding of health in the contexts of multiple health determinants that influence our day-to-day activities.

The Lalonde Report (1974), the meeting at Alma-Ata (WHO, 1978), and the Ottawa Charter for Health Promotion (WHO, 1986) are examples of efforts that influenced a paradigm shift beyond the biomedical paradigm (clinical and curative services) toward "an expanded mandate which is sensitive and respects cultural needs" (WHO, 1986, p. 3). This expanded mandate identified the needs of individuals and communities through a broad lens of health that acknowledged social, political, economic, and physical components. The goal was the creation of a more inclusive health care strategy within a more effective health care system. Interestingly, in Canada, the largest proportion of health care funding goes to treatment services (i.e., hospitals, physicians, and pharmaceuticals) rather than to disease and injury prevention and health promotion services, even though the Lalonde Report declared that health services contributed only 10 percent to population health as compared to lifestyle and the environment that together contributed 80 percent. Health care does not equal *health*—the Lalonde Report challenged the fundamental precept that a hospital- and physician-based treatment system should dominate health services. Such services are necessary for illness care, but a health system that also integrates health promotion and injury prevention and advocates for improvements in the way we collectively address the broad factors that affect health is what is called for by the Ottawa Charter and the strategy to reorient health services.

Canada's movement toward an integrated approach to health care delivery has included responding to shifts in how and why people access health services (Health Canada, 1997), including an increased emphasis on approaches that enhance communities' ability and capacity to deliver services. The move toward an integrated health model has not been without challenges. For example, despite increased efforts in health promotion, the traditional biomedical model continues to dominate the health care system. As a result, health promotion efforts in Canada's health care reform have played a secondary role. According to Health Canada (1997), health promotion efforts have been "positioned as a complementary effort" (p. 24). This is reflected in the limited investment by government toward health promotion activities. However, literature and evidence to support comprehensive approaches have gained support along with the commitment of various health sectors to enhance health promotion efforts.

In order to move health promotion efforts to the forefront of the health care agenda, Health Canada (1997) identified core strategies toward an integrated health care system. Health care systems should "be advocates for health promoting policies and programs in non-health sectors; identify and address the environmental, social and economic determinants of health in their community, in partnership with other key stakeholders; ensure their own facilities and operations are environmentally sustainable and healthy for patients and staff; work with others in the community to strengthen community action while training and supporting community members to participate in the governance of their health care system; and work with others to support people in the development of personal skills for health, including patients and staff of the health care system" (Health Canada, 1997, p. 34). In order to address these core strategies, there has been an increased effort to explore the preventive and health promotion services in the context of other services.

Politicians and governments respond to the demands of their constituents. At present, Canadians are demanding hospital beds and health care services. Health promotion proponents need to better communicate to the public at large the links between determinants of health (e.g., income, education, food security, safe housing) and population health. The public's preoccupation with eating and exercise must be expanded to include issues of social justice and equity so that inequalities in health status between the wealthy and the poor can be addressed and that people suffering from disease caused by tobacco or obesity will not suffer blame in addition to their illnesses. As we reorient health services in Canada, we need to consider redirecting services toward community-based health care delivery models that focus on accessibility, affordability, acceptability, and appropriateness of services to the groups that use them. In other words, the health system must recognize that health is created and sustained in places where people live, learn, work, play, and worship and must embrace and involve community agencies and institutions in population health efforts.

The reorientation of health services has included a process of health care reform, including a re-examination of the role that institutions and professionals play in our communities (Hancock, 1999). In the mid-1980s, the Ottawa Charter led to "the development of a series of 'settings-based' health promotion strategies, where specific health-related settings were designated special attention" (Whitehead, 2005, p. 21). Examples of these settings include schools, communities, workplaces, and families (Whitehead, 2005). These health promotion and prevention strategies were key to the enhancement of health services beyond the existing treatment- and cure-based efforts (Hancock, 1999). Thus, the traditional biomedical model became recognized as one option among many in the broad health spectrum. Subsequently, broad frameworks (e.g., socioecological) and approaches (e.g., population health) have expanded the ways in which we view health (Hancock, 1999). The broadened focus has allowed for a re-examination of approaches to improve health, well-being, and quality of life for communities (Hancock, 1999).

The reorientation of health services to include sociopolitical and environmental approaches to health promotion has provided the principal basis for the settings approach (Hancock, 1999). The concept of healthy settings was founded during the Healthy Cities movement (WHO, 2006). This concept "aims at establishing more effective work relations between the health sector and other sectors to create a healthier environment by solving health and related problems closer to their source" (WHO, 2006, p. 1). The health settings concept includes external factors that are "caused by existing social, physical and economic environment surrounding the individuals" (WHO, 2006, p. 1).

THE SETTINGS APPROACH TO HEALTH

The settings approach has been one of the most successful strategies to emerge from the call for action on reorienting health services as outlined in the Ottawa Charter (Hancock, 1999). This includes a focus on the multiple settings in which we operate, including where we work, live, and participate in daily activities (Hancock, 1999). A hospital is one *setting* in which health promotion activities occur. Hospitals have dual roles—employers and providers of health services (Hancock, 1999); they are also physical and social settings. Similarly, health–education–social services sector collaborations in school settings have potential for health promotion and community development. On a larger scale, the Healthy Cities movement is instrumental in fostering healthy local environments.

The Health Promoting Hospital Movement

The notion of health promoting hospitals (HPH) stems from a hospital development strategy created in response to the Ottawa Charter's strategy for action reorienting health services (Aujoulat et al., 2006; Pelikan et al., 2001; WHO, 1986).

The WHO launched the HPH movement in 1988, including the establishment of an International Network of HPH in 1990 (Bakx et al., 2001). Between 1993 and 1997, WHO launched a European Pilot Hospital Project on the role of HPH (Bakx et al., 2001). According to Groene et al. (2005), the aim of the HPH network was "to strengthen health promotion, disease prevention, and rehabilitation services and enhance a reorientation of the hospitals" (p. 301). The European Pilot Project on HPH led to the development of regional networks (Pelikan et al., 2001).

A HPH approach is one that enables health professionals to recognize that the major factors that contribute to health lie beyond the health care sector in the broad environmental, social, political, economic, and cultural conditions of the community (Hancock, 1999). The HPH movement was designed to assist hospitals to steer toward the reorientation of service delivery by incorporating the principles of capacity building and organizational change in order to promote health within and outside its physical boundaries (Whitehead, 2005). A HPH approach includes efforts to use available resources to influence health by narrowing the health status gap of those living in the community (Hancock, 1999). The movement, which became active in 1991, now includes more than 700 hospitals in Europe and growing interest worldwide and has resulted in the development of coherent direction, standards, and effectiveness measures. There are five standards to assess quality of HPH: management policy, patient assessment, patient information and intervention, promoting a healthy workplace, and continuity and cooperation (Box 8-1).

BOX 8-1

Standards for Health Promotion in Hospitals

1. The organization has a written policy for health promotion. The policy is implemented as part of the overall organizational quality improvement system, aiming at improving health outcomes. This policy is aimed at patients, relatives, and staff.
2. The organization ensures that health professionals, in partnership with patients, systematically assess needs for health promotion activities.
3. The organization provides patients with information on significant factors concerning their disease or health condition and health promotion interventions are established in all patient pathways.
4. The management establishes conditions for the development of the hospital as a healthy workplace.
5. The organization has a planned approach to collaboration with other health service levels and other institutions and sectors on an ongoing basis.

World Health Organization European Office for Integrated Health Care Services. (2004). *Standards for health promotion in hospitals*. Geneva, Switzerland: Author. Retrieved June 7, 2007 from **www.euro.who.int/document/e82490.pdf.**

Hospitals are critical settings for the delivery of health care services and health promotion activities (Aujoulat et al., 2001). Pelikan et al. (2001) identified several key hospital development components that HPH offers, including: physical and social settings; health promoting workplaces; provider of health services; sites for training, education, and research; advocacy and agent of change in its community/ environment; and healthy hospital governance with a focus on quality.

Groene and Jorgensen (2005) noted that HPH can include interventions that are directed at "structures and processes, as well as interventions directed at individuals" (p. 7). As a physical setting, such activities as waste disposal, architecture, and healthy policies (e.g., nonsmoking) can be either destructive or health promoting. Participatory governance and strong policies against sexual, racial, and other forms of harassment are activities that foster a healthy social environment. As a workplace, there are empowerment measures and risk reduction measures (e.g., against stress and injury) that make a hospital a healthy work environment. Examples of integrating principles of health promotion into service provision include: quality assurance measures; patient participation in service planning, delivery, and evaluation decisions; and reorienting in-service education so that personnel develop an appreciation of nonmedical factors that affect health and well-being. Hospitals are situated in communities and can be powerful advocates for healthy public policy and population-level behaviour change through social marketing activities and partnerships with other community agencies. According to Aujoulet et al. (2001), HPH can work at the program level through the fostering of community action during intersectoral work and collaboration. This includes the opportunity for communities to identify their own health promotion needs, to develop personal skills, and to improve control over their determinants of health.

School Health Promotion

School health promotion is based on the premise that health is a prerequisite for learning. Healthy children in safe and health promoting school environments are ready to learn and learn more effectively than students who are ill, hungry, or under stress (Public Health Agency of Canada [PHAC], 2003). In a program called "Voices and Choices: Health and Participation," students are actively involved in their school community through a democratic process, enabling them to have greater influence over their school environment and health practices. Schools are uniquely positioned to inspire action on many determinants of healthy child and adolescent development because they have a "captive" population (including parents), are situated in the community, and have connections to health-related services and personnel (e.g., public health unit, social services, justice). If students view the school as a positive place to be, absentee rates and violence (e.g., bullying, racism) will be minimized, and mutual respect, social engagement, and positive relationships will be fostered, resulting in resilient children in a health promoting environment (PHAC, 2003).

The comprehensive school health model (developed by the Canadian Association for School Health [CASH]) is based on the principle that administration, staff, faculty, and students must act on several fronts simultaneously to develop healthy young people: instruction, psychosocial environment, physical environment, and support services. To become responsible for their own health, students need age-appropriate instruction to acquire the knowledge, skills, and values to acquire lifelong positive personal health practices. These practices include media literacy, problem-solving, and communication. Social support can be informal (e.g., peers, teachers) or formal (e.g., rules, clubs). Social support is also demonstrated by the respectful application of school policies to foster students' sense of belonging to the school community. For optimal growth and development, children need safe and violence-free physical environments. Clean air and water, ergonomic facilities, safe places to play, and safe transportation to school are important aspects of the environment. The school can be a convenient and economical access point for support services (e.g., early diagnosis and treatment) to help students and families who are experiencing difficulties.

Universities are also recognising the importance of healthy environments for learning, and a health promoting university approach is developing across Canada. In October 2005, a second international conference for health promoting universities was held in Edmonton, Alberta. This was a follow-up to the "Constructing Healthy Universities" conference held in Santiago, Chile, in October 2003. The focus of the Edmonton conference—"Vitamin C for Health Promoting Universities"—promoted a comprehensive approach to the creation and maintenance of health promoting universities and colleges from the perspective of people in all areas of campus life by focusing on the development of healthy work and study environments, healthy lifestyles, and organizational health (Pan American Network for Health Promoting Universities, 2005) (Box 8-2).

> **BOX 8-2**
> ### Health Promoting Universities
>
> Health promoting universities/institutions of higher education look internally at their own systems, processes, and culture and the influence that these have on individual and organizational health and well-being. Also, they accept responsibility for assuming a leadership role to contribute to increasing the health and well-being of society at large through collaboration and networking. As academic institutions, they have collegial governance processes that are unique from other organizations.
>
> Health promoting universities/institutions of higher education strive to:
>
> - Institutionally model a health promoting culture and a sustainable working, living, and learning environment
> - Take action to improve the learning, working, and living environments of staff and students
> - Enable and support individuals to live a purposeful life and make healthy lifestyle choices
> - Improve health services for staff and students
> - Encourage staff and students to accept responsibility for their own health and well-being
> - Encourage alumni to participate in advocacy of health promoting concepts and to be involved in institutional life
> - Prepare students as citizens committed to promoting health in their organizations and communities
> - Support health promotion in the community—locally, regionally, and globally
>
> Pan American Network for Health Promoting Universities (2005). Draft Charter for Health Promoting Universities and Institutions of Higher Learning (2006) proposed from the second international conference devoted to the creation and maintenance of health promoting universities. *Vitamin C for health promoting universities: Community, culture, creativity and change* held October 3–6, 2005, in Edmonton, AB. Available at **http://www.healthyuconference.ualberta.ca/docs/Charter4.pdf.**

Healthy and Safe Communities

The healthy community approach is described by Hancock (1999) as "perhaps the most concrete and practical expression of health promotion" (p. xiv). The premise of the healthy community approach is "if people are to have more control over their health, they must have more control over all the different factors in the community that affect their health" (Hancock, 1999, p. xiv). The reorientation of health services and systems includes models that are conducive to building and enhancing the capacity of communities to improve their health and embraces efforts that focus on building leadership and capacity of local organizations, business, hospitals, and governments (Hancock, 1999).

In the years following the release of the Ottawa Charter, the Canadian government targeted specific issues and groups in order to strengthen health promotion programs, establish health councils, guide health care reforms, create healthy communities, and strengthen community health projects (Health Canada, 1997). Given these priorities, Canada played a critical role in the birth of the international healthy cities/communities movement (Health Canada, 1997). This movement originated in Canada and was implemented in 1986 by WHO Europe in consultation with Health and Welfare Canada (Health Canada, 1997). In the early stages, a Canadian Healthy Communities Project (CHCP) was created and was supported federally through sponsorship from the Canadian Institute of Planners, the Federation of Canadian Municipalities, and the Canadian Public Health Association (CPHA) (Health Canada, 1997). This was followed-up by CPHA's establishment of the Strengthening Community Health Project (SCHP) in 1988 with funding from the Health Promotion Directorate (Health Canada, 1997). The SCHP focused on collaborative health partnerships by forming partnerships between organizations and agencies (Health Canada, 1997). Despite early efforts in Canada to advance the healthy cities/communities movement, the majority of work on this front has been conducted within the European context.

A reorientation of health services means embracing movements that are outside the traditional health purview, such as the programs that are developing to ensure the cities, towns, and neighbourhoods in which we live are safe and healthy. Coalitions form that bring together municipal, provincial/territorial, and national organizations (private, public, and nonprofit) with individual citizens to better understand and address priority health and quality of life issues. Collaborative action and efficient use of resources from multiple sectors are mobilized to produce positive community-focused long-term solutions and build foundations for healthier physical and social environments. Actions are built on an assets approach that promotes public policy as well as structural and systemic change that results in quality of life improvements for the community as a whole.

In these instances, reorienting health services to include community health intersects with Ottawa Charter strategies that create supportive environments, strengthen community action, and foster the development of personal skills and capacities.

CAPACITY BUILDING AND THE REORIENTATION OF HEALTH SERVICES

Including approaches that are supportive of health promotion methods as health services are reoriented requires that individuals, groups, communities, organizations, and populations have the capacity to facilitate change (Yeatman & Nove, 2002). *Capacity building* is defined by Hawe et al. (1997) as a process "to enhance the capacity of the system to prolong and multiply health effects [and] thus represents a value-added dimension offered to health outcomes offered by a particular health promotion program" (p. 29). Hawe et al. (1997) created a capacity building framework to identify indicators for success at individual, program, and organizational levels. Within this framework, the importance of building health promotion frameworks into organizational structures was highlighted (Hawe et al., 1997). This includes incorporating components into the policies, procedures, and structures that exist within organizations (Hawe et al., 1997).

Internationally, community capacity building is a critical component to health promotion activities (Casebeer et al., 2000; Crisp et al., 2000; Ebbesen et al., 2004; Elliott et al., 1998; Goodman et al., 1998; Hawe et al., 1997; Smith et al., 2001). Capacity building is commonly linked with an enhanced ability to "develop, implement and sustain health promotion programs and, ultimately, health changes" (Ebbesen et al., 2004, p. 86). According to Ebbesen et al. (2004), health promotion capacity building includes a process of "increasing knowledge, improving skills, creating infrastructure, and garnering human and financial resources" (p. 89). The process of building community capacity is central to community development (Goodman et al., 1998). Community capacity is "a necessary condition for the development, implementation, and maintenance of effective, community-based health promotion and disease prevention programs" (Goodman et al., 1998, p. 259). Although terms such as *community empowerment*, *competence*, and *readiness* are often used interchangeably with community capacity, Goodman et al. (1998) cautions that capacity is a broader construct.

Australian health policy commonly refers to capacity building as either "a strategy for achieving a healthy society or as an objective in its own right" (Crisp et al., 2000, p. 99). Four main approaches to capacity building strategies, as summarized by Crisp et al. (2000), include:

1. A top-down, hierarchical organization approach, such as policy and procedures
2. A bottom-up approach within organizations, such as skills development
3. A partnership approach, such as the strengthening of relationships
4. A community organizational approach, such as the formation or joining of structures to improve the health of communities (p. 100)

In general, the notion of capacity building can include changed or new initiatives by communities to address health issues (Crisp et al., 2000).

Yeatman and Nove (2002) evaluated a case study that applied the work of Hawe et al. (2000) to a capacity building project, describing the actions taken to build organizational support for a health promotion program in New South Wales (NSW), Australia. They found three key elements to capacity building and achieving desired change in health organizations: partnership, leadership, and commitment. A critical component to capacity building is the development and enhancement of partnerships between different sectors in the health system (Crisp et al., 2000). These elements can be useful in the application of capacity building within the Canadian context.

HEALTH SECTOR REFORM

Recent reports from several provinces call for the reorientation of services from institutions to the community. Two national reports, "The Health of Canadians—The

Federal Role" of the Standing Senate Committee on Social Affairs, Science and Technology (Kirby, 2002) and "Building on Values: The Future of Health Care in Canada" (Romanow, 2002), have also been published that deal with health care in Canada. There is a common message in all reports: Canadians value the health care system and Medicare, but changes are needed to make service delivery more efficient, effective, and affordable. To do this, the various reports recommend sweeping changes in how services are organized, funded, and resourced (in terms of personnel and technology). In most instances, people, and keeping people well, are the highest priority and competition, choice, and accountability are key concerns in service delivery to maintain health and care for those who need care. Improving access to services, shortening waiting lists, maintaining an adequate number and variety of health care staff, and supporting health promotion and increasing the prevention effort are the means suggested for achieving the results needed to sustain the Canadian health care system. It is also clear from the reports that the health system cannot be held solely responsible for the health of the nation's people; cooperation and collaboration are required with other sectors and governments to align services, policies, and programming.

Hence, we see increasing examples of education, health, and social service sectors collaborating in order to address gaps and reduce duplication of population health services. In addition, community involvement in making policy decisions around education, health, and social services is increasingly more apparent as agencies deal with lower levels of funding, high consumer expectations, and changing demographics. For this purpose, community-based professionals are interested in building skills that foster community capacity. These skills are outlined in detail in Part II of this book: community assessment; problem analysis and asset identification; program planning and intervention; and evaluation using the principles and processes of public participation, partnership, and health promotion.

SUMMARY

The reorientation of health systems as a process is adaptive to the shifts that occur among individuals, communities, organizations, and populations on multiple levels. Since the origins of the PHC approach in the 1978 Declaration of Alma-Ata, there have been rapid shifts in trends, demographics, priorities, and ways of working. No single approach to health care delivery is equipped to address the broad health experiences in our communities. The traditional biomedical model has played a critical role in the delivery of health services to date. However, today this model needs to be more encompassing in order to be effective. The healthy community and healthy settings movements have informed the reorientation of health services. The HPH is a movement that has been well documented with measurable standards and demonstrable outcomes. Workplace health promotion, school health promotion, healthy communities programs, faith-based health promotion projects, and community capacity building play integral roles in the implementation of strategies that are meaningful and relevant for the communities in which we live, work, learn, play, and worship. PHC as envisioned by the Declaration of Alma-Ata (WHO, 1978) plays an important role in the reorientation of health services today and in the future. Building on the lessons learned in the last century, health promotion principles can be applied to future health care reform efforts.

References

Aujoulat, I., Le Faou, A. L., Sandrin-Berthon, B., Martin, F., & Deccache, A. (2001). Implementing health promotion in health care settings: Conceptual coherence and policy support. *Patient Education and Counseling, 45*(4), 245–254.

Aujoulat, I., Simonelli, F., & Deccache, A. (2006). Health promotion needs of children and adolescents in hospitals: A review. *Patient Education and Counseling, 61*, 23–32.

Bakx, J., Dietscher, C., & Visser, A. (2001). Health promoting hospitals (editorial). *Patient Education and Counseling, 45*, 237–238.

Canadian Association for School Health. (n.d.). Consensus Statement on Comprehensive School Health. Retrieved June 6, 2007 from **http://www.schoolfile.com/cash/consensus.htm**.

Casebeer, A., Scott, C., & Hannah, K. (2000). Transforming a health care system: Managing change for community gain. *Canadian Journal of Public Health, 91*(2), 89–93.

Crisp, B. R., Swerissen, H., & Duckett, S. J. (2000). Four approaches to capacity building in health: Consequences for measurement and accountability. *Health Promotion International, 15*(2), 99–107.

Ebbesen, L. S., Heath, S., Naylor, P.-J., & Anderson, D. (2004). Issues in measuring health promotion capacity in Canada: A multi-province perspective. *Health Promotion International, 19*(1), 85–94.

Elliott, S. J., Taylor, S. M., Cameron, R., & Schabas, R. (1998). Assessing public health capacity to support community-based heart health promotion: The Canadian Heart Health Initiative, Ontario Project (CHHIOP). *Health Education Research, 13*(4), 607–622.

Goodman, R. M., Speers, M. A., McLeroy, K. R., Fawcett, S., Kegler, M., Parker, E., et al. (1998). Identifying and defining the dimensions of community capacity to provide a basis for measurement. *Health Education and Behavior, 25*(3), 258–278.

Groene, O., & Jorgensen, S. J. (2005). Health promotion in hospitals—A quality issue in health care. *European Journal of Public Health, 15*(1), 6–8.

Groene, O., Jorgensen, S. J., Fugleholm, A. M., Møller, L., & Garcia-Barbero, M. (2005). Standards for health promotion in hospitals: Development and pilot test in nine European countries. *Leadership in Health Services, 18*(4–5), 300–307.

Hancock, T. (1999). Creating health and health promoting hospitals: A worthy challenge for the twenty-first century. *Leadership in Health Services, 12*(2–3), viii–xix.

Hawe, P., King, L., Noort, M., Jordens, C., & Lloyd, B. (2000). *Indicators to help with capacity building in health promotion*. Sydney, Australia: NSW Health.

Hawe, P., Noort, M., King, L., & Jordens, C. (1997). Multiplying health gains: The critical role of capacity building within health promotion programs. *Health Policy, 39*, 29–42.

Health Canada. (1997). Health promotion in Canada—A case study. Ottawa: Author.

Kekki, P. (2003). *Primary health care and the Millennium Development Goals: Issues for discussion* (Discussion paper). Helsinki, Finland: University of Helsinki.

Kirby, M. (2002). The health of Canadians—The federal role. Retrieved June 6, 2007 from **http://www.parl.gc.ca/37/2/parlbus/commbus/senate/com-e/soci-e/rep-e/repoct02vol6-e.htm**.

Labonté, R. (1995). Population health and health promotion: What do they have to say to each other? *Canadian Journal of Public Health, 86*(3), 165–168.

Lalonde, M. (1974). *A new perspective on the health of Canadians*. Ottawa, ON: Health and Welfare Canada.

Pan American Health Organization & World Health Organization. (2003). *Global meeting on future strategic directions for primary health care: Primary health care and human resources development*. Madrid, Spain: World Health Organization.

Pan American Network for Health Promoting Universities (2005). Draft Charter for Health Promoting Universities and Institutions of Higher Learning (2006) proposed from the second international conference devoted to the creation and maintenance of health promoting universities. *Vitamin C for health promoting universities: Community, culture, creativity and change* held October 3–6, 2005, in Edmonton, AB. Available at **http://www.healthyuconference.ualberta.ca/docs/Charter4.pdf**.

Pelikan, J. M., Krajic, K., & Dietscher, C. (2001). The health promoting hospital (HPH): Concept and development. *Patient Education and Counseling, 45*, 239–243.

Public Health Agency of Canada. (2003). Voices and Choices: Planning for School Health. Ottawa: Author. Retrieved June 6, 2007 from **http://www.phac-aspc.gc.ca/vc-ss/bg_e.html**.

Romanow, R. (2002). Commission on the future of health care in Canada. Retrieved June 6, 2007 from **http://www.hc-sc.gc.ca/english/care/romanow/hc0086.html**.

Smith, N., Littlejohns, L. B., & Thompson, D. (2001). Shaking out the cobwebs: Insights into community capacity and its relation to health outcomes. *Community Development Journal, 36*(1), 30–41.

Whitehead, D. (2005). Health promoting hospitals: The role and function of nursing. *Journal of Clinical Nursing, 14*, 20–27.

World Health Organization. (1978). *Alma-Ata declaration on primary health care*. Geneva, Switzerland: Author.

World Health Organization. (1986). *Ottawa charter for health promotion*. Geneva, Switzerland: Author.

World Health Organization. (2000). The World Health Report 2000—Health Systems: Improving Performance. Geneva: Author.

World Health Organization. (2003a). Chapter seven. Health systems: Principled integrated care. In *The World Health Report 2003* (pp. 103–131): Author.

World Health Organization. (2003b). *Primary health care: A framework for future strategic directions*. Geneva, Switzerland: Non-communicable Disease and Mental Health Evidence and Information for Policy, World Health Organization.

World Health Organization. (2006, May 5). *Healthy settings: The concept, the settings, framework for action*. Retrieved September 24, 2006 from **http://www.searo.who.int/en/Section23/Section24/Section25.htm**.

Yeatman, H. R., & Nove, T. (2002). Reorienting health services with capacity building: A case study of the Core Skills in Health Promotion Project. *Health Promotion International, 17*(4), 341–350.

Internet Resources

http://www.euro.who.int/healthpromohosp
Health Promoting Hospitals—Backgrounder

http://www.camh.net/About_CAMH/Health%20Promotion/
Centre for Addiction and Mental Health—Health Promotion Page

http://web.uvic.ca/chpc/whatwedo/educationtraining/2006institutes.htm
University of Victoria—Centre for Health Promotion (summer institutes)

http://www.searo.who.int/en/Section23/Section24/Section25.htm
Health Settings Backgrounder

http://www.cpha.ca/english/policy/pstatem/ounce/Ounce_e.pdf#search=%22
    reorienting%20health%20services%20and%20canada%22
Canadian Public Health Association—Paper 2000 (ounce of prevention)

http://www.health.vic.gov.au/healthpromotion/environ_settings/hume_reg2002_
    forum.htm
Health Promoting Health Services—Hume Region 2002 Forum

http://www.paho.org/English/D/OD302_04.pdf
Health Systems and Services Development (annual report)

http://www.phac-aspc.gc.ca/hp-ps/index.html
Public Health Agency of Canada—Health Promotion

Honouring Culture and Diversity in Community Practice

FRANCES E. RACHER

ROBERT C. ANNIS

Chapter Outline

Introduction

The Cultural Landscape of Canada

Key Concepts Related to Culture
  and Ethnicity

Multiculturalism in Canada

The Canadian Mosaic and the
  American Melting Pot

Barriers to Multiculturalism

Facilitators of Multiculturalism

Community Practice in Multicultural
  Environments

Summary

Learning Objectives

After studying this chapter, you should be able to:

❖ Describe the cultural composition of Canada

❖ Define key concepts related to culture and ethnicity

❖ Discuss multiculturalism in Canada, including the benefits

❖ Differentiate between the Canadian Mosaic and the American Melting Pot and implications for practice

❖ Outline barriers and facilitators related to multiculturalism in community practice

❖ Develop cultural attunement and apply cultural humility in working with groups and organizations in the community

Introduction

Canada is a country of ethnic and cultural diversity. The Aboriginal peoples, the British and French founding peoples, and a wide variety of other ethnic groups create the cultural mosaic that is Canada. Health professionals work with individuals, families, groups, and communities whose lives are both enriched and challenged by the cultural diversity that exists across this country. In this book, the focus is "community as partner," which denotes work with groups, organizations, populations, and the community as a whole. Therefore, this chapter will diverge from the traditional nursing and health professional practice of working with individuals to discussions related to working with collectives and to community practice beyond individuals and families, beyond community as context. Health professionals are more frequently turning their attention and contributing their knowledge and skills to this focus of community as partner.

Culture is identified as one of the 12 determinants of health. These determinants do not act in isolation but are known to be complex and interrelated, creating an intricate web. For example, culture affects people's opportunities for education and occupation, which in turn has considerable consequences for income, knowledge of support structures, access to informal support in social networks, and personal coping skills.

The chapter begins with a description of the cultural landscape of Canada and the composition of the Canadian population. Key concepts, related to culture and ethnicity, are defined to set the stage for discussions of theory and the application of theory to practice. A dialogue on the history of multiculturalism in Canada and its benefits provides a context for community practice. Multiculturalism offers a theoretical and ethical framework for working toward the improvement of human rights and social conditions in Canada, its communities, and the lives of its citizens. Theory on acculturation is explored through comparisons of the Canadian mosaic and the American melting pot. Given the paucity of nursing or health care literature on matters of racism, marginalization, and inequities in health and health care (Kirkham, 2003), challenges to multiculturalism including prejudice, ethnocentrism, stereotyping, and racism are incorporated. Cultural competence, cultural attunement, and cultural humility are examined and thoughts about effective community practice in working with groups and organizations are shared.

THE CULTURAL LANDSCAPE OF CANADA

In 2001, some 29,639,030 people comprised the diverse cultural landscape of Canada. Three particular influences contributed to that diversity, including (1) the various cultures of Aboriginal peoples, (2) the heritage of the British and French founding nations, and (3) the diverse cultures of immigrants to this country.

Aboriginal Peoples

In 1996, the population of Canada included 799,010 Aboriginal people, who comprised less than 1.7% of the population (Driedger, 2003). However, according to the 2001 census, this population had risen considerably to 976,305 or 3.3% of the population of Canada (Table 9-1). These population changes may reflect not only

TABLE 9-1				
Aboriginal Identity Population, 2001 Counts for Canada, Provinces and Territories				
	NORTH AMERICAN INDIAN	MÉTIS	INUIT	ABORIGINAL POPULATION[a]	
	(#)	(#)	(#)	(#)	(%[b])
Canada[c]	608,850	292,305	45,070	976,305	3.3
Newfoundland and Labrador	7,040	5,480	4,560	18,775	3.7
Prince Edward Island	1,035	220	20	1,345	1.0
Nova Scotia	12,920	3,135	350	17,010	1.9
New Brunswick	11,495	4,290	155	16,990	2.4
Quebec[c]	51,125	15,855	9,530	79,400	1.1
Ontario[c]	131,560	48,340	1,375	188,315	1.7
Manitoba[c]	90,340	56,800	340	150,045	13.6
Saskatchewan[c]	83,745	43,695	235	130,185	13.5
Alberta[c]	84,995	66,060	1,090	156,225	5.3
British Columbia[c]	118,295	44,265	800	170,025	4.4
Yukon Territory[c]	5,600	535	140	6,540	22.9
Northwest Territories[c]	10,615	3,580	3,910	18,730	50.5
Nunavut[c]	95	55	22,560	22,720	85.2

[a]Includes the Aboriginal groups (North American Indian, Métis, and Inuit), multiple Aboriginal responses, and Aboriginal responses not included elsewhere. The Aboriginal identity population comprises those persons who reported identifying with at least one Aboriginal group, that is, North American Indian, Métis, or Inuit, and/or who reported being a Treaty Indian or a Registered Indian, as defined by the Indian Act of Canada, and/or who reported being a member of an Indian Band or First Nation.
[b]Includes percentage of total population, including Aboriginal and non-Aboriginal populations.
[c]Excludes census data for one or more incompletely enumerated Indian reserves or Indian settlements.
Statistics Canada. (2005a). *Aboriginal People of Canada: Highlight Tables, 2001 Census.* Cat. No. 97F0024XIE2001007. Retrieved May 30, 2006, from **http://www12.statcan.ca/english/census01/products/highlight/Aboriginal/Index.cfm?Lang=E**.

increases in population but greater involvement in census participation by First Nations people.

In the 2001 census, of the Aboriginal people reporting, 62.4% considered themselves to be North American Indian, 29.9% Métis, and 4.6% Inuit (Statistics Canada, 2005a). Over 85% of the population of Nunavut, 50% of the Northwest Territories, and 23% of the Yukon Territory were comprised of Aboriginal people. Manitoba and Saskatchewan were reported to have the highest proportions of Aboriginal residents, with 13.6% and 13.5% of their populations, respectively. Although proportions of the populations were lower for Ontario and British Columbia, the population counts were the highest in the country, with 131,560 and 118,295 Aboriginal residents, respectively. The Aboriginal population coupled with those of early British and French origin has influenced the composition of the Canadian population from early times.

Founding Nations

In 1871, the first Canadian census identified 3.5 million people living in Canada, with 92% of either British (61%) or French (31%) origin and 6% German

(Driedger, 2003). As this census covered the four original Canadian provinces in the east, an estimated one-half million North American Indians, scattered over the northwestern territories, were not included.

According to the 2001 census, the ethnic origins of the Canadian population had shifted considerably over the ensuing 130 years (Table 9-2). By this time, 38.2% of the Canadian population reported more than one ethnic or cultural group to which their ancestors belonged. Almost 12 million residents, or 39.4%, reported a Canadian

TABLE 9-2
Canadian Population by Selected Ethnic Origins[a]

	TOTAL RESPONSES	SINGLE RESPONSES	MULTIPLE RESPONSES[b]
Canada			
Total population	29,639,035	18,307,545	11,331,490
Ethnic Origin			
Canadian	11,682,680	6,748,135	4,934,545
English	5,978,875	1,479,525	4,499,355
French	4,668,410	1,060,760	3,607,655
Scottish	4,157,210	607,235	3,549,975
Irish	3,822,660	496,865	3,325,795
German	2,742,765	705,600	2,037,170
Italian	1,270,370	726,275	544,090
Chinese	1,094,700	936,210	158,490
Ukrainian	1,071,060	326,195	744,860
North American Indian	1,000,890	455,805	545,085
Dutch (Netherlands)	923,310	316,220	607,090
Polish	817,085	260,415	556,665
East Indian	713,330	581,665	131,665
Norwegian	363,760	47,230	316,530
Portuguese	357,690	252,835	104,855
Welsh	350,365	28,445	321,920
Jewish	348,605	186,475	162,130
Russian	337,960	70,895	267,070
Filipino	327,550	266,140	61,405
Métis	307,845	72,210	235,635
Swedish	282,760	30,440	252,325
Hungarian (Magyar)	267,255	91,800	175,455
American (USA)	250,005	25,205	224,805
Greek	215,105	143,785	71,325
Spanish	213,105	66,545	146,555
Jamaican	211,720	138,180	73,545
Danish	170,780	33,795	136,985
Vietnamese	151,410	119,120	32,290

[a]Ethnic origin: refers to the ethnic or cultural group(s) to which the respondent's ancestors belong. An ancestor is someone from whom a person is descended and is usually more distant than a grandparent. Ethnic origin pertains to the ancestral "roots" or background of the population and should not be confused with citizenship or nationality.
[b]Multiple ethnic response: occurs when a respondent provides two or more ethnic origins. As a result of increasing intermarriage between persons of different ethnic backgrounds, an increasing proportion of the population of Canada report two or more ethnic origins.
Statistics Canada. (2005b). *Population by selected ethnic groups by province and territory*. Retrieved June 9, 2006, from **http://www40.statcan.ca/l01/cst01/demo26a.htm**.

ethnic origin; 48.3% reported British (English, Irish, Scottish, Welsh) ancestry; and 15.6% reported French ancestry. Ethnic origins from other European countries, Asia, Africa, and Latin America are noted in Table 9-2. In 2001, 18% of Canadians were immigrants, and 39% of the population reported being either first or second generation immigrants, which include persons born outside Canada or having at least one parent born outside Canada (Statistics Canada, 2005b).

Immigrants

During the 1990s, an average of 220,000 people emigrated to Canada each year, well above the annual average for the 1980s at 125,000 per year (Canadian Labour & Business Centre, 2004). According to Citizenship and Immigration Canada (2005), those numbers continued to rise to 235,824 in 2004, exceeded only in 2001 with over 250,000 immigrants.

People from all over the world immigrate to become Canadians. Table 9-3 illustrates the top 10 source countries that generated the immigrant population of Canada in 2004 and the immigration trends for these 10 source countries for the 4-year period from 2001 to 2004. For each of these 4 years, the majority of immigrants came from the People's Republic of China, followed by India, with the Philippines and Pakistan being ranked third or fourth. Immigrants from the United States rank fifth for 2004 and are notably in the top 8 countries for the past 4 years.

Immigrant population by place of birth, province, and territory is provided in Table 9-4. The term *immigrant population* is defined as people who are or who have ever been landed immigrants, with landed immigrants being people who have been permitted by immigration authorities to live in Canada permanently. Some immigrants will have lived in Canada for many years, while others will have arrived recently.

Within the 2001 census, 5,448,480 individuals, or 18.4% of respondents, identified themselves as permanent immigrants (Statistics Canada, 2005c). Of these permanent immigrants, 42.0% came from Europe and 36.5% came from Asia. While 55.6% reside in Ontario, 18.5% live in British Columbia, 13.0% in Quebec, and 8.0% in Alberta.

Some 3,983,845 census respondents, or 13.4% of Canadians, identified themselves as members of a visible minority (Statistics Canada, 2005d). In Canada, the official definition of *visible minority population* is derived from the Employment Equity Act. Members of visible minorities are persons, other than Aboriginal persons, who are not white in race or colour. Under this definition, regulations specify the following groups as visible minorities: Chinese, South Asians, Blacks, Arabs, West Asians, Filipinos, Southeast Asians, Latin Americans, Japanese, Koreans, and other visible minority groups such as Pacific Islanders (Statistics Canada, 2005d).

Eighty percent of immigrants who arrived in Canada between 1991 and 2001 resided in Canada's five largest urban centres. Forty-three percent of all recent

TABLE 9-3

Immigrant Population of Canada by Top 10 Source Countries for 2004

SOURCE COUNTRIES	2004 Rank	(#)	(%)	2003 Rank	(#)	(%)	2002 Rank	(#)	(%)	2001 Rank	(#)	(%)
China, People's Republic	1	36,411	15.4	1	36,236	16.4	1	33,294	14.5	1	40,363	16.1
India	2	25,569	10.8	2	24,589	11.1	2	28,838	12.6	2	27,906	11.1
Philippines	3	13,301	5.6	4	11,986	5.4	4	11,011	4.8	4	12,927	5.2
Pakistan	4	12,796	5.4	3	12,351	5.6	3	14,169	6.2	3	15,353	6.1
United States	5	7,494	3.2	6	5,992	2.7	8	5,293	2.3	6	5,911	2.4
Iran	6	6,063	2.6	7	5,652	2.6	5	7,889	3.4	7	5,746	2.3
United Kingdom	7	6,058	2.6	9	5,196	2.4	10	4,724	2.1	10	5,358	2.1
Romania	8	5,655	2.4	8	5,465	2.5	7	5,688	2.5	8	5,588	2.2
Korea, Republic of	9	5,337	2.3	5	7,088	3.2	6	7,334	3.2	5	9,608	3.8
France	10	5,026	2.1	12	4,127	1.9	13	3,962	1.7	12	4,424	1.8
Top 10 Source Countries		123,710	52.5		119,003	53.8		123,206	53.8		134,279	53.6
Other Countries		112,114	47.5		102,352	46.2		105,834	46.2		116,359	46.4
TOTAL		235,824	100.0		221,355	100.0		229,040	100.0		250,638	100.0

Citizenship and Immigration Canada. (2005). *Facts and figures: Immigration overview*. Cat. No. CiI-8/2004E-PDF. Ottawa: Author.

TABLE 9-4

Immigrant Population by Place of Birth, Province, and Territory (2001 Census)

	CANADA	NL	PE	NS	NB	QC	ON	MB	SK	AB	BC	YT	NT	NU
TOTAL	5,448,480	8,030	4,140	41,315	22,465	706,965	3,030,075	133,660	47,825	435,335	1,009,820	3,020	2,355	450
United States	237,920	1,600	1,310	8,065	7,955	25,255	98,195	6,905	5,865	27,510	54,410	580	215	55
Central and South America	304,650	50	70	760	535	53,750	184,075	13,145	2,140	22,300	27,670	65	60	15
Caribbean and Bermuda	294,050	105	70	880	390	69,895	199,800	4,580	685	9,010	8,500	50	60	30
Europe	2,287,555	4,220	2,195	21,060	10,160	284,745	1,336,015	63,430	24,715	185,760	352,325	1,640	1,065	225
United Kingdom	606,000	2,590	1,050	10,800	5,300	17,590	342,895	15,305	8,450	59,515	141,375	555	460	125
Other Northern and Western Europe	494,825	910	755	6,320	3,325	83,625	220,325	15,340	6,585	54,485	101,905	870	335	50
Eastern Europe	471,365	350	135	1,790	625	54,545	289,305	19,135	6,505	43,675	54,965	165	135	20
Southern Europe	715,370	365	255	2,150	915	128,985	483,485	13,650	3,175	28,095	54,085	60	140	25
Africa	282,600	405	45	1,285	820	81,265	137,755	4,365	2,310	22,965	31,125	95	130	35
Asia	1,989,180	1,520	410	8,710	2,305	190,420	1,061,935	40,550	11,660	163,075	507,285	460	785	75
West Central Asia and Middle East	285,585	205	135	3,945	485	67,030	163,965	1,870	1,220	17,085	29,560	30	60	0
Eastern Asia	730,600	365	155	1,980	720	36,555	348,555	6,220	4,150	55,690	275,945	120	130	10
South East Asia	469,105	355	55	1,200	555	50,965	226,275	26,025	4,595	58,080	100,245	210	515	40
Southern Asia	503,895	600	65	1,590	540	35,870	323,145	6,440	1,700	32,220	101,535	100	80	15
Oceania and other countries	52,525	135	45	555	295	1,640	12,300	685	445	7,715	28,505	130	60	15

From Statistics Canada. (2005c). *Immigrant population by place of birth, by province and territory.* Retrieved June 9, 2006, from **http://www40.statcan.ca/l01/cst01/demo34a.htm.**

immigrants resided in the Toronto metropolitan area (79% visible minority), 17.7% in Vancouver (86% visible minority), 11.8% in Montreal (69% visible minority), 3.8% in Calgary (72% visible minority), and 3.5% in Ottawa (74% visible minority) (Canadian Labour & Business Centre, 2004). This diverse cultural landscape of Canada demonstrates the rationale for multiculturalism, including the development and implementation of practices, programs, and policies to support the quality of life and well-being of people and groups who comprise the Canadian mosaic.

KEY CONCEPTS RELATED TO CULTURE AND ETHNICITY

Clarification of key concepts related to culture and ethnicity will enhance understanding of cultural diversity and assist in building knowledge and skills for working with people from different cultures. Differentiation among the terms *culture*, *ethnicity*, and *race* is followed by a discussion of cultural pluralism, universality, and multiculturalism.

Culture refers to the integrated lifestyle, the learned and shared beliefs, values, worldviews, knowledge, artifacts, rules, and symbols that guide behaviour of a particular group of people. Culture is transmitted intergenerationally, explains patterns of thought and action, and contributes to the group's social and physical survival. Culture is continuous, cumulative, and progressive (Fleras & Elliott, 2002; Leininger, 2002).

Individuals are the primary building blocks upon which cultural groups are based. Individuals bring with them their past experiences based on socialization and knowledge that have been reinforced by influential others such as coworkers, peers, social groups, and family members (Goto & Chan, 2003). When commonalities along these lines exist in an aggregate of people, it is often identified as a culture. Although culture is most commonly related to ethnicity, a culture may develop within an organization, a workplace, a profession, across a population or group, or within a community. Although this chapter will concentrate on culture related to ethnicity, much of the content may be applied to other cultural aspects and environments.

Ethnicity involves cultural, organizational, and ideational values, attitudes, and behaviours. In its broadest sense, ethnicity refers to groups whose members share a common social and cultural heritage passed on to successive generations. Members of an ethnic group feel a sense of identity, as people are defined, differentiated, organized, and rewarded on the basis of commonly shared physical or cultural characteristics (Driedger, 2003; Fleras & Elliott, 2002).

Race refers to the biological status of a group and distinguishing physical features such as skin colour, bone structure, or blood group. The term *race* may be sociobiological or socially constructed. From a sociobiological perspective, the primary divisions of humans include Caucasoid (white), Mongoloid (yellow), and Negroid (black). Stratification by race, however, is socially constructed and has been perpetuated by white Europeans and their ancestors for purposes of claiming superiority (Driedger, 2003).

Cultural pluralism or *cultural relativism* is the view that beliefs are influenced by and best understood within the context of culture. This theory developed by anthropologists is used to prevent the natural tendency to judge other cultures in comparison with one's own and to promote the collection and analysis of information about other cultures without this bias (Birx, 2006). Cultural pluralism cautions against unfairly condemning another group for being different and promotes respect for the right of others to have different beliefs, values, behaviours, and ways of life. Cultural relativism fosters awareness and appreciation of cultural differences, rejects assumptions of superiority of one's culture, and averts ethnocentrism. While cultural convergence or assimilation involves merging cultures and creates a cultural melting pot, cultural relativism involves respecting culture and honouring diversity, thus generating a cultural mosaic.

Cultural pluralism and the cultural relevance of moral, ethical, and legal positions may suggest that morality and ethics are depicted by each culture and society. Although differences exist, so do similarities or universals across cultures. According to Cameron-Traub (2002), "Condemnations of some societal actions with moral implications of universal significance (e.g. persecution, torture, victimization, war crimes, and ethnic cleansing) in many ways transcend culture-specific views of morality and judgments about right or wrong" (p. 170). She recognized that common or *universal principles* that guide moral action or resolve moral problems across cultures (1) consider more than the interest of individuals and their self-interest, (2) are applicable across all such cases or situations, and (3) are based on culturally shared reasons for supporting or defending decisions or actions. Health professionals are challenged to be open and responsive to cultural differences, while respecting, protecting, and promoting the rights and well-being of those people and groups with whom they work.

For the purposes of this chapter, *multiculturalism* is considered to be a set of ideas and practices for engaging cultures, as different yet equal, for the purposes of living together with those differences (Fleras & Elliott, 2002). Canada as a multicultural society is ethnically diverse, espouses to a set of ideals that celebrate diversity, and advances a social movement that challenges the privileging of any culture over any other. From a political stance, official multiculturalism represents a doctrine and set of practices that officially acknowledge and promote diversity as legitimate and integral to the composition of the country.

MULTICULTURALISM IN CANADA

The history of multiculturalism in Canada begins with the early periods of the country; however, its official beginnings start with the multicultural policy adopted by the Canadian government in 1971. The policy *Multiculturalism within a Bilingual Framework* sought to support integration and affirm multiculturalism as the official position of the Canadian government and the people of Canada. In 1982, the *Canadian Charter of Rights and Freedoms* situated multiculturalism within the framework of Canadian society and enshrined the rights of all Canadians regardless of race or national or ethnic origin. In 1988, parliament adopted *An Act for the Preservation and Enhancement of Multiculturalism in Canada*, acknowledging multiculturalism as a fundamental characteristic of Canadian society. Multiculturalism offers a theoretical, ethical, and practical framework for community practice and working toward the improvement of human rights and social conditions in Canadian communities.

Multiculturalism Within a Bilingual Framework

In 1971, Canada officially became the first country to adopt a multicultural policy, a policy that has been touted as a model taken up by other countries seeking a pluralist route. In his affirmation of multiculturalism and rejection of the monocultural or assimilation model, Prime Minister Trudeau (1971) declared:

> . . . there cannot be one cultural policy for the Canadians of British and French origin, another for the original peoples and yet a third for all others. For although there are two official languages, there is no official culture, nor does any ethnic group take precedence over any other. (p. 1)

The concept of Canada as a multicultural society can be interpreted descriptively as a sociological fact, prescriptively as ideology, politically as policy, and practically as a set of dynamic intergroup processes and actions (Leman, 1999). The policy of *Multiculturalism within a Bilingual Framework* involved four elements (Berry, 1991):

1. The policy seeks to avoid assimilation by encouraging ethnic groups to maintain and develop themselves as distinctive groups within Canadian society.
2. A fundamental goal of the policy is to increase intergroup harmony and the mutual acceptance of all groups that maintain and develop themselves.
3. The policy argues that own-group development by itself is not sufficient to lead to other-group acceptance and that intergroup contact and sharing is also required.
4. Full participation by groups cannot be achieved if common language is not learned, thus the learning of official languages is encouraged by the policy.

Canadian Charter of Rights and Freedoms

In 1982, the *Canadian Charter of Rights and Freedoms* located multiculturalism within the wider framework of Canadian society and empowered the courts accordingly. The Charter stated that its contents should be interpreted in a manner consistent with the multicultural heritage of Canadians and declared the equality of every Canadian, including the right to equal protection and equal benefit of the law without discrimination based on race, national or ethnic origin, colour, religion, sex, or mental or physical disability (Leman, 1999).

During his term as Director General of Multiculturalism, Scott (1988) noted that equality, diversity, and community were the essence of Canadian citizenship. In updating the intention of Canada's multiculturalism policy, 15 years after its inception, he identified three primary goals including (1) *societal adaptation*, to foster within Canadian society, respect for the multicultural/multiracial nature of the nation and capacity to serve and reflect Canadians of all cultures; (2) *heritage enhancement*, to promote the enhancement of ethnocultural heritages as integral and evolving forms of the Canadian experience; and (3) *integration*, to assist immigrants and members of ethnocultural and racial groups to function effectively as Canadians.

Canadian Multiculturalism Act

In 1988, the Canadian Multiculturalism Act, formally entitled *An Act for the Preservation and Enhancement of Multiculturalism in Canada*, was adopted by parliament, making Canada the first country in the world to pass a multiculturalism law. The Act acknowledged multiculturalism as a fundamental characteristic of Canadian society and sought to (1) assist in the preservation of culture and language, (2) to reduce discrimination, (3) to enhance cultural awareness and understanding, and (4) to promote culturally sensitive institutional change at the federal level (Leman, 1999). While many espouse the benefits and achievements of multiculturalism, others extol its shortcomings and disappointments; most, however, will agree that much has been achieved and much remains to be done. A discussion of the benefits of multiculturalism is introduced, followed by a delineation of the differences between the multicultural Canadian Mosaic and the monocultural American Melting Pot.

Benefits of Multiculturalism

In his working paper for the Economic Council of Canada, cross-cultural psychologist John Berry (1991) identified the social benefits of multiculturalism. Berry articulated the goal of the multiculturalism policy as the support and encouragement of groups and individuals to adopt an integration strategy, following a midcourse between the alternatives of assimilation and separation, and moving away from the social and psychological pathologies associated with marginalization. The policy emphasizes human rights, social participation, and equity, in addition to group maintenance and intergroup tolerance, thus demonstrating concern for individual as well as group choices and freedoms. Berry identified the balancing act between collective rights and individual rights as well as between two sets of collective rights, those of the dominant society and those of the various constituent groups.

Benefits of multiculturalism identified by Berry (1991) include:

◆ The existence of the policy demonstrates concern for the quality of human relations in Canada and makes people aware that their ethnocultural and individual needs are not being ignored, psychologically contributing to morale, self-esteem, and positive group relations.

◆ The policy is a primary prevention program with the intention of giving every individual and ethnocultural group a place and a sense of belonging in Canadian society.

◆ Diversity is a resource: The greater the variance in a population, the greater the capacity of that population to deal effectively with changing circumstances. The maintenance of ethnocultural diversity at home may be seen as important in Canadian ability to participate abroad. Advantages can be seen at a national level related to international trade and at an individual level as people grow through experience in a multicultural environment.

◆ Multiculturalism, in principle, permits Canada to better meet her national and international obligations with respect to human rights. While most agree with the need for improvement (Aboriginal rights, culturally sensitive health and education, reduction of bias in policing and delivery of justice), this policy offers an ethical framework for working toward the improvement of human rights and social conditions in Canada.

◆ Multiculturalism has potential to promote social and psychological well-being of Canadians. Potential benefits of multiculturalism and integration must be judged in relation to potential costs of the alternatives, including the denial of the right to be different (assimilation), the rejection of persons who pursue that right (segregation), or both (marginalization).

THE CANADIAN MOSAIC AND THE AMERICAN MELTING POT

Acculturation, although first coined as occurring at a cultural level, is known also to occur at an individual level. At a cultural level, acculturation refers to cultural change that results from contact between autonomous cultural groups. Although change is recognized to occur within both groups, in reality, more change occurs in the nondominant group than in the dominant group. At an individual level, acculturation requires individual members of both the larger society and various acculturating groups to engage in new attitudes and behaviours and to develop new forms of relationships in their daily lives. *Voluntary acculturation* occurs with ethno-cultural groups and immigrants, who are in voluntary contact with other groups, while *involuntary acculturation* is applicable to indigenous peoples and refugees, who have not made a free choice to be in contact with another culture.

Berry (2001, 2003, 2004) recognized two issues that predominate in the lives of acculturating individuals and their groups: (1) the maintenance and development of ethnic distinctiveness in society and the decision of whether or not cultural identity and customs are of value and to be retained; and (2) the desirability of interethnic contact, and the decision of whether or not relations with other groups are of value and are to be sought. In consideration of these two issues, Berry identified four group-level acculturation strategies, including integration, assimilation, separation, and marginalization, and four dominant larger societal level acculturation strategies, including multiculturalism, melting pot, segregation, and exclusion.

When members of the nondominant group wish to maintain their original culture during their daily interactions with other groups, while seeking to participate in the larger society, they use integration as the group-level strategy. When members of the nondominant group seek daily interactions with other cultures but do not wish to maintain their cultural identity, assimilation is the strategy used. In contrast, when members of the nondominant group wish to maintain their cultural identity but wish to avoid interacting with others, separation is the strategy used. Finally, when members of the nondominant group have little interest in maintaining their culture of origin or in interacting and having relationships with other groups, marginalization is the acculturation strategy that is used.

Figure 9-1 is an adaptation of Berry's work and demonstrates these four strategies graphically. The italicized terms refer to strategies of groups (integration, assimilation, separation, marginalization), while the standard text denotes strategies of the dominant society (multiculturalism, melting pot, segregation, exclusion). The integration strategy can be pursued effectively only in societies that are explicitly multicultural and where four preconditions exist. These preconditions include (1) a widespread acceptance by a society of the value of cultural diversity; (2) relatively low levels of prejudice, with minimal ethnocentrism, racism, and discrimination; (3) positive mutual attitudes among cultural groups; and (4) a sense of attachment to or identification with the larger society by all individuals and groups (Berry, 2003). For ethnocultural groups, immigrants, indigenous peoples, and refugees in Canada, the preferred option has become integration as evidenced and supported by Canada's multiculturalism policy and the resulting Canadian mosaic.

In the United States, the motto 'e pluribus unum', meaning 'one from many', is indicative of an American society that is derived from many cultures to become one culture. Positive intergroup relations and participation are sought, while maintaining

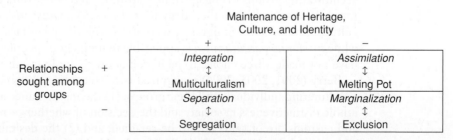

FIGURE 9-1 ◆ Intercultural strategies between groups and the dominant society. (Adapted from Berry, J. W. [2001]. A psychology of immigration. *Journal of Social Issues*, *57*[3], 615–631.)

the culture and heritage of diverse groups is not desired. Acculturation in the United States takes the form of assimilation of cultural groups to create the familiar metaphor of a 'melting pot' (Bossman, 2000). If assimilation is freely selected by individuals and groups of diverse cultural origins, a 'melting pot' may result; however, if assimilation is forced by the dominant society, a 'pressure cooker' may be the outcome (Berry, 2003). In multiculturalism, the nondominant groups adopt the basic values of the larger society, while the dominant group is prepared to adapt its national institutions such as education, health, and labour. Change occurs within the nondominant group and the dominant society. In the melting pot scenario, acculturation requires much adaptation of the nondominant group and no accommodation or change of the dominant society. As a result of expectations of adaptation held by the dominant society, acculturation stress is experienced by individuals (Berry, 2003). Adaptation may involve resistance and attempts to change the environment or to become separated from it completely. Assimilation and its required degree of adaptation has become a more frequent source of conflict both within and between cultural groups residing in the United States.

These fundamental differences in national philosophy and policy related to integration and multiculturalism in Canada and the melting pot strategy of assimilation in the United States contribute to two very different approaches to creating the fabric of these two societies. Divergent theory and practice have ensued and continue to evolve. Barriers to multiculturalism continue to challenge this work. Health professionals working in and with community groups and organizations will increase their skills by taking time to reflect on these barriers in order to be able to recognize their existence while working to reduce their impact and to prevent their occurrence. In efforts to facilitate multiculturalism, the federal and provincial governments in Canada have developed various policies and programs over the years. Organizations, communities, and practitioners have taken action to support its successful advancement.

BARRIERS TO MULTICULTURALISM

The focus of the traditional transcultural nursing theory and relationships with the individual client renders less visible and less apparent for discussion the broader context and social practices that perpetuate racism, sexism, and other systematic oppressions (Gustafson, 2005). Discussion of the barriers to multiculturalism opens that dialogue and encourages health professionals to expand their thinking as they extend their work to the broader community.

Prejudice

Prejudice involves negative and preconceived notions about others. Though often unconscious, these attitudes are irrational, unfounded, and run counterproductive to existing evidence. Refusal to modify beliefs in the face of contrary evidence distinguishes prejudice from ignorance (Fleras & Elliott, 2002). Prejudice is a deep and visceral dislike of those whose appearances or customs threaten the status quo. Fleras and Elliott identified variations of prejudice, seeing it as (1) based on fear of those who are different or who challenge certitudes and values; (2) linked with feelings of superiority, perceptions of subordinate groups as inferior, a belief in white privilege and power, and a reluctance to share scarce resources; or (3) a projection of mainstream fears and fantasies onto the 'other'. Prejudice is a function of group dynamics, with social and historical roots and dimensions of ethnocentrism and stereotyping.

Ethnocentrism

Ethnocentrism is a tendency to see reality through one's own cultural perspective—a culture, which is deemed necessary, normal, and desirable. With this preferred cultural lens comes a faith in the superiority of one's ethnic or cultural group and a privileging of its values and views, beliefs, and behaviours (Fleras & Elliott, 2002). Ethnocentrism involves a strong in-group preference or glorification and out-group rejection. While some form of ethnocentrism likely characterizes all groups of people, in an extreme form ethnocentrism is a generalized prejudice (Kalin, 1984). *Cultural bias* is a firm stance that one's own values and beliefs must govern the situation, and *cultural imposition* is the tendency of individuals or groups to impose their beliefs, values, and ways on another culture (Leininger, 2002). The existence of ethnocentrism in people's lives, the books they read, and the television shows they watch perpetuate the influences of ethnocentrism as a social norm and value. Replacing ethnocentrism with tolerance has potential to facilitate multiculturalism and respect for all cultural groups.

Stereotyping

Categorization of things has been considered characteristic of the thinking of all people. Categorizing of people or stereotyping may reflect prejudice, although it need not (Kalin, 1984). Stereotyped thinking can be functional for the person who uses it to organize and simplify a wealth of information, leading to accurate predictions about others to the extent that the stereotypes contain accurate generalizations. Even innocuous and accurate stereotypes can be dysfunctional. Kalin stated that suspending stereotypes is important and that stereotypical beliefs must be replaced by relevant information retrieved from the current situation. Tolerant individuals suspend stereotypes when appropriate, while intolerant ones probably do not.

Ethnocentrism may lead to stereotyping, or the universal tendency to assign simplistic explanations to complex phenomena and to generalize those explanations to an entire category in such a way that individual differences are rejected (Fleras & Elliott, 2002). Like prejudices, stereotypes are not supported by available evidence. Problems arise when preconceived mental images give way to discriminatory practices. Through experience, growth of logical thinking, and maturity in moral reasoning, stereotyping becomes less pervasive, while differentiation and the recognition of individuality grow (Kalin, 1984).

Racism

Racism is an ideology that ascribes beliefs of inferiority to physical and cultural differences among people, places people in a hierarchy, and perpetuates inequality and privilege. Racism involves ideas and ideals of normalcy or superiority of one social group over another because of perceived differences, together with the institutionalized power to put these beliefs into practice with the intent or effect of denying or excluding (Fleras & Elliott, 2002). Racism can be expressed in terms of race, culture, and power. Racism related to race projects a doctrine that behaviour is determined by stable inherited characteristics, derived from racial stocks, with distinctive attributes that can be ranked as superior or inferior (Driedger, 2003). Racism related to culture emphasizes cultural superiority and uniformity beneath a mask of citizenship, patriotism, and heritage. Dominant groups are considered culturally appropriate, and minorities are dismissed as culturally inappropriate and incompatible (Fleras & Elliott, 2002). Racism as an expression of privilege and power is part of the very structure of society and can be defined as any exploitation or process of exclusion that institutionalizes and privileges the dominant group at the expense of others.

Systemic racism refers to an impersonal, largely unconscious form of bias, built into systems without people being aware of its processes or consequences. An example is the plight of foreign-born professionals who experience the Canadian immigration policy that strips away the validity of their credentials in Canada. Professional bodies may have rationale for insisting on retraining, but the consequences are systematically discriminatory (Fleras & Elliott, 2002).

The recently constructed term *democratic racism* depicts the resistance to provide members of minorities equal access to opportunities in Canada and is carried out under the pretext of difference. Democratic racism is an ideology where two conflicting sets of values are positioned congruently. Commitments to democratic principles with egalitarian values of justice, equality, and fairness are juxtaposed yet in conflict with negative attitudes, feelings, and behaviours toward minority groups, resulting in potential for differential treatment or discrimination against them (Driedger, 2003). According to Kirkham (2003), these conflicting ideologies come together as a powerful force in sustaining racism.

Discrimination occurs when individuals or groups of people are denied equality of treatment because of race, ethnicity, gender, or disability and is often viewed as the behavioural counterpart of prejudice that is considered attitudinal. A popular equation summarizes the components of racism: racism = prejudice + discrimination + power (Fleras & Elliott, 2002). Four levels that demonstrate a continuum of prejudice and discrimination include differential treatment, prejudicial treatment, disadvantageous treatment, and denial of desire. The differential end of the continuum refers to a predisposition to prejudice, and disadvantageous treatment represents blatant discrimination (Driedger, 2003). Differential treatment might include ethnic jokes, while vandalism is disadvantageous treatment. Denial of the desire for equality may be apparent in housing or employment opportunities.

FACILITATORS OF MULTICULTURALISM

Federal, provincial, and local governments as well as organizations, agencies, and individuals take action to promote multiculturalism and integration among people of all cultural groups. Programs and activities that support knowledge exchange and the development of understanding and participation across cultures are valuable resources for health professionals engaged in community practice. Building skills that facilitate knowledge exchange and cultural awareness encourage inclusion and participation and assist in developing projects and initiatives with people from across different cultures.

Government Programs and Policies

In support of the national policy on multiculturalism, programs are offered by federal and provincial governments (Government of Canada, 2006) to provide English and French language education and training, Aboriginal languages maintenance and revitalization, and interpretation and translation services. Young people learn about and share in the cultural diversity of Canada through government-sponsored youth forums and youth exchange programs. Governments offer grants designed to increase access for Canadians to performing, visual, and media arts; museum collections; and heritage displays. Research funding is provided to identify socioeconomic and cultural barriers and to inform the development of policies and practices intended to foster and promote an inclusive society.

Community and Organizational Initiatives

Many communities have multicultural groups and organizations that undertake activities and sponsor events designed to celebrate diversity and promote cultural understanding. For example, Folklorama, sponsored for 2 weeks each year by the Folk Art Council of Winnipeg, Manitoba, boasts of being the largest and longest-running multicultural event of its kind in the world, with more than 40 cultural pavilions spread throughout the city's school auditoriums, arenas, curling rinks, and cultural centres (Folk Arts Council of Winnipeg, 2006). First Nations often host cultural events to celebrate and share their cultures through sports competitions, native art festivals, and Pow-wows.

Organizations are striving to be culturally sensitive in reviewing their structures, policies, and practices. For example, the Pan West Community Futures Network (2005) has developed and continues to refine a board training module on cultural awareness. Communities are using such tools as *An Inclusion Lens: Workbook for*

Looking at Social and Economic Exclusion and Inclusion (Shookner, 2002) in an effort to foster inclusion and participation of residents through a philosophy of valuing members of all cultures and their contributions.

Professional and Individual Responsibilities

Community practice built on ethical foundations facilitates multiculturalism. The *Ethical Foundations of Public Health and Community Practice* as discussed in Chapter 2 include participation, diversity, inclusion, empowerment, social justice, advocacy, and interdependence. These ethical foundations facilitate multiculturalism when health professionals incorporate them into the values that underpin their practice and apply them consistently in the work they do. Practitioners must identify and work to redress prejudice, ethnocentrism, stereotyping, racism, and discrimination as barriers to multiculturalism.

Health professionals have a responsibility to encourage and actively support integration and multiculturalism in the organizations that employ them and the agencies and communities with which they work. As health professionals demonstrate a thirst for knowledge, an open and enduring curiosity, and consummate critical reflection as a "way of being" (Will, 2001), they facilitate respect for the culture of all Canadians and foster participation in Canadian society.

COMMUNITY PRACTICE IN MULTICULTURAL ENVIRONMENTS

Theory that underpins community practice in multicultural environments continues to evolve. Cultural competence, conceptualized as a commendable goal for health professionals, is viewed from an organizational perspective. Cultural attunement, a more recently developed approach, and cultural humility are explored concerning their application in community practice.

Cultural Competence in Community Practice

Cultural competence is a common goal sought by health professionals as they work with individuals from cultures that differ from their own. Unlike traditional definitions of cultural competence that function at an individual level, the National Centre for Cultural Competence (NCCC) has developed the *Cultural Competence Continuum* (Goode, 2004) to generate guidelines for achieving cultural competence at a systems or organizational level (Pumariega, Rogers, & Rothe, 2005; Schim, Doorenbos, & Borse, 2005). More recent considerations of cultural competence look at the concept more as a process in addition to an outcome and recognize that achievement is a lifelong struggle. According to the NCCC definition, "Cultural competence requires that organizations:

◆ Have a defined set of values and principles, and demonstrate behaviors, attitudes, policies and structures that enable them to work effectively cross-culturally

◆ Have the capacity to (1) value diversity, (2) conduct self-assessment, (3) manage the dynamics of difference, (4) acquire and institutionalize cultural knowledge and (5) adapt to diversity and the cultural contexts of the communities they serve

◆ Incorporate the above in all aspects of policy making, administration, practice, service delivery and involve systematically consumers, key stakeholders and communities" (Goode, 2004, p. 2).

Six levels span the *Cultural Competence Continuum* (Table 9-5), from very negative circumstances of cultural destructiveness and cultural incapacity, through cultural blindness and cultural precompetency, to positive circumstances of cultural competence and cultural proficiency. When an organization reaches cultural proficiency, it is seen to hold culture in high esteem and use this perspective as a foundation to guide all of its work: endeavours including practice, research, advocacy, and partnerships. Health professions have responsibilities and opportunities to influence the agencies and systems within which they work, and the groups and organizations within their community practice, to strive to reach these laudable goals.

Cultural Attunement

Cultural competence can be viewed as content knowledge, as practitioners learn about unique customs, rules, rituals, and norms of specific ethnic groups—the concrete

---

TABLE 9-5
Cultural Competence Continuum for Systems and Organizations

LEVEL OF COMPETENCE	APPLICATION
Cultural destructiveness	The organization is characterized by system attitudes, policies, structures, and practices that are destructive to a cultural group.
Cultural incapacity	The organization demonstrates a lack of capacity to respond to needs, interests, and preferences of culturally and linguistically diverse groups.
Cultural blindness	The organization exhibits a philosophy of viewing and treating all people as the same, encourages assimilation, and ignores cultural strengths.
Cultural precompetency	The organization demonstrates awareness within the system of strengths and areas for growth to respond effectively and values the delivery of high-quality services to culturally and linguistically diverse populations. Hiring practices support a diverse workforce.
Cultural competence	The organization demonstrates acceptance and respect for cultural differences; works effectively cross-culturally; values diversity; and advocates for and is culturally sensitive in community engagement that results in reciprocity between all collaborators, partners, and stakeholders.
Cultural proficiency	The organization holds culture in high esteem and uses this foundation to guide all endeavours, including research, organizational practices, knowledge transfer, resource development, employment practices, advocacy, and partnership development.

Adapted from Goode, T. (2004). *Cultural Competence Continuum.* Washington: National Centre for Cultural Competence. Retrieved November 30, 2006, from **http://www11.georgetown.edu/research/gucchd/nccc/projects/sids/dvd/continuum.pdf.**

knowledge passed from one generation to the next (Hoskins, 1999). While continuous learning about groups, their beliefs, and customs is important, Hoskins warns about this kind of objectification of groups leading practitioners onto dangerous ground. Not all Chinese people have the same values, beliefs, and experiences, neither do all Pakistani or all Cree, Dene, or Mohawk. Health professionals, educators, and others must move beyond the superficial knowledge of a culture to seek and consider the personal meanings that individuals ascribe to their own ethnicity. Carefully 'attuned' listening is required to understand meaning; 'cultural attunement' is a way of 'being' in relation to the 'other'. Kirkham (2003) adds that feminist and critical social theory can assist in moving analytical lenses beyond culturalist approaches that focus on cultural meanings and ethnicity. She supports an intersectoral analysis of the shifting and contradictory nature of intergroup relations and the inclusion of the perspectives and experiences of each individual.

Hoskins (1999) encourages movement from content knowledge to relational processes. Out of these relational processes, she offers principles to use "when entering into the spaces between self and other, particularly when they, us, and we, are worlds apart" (p. 77). From her experience as a teacher, she generated five principles to assist people in working toward cultural attunement including:

1. Acknowledging the pain of oppression
2. Engaging in acts of humility
3. Acting with reverence
4. Engaging in mutuality
5. Maintaining a position of 'not knowing'

ACKNOWLEDGING THE PAIN OF OPPRESSION

Although there are aspects of Canadian history such as Canadian Residential Schools, The Chinese Head Tax and Exclusion Act, and Internment of Japanese Canadians that many would prefer to deny or forget, acknowledging the pain of oppression is essential. Such misuses of power, often perpetuated through a reluctance to share power, must be acknowledged in order for people to be able to take responsibility for their contributions, seek to grow from them, and change oppressive tendencies. Recognizing that privilege, particularly white privilege, is constantly operating to some degree and creating situations of power imbalance (Chavez et al., 2003) is crucial in honest communication that builds trust and respect.

ENGAGING IN ACTS OF HUMILITY

Humility is an act of control, restraint, temperance, and modesty. Practitioners strive to resist the inclination to privilege their own cultures, their own perspectives in their work. Hoskins (1999) challenges those who seek to achieve cultural attunement to engage in acts of humility. She challenges them to allow themselves to be vulnerable in reaching into the space between self and other, although that effort may not be well received by those who have been marginalized by the dominant culture. She urges those who work across cultures to recognize that reaching toward others without a guarantee of reciprocity requires courage and willingness to abandon a position of social comfort. Reaching forward effectively requires acquiescence to the other and surrender of cultural perspectives, biases, and expectations of specific behaviour.

ACTING WITH REVERENCE

Respect for difference is a common quality espoused by health professionals. Hoskins (1999) argues that movement beyond acting with respect for difference (which implies judgment) to acting with reverence, honour, and regard is preferred. "Homage can be paid to courageous lives, and people's initiatives to fight poverty, sexism, and racism can be honoured and discussed. Reverence can be lived, modeled, and taught so that when differences arise a deeply felt sense of awe moves one beyond basic 'respect for difference' to nurture souls and spirits" (p. 80).

ENGAGING IN MUTUALITY

When similarities are shared in the development of a relationship, feelings of connection emerge. Kirkham (2003) found that seeking common ground and emphasizing shared humanity were common practices used by nurses in intergroup interactions. Engaging in mutuality, identifying similarities, and sharing likenesses from one's own world are effective in building connections and establishing meaningful relationships. These meaningful relationships become the foundations on which partnerships are developed and groups work together to achieve mutually determined outcomes. Connections through difference can thus become the ideal that shapes a revisioning of intergroup relationships.

MAINTAINING A POSITION OF 'NOT KNOWING'

Cultural competence often conjures up visions of knowing, competency, proficiency, and mastery. Such is not the case with culture (Chavez et al., 2003). Assumptions of knowing can lead to decreased efforts to learn. Rather, effective learning in relationships is facilitated when coming from a place of 'not knowing'. Abandoning a desire for certainty, closure, and control in relationships and replacing it with efforts to be tentative, experimental, and open-ended is useful in community practice. The desire 'to learn' and 'to understand' replaces the desire 'to know' and 'be proficient'. Competence may also be problematic if it implies that certain skills can be learned in order to deal with certain situations. Building bridges to connect diverse worlds is not merely a set of strategies but is an all encompassing 'way of being' that comes from an ethic of care, an ethic of cultural attunement (Hoskins, 1999). The most critical role of the community practitioner is that of learner: learner seeking to gain understanding when working with community members to facilitate change (Gutierrez & Lewis, 2005).

Cultural attunement begins with self-exploration and self-awareness. As practitioners gain personal self-awareness, and professional self-awareness, they are able to engage with organizations and communities to raise cultural awareness and sensitivity. A series of questions for personal reflection are offered in Box 9-1. Reflection on these questions will assist professionals in determining how they choose 'to be' as they engage with others in their community practice. The exercise offers questions about organizations that employ health professionals and their efforts at cultural attunement. These same questions can be useful for any organization to explore. Questions are also offered for communities to consider as they strive to build capacity for social change and sustainability.

BOX 9-1

Questions for Reflection and Building Awareness in Community Practice

Personal Self-Awareness

- What is my ethnic background? How does my knowledge of my ethnicity affect my identity? What meaning do I ascribe to my ethnic origins? How have they shaped who I am today? What cultural groups do I belong to? What are the rules, customs, and rituals that have been passed on to me? That I will pass on to the next generation of my family? How were these passed on to me and what meaning do I give to them now? How do the rules and customs passed on to me inform how I engage with others?

Professional Self-Awareness

- In my work, how do I relate to others of different cultures? What taken-for-granted assumptions am I prepared to make in the name of efficiency and time constraints? What stereotypes do I hold? How do these beliefs influence my practice? How do I maintain an attitude of cultural attunement in my work with groups and organizations? How do I bridge the differences between ethnic backgrounds in my work? What action might I take to improve my cultural attunement?

Organizational Awareness

- What are the values and principles of my organization for working cross-culturally? How does my organization demonstrate behaviours, attitudes, policies, and structures when working cross-culturally? How does my organization value diversity, manage the dynamics of difference, acquire and institutionalize cultural knowledge, and adapt to diversity and the cultural contexts of the communities it serves?

Community Awareness

- How do the dynamics of the community, such as racial tensions, enter into my work with community groups and organizations? When does difference make a difference? How does this community influence feelings of belonging among its residents? What actions do we take to be inclusive? How do we celebrate and honour cultural diversity? What do we need to do differently to be more inclusive and generate feelings of belonging among residents from all cultures?

Adapted from Hoskins, M. L. (1999). Worlds apart and lives together: Developing cultural attunement. *Child and Youth Care Forum, 28*(2), 73–85; Kirkham, S. (2003). The politics of belonging and intercultural health care. *Western Journal of Nursing Research, 25*(7), 762–780; and Goode, T. (2004). *Cultural Competence Continuum.* Washington: National Centre for Cultural Competence. Retrieved November 30, 2006, from **http://www11.georgetown.edu/research/gucchd/nccc/projects/sids/dvd/continuum.pdf.**

Cultural Humility

Minkler (2005) contributes to this dialogue on cultural attunement with a definition and discussion of 'cultural humility' and its application at the community level. She defines cultural humility as a lifelong commitment to self-evaluation and self-critique

---

BOX 9-2

Touchstones for Working with Diverse Communities

- *Reframing cultural diversity as a benefit* and understanding the multiple and varied cultural contributions to community and society decreases the potency and counters the negative conceptualization of cultural diversity.
- *Creating spaces for voices to be heard and groups to be represented* produces opportunities to break down resistance and facilitate social change. Health professionals have both opportunity and responsibility to take action in creating such spaces.
- *Understanding concepts of health, health practices, and health promotion used by different cultures* expands the knowledge base of health professionals. Sharing knowledge across cultures creates a foundation for new ideas and the evolution of effective strategies to achieve and sustain health.
- *Health professionals have the responsibility to facilitate alliances and partnerships across different cultures* in order to develop needed programs, confront exclusionary practices and marginalization, and advocate for integration and the promotion of full participation by all cultural groups in the larger society.
- *Effective community practice requires the ability to differentiate* between (1) facilitating discussion between people with diverse perspectives to reach a single outcome and (2) facilitating acceptance of multiple different cultural perspectives within an inclusive framework so that outcomes do not require the relinquishing of cultural ideologies by participants nor do they privilege one culture over another.
- *Knowledge of language is necessary but is not sufficient* for effective communication; practitioners have the opportunity to develop programs that involve interpreters who have knowledge of language and culture rather than translators of language only.
- *Practitioners working with Aboriginal communities need to share their experiential learning*, speak about their work, and publish it. The capacity of health professionals to facilitate and support change is growing; education and training to support work with Aboriginal communities is early in its development, and advocacy for its extension is pivotal.
- *Examining the cultural awareness and sensitivity of organizations* within the health care system and beyond offers opportunity for change and growth. Recognizing democratic racism, action from positions of exclusion, or unequal power relations within systems is an important step toward change. Self-assessment by organizations builds organizational commitment to be inclusive, open, and progressive in meeting the needs of clients from different cultures. Health professionals are advocates and resources for this work.
- *Effective, committed community practitioners examine their cultural attunement and humility*; grow as lifelong learners and reflective practitioners; and critically determine how they chose 'to be' in their relationships with individuals, groups, and communities of multiple cultures.

to redress power imbalances and develop and maintain mutually respectful and dynamic partnerships with communities. She challenges those who work with communities to recognize and confront the many courses of white privilege and invisible systems of conferring dominance. Minkler suggests that although practitioners can never become truly competent in another's culture, demonstrating humility in one's outsider status, along with openness to learning and making one's best effort, can be quite effective in cross-ethnic group interactions. From their experience, El-Askari and Walton (2005) learned that "being willing to hold back your ideologies, or your truth, or your personal and national narrative, and make room in yourself for the truth and the narrative of the other was vital to [community] project success" (p. 267). Building culturally sensitive relationships of mutual respect and trust is essential before becoming immersed in collaborative planning and decision making related to community initiatives. Refer to Box 9-2 for touchstones of working with diverse communities.

SUMMARY

Embracing the value of diverse cultures, along with the perspectives and insights they generate, builds new ways to achieve social change and community well-being. Capacity building, civic engagement, inclusion, and participation are keys to health promotion and social transformation within communities. The lens through which individuals, organizations, and communities see each other informs their response to health and social problems as well as their action in building community.

Cultural pluralism, as it honours culture and diversity, generates the cultural mosaic that is Canada. Multiculturalism acknowledges and promotes diversity as legitimate and integral to the composition of the country. Discussion of prejudice, racism, and discrimination opens a dialogue that encourages practitioners to expand their thinking as they extend their work to community and the broader society.

In response to this open dialogue, an increasing number of community organizations are striving to establish processes of cultural competence and proficiency, while more community practitioners are seeking cultural attunement and humility. Social change is becoming more apparent as health professionals grow in their emphasis of shared humanity and reverence for cultural diversity. Practitioners are pursuing new visions of intergroup relationships and building bridges to connect diverse worlds. For more and more health professionals, cultural attunement and cultural humility are becoming an encompassing 'way of being' situated within the ethic of a caring community practice.

References

Berry, J. W. (1991). *Sociopsychological costs and benefits of multiculturalism.* Working Paper No. 24. Ottawa: Economic Council of Canada.

Berry, J. W. (2001). A psychology of immigration. *Journal of Social Issues, 57*(3), 615–631.

Berry, J. W. (2003). Conceptual approaches to acculturation. In K. M. Chun, P. B. Organista, & G. Marin (Eds.), *Acculturation: Advances in theory, measurement, and applied research.* Washington: American Psychological Association.

Berry, J. W. (2004). Psychology of group relations: Cultural and social dimensions. *Aviation, Space, and Environmental Medicine, 75*(7), C52–C57.

Birx, H. J. (2006). *Encyclopedia of anthropology.* Thousand Oaks: Sage.

Bossman, D. M. (2000). Teaching pluralism: Values to cross-cultural barriers. In M. L. Kelley & V. M. Fitzsimmons (Eds.), *Understanding cultural diversity: Culture, curriculum, and community in nursing* (pp. 55–66). Sudbury, MA: Jones & Bartlett.

Cameron-Traub, E. (2002). Western ethical, moral, and legal dimensions within the Culture Care Theory. In M. Leininger & M. McFarland (Eds.), *Transcultural nursing: Concepts, theories, research and practice* (3rd ed., pp. 169–177). New York: McGraw-Hill.

Canadian Labour and Business Centre. (2004). *CLBC handbook—Immigration and skills shortages.* Ottawa: Author. Retrieved June 9, 2006, from **http://www.clbc.ca/files/Reports/Immigration_Handbook.pdf**.

Chavez, V., Duran, B., Baker, Q. E., Avila, M. M., & Wallerstein, N. (2003). The dance of race and privilege in community based participatory research. In M. Minkler & N. Wallerstein (Eds.), *Community-based participatory research for health* (pp. 81–97). San Francisco: Jossey-Bass.

Citizenship and Immigration Canada. (2005). *Facts and figures: Immigration overview.* Cat. No. Cil-8/2004E-PDF. Ottawa: Author.

Driedger, L. (2003). *Race and ethnicity: Finding identities and equalities* (2nd ed.). Don Mills, ON: Oxford University Press.

El-Askari, G., & Walton, S. (2005). Local government and resident collaboration to improve health. In M. Minkler (Ed.), *Community organizing and community building for health* (2nd ed., pp. 254–271). New Brunswick, NJ: Rutgers University Press.

Fleras, A., & Elliott, J. (2002). *Engaging diversity: Multiculturalism in Canada* (2nd ed.). Toronto: Nelson Thomas Learning.

Folk Arts Council of Winnipeg. (2006). *Folklorama.* Winnipeg: Author. Retrieved June 11, 2006, from **http://www.folklorama.ca/folklorama.php**.

Goode, T. (2004). *Cultural Competence Continuum.* Washington: National Centre for Cultural Competence. Retrieved November 30, 2006, from **http://www11.georgetown.edu/research/gucchd/nccc/projects/sids/dvd/continuum.pdf**.

Goto, S. G., & Chan, D. K. (2003). Are we the same or are we different? In N. A. Boyacigiller, R. A. Goodman, & M. E. Phillips (Eds.), *Crossing cultures: Insights from master teachers* (pp. 13–19). New York: Routledge.

Government of Canada. (2006). *Culture, heritage and recreation: Government-wide programs and services.* Ottawa: Author. Retrieved June 15, 2006, from **http://www.culturecanada.gc.ca/index_e.cfm**.

Gustafson, D. (2005). Transcultural nursing theory from a critical cultural perspective. *Advances in Nursing Science, 28*(1), 2–16.

Gutierrez, L. M., & Lewis, E. A. (2005). Education, participation, and capacity building in community organizing with women of color. In M. Minkler (Ed.), *Community organizing and community building for health* (2nd ed., pp. 240–253). New Brunswick, NJ: Rutgers University Press.

Hoskins, M. L. (1999). Worlds apart and lives together: Developing cultural attunement. *Child and Youth Care Forum, 28*(2), 73–85.

Kalin, R. (1984). The development of ethnic attitudes. In R. J. Samuda, J. W. Berry, & M. Laferriere (Eds.), *Multiculturalism in Canada: Social and educational perspectives* (pp. 114–127). Toronto: Allyn & Bacon.

Kirkham, S. (2003). The politics of belonging and intercultural health care. *Western Journal of Nursing Research, 25*(7), 762–780.

Leininger, M. (2002). Essential transcultural nursing care concepts, principles, examples, and policy statements. In M. Leininger & M. McFarland (Eds.), *Transcultural nursing: Concepts, theories, research and practice* (3rd ed., pp. 3–43). New York: McGraw-Hill.

Leman, M. (1999). *Canadian multiculturalism.* Current Issue Review 93-6E. Ottawa: Parliamentary Research Branch, Library of Parliament.

Minkler, M. (2005). Introduction to community organizing and community building. In M. Minkler (Ed.), *Community organizing and community building for health* (2nd ed., pp. 1–21). New Brunswick, NJ: Rutgers University Press.

Pan West Community Futures Network. (2005). *Community Futures Board development: Module 10—Cultural awareness*. Cochrane, AB: Community Futures Development Associations of Western Canada.

Pumariega, A. J., Rogers, K., & Rothe, E. (2005). Culturally competent systems of care for children's mental health: Advances and challenges. *Community Mental Health Journal, 41*(5), 539–555.

Schim, S. M., Doorenbos, A. Z., & Borse, N. N. (2005). Cultural competence among Ontario and Michigan healthcare providers. *Journal of Nursing Scholarship, 37*(4), 354–360.

Scott, G. H. (1988). Multicultural policy and practice in Canada. In J. W. Berry & R. C. Annis (Eds.), *Ethnic psychology: Research, practice with immigrants, refugees, native peoples, ethnic groups and sojourners* (pp. 7–12). Amsterdam: Swets & Zeitlinger.

Shookner, M. (2002). *An inclusion lens: Workbook for looking at social and economic exclusion and inclusion*. Halifax, NS: Health Canada, Population and Public Health Branch. Retrieved June 11, 2006, from **http://www.phac-aspc.gc.ca/canada/regions/atlantic/Publications/Inclusion_lens/inclusion_e.html**.

Statistics Canada. (2005a). *Aboriginal People of Canada: Highlight Tables, 2001 Census*. Cat. No. 97F0024XIE2001007. Retrieved May 30, 2006, from **http://www12.statcan.ca/english/census01/products/highlight/Aboriginal/Index.cfm?Lang=E**.

Statistics Canada. (2005b). *Population by selected ethnic groups by province and territory*. Retrieved June 9, 2006, from **http://www40.statcan.ca/l01/cst01/demo26a.htm**.

Statistics Canada. (2005c). *Immigrant population by place of birth, by province and territory*. Retrieved June 9, 2006, from **http://www40.statcan.ca/l01/cst01/demo34a.htm**.

Statistics Canada. (2005d). *Visible minority population, by province and territory*. Retrieved June 9, 2006, from **http://www40.statcan.ca/l01/cst01/demo52a.htm**.

Trudeau, P. E. (1971, October). *Federal government's response to book IV of the Royal Commission on bilingualism*. Ottawa: House of Commons.

Will, C. I. (2001). Knowledge in nursing: Contemplating life experience. *Canadian Journal of Nursing Research, 33*(3), 107–116.

Internet Resources

http://laws.justice.gc.ca/en/charter/index.html
Canadian Charter of Rights and Freedoms

http://www.pch.gc.ca/index_e.cfm
Canadian Heritage

http://www.pch.gc.ca/progs/multi/policy/act_e.cfm
Canadian Multiculturalism Act

http://www.cp-pc.ca/english/
Cultural Profiles Project

http://www.culturecanada.gc.ca/index_e.cfm
Culture, Heritage, and Recreation

http://www.culture.ca/
Culture on Line: Made in Canada

http://www.culturescope.ca/ev_en.php
Culturescope: Canadian Cultural Observatory

http://www11.georgetown.edu/research/gucchd/nccc/foundations/need.html
National Center for Cultural Competence

10

Community Health Informatics

TRACY HALBERT

Chapter Outline

Introduction

Community-Based Health
   Informatics

Health Status: Health Determinants,
   Services, and Choices

Community Health Policy
   Development

Health Informatics Methods and
   Requirements

Summary

Learning Objectives

After studying this chapter, you should be able to:

❖ Define the key concepts in community health informatics

❖ Outline the key purposes of community health informatics

❖ Access Internet sites to acquire information to inform practice

❖ Assess your personal level of e-health literacy

Introduction

*W*e are in the midst of a health information explosion. A quick Google Canada Internet search using the key words 'community health informatics', 'health informatics', and 'informatics' resulted in a return of 237,000; 461,000; and 982,200 hits respectively (Table 10-1). Repeated 8 weeks later, the same search produced 14% more results for community health informatics (270,000) and health informatics (526,000) and 35% more for a search of informatics (1,330,000).

Past precedents related to difficulties in accessing health and health-related information are now surpassed by the need to filter masses of information into meaningful and usable fragments. If harnessed and managed adeptly, community health informatics has interminable potential to advance population health status

TABLE 10-1			
Informatics Key Word Search			
GOOGLE SEARCHES			
Key Words	Time 1	Time 2	Variance (%)
Community health informatics	237,000	270,000	14
Health informatics	461,000	526,000	14
Informatics	982,200	1,330,000	35

and promote effective and efficient health systems through the application of information technologies and methods.

Community health informatics can serve to channel a course toward the attainment of population-based health goals, recognizing susceptibilities inherent to a broad range of health determinants, behaviours, and services. The advancement of population health informatics through the application of information sciences has promised communities and health and health-impacting sectors enhanced means of communication, knowledge, and support. As health information technologies improve, we can anticipate intensified production and dispersal of health information. New complexities will challenge, motivate, and necessitate continuous improvements in the competencies of users.

COMMUNITY-BASED HEALTH INFORMATICS

The focus of community practice is population based, with population health status reflecting an interplay of multiple and complex determinants. Equally diverse are opportunities and strategies for promoting and improving positive health outcomes. Conceivably, integration of health promoting practices and information technologies creates potential to make considerable and positive gains in the health status of populations.

A proposed interface between population health and community informatics is shown in Figure 10-1. The model suggests the potential for single or clustered client and/or provider participants and brings complementary and interrelated stances into play, including research and awareness, knowledge translation and understanding, and information application and action and access.

Determinants of health, health-related behaviours and choices, and health services integrate to influence population health status. Convergence of these concepts provides the basis for community health policy development. Health information methodologies then provide a means for action, further contextualized by functional and structural dependencies requisite for the implementation of information systems that best support community health practice.

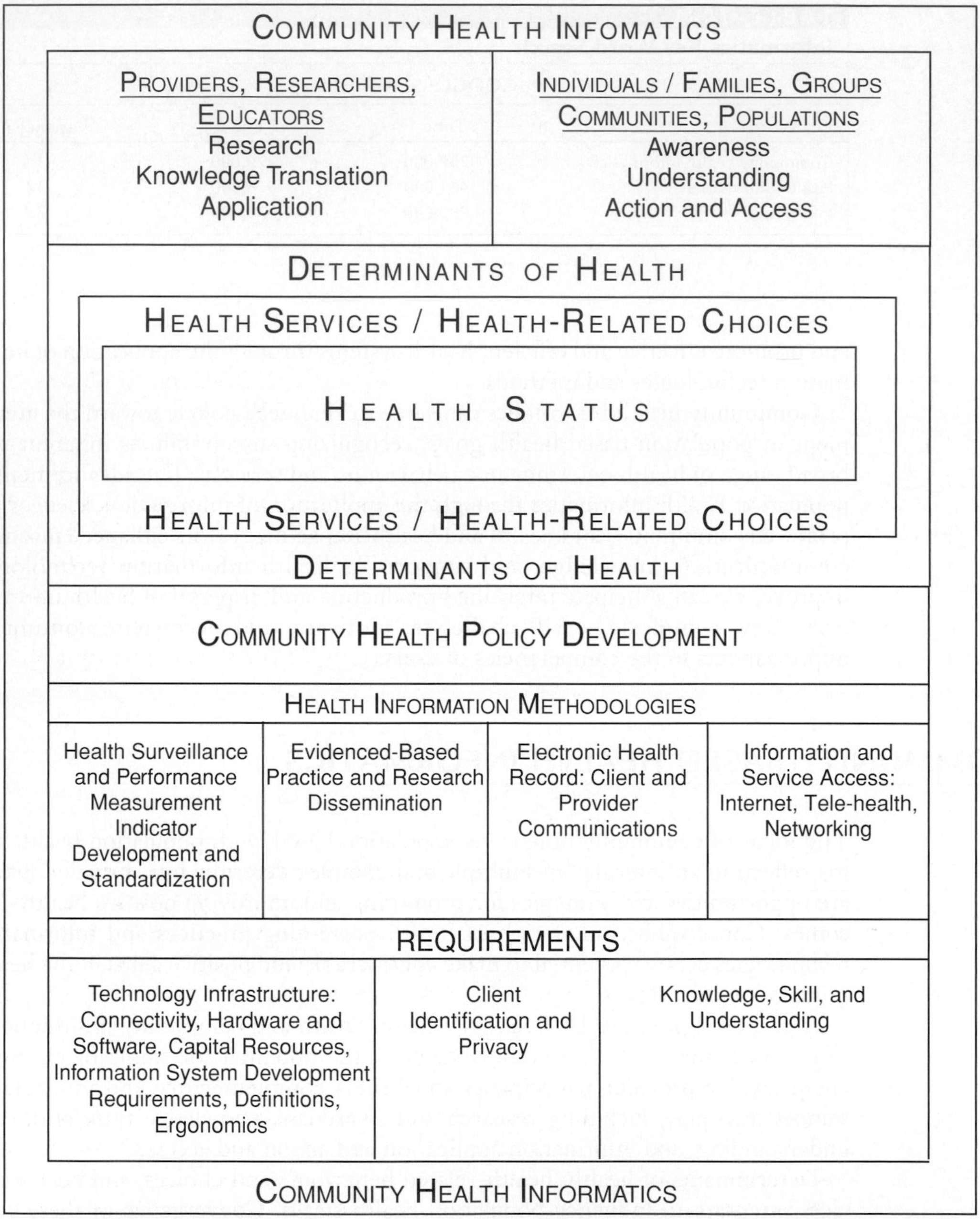

COMMUNITY HEALTH INFOMATICS

PROVIDERS, RESEARCHERS, EDUCATORS	INDIVIDUALS / FAMILIES, GROUPS COMMUNITIES, POPULATIONS
Research Knowledge Translation Application	Awareness Understanding Action and Access

DETERMINANTS OF HEALTH

HEALTH SERVICES / HEALTH-RELATED CHOICES

HEALTH STATUS

HEALTH SERVICES / HEALTH-RELATED CHOICES

DETERMINANTS OF HEALTH

COMMUNITY HEALTH POLICY DEVELOPMENT

HEALTH INFORMATION METHODOLOGIES

Health Surveillance and Performance Measurement Indicator Development and Standardization	Evidenced-Based Practice and Research Dissemination	Electronic Health Record: Client and Provider Communications	Information and Service Access: Internet, Tele-health, Networking

REQUIREMENTS

Technology Infrastructure: Connectivity, Hardware and Software, Capital Resources, Information System Development Requirements, Definitions, Ergonomics	Client Identification and Privacy	Knowledge, Skill, and Understanding

COMMUNITY HEALTH INFORMATICS

FIGURE 10-1 ◆ Conceptual model for community health informatics.

HEALTH STATUS: HEALTH DETERMINANTS, SERVICES, AND CHOICES

It is widely accepted that population health status is the compilation of individual, family, group, and aggregate health determined through the intersection of a range of social circumstances, biological attributes, and personal experiences. Key health determinants go far beyond physical attributes and heredity to include diverse social, environmental, and economic conditions; individual lifestyle and behavioural choices; and finally, the availability and accessibility of appropriate health services.

At this time, and in the predicted future, population health status in Canada is dominated by the effects of an increasing burden of disease related to the development and progression of chronic health conditions. The Health Council of Canada (2006) has recommended the modernization of the management of chronic diseases by ensuring that service providers have access to information tools to help prevent and manage complex diseases in the safest, most effective, and most appropriate way possible. The prospect of chronic disease epidemics and communicable disease outbreaks in Canada and the world have provided the impetus and urgency needed to improve (and develop new) proactive response plans for identifying and managing future public health outbreaks. Broad-based information systems are being established to ensure accurate information sharing and timely public health response.

COMMUNITY HEALTH POLICY DEVELOPMENT

Government is largely accountable for sound and efficient allocations of public resources that are responsive to population needs as well as program sustainability. Central to the achievement of these mandates is development and implementation of available and accessible information systems to support policy development. The use of research evidence to support community health system and policy development has been meaningfully advanced through the availability of electronic communication technologies. Given the broad reach of policy influence necessary to promote population health, means to integrate and collaborate across government sectors have spurred the establishment of several Canadian policy development and information networks (see this chapter's Internet Resources). A study of the use of systematic reviews evaluating the effectiveness of public health interventions in the development of provincial policies for public health practice in Ontario concluded that decision makers had very positive perceptions related to the application and usefulness of the reviews (Dobbins et al., 2004). A similar study was undertaken to assess the usefulness of systematic reviews for health care managers and polic makers. Results found that managers and policy makers would benefit from receiving highlighted information relevant for decision support, in rapid scanning format for relevance as well as graded entry (Lavis et al., 2005).

HEALTH INFORMATICS METHODS AND REQUIREMENTS

The practice of population health promotion includes the use of health surveillance, performance measurement, evidence for best practice, electronic health record, and information and service access structures and processes. These health information methods and strategies inform and direct community and provider activities across the health continuum; optimizing potential gains in health status will require implementation of information management strategies.

Health Surveillance and Performance Measurement

Recent population health trends in Canadian, North American, and global communities have included the emergence of biological and environmental threats. Efforts to identify, understand, and mediate the actual and potential effects of these occurrences have been in the forefront of public health preparedness efforts. These efforts are grounded primarily in scientific theory as well as in new information communication methods. Proficiency in the early detection of public health threats and the assurance of valid and reliable programs and services will positively impact population health outcomes. Failure to meet this challenge will have results burdened with high risk and costly, ineffective, and inefficient prevention scenarios.

Performance management processes and systems are required to meet the demands for high-quality and safe health care systems as well as financial accountability. Integral to performance management is the identification and measurement of structure, process, and outcome indicators, enhanced by the use of electronic surveillance and performance measurement systems. Automation of these processes secures real-time access to program and service goals, objectives, strategies, targets, and results. For example, the public health and community services area within the Calgary Health Region has developed and implemented an information system that has been used to support the development, documentation, and reporting of business plans as well as contributions to the regional "balanced scorecard" report. This information system results in a single document that is accessible to program and service areas through the regional intranet. Direct access of this system by service area directors has eliminated the need for the circulation of multiple copies of annual business plans as well as duplication of data entry effort that occurred in the past to consolidate reports from various program and service areas into a single portfolio plan. This system also terminated the duplication of multiple versions of reports and data reporting for differing audiences, resulting in less opportunity for errors and enhanced the ability for timely data access, reporting, and analysis.

Related to but beyond business planning and performance reporting is the need to accommodate, track, and report surveillance and performance data. The Calgary Health Region public health and community services area has worked to develop an indicator database responsive to both surveillance and performance reporting. Key to the success of this system is accessibility and development of multiple standardized reporting templates responsive to individual program requirements. This information system will provide further advantage as it is integrated with a geographic information system (GIS) application, as in other Canadian provinces (Manitoba Centre for Health Policy, 2004; Mcgrail, Schaub, & Black, 2004). GIS visual representations use spatial analyses to link health status, utilization, and health determinant data. The WHO Collaborating Center for Health Technology Assessment (2006) promotes four primary uses of spatial data: data collection and storage, data management, modeling, and infectious disease support.

The Canada Health Infoway announced the approval of an investment strategy providing a total of $100 million for the enhancement of pan-Canadian public health surveillance. The aim is to help public health professionals better detect and respond to outbreaks of communicable diseases such as severe acute respiratory syndrome (SARS).

Evidenced-Based Practice and Research Dissemination

The potential for providers and consumers to access current research, education, and practice documentation has accelerated as information technologies have become customary and accessible within most communities and organizations. The Canadian Health Services Research Foundation (CHSRF) defines *evidence* as "information that comes closest to the facts of a matter. The form it takes depends on context. The findings of high-quality, methodologically appropriate research are the most accurate evidence. Because research is often incomplete and sometimes contradictory or unavailable, other kinds of information are necessary supplements to or stand-ins for research. The evidence base for a decision is the multiple forms of evidence combined to balance rigor with expedience—while privileging the former over the latter" (Canadian Health Services Research Foundation (n.d). *Conceptualizing and Combining Evidence — The Foundation's definition of evidence*. Retrieved June 7, 2007 from http://www.chsrf.ca/other_documents/evidence_e.php).

Access to research-based evidence is expedited with the availability of open access scientific/scholarly literature, where (with or without a fee) information retrieval is granted without a subscription to the publishing journal. In a longitudinal cohort study of open access and nonopen access reporting, Eysenbach (2006) proposed and found that open access accelerated recognition and dissemination of research results as measured by the average number of times a published article was subsequently cited. The University of British Columbia Library has amassed an inventory of greater than 60 open and closed evidenced-based health information access websites. Each website is coded for type of evidence provided.

As identification, access, and review of individual publications are not always feasible, summaries of analyzed and graded research literature provide an alternative decision support resource. Systematic reviews are generated through the application of rigorous scientific review criteria. These publications serve to provide rapid and undemanding access to information that can be used for decision making and policy development. Expediency is compounded through Internet postings of these reviews.

Evidence is also used to develop clinical practice guidelines. These clinical decision support aids provide standard research-based interventions that can be integrated with electronic health records and adapted to suit unique and varied circumstances. Once operational, gains such as increased clinical safety and time savings are realized as the health team spends less time searching, accessing, and retrieving information.

Electronic Health Records

Community practice has been, and for the most part remains, operational without benefit of point of care access to clinical records when services are provided at more than one geographic location. For example, a child attending a vaccination clinic could have a clinical record at the point of care as well as records at the office of her family physician, paediatrician, medical specialist, hospital of birth, and/or walk-in medical clinic. Communications between and among care providers, when they occur at all, are managed through fax, mail, and/or by telephone, creating clinical risk scenarios due to miscommunications and/or discontinuous care.

Advancement of the electronic health record has the promise of increased service quality and reduced harmful outcomes as real-time access to clinical documentation across community and acute care sectors is realized. At this time, there is widespread endorsement of the electronic health record in principle, and public funds have been allocated to support related hardware and software investments. The Health Council of Canada (2006) defines the *electronic health record* as a "health record that integrates information from many sources into a single patient record to provide a secure, private, lifetime record of an individual's key health history and care, including test results, medications and past treatment" (P-2) The Canada Health Infoway is a 10-year federal/provincial/territorial partnership promoting the acceleration of networked electronic health records. This strategy will result in the connection of disparate information systems through nine targeted investment programs, including: electronic registries, laboratory information systems, interoperable electronic health records, diagnostic imaging, telehealth, innovation and adoption, drug information systems, public health surveillance, and infrastructure development.

Technology Infrastructure Requirements

Successful integration of community health informatics is dependent on the existence of appropriate, sound, and reliable technologies and infrastructures. Significant barriers can exist to sabotage the feasibility and functioning of an information system, even when targeted users have been fully involved and supportive. In the community environment, it is essential to ensure that potential risks are identified, considered, and mitigated prior to implementation. This process can be best served through the conduct of projects using project management methodologies, with full collaboration of all stakeholders. Stakeholders include researchers, vendors, systems integrators, standards development organizations, Canada Health Infoway, Canadian Institute for Health Information, providers, patients, service delivery organizations, provinces and territories, and educators.

Conscious attention must be given to all information technology directives regardless of any overt appearances of simplicity. Users must be involved in defining and mapping business requirements for which information systems can be adapted or developed. In general, any health services information technology development is initiated with a request for information (RFI) to potential vendors that is followed with a request for proposal (RFP). Both of these requests include details of system needs and functionality that are used to grade and select potential solutions. Leonard (2004) suggested five guidelines for successful adoption of new health care technologies: clear objectives communicated to all parties, controls and measures put in place at the outset to allow evaluation to take place, positive and negative consequences considered and communicated, taking advantage of opportunities that overcome obstacles to implementation, and abandon ideas of information technology as a cost saviour (p. 79). There are three imperatives for successful information technology programs: keep data and information secure, use data to support decision making, and collect and manage information. Security means policies that govern confidentially, destruction of confidential records, management of software, and access.

Knowledge, Understanding, and Skills

A considerable barrier to realizing the potential of community informatics is the level of provider preparedness to give up traditional means of clinical practice documentation, communication, and networking. Discomfort and distrust of information systems and hardware limit momentum and success in making the transition to electronic structures and processes. Experienced practitioners, administrators, and educators are challenged to adopt new technologies regardless of personal comfort levels and scepticism.

At this time, there are several Canadian educational institutions, journals, and magazines and other general supports available to individuals pursuing a career in community health informatics or aiming to develop skills to enable professional application of related technologies within their positions (Canadian Nursing Informatics Association, 2006). Results of a survey of health informatics programs in Canada, undertaken through the University of Waterloo (2006), provides an extensive listing of health informatics programs in Canada, with detailed contact and program information. The website provides information on 29 existing programs and 4 programs under development. Competencies, challenges, and day-to-day management of information technology/information management resources relevant to the application of computer technologies in health-related fields of practice are required for success.

Information and Service Access

While relative access to information for all population groups continues to increase, gaining access to valid and reliable health information and health services can be a discouraging and risky course of action. Health team members are challenged to find their way into and through information systems, filter results to include only valid and relevant data, and then retrieve and assemble the information into a meaningful resource.

Historically, Internet penetration in Canada was rapid, with home access increasing to 55% and access from any location reaching 64% in 2003. Computer and Internet use and intensity of use has been positively associated with income, education, literacy, and health status and inversely associated with age (Veenhof, Clemont, & Sciadas, 2005).

e-Health

e-Health, the application of communications technology within the field of population health, emerged in the literature in the year 2000, with far-reaching implications (Pagliari et al., 2005). e-Health is an emerging field, traversing medical informatics, public health, and business. Health services and information are provided through on-line technologies, characterizing technical development as well as behaviours and attitudes demonstrating commitment to networked, global thinking supporting the improvement of health care at all levels by using information and communication technology (Eysenback, 2001).

Information and communication technology (ICT) literacy comprises cognitive and technical proficiency to access, manage, integrate, evaluate, and create information.

Norman & Skinner (2006) cited six process-oriented literacy skills needed to optimize e-health. These skills evolve over time as new technologies are introduced and personal, social, and environmental contexts change. Like other literacy types, e-health literacy endeavours to uncover the ways in which meaning is produced and the organization of thinking and action. It aims to empower individuals and enable them to fully participate in health decisions informed by e-health resources.

The establishment of e-health practices and consumer access to health-related information and services have the potential to realize gains in the promotion of

TABLE 10-2	
A Model to Assess e-Health Literacy Competence	
Analytic Literacy	Foundational skills that are required to participate in daily informational life.
Traditional Literacy and Numeracy	Ability to read simple language, and to understand printed materials in day-to-day interactions (e.g., street signs).
	Ability to perform basic mathematical functions with small whole numbers (e.g., balance a cheque book).
	Able to read maps and understand simple charts.
Media Literacy	Aware of media bias or perspective; ability to discern both explicit and implicit meaning from media messages.
Information Literacy	Able to see connections between information from various sources such as books, pamphlets, or Internet websites.
	Familiar with libraries and other information repositories available in the community.
	Able to frame search questions in a manner that produces desired answers.
Context-Specific Literacy	Context-specific literacy skills are centered on specific issues, problem types, and environments.
Computer Literacy	Familiar with basic computer terms such as *e-mail, mouse*, and *keyboard*.
	Able to use a mouse or other input devices.
	Exposed to computers in everyday life.
Science Literacy	Understands the cumulative impact of scientific knowledge.
	Aware that science can be understood by lay persons.
	Familiar with science terms, the process of discovery, and the application of scientific discoveries to everyday life.
Health Literacy	Can follow simple self-care directions or prescription instructions.
	Able to confidently take medications without assistance.
	Familiarity with and understanding of basic health care terms.

population health and the management of disease. Eysenbach (2001) recognized and qualified this potential in proposing 10 promising attributes of e-health: efficiency, enhanced quality, evidence-based, empowering, encouragement, education, enabling, extending scope of health care, ethics, and equity.

Understanding types of literacy issues will assist in the determination of appropriate resource development and/or potential means or methods of remediation. A framework to assess e-health literacy competencies is summarized in Table 10-2 (Norman & Skinner, 2006).

In an effort to validate the usefulness of e-health, Ahern, Kreslake, and Phalen (2006) conducted semistructured qualitative interviews with 38 e-health stakeholders. This research reported the following themes:

1. Consensus and standardization: Most stakeholders expressed a strong desire for a more coordinated, rigorous effort to define and integrate the field.
2. Evaluation methods and challenges: Demonstrating outcomes is required to establish e-health quality and efficacy, but stakeholders were not satisfied with the sensitivity, validity, and reliability of existing outcome measures.

BOX 10-1

Factors That Prevent Uptake and Increase Attrition in the Use of e-Health Interventions

1. Quantity and appropriateness of information given before the project; expectation management: Inappropriate information leads to unrealistic expectations, which in turn leads to disenchantment, nonuse, and discontinuance.

2. Ease of enrolment (e.g., with a simple mouse-click as opposed to personal contact, physical examination, etc.), recruiting the "right" users, degree of pre-enrolment screening: Enrolling the "wrong" participants (i.e., those who are less likely to use it, unwilling to invest time, and for whom the intervention does not "fit").

3. Ease of drop out: The easier it is to stop using the application and to leave the project, the higher the attrition rate will be.

4. Usability and interface issues: User-friendliness issues affect usage.

5. "Push" factors (reminders, "chasing" participants): Participants may feel obliged to continue usage if reminded and may feel obliged to stay in the project.

6. Personal contact (on enrolment and continuous contact) via face-to-face or phone as opposed to virtual contact: The more "virtual" is the contact with the research team, the more likely that participants will drop out.

7. Positive feedback, buy-in, and encouragement from change agents and from health professionals/care providers: Participants may discontinue usage without buy-in from change agents. In particular, patients may stop using e-health applications if discouraged (or not actively encouraged) by health professionals.

8. Tangible and intangible observable advantages in completing the project or continuing to use services (external pressures such as financial disadvantages, clinical/medical/quality of life/pain): Impact nonusage and dropout attrition rate.

9. Payment options for out-of-pocket expense: If individuals have paid for an innovation upfront, they are less likely to abandon it (as opposed to interventions paid on a fee-per-usage basis).

10. Workload and time required: To fill in the follow-up questionnaires may create such a burden that participants drop out.

11. Competing interventions: Replacement discontinuance if similar interventions on the web or off-line are available.

12. External events: May lead to distractions and discontinuance, especially if the intervention is not essential.

13. Networking effects/peer pressure, peer-to-peer communication, and community-building (open interactions between participants): Communities may increase or slow the speed with which an innovation is abandoned or may increase or slow dropout attrition.

14. Experience of the user (or being able to obtain help): As most e-health applications require an initial learning curve and organizational change, users have to overcome initial hurdles to make an application work. Experience/external help can contribute to overcoming these initial hurdles and help to see the "light at the end of the tunnel."

Eysenbach, G. (2005). The law of attrition. *Journal of Medical Internet Research, 7*(1), e11.

3. Quality, value, and future potential: The intersection between e-health's potential cost-effectiveness, efficiency, and improved clinical status among users generated a high degree of interest.
4. Health disparities: Many stakeholders contended that traditionally underserved populations will particularly benefit from e-health applications, although others argued that the underserved are also disadvantaged in terms of access to technology.

Recommendations included the need for improvement and formalization of development and evaluation standards across private and public sectors, additional research on the technology needs and preferences of traditionally underserved populations, and long-term epidemiologic studies of the impact of e-health on outcomes and cost-effectiveness.

A systematic review of health-related interventions delivered over the Internet cautioned that while issues of isolation, time, mobility, and geography can be overshadowed, interventions could result in the inadvertent reinforcement of the issues that the intervention was intended to help and that e-health may not be a good replacement for direct contact (Griffiths et al., 2006).

Subsequent to the emergence and development of e-health, issues related to individual use and attrition have been identified and require further study. A sampling of several factors that prevent uptake and increase attrition in the use of e-health interventions can be found in Box 10-1.

SUMMARY

As consumers, students, educators, practitioners, and leaders interacting and connecting to access and interpret masses of health-related and health-impacting information and resources, insight and appreciation of the complexities inherent in community health informatics will serve us well. Some will choose to indulge, and others, at best, will tolerate these technologies. This knowledge will help to thwart intimidation, as points of access and means of support are as many and varied as any perceived obscurities to be encountered with the certain and continued growth in information technologies.

References

Ahern, D. K., Kreslake, J. M., & Phalen, J. M. (2006). What is e-health? (6): Perspectives on the evolution of e-health research. *Journal of Medical Internet Research, 8*(12), e4.

Canadian Nursing Informatics Association. (2006). *Resources*. Retrieved September 30, 2006, from **http://www.cnia.ca/resources.htm**.

Dobbins, M., Thomas, H., O'Brien, M. A., & Duggan, M. (2004). Use of systematic reviews in the development of new provincial public health policies in Ontario. *International Journal of Technology Assessment in Health Care, 20*(4), 399–404.

Eysenbach, G. (2001).What is e-health? *Journal of Medical Internet Research, 3*(2), e20.

Eysenbach, G. (2006). Citation advantage of open access articles. *PLoS Biology, 4*(5), 157.

Griffiths, F., Lindenmeyer, A., Powell, J., Lowe, P., & Thorogood, M. (2006). Why are health care interventions delivered over the internet?: A systematic review of the published literature. *Journal of Medical Internet Research*, *8*(2), e10.

Health Council of Canada. (2006). *Health care renewal in Canada: Clearing the road to quality*. Toronto: Author.

Lavis, J., Davies, H., Oxman, A., Denis, J. L., Golden-Biddle, K., & Ferlie, E. (2005). Towards systematic reviews that inform health care management and policy making. *Journal of Health Services Research & Policy*, *10*[Suppl 1], 35–48.

Leonard, K. J. (2004). Critical success factors relating to healthcare's adoption of new technology: A guide to increasing the likelihood of successful implementation. *Electronic Healthcare*, *2*(4), 72–81.

Manitoba Centre for Health Policy. (2004). *Manitoba Child Health Atlas*. Winnipeg: Author.

Mcgrail, K., Schaub, P., & Black, C. (2004). *British Columbia Health Atlas*. Vancouver: Centre for Health Services & Policy Development.

Norman, C. D., & Skinner, H. A. (2006). eHealth literacy: Essential skills for consumer health in a networked world. *Journal of Medical Internet Research*, *8*(2), e9.

Pagliari, C., Sloan, D., Gregor, P., Sullivan, F., Detmer, D., Kahan, J. P., et al. (2005). What is Ehealth (4): A scoping exercise to map the field. *Journal of Medical Internet Research*, *7*(1), 69–86.

University of Waterloo. (2006). *Survey of health informatics programs in Canada*. Retrieved September 30, 2006, from **http://hi.uwaterloo.ca/hi/HI_Programs_Survey_2006.pdf.**

Veenhof, Y., Clemont, Y., & Sciadas, G. (2005). *Literacy and digital technologies: Linkages and outcomes*. Ottawa: Statistics Canada. Catalogue No. 56F0004Mie–No. 12.

WHO Collaborating Center for Health Technology Assessment. (2006). *Geographical Information Systems*. Retrieved September 30, 2006, from **http://www.iph.uottawa.ca/who-hta/projects/eo_toolkit/chpt4/t_gis_EOT.htm.**

Internet Resources

http://www.chsrf.ca/home_e.php
Canadian Health Services Research Foundation

http://www.cprn.org/
Canadian Policy Research Networks

http://www.chspr.ubc.ca
Centre for Health Services and Policy Research, University of British Columbia

http://www.policyalternatives.ca
Canadian Centre for Policy Alternatives

http://secure.cihi.ca/cihiweb/dispPage.jsp?cw_page=home_e
Canadian Institute for Health Information

http://www.cihr.ca
Canadian Institutes of Health Research

http://www.cma.ca
Canadian Medical Association

http://www.hc-sc.gc.ca
Health Canada

http://www.ices.on.ca
Institute for Clinical Evaluative Sciences

http://www.pre.ethics.gc.ca
Interagency Advisory Panel on Research Ethics

http://www.umanitoba.ca/centres/mchp
Manitoba Centre for Health Policy

http://www.naho.ca
National Aboriginal Health Organization

http://www.phru.medicine.dal.ca
Population Health Research Unit

http://www.phred-redsp.on.ca
Public Health Research, Education, and Development (PHRED)

http://www.privcom.gc.ca
Privacy Commissioner of Canada

11

Emerging Threats to Community Health

MONIQUE STEWART

Chapter Outline

Introduction

Identification of Emerging Public
 Health Issues

Influenza Pandemic

Environmental Health

Infectious Diseases

Chronic Diseases

Mental Health

Summary

Learning Objectives

After studying this chapter, you should be able to:

❖ Describe a process for identifying emerging issues in public health

❖ Appreciate the complexities of the interaction of social determinants of health with respect to emerging public health issues

❖ Discuss various emerging and re-emerging public health issues from a social determinants of health perspective

❖ Understand the impact of emerging issues on the health of the population

❖ Describe practice implications for addressing various emerging public health threats

Introduction

The health of the population is not static. There are continuously emerging and re-emerging threats to the health of the public. Public health practitioners must diligently scan the environment to forecast future public health issues in order to prepare action plans to mitigate their impact on the population.

This chapter will briefly describe a process for identifying emerging public health threats and present some of the anticipated emerging issues that public health must prepare to address for the 21st century. This discussion will also include implications for practice in addressing the emerging issues. The public health issues that will be discussed include influenza pandemic, environmental health, new and re-emerging infectious diseases, chronic diseases, and mental health.

IDENTIFICATION OF EMERGING PUBLIC HEALTH ISSUES

In order to identify, characterize, and assess for potential emerging and re-emerging public health threats, public health practitioners must engage continuously in environmental scans. While several national and international public health organizations (e.g., World Health Organization, U.S. Centers for Disease Control and Prevention, Public Health Agency of Canada, Canadian Public Health Association, American Public Health Association) assume this role, it is still imperative that all practitioners participate in the scanning of public health issues as part of delivering effective, efficient, and relevant public health services.

An environmental scan should include the examination and monitoring of:

◆ Epidemiological trends
◆ Social determinants of health
◆ Historical review
◆ Literature review
◆ Societal factors

Epidemiology provides a richness of data on an array of indicators that measure the current health status of the population (see Chapter 3). Additionally, the tracking of health measures over time highlights new emerging or re-emerging health threats. Monitoring epidemiological trends assists in identifying significant changes in disease incidence and prevalence rates, population demographics, behavioural risk factors, and other population-level metrics.

To conduct a comprehensive scan of the environment, the critical role of the social determinants of health must be considered, and the political and economic factors must also be taken into account. Since the health of the population is impacted by the interconnectedness of the determinants of health, it is critical that the effects of all the determinants be considered in the thorough analysis of any given issue.

A historical review of public health issues helps to forecast a resurgence of potential public health threats. For example, the prediction of an upcoming influenza pandemic can be based on an analysis of the triggers and catalysts of previous pandemics (e.g., radical changes in the influenza virus).

Conducting a literature review will highlight current or escalating issues that public health is encountering either locally or abroad. The identification of public health issues that others are experiencing can serve as an early warning system, permitting the establishment of the interventions necessary to minimize the impact of the potential threats on the home front.

Being cognizant of societal factors is another key component in the identification of public health issues. For example, societal factors that are currently creating a significant impact on the population's health include terrorism, increased global mobility, cultural diversity, and use of technology.

A comprehensive process that encompasses all of the elements listed previously must be undertaken to effectively anticipate issues that will have or currently have the potential to compromise the health of the public. All public health practitioners must be diligent in this area.

INFLUENZA PANDEMIC

A well-publicized and anticipated threat to the health of the population is the forecast of a future influenza pandemic as a result of the appearance of the virulent avian influenza viruses. Although the avian virus is found in birds, the natural close proximity between animals and humans creates opportunity for the evolution of the virus and facilitates its spread to other species. Of increasing concern, therefore, is the potential for transmission of viruses to humans. It should be noted that the pandemic influenza differs from the seasonal influenza viruses that circulate yearly. Whereas the seasonal influenza virus is relatively static (only experiencing minor antigenic changes), the pandemic influenza virus has undergone a dramatic antigenic shift. Without previous exposure to this new strain, any particular natural immunity to the virus will be limited or nonexistent in the human population. This lack of an established immunological defense system will permit the unabated spread of the virus within the human population (Fauci, 2006; Gostin, 2006; Sheff, 2006).

Implications for Practice

In the development of pandemic preparedness and response plans, public health practitioners need to establish approaches that minimize the spread of the virus and curtail the associated societal disruption. International and national centres for disease control have established guidelines for emergency preparedness that facilitate the development of local public health response plans. Pandemic preparedness plans should also address community hygiene measures (e.g., hand-washing), hospital infection control, social mixing, border controls, and isolation and quarantine (Gostin, 2006).

In terms of current pandemic preparedness activities, public health practitioners are monitoring the spread of the avian virus in animals and humans and are being especially alert to any dramatic changes that would increase the virulence or transmissibility of the virus. In addition, scientists are preparing for the development of potential vaccines or antivirals to counter the spread and impact of the virus (Fauci, 2006; Sheff, 2006). The Canadian Pandemic Influenza Plan (Health Canada, 2004)

> **BOX 11-1**
>
> **Websites for Pandemic Preparedness Information**
>
> World Health Organization   www.who.int
> British Columbia Centre for Disease Control   www.bccdc.org
> Public Health Agency of Canada   www.phac-aspc.gc.ca
> U.S. Centers for Disease Control and Prevention   www.cdc.gov
> Canadian Public Health Association   www.cpha.ca
> American Public Health Association   www.apha.org

includes recommendations for priority pandemic vaccine use in the event of a vaccine shortage. Five priority groups have been identified with frontline health care providers (e.g., doctors, nurses, paramedics, public health workers) and essential service providers (e.g., police, fire fighters, funeral service personnel) receiving the highest priority. A coordinated global response will be required and will have a critical role in minimizing the impact of an influenza pandemic. For further information on pandemic preparedness, refer to the websites listed in Box 11-1.

ENVIRONMENTAL HEALTH

The increasing evidence relating to the profound effect of the environment on the health of the population is garnering national and international attention from health professionals, politicians, media, and the public. In 2006, the World Health Organization released a report, *Preventing Disease Through Healthy Environments—Towards an Estimate of the Environmental Burden of Disease*, which examined the causal relationship of specific environmental factors and various diseases and injuries. The report indicates that approximately 24% of global disease is a result of environmental exposure. Furthermore, about 25% of these diseases are caused by preventable environmental factors (Prüss-Üstün & Corvalán, 2006). The diseases that have experienced the greatest impact from environmental factors include diarrhea, lower respiratory infections, unintentional injuries, malaria, road traffic injuries, chronic obstructive pulmonary disease, and perinatal conditions. In developing countries, the health of children is most affected by environmental-related diseases, particularly communicable diseases and injuries. Although these environmentally caused diseases and injuries have a larger influence in developing countries, the per capita disease burden of specific noncommunicable diseases is more prevalent in developed countries. For example, the dramatic decrease in physical activity levels (and consequent obesity) has been shown to have a significant negative impact on cardiovascular disease and some cancers. Some additional examples of environment-induced negative health effects include heat stress, air pollution–related morbidity and mortality, spread of infectious diseases from weather disasters, mosquito-borne diseases, and water/food-borne diseases (Galea & Vlahov, 2005; Prüss-Üstün & Corvalán, 2006).

The effect of global climate change is escalating awareness worldwide. The increase of carbon dioxide and other greenhouse gases in the atmosphere as a result of the expanding use of fossil fuels has contributed to a negative effect on climate. Such climatic phenomena as floods, droughts, and elevated levels of airborne pollutants have been attributed to the effects of global warming. These negative climate changes in turn can lead to health-related conditions such as respiratory illnesses (e.g., asthma, chronic obstructive pulmonary disease), heat stroke, and heat-related morbidity. Monitoring the impact of climate change on the health of the population takes several years (perhaps decades) of data collection (Kovats, Campbell-Lendrum, & Matthies, 2005; Plotnikoff, Wright, & Karunamuni, 2004; Roberts & Hillman, 2005).

Implications for Practice

Recognizing the relationship between environmental factors and health facilitates the identification and implementation of public health interventions (e.g., policy development, preventive measures). Health professionals must engage the non-health sector to work collaboratively to identify and implement programs that eliminate or alleviate these environmental factors. For instance, public health practitioners can work with urban planners to design safe neighbourhoods with more green space and closer proximity to retail markets to create and foster opportunities for increased physical activity (Galea & Vlahov, 2005; Prüss-Üstün & Corvalán, 2006).

Public health has a substantial role in championing healthy public policy that is engineered to reduce or eliminate factors that are responsible for creating negative health effects. Additionally, the development of population-level strategies to influence behavioural change can be an effective way to ameliorate or reverse the effects of the negative environmental factors. For example, a strategy that could have a positive effect on environmental change and yield associated health benefits would be to significantly reduce energy consumption through such means as the decreased use of air conditioners, the use of programmable thermostats, the use of energy-efficient appliances, and use of public transportation.

The effects of the environment on health are a global issue, and therefore interventions, programs, and policies must be developed and implemented with the collective involvement of all countries. Health professionals must traverse political and geographical boundaries in hopes of confronting this critical issue.

INFECTIOUS DISEASES

The escalating focus on infectious disease is a consequence of multitude factors, including the evolution of new emerging infectious diseases, the resurgence of previously eradicated infectious diseases, globalization, and increasing number of natural disasters. The spread of infectious disease has the potential to be one of the most significant threats to the public's health. Infectious disease crosses all geographical boundaries, socioeconomic levels, ethnicities, and sexes. One has only to look at the recent severe acute respiratory syndrome (SARS) outbreak in 2003, which infected over 8,000 people worldwide and resulted in approximately 800 deaths, to comprehend the far-reaching impact of an infectious disease (Sakaguchi, 2005).

Our rapidly changing environment has led to the emergence of diseases. Public health centres for disease control must continually monitor new diseases and assess the associated risks in order to respond quickly to inhibit their progression. For example, the increasing appearance of antibiotic-resistant pathogens are resulting in "superbugs" that are difficult to treat (Sakaguchi, 2005; World Health Organization, 2003).

Health professionals are witnessing the re-emergence of diseases that were previously eradicated through immunizations. However, many of these diseases still exist in developing countries and can be reintroduced into other countries through intercontinental travel and immigration. In addition, once vaccinations have been suspended for a specific disease threat that has been eliminated (e.g., smallpox, polio), the disease can reappear many years later as a more virulent strain. Other factors that are linked to the re-emergence of infectious diseases include the creation of new environments (such as the deforestation of the Amazon), advances in science and technology, and changes in human behaviour (Sakaguchi, 2005; World Health Organization, 2003).

The spread of infectious diseases is compounded by the effects of globalization. People are more able to travel readily across continents. Urbanization has led to an increasing number of megacities, especially in developing countries, which produce an optimal environment for pathogens to multiply. These overpopulated areas, often with below-standard water and sewage infrastructure, foster the rapid spread of disease. Agricultural products are shipped internationally, thereby creating an opportunity for the transmission of pathogens (e.g., unsafe food-handling practices). Bovine spongiform encephalopathy (BSE) ("mad cow disease") is an example of an infectious disease that was transmitted to humans through the consumption of prion-infected beef (Campbell, 2004; Sakaguchi, 2005; World Health Organization, 2003).

The spread of infectious disease is an issue of paramount importance, especially in light of the numerous natural disasters witnessed during the last few years (e.g., tsunamis in Sri Lanka, Thailand, and Indonesia; hurricanes in New Orleans and Texas; volcanic eruptions in El Salvador; drought in Africa). These natural disasters displace large numbers of people, often relocating them into overcrowded temporary emergency shelters. This situation creates opportunities for infectious disease to proliferate due to the contamination of the water and food supplies, the incapacitation of sewage systems, pooling of standing water that creates a breeding site for vector and insect-borne diseases, and difficulty maintaining optimal personal nutrition and hygiene practices. Public health will need to monitor and respond rapidly to such infectious diseases as respiratory infections, cholera, diarrheal diseases, hepatitis A, hepatitis E, parasitic diseases, rotavirus, shigellosis, typhoid fever, rabies, West Nile virus, and malaria (Ligon, 2006; Waring & Brown, 2005).

Implications for Practice

Managing the spread of infectious disease is the most critical element of an effective mitigation program. The ongoing collection of baseline epidemiological data on various infectious diseases helps to identify potential changes in disease rates. Anomalous deviations from baseline data can guide the public health sector in the implementation of strategies to prevent outbreaks. Public health practitioners must be aware of the various situations and factors that contribute to the presence of infectious disease. Controlling the transmission of infectious disease requires ongoing and vigilant surveillance and the ability to respond promptly and appropriately. For example, the public health sector needs to complete a rapid community assessment of health threats following a disaster. Furthermore, public health practitioners play a pivotal role in the provision of various strategies that prevent epidemics, including the identification of adequate shelters, supplying clean water and food, and providing health information to the public.

CHRONIC DISEASES

Chronic diseases have emerged as a global noncommunicable disease threat to the population. Over the past 50 years, the rate of obesity in adults has risen significantly, making it a health issue of almost epidemic proportions in developed countries. In Canada, the 2005 Canadian Community Health Survey (CCHS) showed a *self-reported* adult body mass index (BMI) overweight rate of 33.4% and an obese rate of 15.5%. However, the *measured* adult BMI overweight rate was actually 34.9%, and the obese rate was 24.3%. The disparity between the self-reported and the measured BMI rates is due to the fact that people tend to overestimate their height and underestimate their weight (Statistics Canada, 2005). This health issue affects both males and females in all ethnic groups, at all age groups, and of all educational levels. Being overweight or obese contributes to an array of metabolic and musculoskeletal problems, including cardiovascular disease, hypertension, diabetes, osteoarthritis, and some cancers, and both the length and quality of life are substantially decreased (Choi et al., 2005; Jakicic & Otto, 2006; Katzmarzyk & Mason, 2006; Prentice, 2006; Swinburn, Gill, & Kumanyika, 2005; Tao, 2005; Wyatt, Winters, & Dubbert, 2006). Chronic diseases, particularly obesity and its effects, result in increased financial burden to medical and public health costs. Obesity requires a greater need for treatment that in turn increases the use of health services. Work absenteeism and premature death are examples of indirect costs associated with obesity.

At the same time as the population faces an epidemic in obesity, it is encountering a rise in the incidence of malnutrition, which is particularly prevalent in children and seniors. Malnutrition is primarily associated with physical, social, and psychological issues (Dinsdale, 2006; Prentice, 2006). This contradictory situation underscores the need to take a comprehensive population-based approach to interventions targeted at nutrition.

Implications for Practice

Targeted interventions must be developed in order to reverse the trend of escalating obesity. In order to be successful in reversing this trend, greater financial investment in public health is required to alleviate this critical health issue. Also, public health practitioners must comprehend the causative factors that contribute to weight gain. Policies and program development directed at societal and environmental causal factors are needed, particularly those with respect to food intake and physical activity. Several researchers recommend interventions directed at the whole population, focusing on personal behaviours that relate to all segments of the population (Choi et al., 2005; Swinburn, Gill, & Kumanyika, 2005; Tao, 2005).

MENTAL HEALTH

Mental illness is a public health issue that has been hidden for decades. However, it is now attracting the attention of politicians, the public, and the media due to the recent release of alarming statistical data. With global suicide rates topping 900,000 deaths per year (a figure that is considered to be an underestimation and does not include the significant number of suicide attempts, many of which go unreported), it is not surprising that mental health has become a profound public health problem (Bertolote et al., 2006; Cole & Glass, 2005).

Although it is difficult to collect population-level statistics on mental health, there are some proxy measures that are included in the 2005 CCHS. For instance, 23.2% of the survey respondents reported they experienced *quite a lot of life stress*. In addition, using a self-rated mental health scale with values of poor, fair, good, very good, and excellent, over 25% of respondents rated their mental health as poor, fair, or good. Another indicator captured in the 2005 CCHS is the sense of belonging to the local community. Research studies have demonstrated a strong correlation between a sense of belonging to the local community and mental and physical health. In this survey, 25.2% of respondents said they had *somewhat weak sense of belonging to the local community*, while 9.3% reported a *very weak sense of belonging to the local community* (Statistics Canada, 2005).

Unfortunately, stigma associated with mental illness has been a significant barrier to addressing this issue. The financial burden on the health care system is considerable, as mental health disorders usually begin at an earlier age than other chronic or infectious diseases and typically exist for a long time, thereby requiring long-term treatment (Miller, 2006). One of the leading childhood health problems involves mental health issues. In Canada, approximately 14% of children aged 4 to 17 experience mental illnesses. Furthermore, less than 25% of them have access to specialized treatment. This lack of access to effective treatment can result in these problems persisting throughout adolescence and into adulthood. The severity of mental illness interferes with childhood growth and development and can produce emotional and behavioural consequences. Untreated childhood mental illness often leads to mental health issues in adolescence, which can lead to acts of violence either toward oneself or others (Kulig et al., 2005; Waddell et al., 2005).

Although issues surrounding homelessness are quite complex and are interconnected with various determinants of health, mental health disorders are a significant contributing factor. Characterizing and thus assessing the magnitude of the impact of homelessness can be extremely challenging. It is difficult, for example, to obtain an accurate number of homeless individuals. Canadian census data is only able to collect the number of individuals staying in a shelter at one point in time. Furthermore, rates of homelessness are affected by seasonal variation (e.g., more people in shelters during winter months than during the summer months) and also exclude individuals who are in hostels or other temporary shelters (Werapitiya, 2002).

Homelessness can be categorized as either a temporary situation or a chronic situation. Several factors lead to temporary homelessness. For instance, individuals who experience family violence, in particular women and children, often spend a period of time in family shelters. Other population groups that experience temporary homelessness include new immigrants and urban Aboriginals. This is principally due to a shortage of affordable or subsidized housing.

Chronic homelessness refers to individuals who use shelters regularly; they often suffer from mental illness or substance abuse. Mental health patients who have been recently discharged from a hospital often suffer chronic homelessness due to a lack of appropriate and adequate housing. It has been shown that the increased stress and anxiety they experience due to the lack of housing only exacerbates their mental illness (Andresen, 2006; Hargrave, 2006). It has also been shown that youth living on the streets have a higher prevalence of mental health problems, especially with respect to depression and substance abuse (Boivin et al., 2005).

Implications for Practice

A global public health strategy to address lifelong mental health issues is long overdue. Not only must this strategy focus on promotion and prevention initiatives, public health must advocate for increased specialized treatment programs (Miller, 2006; Waddell et al., 2005). Public health interventions must also be tailored to and address the various factors that create both temporary and chronic homelessness. Investment in mental health is a necessity, with interventions targeted at a population level in order to effectively address this serious public health issue. Increased public awareness, supportive environments that include better housing and less stigma, and healthy public policy are key foci for intervention.

SUMMARY

Public health has a leadership role in the monitoring and identification of emerging public health issues. The complexity of these issues mandates the implementation of a comprehensive surveillance approach that entails a detailed examination of the environment both locally and globally.

In this chapter, several key public health issues that require urgent population level interventions were discussed, and the multiple and interconnected factors that influence these issues were highlighted. The complex nature of emerging public health issues illustrates and underscores the necessity for intersectoral and interdisciplinary collaboration in monitoring issues affecting the population as well as in the development and implementation of effective programs and policies. Decreasing public health capacity and shrinking resources (e.g., staffing, funding) will be future challenges that public health will need to manage in order to respond to emerging issues. This anticipated situation will require innovative approaches for public health practice with an ever-increasing need for collaboration with community-based partners, policy makers, funders, nongovernmental organizations, faith-based and educational institutions, the media, and governments.

The development of population-level interventions (e.g., healthy public policy) must consider the global nature of public health issues in order to ensure that the strategies address health inequities across the world. Additionally, the social determinants of health provide a population-level framework in which to assess public health issues and identify innovative, effective, and timely interventions.

References

Andresen, M. (2006). Mental health moves up the agenda. *Canadian Medical Association Journal*, *175*(2), 139.

Bertolote, J. M., Fleischmann, A., Butchart, A., & Besbelli, N. (2006). Suicide, suicide attempts and pesticides: A major hidden public health problem. *Bulletin of the World Health Organization*, *84*(4), 260.

Boivin, J-F., Roy, E., Haley, N., & Galbaud du Fort, G. (2005). The health of street youth: A Canadian experience. *Canadian Journal of Public Health*, *96*(6), 432–437.

Campbell, K. (2004). The veterinarian and human public health. *Canadian Veterinarian Journal*, *45*, 723–725.

Choi, B. C. K., Hunter, D. J., Tsou, W., & Sainsbury, P. (2005). Diseases of comfort: Primary cause of death in the 22nd century. *Journal of Epidemiology and Community Health*, *59*, 1030–1034.

Cole, T. B., & Glass, R. M. (2005). Mental illness and violent death: Major issues for public health. *Journal of American Medical Association*, *294*(5), 623–624.

Dinsdale, P. (2006). Malnutrition: The real eating problem. *Nursing Older People*, *18*(3), 8–11.

Fauci, A. S. (2006). Pandemic influenza threat and preparedness. *Emerging Infectious Diseases*, *12*(1), 73–77.

Galea, S., & Vlahov, D. (2005). Urban health: Evidence, challenges, and directions. *Annual Review of Public Health*, *26*, 341–365.

Gostin, L. (2006). Public health strategies for pandemic influenza. *JAMA*, *295*(14), 1700–1704.

Hargrave, C. (2006, July). *Homelessness in Canada: From housing to shelters to blankets.* Share International Archives. Retrieved July 26, 2006, from **www.shareintl.org/archives**.

Health Canada. (2004). *Canadian Pandemic Influenza Plan.* Ottawa: Her Majesty the Queen in Right of Canada. Retrieved August 8, 2006, from **www.phac-aspc.gc.ca/cpip-pclcpi**.

Jakicic, J. M., & Otto, A. D. (2006). Treatment and prevention of obesity: What is the role of exercise? *Nutrition Reviews*, *64*(2), S57–S61.

Katzmarzyk, P. T., & Mason, C. (2006). Prevalence of class I, II and III obesity in Canada. *Canadian Medical Association Journal*, *174*(2), 156–157.

Kovats, R. S., Campbell-Lendrum, D., & Matthies, F. (2005). Climate change and human health: Estimating avoidable deaths and disease. *Risk Analysis*, *25*(6), 1409–1418.

Kulig, J. C., Nahachewsky, D., Hall, B. L., & Kalischuk, R. G. (2005). Rural youth violence. *Canadian Journal of Public Health*, *96*(5), 357–359.

Ligon, L. (2006). Infectious diseases that pose specific challenges after natural disasters: A review. *Seminars in Pediatric Infectious Diseases*, *17*, 36–45.

Miller, G. (2006). The unseen: Mental illness's global toll. *Science*, *311*, 458–461.

Plotnikoff, R. C., Wright, M-F., & Karunamuni, N. (2004). Knowledge, attitudes and behaviours related to climate change in Alberta, Canada: Implications for public health policy and practice. *International Journal of Environmental Health Research*, *14*(3), 223–229.

Prentice, A. M. (2006). The emerging epidemic of obesity in developing countries. *International Journal of Epidemiology*, *35*, 93–99.

Prüss-Üstün, A., & Corvalán, C. (2006). *Preventing disease through healthy environments— Towards an estimate of the environmental burden of disease.* Geneva: World Health Organization Publication.

Roberts, I., & Hillman, M. (2005). Climate change: The implications for policy on injury control and health promotion. *Injury Prevention*, *11*, 326–329.

Sakaguchi, A. (2005). Emerging and reemerging diseases and globalization. *Journal of Health Politics, Policy and Law*, *30*(6), 1162–1178.

Sheff, B. (2006). Avian influenza: Poised to launch a pandemic? *Nursing*, *36*(1), 51–53.

Statistics Canada. (2005). *Canadian Community Health Survey* (CCHS 3.1). Ottawa: Her Majesty the Queen in Right of Canada.

Swinburn, B., Gill, T., & Kumanyika, S. (2005). Obesity prevention: A proposed framework for translating evidence into action. *Obesity Reviews*, *6*, 23–33.

Tao, H. (2005). Obesity: From a health issue to a political and policy issue. *Online Journal of Issues in Nursing*, *10*(2), 1091–1096.

Waddell, C., McEwan, K., Shepherd, C. A., Offord, D. R., & Hua, J. M. (2005). A public health strategy to improve the mental health of Canadian children. *Canadian Journal of Psychiatry*, *50*(4), 226–233.

Waring, S. C., & Brown, B. J. (2005). The threat of communicable diseases following natural disasters: A public health response. *Disaster Management & Response*, *3*(2), 41–47.

Werapitiya, M. (2002). Statistics just a first step in helping the homeless. *Capital News Online*, *11*(5), 1–4.

World Health Organization. (2003). *Emerging issues in water and infectious disease.* Geneva: World Health Organization Publication.

Wyatt, S. B., Winters, K. P., & Dubbert, P. M. (2006). Overweight and obesity: Prevalence, consequences, and causes of a growing public health problem. *The American Journal of the Medical Sciences*, *331*(4), 166–174.

Internet Resources

http://www.phac-aspc.gc.ca/ccdpc-cpcmc/index_e.html
Centre for Chronic Disease Prevention and Control

http://www.who.int/chp/en/
WHO Chronic Diseases and Health Promotion

http://www.phac-aspc.gc.ca/cidpc-cpcmi/
Centre for Infectious Disease Prevention and Control

http://www.phac-aspc.gc.ca/cepr-cmiu/
Centre for Emergency Preparedness and Response

http://www.bt.cdc.gov/
CDC Emergency Preparedness and Response

http://www.cdc.gov/nceh/
CDC National Center for Environmental Health

http://www.who.int/topics/environmental_health/en/
WHO Environmental Health

http://www.who.int/phe/en/
WHO Public Health and Environment

http://www.who.int/topics/mental_health/en/
WHO Mental Health

http://www.homelessness.gc.ca/home/index_e.asp
Homelessness Partnering Strategy

Part 2

The Process of Community as Partner

Chapter 12
A Model to Guide Practice / 218

Chapter 13
Community Assessment / 238

Chapter 14
Community Analysis and Diagnosis / 280

Chapter 15
Planning a Community Health Program / 306

Chapter 16
Implementing a Community Health Program / 327

Chapter 17
Evaluating a Community Health Program / 346

A Model to Guide Practice

ARDENE ROBINSON VOLLMAN

Chapter Outline

Introduction
Models
Assessment
Analysis, Diagnosis, and Planning
Intervention

Evaluation
Partnership Planning and
   Teamwork
Summary

Learning Objectives

Models that serve as guides for practice, education, and research have become important tools for community health workers. This chapter, in which we begin our examination of the process as applied to the community as partner, focuses on the use of one model to guide practice.

After studying this chapter, you should be able to:

❖ Define *model*

❖ Describe the purposes of a model

❖ Describe selected models relevant to community practice

❖ Define *community* and the aspects of a healthy community

❖ Begin to apply a model to community practice

❖ Understand the interprofessional multidisciplinary nature of community work

Introduction

              ealth disciplines have developed models for practice that provide processes and structures to identify issues and work across disciplines and with communities. Conceptual maps are useful guides for action, particularly when practice focuses on entire communities. The community-as-partner model provides us with processes, structures, and a conceptual map that will be used throughout this chapter. While a model might look structural, it encompasses also the processes by which the model is enacted. Throughout, we will refer to these processes as well as to the values and assumptions that underpin the practice of working with community as partner.

MODELS

A *conceptual model* is the synthesis of a set of concepts and the statements that integrate those concepts into a whole. A *community process model* can be defined as a frame of reference, a way of looking at a community, or an image of what working in and with a community encompasses. A model is a representation of practice, not a reality. Other types of models that are used to represent realities are model airplanes, blueprints, chemical equations, and anatomic models.

A model with which health workers identified for many years was the medical model, that is, a disease-oriented, illness- and body system–focused approach to patients, with an emphasis on pathology. This model has served us well in our quest to eliminate childhood communicable diseases and common preventable illness. However, reliance on the medical model that focuses on individuals excludes health promotion and the holistic focus that is central to population/public health and community well-being. Additionally, important aspects of care, such as psychological, sociocultural, and spiritual areas, are not explicitly included in the medical model. Thus, a community-as-partner model should encompass all aspects of health and incorporate long-range goals and planning.

As a representation of reality, a model can take numerous forms. Because they describe professional practice, all models are narrative; that is, words are the symbols that are used by workers (e.g., nurses, social workers, nutritionists, etc.) to define how they view their practice. And although all models are described in words, many are clarified further through the use of diagrams or illustrations. Diagrams are an efficient and effective way of depicting models; the use of such images allows the model builder to show relationships and linkages among the concepts in the model. The diagram is often thought of as the model itself, with the accompanying text seen as the elaboration or explanation of the model.

The method chosen to depict a model reflects the model builder's own philosophy and preference; no one method is accepted as the best. Certain components, however, must be included in any health-related model. Table 12-1 presents these essential elements. General agreement exists that four concepts are central to health disciplines: person, environment, health, and the defining characteristics of the specific health discipline (e.g., nursing, social work, medicine, nutrition). *Concepts* are defined as general notions or ideas and are considered the building blocks of models. How each of the four concepts is defined will both dictate the organization of the model and be illustrated in that model. For example, health may be

TABLE 12-1	
Essential Units of a Health Model	
UNIT	**DESCRIPTION**
Goal of action	The mission or ideal goal expressed as the end product desired (a state, condition, or situation)
The population or community	A description that best describes the population and the processes of inclusion to involve the population to identify issues, set goals and plan interventions
The health team's role	As facilitators, catalysts, advocates and resources to collaborate with populations or communities
Source of difficulty, dysfunction	The origins of deviations from the desired state, stressors
Intervention focus, strategies for action	The means for achieving the desired goal
Consequences	Intended and unexpected outcomes (desired and not) that result from the interventions and strategies implemented.

Adapted from Anderson, E. & McFarlane, J. (2008). *Community as Partner: Theory and practice in nursing*, 5th ed., p 203.

defined on a continuum with wellness at one end and death at the other; as a dichotomy wherein one is seen as well or ill; as the outcome of numerous biopsychosocial and spiritual forces; or as the interaction of these same forces. In the medical model, *health* has been defined traditionally as the absence of disease. Figure 12-1 depicts one way to view health and illustrates these definitions. Labonté (1993) argues that health is not a continuum but is a domain that overlaps in varying degrees with the domains of illness and disease. In the figure, health and wellness (circle A) represents people (population, aggregate) who would describe themselves as healthy or well—they would have a commitment to important values, feel a sense of control over their lives, view change as a challenge rather than a threat, and are not experiencing illness and do not have a medically diagnosed condition. If we are talking about a geopolitical community, this community would see itself as one where its members were productive, supportive, and took pride in their physical community setting. Illness (circle B) represents people who have subjective senses of feeling "not quite right" but do not have specific diagnoses (as a population group), or they have a feeling that something is "off" about the community in which they live, learn, work, and the like. Disease (circle F) represents people with diagnosed or "silent" (undiagnosed) pathologies; it might also represent a community that is in dysfunction but that is as yet not showing symptoms. Sickness (area D) represents those people who have diagnoses and actually feel sick; it also represents the community that is demonstrating signs of malfunction (e.g., graffiti, low morale, violence, disrepair). Area E represents people who feel sick as a result of being diagnosed or a community that begins to see dysfunction escalate as a result of being labelled a problem. Area G represents those people who have been diagnosed with a disease but consider themselves to be quite healthy or communities that know they suffer many challenges to health and well-being but nevertheless focus on strengths and community assets and pride. Area C represents the transition between feeling well and healthy or feeling ill as either a population or

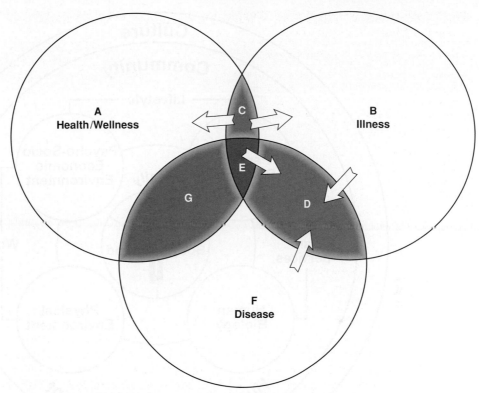

FIGURE 12-1 ◆ Labonté model of health, illness, and disease.

as a community. It is important to understand that the Labonté (1993) model can be applied to multiple units of the population (individuals, families, communities, groups and aggregates, systems and structures, or society as a whole) and to "diagnoses" that are biomedical, social, cultural, psychological, emotional, or spiritual. You are encouraged to apply this model as we work through this part of the book using your professional perspective on health and well-being.

The Labonté model is a model of health and does not include consideration that people live in a complex environment that influences experiences and perceptions. Hancock and Perkins (1985) and Hancock (1993) address this limitation in their model of the Mandala of Health (Fig. 12-2). The Mandala resonates with the concepts presented in earlier chapters. It is based in part on an understanding of human ecology as the interaction of culture (including politics) with the natural environment (biosphere) depicted in the outer circle and represents the living planet. Health is understood in a holistic sense, so the health of the population is seen as having body, mind, and spiritual dimensions. The system levels or shells extend outward from the individual and comprise the family, the community, the built environment, and include also the natural environment as exemplified by the

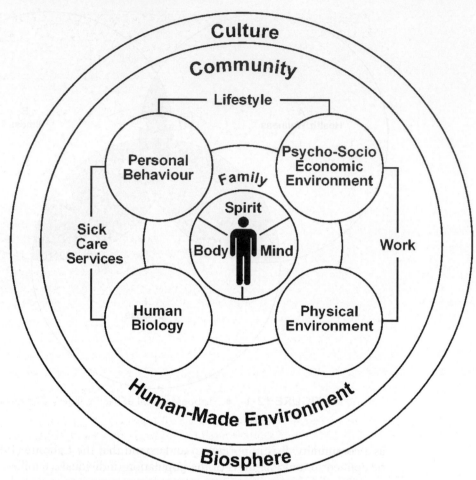

FIGURE 12-2 ◆ The Mandala of Health: A model of the human ecosystem.

culture/biosphere shell. The social sciences (psychology, sociology, economics, anthropology) are integrated in the upper half of the model (personal behaviour and psycho-social-economic environment), while the physical sciences (physics, chemistry, biology, engineering) are integrated into the lower half of the model with human biology and physical environments as factors that influence health. *Lifestyle* is defined as "personal behaviour as influenced and modified by, and constrained by, a lifelong socialization process and by the psycho-social environment, including cultural and community values and standards" (Hancock & Perkins, 1985, p. 8). The health care system is rightfully given the title "sick care services," a determinant of health that attempts to integrate the physical and social sciences (Hancock, 1993). The Mandala should be viewed as a three-dimensional model in

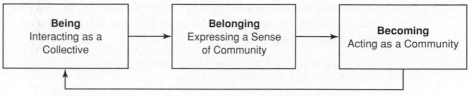

FIGURE 12-3 ◆ Being, belonging, and becoming model for health.

which various components shift in shape and size according to their relative importance over time and in different settings.

Neither of the above models has an action component, however. For this, we go to a model developed by the Rural Development Institute (Rural Development Institute [RDI], 2005) in Brandon MB (Fig. 12-3). It illustrates the goal of action (becoming) and the steps along the process—being and belonging.

Being represents those actions that people undertake and involves their interactions with others as they form a collective unit. These interactions lead to a sense of *belonging* or expression by the group of a "sense of community." McMillan and Chavis (1986; cited in RDI, 2005) identify four elements of sense of community: membership, influence, need fulfillment, and shared connections. Belonging leads to *becoming* through the collective action of the community. This community action entails the processes of assessing the community, settings goals and planning for change, implementing change processes, and evaluating both the processes and the outcomes of the actions taken (RDI, 2005). The goal of action is to improve community health. Action relates to community development with the outcome being healthy people in healthy settings.

Health is one of the four concepts central to health disciplines and is defined for the purposes of this book as "a resource for everyday life, not the objective of living. [It is] a positive concept emphasizing social and personal resources as well as physical capacities" (World Health Organization, 1986). *Person*, in this book, refers to collectives rather than individuals or families; that is, populations, aggregates, systems, structures, and society. The *environment* is conceived as an encompassing concept that includes biological, psychological, social, emotional, and spiritual dimensions and the contexts or settings where people live, love, learn, work, play, and pray. The mandate of the action of *health disciplines* is preventive, aimed at reducing stressors and building capacity and enhancing resilience. As we proceed through the action components of the community process in this section of the book, you will encounter other models to guide your community practice. What, then, are the purposes of a model of practice? Think for a moment of what a model is to you and how a model might be useful in your practice. Although you may not have formulated your own model of practice, you have been influenced greatly in your education by the model or models on which your professional curriculum is based. Does your faculty or organization subscribe to one particular model? Just as the choice of a model creates a basis for curriculum planning and decisions, a model can also provide a basis for practice.

What does professional practice mean to you? If you can express an answer to that question, you have begun to describe your model of practice. A model serves the following purposes:

◆ Provides a map for the problem-solving process
  ◆ Gives direction for assessment
  ◆ Guides analysis
  ◆ Dictates community diagnoses
  ◆ Assists in planning
  ◆ Facilitates evaluation
◆ Provides a curriculum outline for education
◆ Represents a framework for research
◆ Provides a basis for development of theory

A model is nothing more or less than an explication of practice. A model not only describes what is but also provides a framework for making decisions about what could be.

Community-as-Partner Model

Based on Neuman's 1972 Systems Model (Neuman, 1995) of a total-person approach to viewing client problems, the community-as-client model was developed by Anderson and McFarlane in 1986 to illustrate the definition of community health nursing as the synthesis of public health and nursing. The model has been renamed the community-as-partner model to emphasize the underlying philosophy of multidisciplinary and interprofessional primary health care and the evolving respect for public participation in health decision-making. Beddome (1995) expanded the utility of the model to aggregates within the community as well as to the geopolitical community itself. Mill (1997) applied it in a Canadian setting with issues related to HIV.

The phenomena of interest are the community system and its related environment. The environment can be internal, external, or created. It is based on a social ecological foundation. The objective of the care provider (community worker) is to prevent fragmentation of services to the population and the community. The community health team's goal is to intervene to either (1) decrease the potential of the community system to encounter stressors, (2) limit the impact or effects of stressors on the community through prevention interventions, or (3) build the capacity of the community to act on its own behalf.

CRITICAL THINKING EXERCISE 12-1

Before you read this section, write down on a piece of paper what you think community is. Do this again after you have read this section. Are there any differences?

What is community? When we think about community, we think about geographical locations such as towns or neighbourhoods. We think also of settings where people congregate to carry out their daily lives (e.g., workplaces, schools, places of worship) as communities. But groups of people (populations, aggregates) are also referred to as communities (e.g., ethnic communities, farm communities, gay community, professional community, virtual community). When we use the term *community*, we are placing a boundary (real or symbolic) around a group of people that demarcates who is in and who is out of that group. It refers to people who have a common bond that identifies participants and their degree of adhesion to the group. Communities can be consciously built through creating a shared story and consensual decision-making built on respect for the diversity in the group (Peck, 1987). A healthy community, according to the Ontario Healthy Communities Coalition:

◆ Provides a clean, safe physical environment
◆ Meets the basic needs of all its residents
◆ Has residents who respect and support each other
◆ Involves the community in local government
◆ Promotes and celebrates its historical and cultural heritage
◆ Provides easily accessible health (and social) services
◆ Has a diverse, innovative economy
◆ Rests on a sustainable ecosystem

Additional attributes might include a sense of unity, effective collaboration and communication, judicious balance between utilization and conservation of resources, problem-solving orientation, and the ability to handle crises and conflict (Allender & Spradley, 2005).

Consider the community-as-partner model (Fig. 12-4). Two central factors comprise this model: a focus on the community as partner (represented by the community assessment wheel at the top, which incorporates the community's people as the core) and the use of the problem-solving process. The model is described in some detail to assist in understanding its parts and guiding practice in the community.

The *core* of the assessment wheel represents the people who make up the community. Included in data to describe the community's core are the population's social demographics (e.g., age, sex and ethnic distribution, culture, education and employment levels, socioeconomic status) and the community values, beliefs, and history. Understanding this core is essential in community planning, and changes in the community demographics must be identified and considered over time as development and change are facilitated by working with a community.

As residents of the community, people are affected by and, in turn, influence the eight *subsystems* of the community. These subsystems, consistent with the broad determinants of health, are physical environment, education, safety and transportation, politics and government, health and social services, communication,

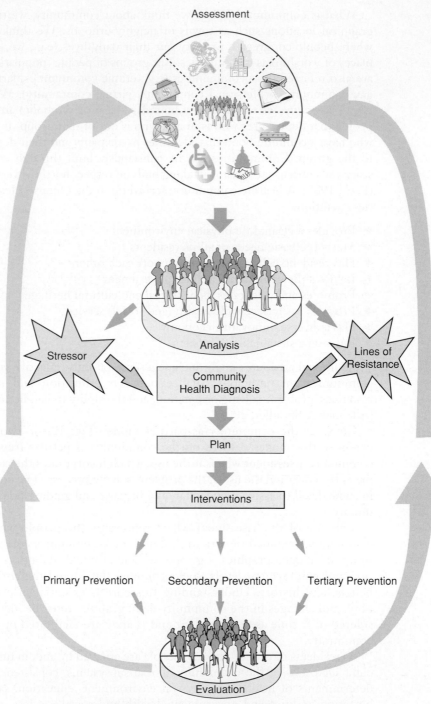

FIGURE 12-4 ◆ Community-as-partner model.

economics, and recreation. The eight subsystems are divided by broken lines to remind us that they are not discrete and separate but influence (and are influenced by) one another and the core (people). One of the principles of ecology (Chapter 4; Fig. 4-2) is that everything is connected to everything else. This premise also applies to the community as a whole. The eight divisions both define the major subsystems of a community and provide the community health worker and those community members involved in the process with a framework for assessment.

The solid line surrounding the community core and its subsystems represents its *normal line of defence* (NLD), or the level of health (health status) the community/population has reached over time. The NLD may include epidemiologic and health status measurements such as birth, mortality, and morbidity rates; incidence and prevalence of disease and injury; presence and prevalence of risk factors; community capacity; social capital; and other health-related statistics. The NLD also includes usual patterns of collective coping and problem-solving capabilities in each of the subsystems; when the NLD is drawn around the outside of the assessment wheel, it represents the health of the community. The NLD may instead be drawn around the core if the interest in the assessment is the people (population) and their collective health status. Ideally, we want to achieve healthy people in healthy communities, but to do that may take stepwise approaches—first to an assessment of the community and subsystems and then to assessment of the people or vice versa. To get a complete picture may take time, but we do not want to exclude one part of the assessment for the sake of efficiency or expediency and fail to make adequate diagnoses because we have not captured the full essence of community—the people and the places.

Take Note

Take a moment to examine the selection of subsystems that have been identified. Can you think of any that have been omitted? Think of the community where you live. Would you add faith or spirituality as a subsystem?

The *flexible line of defence* (FLD), shown as a broken line around the community and its NLD, is a buffer zone representing a dynamic level of health resulting from a temporary response to stressors. It prevents stressors from penetrating through the NLD. An example of a temporary response may be that, in the time of an economic crisis, inner-city churches will provide temporary shelter and the food bank will offer food to a wider clientele when the weather suddenly turns cold. Temporary responses are used until more permanent solutions are found (e.g., the economy recovers and people find jobs and housing or the weather improves). The FLD illustrates the community's *resilience* in the face of challenges. A resilient community bounces back from adversity; the people of the community are mutually supportive through a dense network of social supports. Hard times make people angry, alienated, and disengaged; resilient communities reach out to those who are socially isolated and offer support to those who need a hand. Stressors that have affected a Canadian community and some goals for action toward creating resilience are described in an example from Winnipeg MB (Box 12-1).

Within the community are *lines of resistance* (LR), internal mechanisms that act to defend against penetration of the community core by stressors; they are the strengths and *assets* of the community. The LRs exist throughout each of the sub-systems, and their strength influences the degree of reaction to a stressor that a community or population aggregate experiences. The stronger the capacities and assets of the community, the more likely stressors will be fended off. Networks and connections among people, associations, government and nongovernment agencies, faith institutions, and social agencies are examples of community assets that can be mobilized when a stressor threatens the community core. For instance, if

---

BOX 12-1

The Resilient Community

Six years ago, Winnipeg's United Way began a challenging community involvement initiative it calls *Journey Forward*. The exercise is nothing less than an effort to involve all sectors of the city in creating a community agenda for social action. To lay the groundwork for deciding priorities, *Journey Forward* produced an environmental scan assessing the current situation. Among its findings were that the number of teen births per thousand in Manitoba is twice the Canadian average; 50% of households and 80% of Aboriginal households in Winnipeg's inner city live in poverty; gangs, arson, urban decay, drug abuse, and crime are taking their toll; families with the resources to leave are fleeing the inner city for the suburbs; and $1 invested in early intervention with young children and their parents saves $7 later by reducing crime, teen pregnancy, and the number of parents on welfare. Last year, the United Way asked more than 3,000 Winnipeggers what they regarded as their most pressing social issues. From the results of that survey, *Journey Forward* identified five priority issues for community action and, for each, a goal to attain:

- *Marginalization*—to move from a situation where people feel left out to a community of belonging and opportunity
- *Declining feelings of safety and social civility*—to move to a community that builds harmony toward becoming a civil society
- *Poverty*—to move from a situation where people are unable to meet their basic needs to a community that generates choice for all its citizens
- *Barriers to self-sufficiency and independence*—to move to a community of dialogue focussed on people not processes
- *Stressed families, children, and youth*—to move to a community of supportive and nurturing environments

From Canadian Policy Research Network (CPRN/RCRPP). (2002). The resilient community: Winnipeg's exciting experiment. Document Number 30608. Retrieved July 4, 2007 from **http://www.cprn.com/en/doc.cfm?doc=1031&print=true**.

teen pregnancy is an identified stressor, having a community-based teen health clinic accessible near public transit routes can offer culturally attuned sexual and reproductive health services and social services to prevent teen pregnancy from disrupting the community system. These services, as well as the community attitudes that support them, represent community assets and capacity.

Stressors are tension-producing stimuli that have the potential of causing disruption in the system. They may arise from the internal environment, the external environment, or the created environment. Stressors, then, may be intrasystem (originating within the geopolitical community, population, or group), extrasystem (originating outside of the community and its people), or intersystem (originating from interactions among the subsystems).

Let us use the issue of hypertension within a Hutterite colony to illustrate the model concepts (Table 12-2). A stressor (hypertension) has penetrated the flexible and normal lines of defence, resulting in disruption of the community. The *degree of reaction* is the amount of disruption that results from stressors impinging on the community's lines of defence. The degree of reaction may be reflected in changes to mortality and morbidity rates (impact on the community core), unemployment (effect on the economic subsystem), or crime statistics (effect on the safety subsystem), for instance. In the case of the Hutterite colony, the stressor has caused several individuals to experience symptoms and require medication. The community has also been affected because these individuals need to rest during the day and have special diets; because food is prepared and served communally, accommodations need to be made by the cooks and other colony members. The affected individuals need to be treated differently to regain and maintain their health, which counters the prevailing cultural values of colony life.

TABLE 12-2

Application of Community-as-Partner Model Concepts to a Health Problem in a Population Group

MODEL CONCEPT	COMMUNITY RESPONSE
Stressor	Several people diagnosed with high blood pressure
Degree of reaction	Two older residents experienced symptoms needing medication; some midlife adults are too fatigued to work a full day and need to rest in the afternoon; kitchen requested to prepare special diets for those affected
Core	Mature community with three generations living on it. Head Man and Cook have been leaders for many years. Hutterites live communally on a farm with ready access to meat, vegetables, fruit, and milk. Everyone contributes to the life of the colony. Children go to school on the colony until age 16.
Normal line of defence	Increased incidence of hypertension, moderately high mean blood sugar levels among midlife women and men. Cultural practice of sharing prescriptions.
Flexible line of defence	Multidisciplinary health team mobilizes to provide education, screening, and support
Lines of resistance	Nearby community health centre; on-site school; communal living increases social support; cooks willing to try new recipes. Head Man approves the purchase of blood pressure monitors and training in their use.

Stressors and degree of reaction become part of the *community health diagnosis*. To continue the analysis of the exemplar, the problem is the community's adaptation to members of the colony needing special care (a degree of reaction by the community core) related to hypertension (a stressor) caused by a combination of genetic endowment, diet, and physical inactivity. Data that illustrate the health problem may be increased physician visits for hypertension, costs of medications and equipment (*health services subsystem*), and changes to the communal cooking practices and dietary menus (*physical environment subsystem*). When the regular service provided by the community health nurse (*LR*) is supplemented by a monthly blood pressure clinic and wellness activities (healthy weight and healthy activity programs) in response to the alteration in the *NLD* (health status of the people in the community), this service is considered to be an *FLD*, temporarily put in place in response to the colony's need. How might the members of the colony become more aware of the precipitating factors related to hypertension and work together to tackle prevention of hypertension by taking action at a community level?

Take Note

The outcome of a stressor impinging on a community is not always negative. Often, it is positive. For example, in the face of a crisis, people may band together and develop a community group to deal with the crisis. This group may continue to function after the crisis is over, strengthening the community and continuing to contribute to its health. (Advocacy for gun control laws and the implementation of antibullying programs in schools after a shooting at a school are examples of positive outcomes following a stressor.)

ASSESSMENT

The community's core and subsystems comprise assessment parameters. A variety of methods are used to complete a community assessment (described in Chapter 13), and the data are organized in ways to facilitate the understanding of the interdisciplinary community health team and community members regarding the community core (people), its lines of defence (health status and resilience) and LRs (assets and strengths), any stressors, and the community or aggregate response (degree of reaction) to any stressors present or threatening (Fig. 12-5). Because community work is founded on the principles of primary health care, public participation is a critical component of all steps in the community action process. A team that assesses from a distance will not gain the insider knowledge important to making accurate and appropriate interpretations of the collected data. Assessment might begin with a scenario such as this: take a large picture view and then focus (depending on the data and its interpretation) on a population group (aggregate) or

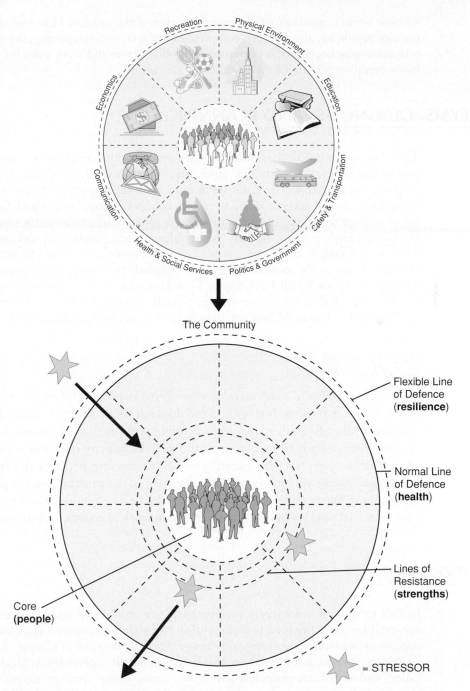

FIGURE 12-5 ◆ The community assessment wheel, featuring lines of resistance and defence within the community structure.

an issue (need or problem) in the planning stage of the process. However, if a community profile has already been completed, or if a crisis is happening, the community team may begin at the aggregate or problem level and work outward to get a more complete picture of the community as a whole.

ANALYSIS, DIAGNOSIS, AND PLANNING

The community health diagnosis (see Chapter 14) is the collaborative determination of the issues of priority that gives direction to both the goal setting and the intervention planning. The goals are derived from the impact of stressors (degree of reaction caused) and are aimed to reduce community encounters with the stressor or to limit the effects of a stressor through prevention activities that strengthen the community's lines of defence. To be relevant, acceptable, and successful, the processes of analysis and diagnosis must include representatives of the population of interest, just as the assessment process included community participants. Planning processes are detailed in Chapter 15 and are built on a comprehension of how people make choices (behaviour change models) so that planning is theory-driven and based on evidence of best practices in health promotion intervention.

Take Note

The term *community health diagnosis* is preferred over a discipline-oriented diagnosis for three reasons: It is holistic and does not imply that only a member of a particular discipline can address the identified problem; it underscores that work in the community is by nature inter- and intradisciplinary (not only confined to health professions but incorporating many others); and it places the emphasis once again on the community, which is the focus of our practice. For the purposes of planning nursing interventions, however, do use a community nursing diagnosis; for social workers, use a community social work diagnosis, and so on.

INTERVENTION

In this model, all community interventions are considered to be preventive in nature. There are three levels of prevention at which interventions are aimed. The process of implementing community interventions is detailed in Chapter 16.

Primary prevention focuses on risk factors and health promotion. Health education and awareness programs that foster social justice, reduce inequities, and encourage healthy lifestyles are examples of primary prevention interventions. These programs assist the community in strengthening its ability to respond to stressors by expanding its FLD. Primary prevention strategies help the community to retain its system stability. Consider the previous exemplar of hypertension among members of a Hutterite colony: Primary prevention could be education about healthy eating and regular exercise for the colony youth at school, an activity program instituted at school or community wide, annual screening of adults for blood pressure and blood glucose levels, and changes in colony food preparation. Often, the most appropriate and relevant ideas come from collaboration with community members to identify strategies that fit with current lifestyles, culture, and adaptation of existing resources.

Secondary prevention is used after a stressor has penetrated the community subsystems. The focus is on treating responses to stressors and focuses on early case finding, symptom management, and correction of maladaptive responses. Such interventions strengthen the LRs by building on the capacities and assets of the community so that it can attain system stability. An example of secondary prevention would be the monitoring of blood pressure and glucose for those with high blood pressure; education about safe and appropriate medication administration; and supportive diet, exercise, and stress reduction programs for those affected. A self-help group offers opportunity for community members to share their concerns and solutions as well as offer support to one another.

Tertiary prevention activities focus on residual consequences of stressor impact by strengthening and re-expanding the FLD to the previous level (or a new level) in an effort to maintain system stability. For instance, weight loss maintenance and healthy activity programs to maintain healthy blood pressure and blood sugar levels of colony residents, development of a cookbook so novice cooks will learn healthy ways of food preparation, and a resulting change in the prevailing diet and activity norms of the colony would be examples of tertiary prevention. Tertiary prevention interventions are aimed at re-establishing equilibrium in the community. An activity program such as one involving an appropriate sport at the community level where all community members can participate offers intervention that benefits residents at primary, secondary, and tertiary levels concurrently. Again, a reminder—community processes challenge the health team to move from the expert model of doing *to* and *for* the community to a model that facilitates the community to build its capacities and strengths from its already-existing assets, connections, and relationships. No intervention should take place without community involvement in all aspects of its planning and delivery.

The outcome desired by interventions relate to both the health of the people and the development of the community. Hancock (1993) presents a model of health and community ecosystem that integrates in a holistic way, the multiple sectors (community, economic, and environment) that must be involved to achieve a healthy population in a healthy world (Fig. 12-6).

The *community* must be convivial—it needs to have social support networks, its members need to participate fully in community life and live harmoniously together. The built *environment* needs to be livable—the urban design must foster a viable human setting and support conviviality and participation. To achieve equity, community members must be treated justly and fairly—their basic needs are met, and they have equal opportunity to achieve their personal potentials.

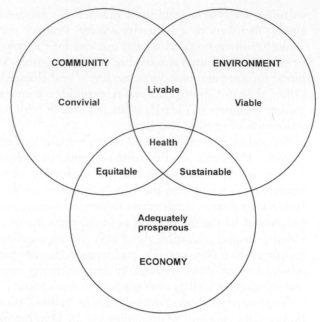

FIGURE 12-6 ◆ Health and community ecosystem (Hancock, 1993).

The *economy* must be adequate to generate enough wealth to enable members of the community to achieve a satisfactory level of health and quality of life while using resources and protect the environment in a responsible manner, ensuring sustainability of the economy and environment over time. The model suggests that health is formed at the conjunction of community, environment, and economy and is best achieved when balance exists among the components.

Take Note

Many single interventions address more than one level of prevention. In the Hutterite community example, tertiary prevention is illustrated, but actions that build trust will have primary preventive qualities as well. The community's capacity to act in concert with the health care providers will be enhanced by improved communication networks and mutual trust should future events occur.

EVALUATION

Feedback from the people in the community provides the basis for evaluation of community interventions (see Chapter 17) just as involvement of community people in all steps of assessment and planning processes ensures relevance to the community and ownership by the community. The community health diagnosis sets the parameters for evaluation (as described in Chapter 14). The population for the intervention is identified by the reaction of the population to the stressors. The goals and objectives of the intervention are related to the stressor that caused the reaction, and indicators for success are established by the manifestations of the reaction as illustrated by a program logic model (see Chapter 15). Such is the process of working with the community as partner. Interconnections, overlap, and interdisciplinary considerations are the rule rather than the exception. While the community-as-partner process appears to be linear, it is in fact iterative. Most health teams analyse the information and data collected on an ongoing basis that informs further data collection. Also, they evaluate "as they go" asking what is going well, what is not, and what needs to be done differently in each of the stages of the process. Left to the end, evaluation suffers because it was not planned for, appropriate data were not collected, and interventions did not match the goals and objectives!

PARTNERSHIP PLANNING AND TEAMWORK

The first step in the community-as-partner process is to establish a working group that includes community members, stakeholders, program participants, program developers, front-line practitioners, and community leaders. Stakeholders have an interest in the problem or program while also holding divergent views; conflicting interpretations of causality; and different values, goals, and life experiences. Community participants can be unaffiliated residents, community organizations, staff members that work in and with communities, managers, and leaders from community groups. The internal systems that link program planners, implementers, and evaluators are also important to include in either steering committee or working group roles.

Green & Kreuter (2005) list six principles of collaboration:

- Community involvement from the beginning and throughout all stages of the project
- Equally shared influence on the direction and activities of the project
- Respect for diversity in values, perspectives, contributions, and confidentiality
- Time and resources to devote to group function
- Compensation for community participants
- Concern for sustainability, long-term benefit, and development of community capacity

Once a work group is composed, it is important to manage it so that it is productive. The group needs to define its responsibilities and decide how it will make decisions. The group will have two key functions: instrumental (tasks) and expressive (group maintenance and team building). Group tasks are the activities that must be accomplished to do the work. The work of the group may suffer if expressive tasks are ignored. Without attention to group maintenance and team building, relationships among members may suffer, group cohesion might be damaged, trust will be eroded, group and cultural norms may be violated, and unpredictability and variable participation may become sources of conflict. Successful work groups have active two-way communication distributed among group members. Leadership and responsibility for group function (e.g., agenda, minutes) are also distributed depending on the task at hand and the readiness of the group members. Acceptance, support, trust, inclusion, and problem-solving ability help to build group cohesion (Johnson & Johnson, 1994).

SUMMARY

Consider the community-as-partner model (see Fig. 12-4) once more. The goal represented by the model is system equilibrium, healthy people in a healthy and resilient community, and includes the preservation and promotion of community health as well as the development of the community and the sustainability of the environment. The model presents a structure but also comprises a process built on participation—working with the population and community in equal partnership.

Take Note

Health may not be a primary goal of the community (although it may be that of the community health worker). It is, however, an important resource for the community to meet its goals. Realizing that we do not always share the same goals is important for anyone working in the community and must at least be considered (if not reconciled) as we plan, implement, and evaluate programs aimed at improving health.

The model views the focus of action as the total community, the population and its aggregate groups, and, as such, includes the individuals and families nested therein. The community worker's role is to assist the community to attain, regain, maintain, and promote health, that is, to act as a facilitator, catalyst, and advocate for health so that the community is empowered to regulate and control its responses to stressors that are the sources of difficulty. The intervention focus is the actual or potential disruption experienced by the community or an inability of the community to function. The intervention mode comprises the three levels of prevention: primary, secondary, and tertiary. The consequences intended in this model include a strengthened NLD, increased resistance to stressors, and a diminished degree of reaction to stressors by the community. Said in other words, the outcomes desired of community interventions are convivial and livable communities that are environmentally viable and sustainable and that treat its members with respect and justice. Congruent with the principles of primary health care, it is the community's competence to deal with its own problems, strengthen its own lines of defence, and resist stressors that dictate the interventions and measure their success. Let us now begin the process.

References _____

Allender, J. A., & Spradley, B. W. (2005). *Community health nursing: Promoting and protecting the public's health* (6th ed.). Philadelphia: Lippincott Williams & Wilkins.

Anderson, E. T., & McFarlane, J. (2006). *Community as partner: Theory and practice in nursing* (5th ed., pp. 201–215). Philadelphia: Lippincott Williams & Wilkins.

Beddome, G. (1995). Community-as-client assessment. In B. N. Neuman (Ed.), *The Neuman systems model* (3rd ed., pp. 567–580). Norwalk, CT: Appleton & Lange.

Green, L. W., & Kreuter, M. W. (2005). *Health program planning: An educational and ecological approach* (4th ed.). New York: McGraw-Hill.

Hancock, T. (1993). Health, human development, and the community ecosystem: Three ecological models. *Health Promotion International, 8*(1), 41–48.

Hancock, T., & Perkins, F. (1985). The mandala of health: A conceptual model and teaching tool. *Health Education, 24*(1), 8–10.

Johnson, D. E., & Johnson, F. P. (1994). *Joining together: Group theory and group skills* (5th ed.). Boston: Allyn & Bacon.

Labonté, R. (1993). *Community health and empowerment.* Toronto: Centre for Health Promotion.

Mill, J. E. (1997). The Neuman systems model: Application in a Canadian HIV setting. *British Journal of Nursing, 6*(3), 163–166.

Neuman, B. N. (Ed.). (1995). *The Neuman systems model* (3rd ed.). Norwalk, CT: Appleton & Lange.

Peck, M. S. (1987). *The different drum: Community-making and peace.* New York: Simon and Schuster.

Rural Development Institute. (2005). *The community health action model.* Brandon, MB: Author.

World Health Organization. (1986). *Ottawa Charter for Health Promotion.* Retrieved 4 July 2007 from www.who.int/hpr/NPH/docs/ottawa_charter_hp.pdf

*Suggested Readings—Model Examples*_____

Clark, M. J. (2003). *Community health nursing: Caring for populations* (4th ed.). Upper Saddle River, NJ: Prentice Hall.

Ervin, N. E. (2002). Exploring frameworks for guiding a community assessment. In N. E. Ervin (Ed.), *Advanced community health nursing practice* (pp. 8–10, 83–108). Upper Saddle River, NJ: Prentice Hall.

Internet Resources _____

http://www.opc.on.ca/
Ontario Prevention Clearinghouse

http://www.healthycommunities.on.ca/about_us/healthy_community.htm
Ontario Healthy Communities Coalition

http://www.unitedwaywinnipeg.mb.ca/uwaytoday/journey.html
Journey Forward Project

http://www.northwestern.edu/ipr/abcd/kelloggabcd.pdf
Community Assets Mapping

http://www.brandonu.ca/rdi
Rural Development Institute

13

Community Assessment

ARDENE ROBINSON VOLLMAN

Chapter Outline

Introduction

The Community Assessment Team

Getting to Know the Community

Planning the Assessment

Methods of Data Collection

Elements of a Community Assessment

Subsystems

Summary

Learning Objectives

Preceding chapters have focused on the foundational concepts for community practice. A model was introduced in Chapter 12 to provide a structure and guide the process of working with communities and populations. This chapter and the four that follow in this section focus on the application of the community-as-partner process in the community. Consequently, the objectives are practice oriented.

After studying this chapter, you should be able to:

❖ Participate with a community to undertake a community assessment using the community-as-partner model

❖ Discuss the challenges of working with communities and populations

❖ Detail the processes that are helpful in overcoming barriers and resistance

❖ Describe the various methods of data collection and their strengths and weaknesses

❖ Begin organizing data for analysis

Introduction

C ommunity assessment is a systematic process; it is the act of becoming acquainted with a community. The people in the community are your partners and contribute throughout the process; the assessment phase is their point of entry into the processes of inquiry, planning, implementing programs, and evaluating their success. The purpose for assessing a community is to identify factors (both positive and negative) that impinge on the health of the people to develop strategies for health promotion. As Hancock and Minkler (1997, p. 140) point out, "For health professionals concerned with . . . community building for health, there are two reasons for [conducting] community health assessments: information is needed for change, and it is needed for empowerment." Haglund, Weisbrod, and Bracht (1990) suggest several additional purposes for community assessment: preintervention planning, developing health risk profiles, evaluating needs for health promotion actions, assessing community readiness and leadership capacity for planned interventions, preparing funding proposals, and setting the stage for ongoing monitoring of processes and progress toward health goals. Put simply, the process of community assessment is useful for:

◆ Developing short- and long-range community plans
◆ Defining and solving community problems
◆ Setting community priorities
◆ Bringing public values, opinions, and traditions to the surface
◆ Developing community awareness and support
◆ Stimulating community action

Assessment is not only a process, it is an outcome. Completing a community assessment project is useful in building community commitment for change; building community capacity with regard to empowerment, knowledge, communication, and conflict resolution; guiding policy development; and acquiring community perspectives and interpretations on issues, needs, and priorities.

In this chapter, we first discuss the community assessment team and how to enter into the community assessment process and then we move into sources and types of data and methods that can be used to collect information. We will use the community assessment wheel (Fig. 13-1) as a framework for the assessment itself and the preparation of the data for the next stage in the process—analysis. (For a specific assessment guide for industry, see Appendix A. Appendix B includes the completed assessment of one industry.)

THE COMMUNITY ASSESSMENT TEAM

Rarely does a professional conduct a community assessment alone; rather, it is a team effort that brings together people with different disciplines, perspectives, agendas, and approaches. It is also critical to have community members on the team to facilitate the processes of the assessment, analysis, planning, implementation, and evaluation. Remember, we work *with* the community. Teams bring people with diverse knowledge and skills together for a common purpose. The same teams may not work on all aspects of a project together—they may re-form with

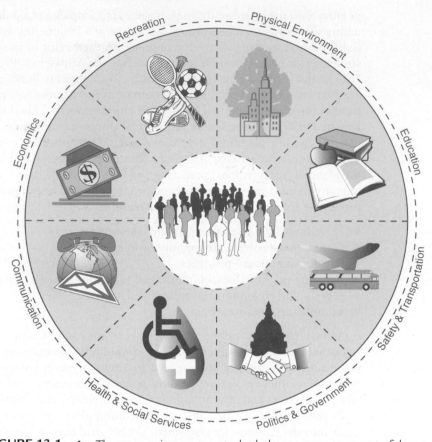

FIGURE 13-1 ◆ The community assessment wheel, the assessment segment of the community-as-partner model.

new members at different stages when different skills are needed. The benefits of teams are that the workload can be shared, more people can be reached, and a project can move ahead more quickly. The capacity of a team is enhanced by members' contacts and networks, and brainstorming exercises can assist with problem solving as the community process proceeds (Diem, 2005).

No matter how well-intended its members may be, the team will likely experience "growing pains" as it evolves and matures. Tuckman (1965; cited in Diem, 2005) found that teams go through four predictable stages as they develop: forming, storming, norming, and performing. Diem (2005) adds a fifth stage: ending (see Table 13-1), and suggests that the process of team development is not linear, and gaining or losing a member, making a major decision, or facing a particular challenge may cause the team to regress in its developmental stage before it can be productive again.

TABLE 13-1	
Five-stage Team Development Process	
STAGE	**CHARACTERISTICS**
Forming	When the team comes together, people are polite and agreeable and tend not to make clear statements of commitment. The primary tasks are to get to know each other, determine leadership, define the purpose of the team and the goals of its work as well as the skills and contributions of each member.
Storming	As the work begins, differences of opinion can arise, causing subgroups to form. At this point, it is natural to have some tension and perhaps conflict that emerges as challenging, detail and procedural haggling, and personal clashes. Conflicts must be brought into the open in helpful ways to avoid negative impacts later in the project.
Norming	As emotions cool down, practical rules of behaviour can be established, and the team can now focus on group cohesion and effective working relationships and processes.
Performing	This stage is a time of team productivity where members have assumed individual and collective responsibility for finishing the work. They agree on tasks ands processes, and most decisions are made by consensus.
Ending	As the project comes to an end, reports are finalized; loose ends and unfinished business are cleared up. Celebrations bring closure to the project, and while some people may mourn the "good times," the team adjourns its work.

Remember, the participation of community members is important at all stages of the community-as-partner process. In fact, assessment is the first stage in building capacity as community members become involved in the various tasks associated with the assessment part of the process. True partnership and full collaboration will evolve as community members gain confidence and competence throughout the process. The ability of community members to contribute will vary at different points in time, by what their formal and informal positions are in the community, by what skills they can contribute, and by what is needed by the team.

The outcome of a community assessment is a realistic profile of the community, its people, and its subsystems that allows a meaningful determination of strengths and capacities as well as an identification of risks to population aggregates and the environment. Assessment goes beyond documenting types of needs—it also helps to examine why the needs are occurring, the prevalence and urgency of concerns, and the capacity of the community to address the issues it faces and may point to some possible solutions.

GETTING TO KNOW THE COMMUNITY

One of the enduring challenges facing the team is the entry into the community and access to people with information. In many cases, team members will be outsiders—they will not live in the community of interest or they may not be "of" the population of interest. It is necessary to get to know the people, how the community is organized formally and informally, and to build rapport and trust. Sometimes, being an agent of an organization is helpful in entering the community; other times, it may be an impediment. For instance, the school nurse may be a valued outsider with a history of positive engagement in the community who will be accepted more readily than a probation officer who may be perceived as a punitive force and a person to be avoided. Building trust and rapport takes time; often, teams do not allow enough time for this important process. How can this process be facilitated?

1. Select a spokesperson or lead agency that already has a relationship with the community.
2. Make contact with the formal community leaders.
3. Be physically present, available, and visible in the community.
4. Engage with people in nonthreatening ways; be open and honest in your actions.
5. Communicate—keep the people involved in decisions and processes.

In particular, sites and moments for informal dialogue can be created through informal, unstructured personal contacts (e.g., at coffee breaks). For this reason, early in the process, personal contacts and interviews are critical to a smooth entry into the community and open access to informants and information sources.

A letter of introduction or a proposal for the assessment may be needed to gain access to formal community leaders (sometimes called *gatekeepers*), reports, and official data. The team needs to have a clear message that states the purpose of the investigation, what it will require of the community, and what benefits it will have to the people involved.

You might also call or participate in formal meetings during the assessment process. An agenda will help the team to keep on task and keep track of items that need to be discussed and who will speak to them. Handouts help attendees follow your presentation and keep track of decisions. Remember to keep lists of contacts from meetings (both formal and informal) with contact information and their relationship to the project for future reference. It is a courtesy to follow meetings with letters of thanks to the chair for giving you time to meet with them or, if you have called the meeting, to attendees for their participation and contribution to your efforts. Remember to file the minutes and make an action list of what you agreed to do by what date; this will be helpful to you when you are trying to remember to whom you promised to send reports at the end of the project!

Role of Team Members in the Community

Will team members be participants in or observers of community life? If present, team members may be asked for their contributions to community decisions, may be requested for advance notice of the assessment findings, or be made to feel somewhat uncomfortable. If any team members are "of" the community or population, they may be perceived to have a privileged position. Regardless, the presence of the assessment team will have an influence on the community; care must be taken to ensure ethical practice and minimize any potential for bias.

TABLE 13-2	
Problems Commonly Encountered in Community Assessment, With Suggested Solutions	
ISSUE	**STRATEGY**
Boundaries for data sets do not match	Making inferences regarding the boundaries used for data and determining their accuracy by interview with key informants
Reluctance to report derogatory data	Emphasize the importance of veracity in the context of assessment
Conflicting opinions among vested-interest groups within the community	Ongoing sharing and analysis of information among team members so that all data are noted and discussed
Insider versus outsider views of various community issues	Make certain that various perspectives are obtained during collection data

Inevitably, something will go wrong. When this happens, it is important to recognize it immediately and take action to rebuild relationships and re-establish the momentum of the assessment. Barton and colleagues (1993) suggest that a systematic analysis of issues related to assessment is needed to avoid pitfalls in the process or to choose strategies that will minimize their impact. Issues related to data generation and strategies to address them are summarized in Table 13-2.

The team may encounter barriers during the entry phase (e.g., resistance to collecting or providing information and impatience about collecting information instead of "doing something"). It is important to cultivate relationships among key community stakeholders, gatekeepers, and champions to ensure a smooth process.

PLANNING THE ASSESSMENT

To be useful for planning, intervention, and evaluation purposes, a community assessment must be based on the best data available—data that are reliable, accurate, and complete. Many methods can be used effectively to gather information; no single method is perfect, so a team will use a variety of means to get a complete picture of a community or an aggregate within the population.

McDevitt and Wilbur (2002) outline three main sources of community data:

1. Sociodemographic and vital statistics data (e.g., census reports, registry reports)
2. Archival materials (e.g., specific reports previously commissioned)
3. Original data collected specifically for the assessment (e.g., windshield surveys, key informant interviews, participant observation, photovoice methods, questionnaire surveys)

Patton (1990) classifies data as numerical or nonnumerical. Numerical data can be analyzed statistically and displayed graphically. It can be used to calculate rates and other measures that have meaning to population health. Although numerical data have many advantages in terms of reliability, validity, understandability, and comparability over time, they do not provide a full picture of the community. Non-numerical data provide depth and detail to statistics and allow us to interpret the beliefs, values, opinions, and culture of the community or population aggregate. They provide the context that situates the numerical data in its unique setting. Used together with community stories and history, both types of data provide a comprehensive community profile that can be used in planning health and social programs.

Edwards and Moyer (2000) provide a summary of health indicators, data sources, and health status reports that can be used in community assessments (p. 425–427). Depending on the purpose of your assessment and the nature of your information needs, the Internet can be an excellent resource along with the published literature and unpublished local reports.

Data are often categorized as primary or secondary. Primary data are composed of information from direct sources specifically for the project—key informant interview data, specific health utilization data, local survey data, and the like. Secondary data on the other hand are data from sources that collect, store, and report certain information on a routine basis—census, vital statistics, notifiable disease reports, social services reports, crime statistics, education system reports, regional social surveys, local research reports, historical documents, and so on. Often, a review of the literature about the topic or population group of interest, using for example the determinants of health as a framework, can help to clarify certain aspects of the project. The review will help the team to see what information already exists in the research literature, policy documents and elsewhere so that appropriate data collection can be planned to address gaps in knowledge and make the assessment locally relevant. Teams run the risk of attempting to find out "everything" about the focus of the assessment rather than determining what is absolutely necessary to learn and what is "nice to know" but not essential. If you had unlimited time and unlimited resources, you could perhaps do and learn more—but more often than not, there are time limits and budget restrictions to be considered. Hence, clearly defining the focus of the assessment, its purpose, and expected outcomes will allow the team to refine a work plan and time line that is realistic and feasible while still allowing time to incorporate community participation.

Before actual data collection begins, the team must prepare itself. It is important that, early in the process, the team agrees on the purposes of the assessment, the goals it wants to achieve, the framework it will use to organize the assessment, and the questions it seeks to answer. Often, team members do not normally work together, so a purposeful team-building process is important to a successful process and outcome. Dimock and Devine (1994) have a series of booklets that suggest how a work team can make itself effective by setting standards of operation and behaviour that allow the group to operate and maintain itself. The team needs to determine how it will function: how often and where it will meet, who will chair or lead, how people will communicate, and how team members will divide the work. A work plan that sets the time lines, delineates responsibilities, and estimates resources required for each activity will guide the team and keep it on track. Minutes of meetings and decisions will remind people of commitments. Occasionally, taking the "pulse" of the group in terms of self-reflection is helpful to minimize conflicts and ensure member satisfaction and enthusiasm.

It is essential in community work that members of the population group of interest are included in the process. Efforts to recruit and retain community people on working teams may be challenging. Community work is not completed quickly, thus making time commitment, travel costs, child care costs, and other considerations important to volunteers. The team must agree to commit resources to supporting and sustaining the involvement of community people in its efforts.

Parks and Straker (1996) caution that much of what is assessed in community work traditionally focuses on problems, barriers, needs, and weaknesses rather than on the strengths or "assets" of a community or its aggregates. We need to be as aware of a community's "possibilities" as we are of its issues to avoid portraying a negative image that can, according to Kretzman and McKnight (1993), have devastating effects on the community.

The key task of the assessment team at this point is to define the scope of the assessment. Will the focus be on a geographic community? Is there evidence of an issue that needs to be further investigated? Or, will the team focus on a particular aggregate? See Table 13-3 for examples of assessment questions for each of these foci. The team will want to understand the rationale for the assessment and the events that lead up to it. The team will also want to understand the goal of the assessment in order to appreciate what others expect from the results—will the report lead to the planning of interventions on the issue, for a population group, or in a community setting? Understanding the purpose for the assessment project will assist the team in clarifying its parameters. Further, understanding the goals and values of the agencies/groups that support the project will often provide some direction for the team with respect to the focus and scope for the assessment.

METHODS OF DATA COLLECTION

Before you begin assessing a community, the team needs to know what information it needs to meet its objectives, where that information can be found, and how it will be collected and organized. All methods of collecting information have strengths and weaknesses. All involve some ethical issues that need to be considered. No one method will give complete information; therefore, multiple methods are recommended, and triangulation of information from one source to another, one type of data to another, and from different methods is needed to ensure the veracity of any inferences or conclusions drawn. Assessment team members are cautioned about jumping to early conclusions without substantiating data. Additional information and specific instructions for each method presented here can be located in Gilmore

TABLE 13-3	
Examples of Community Assessment Questions	
QUESTION	TYPICAL DATA SOURCES
General community profile: What are the characteristics, structure, and history of this community? What geographical features distinguish this community? What are the concerns, agendas, and recent civic actions of this community?	*Secondary sources*: Census, economic development data, social services information, social indicators, historical data, newspapers, minutes of community meetings, or municipal council publications.
Health/wellness assessment: What is the level of health and illness, injury, or disability in the community? What is the wellness level of its residents?	*Secondary sources*: Epidemiologic studies. Health data sources including health status, injury incidence, and health care utilization statistics including pharmaceutical sales.
Health risk profile: What are the behavioural, social, and environmental risks to the population and/or special groups?	*Primary sources*: Targeted surveys, telephone surveys, key informant interviews, and group discussions. *Secondary sources*: National/provincial population health surveys, local health screening surveys, risk factor studies, special registries (e.g., injury, disease specific).
Community health promotion survey: What programs, resources, and provider groups already exist? What is the level of participation in these programs? What are barriers to participation? What possibilities exist for partnership? In what areas are there gaps to be addressed?	*Primary sources*: Key informants from provider organizations and members of the population of interest. *Secondary sources*: National, provincial, and local population health promotion surveys and databases, community resource guides, and local inventories.
Specialized studies: What special target groups exist? Who are the gatekeepers—will they help or hinder the project? Who can facilitate diffusion of program messages? What do these groups want to do?	*Primary sources*: Systematic surveys, key informant interviews, contact (interview, survey) with organizational managers, contact with influential people or groups (champions). Community asset mapping activities.

Adapted from Rissel, C., & Bracht, N. (1995). Assessing community needs, resources, and readiness: Building on strengths. In N. Bracht (Ed.), *Health promotion at the community level: New advances* (p. 65). Thousand Oaks: Sage.

and Campbell (1996) if the team wants to develop and practise the skills and competencies needed for completing a community assessment.

Observation

Observation methods range from being totally unobtrusive to being a full participant in the community. The observer is trying to understand the social setting and lives of the people in the community by observing or participating in events that occur in everyday life. Observation is particularly effective if the team members are outsiders and not familiar with the culture of the community or population group. Obviously, a combined approach allows trust and rapport to build, whereas full observation does not allow for data interpretation. Full participation may not permit an objective distance from which to reflect on meanings. Regardless, preparation is necessary to carry out observational surveys:

1. Establish written guidelines about what to observe.
2. Determine the locations for observations.

3. Decide on the length of observation periods.
4. Assess and determine the methods for recording observations (i.e., some are more obtrusive than others but offer better opportunity for team analysis).
5. Gather equipment to record observations (e.g., audio recorder or video camera, tapes, extra batteries, checklist, writing tools and paper for field notes).
6. Ensure that any required permissions have been obtained.
7. Plan for creating systematic field notes and for their transcription.
8. Plan debriefing sessions with the team.
9. Use an analytic journal for decision-making and interpretation.

Windshield or walking surveys are other observational techniques. Using this type of observation, team members make use of a variety of physical senses to capture the essence of a community, determine areas for further investigation, and sense the tone of the community. It is also useful in observing the physical spaces where population groups of interest meet and interact. Table 13-4 provides a guide for undertaking a windshield survey. In the first column, key points of interest are listed, with suggested questions to ask as you experience the community. Column 2 provides space to capture your observations, and in column 3, space is provided for you to take note of information as you gather it. This chart then becomes part of the raw data that you will analyse in the next step of the process.

Preparation for a walking or windshield survey includes mapping out a route, having a checklist (e.g., Table 13-4) from which to work, finding a means to record findings and reactions (e.g., audiovisual recording), a map to chart locations and make reference to field recordings, and proper equipment for the outdoor conditions (e.g., walking shoes, hats, sunscreen, identification, etc.). It is advisable to conduct walking or windshield surveys in teams of two for safety purposes and to have mobile communication devices available. Refrain from taking pictures of people, particularly children. Observations need to be made at different times of the day and different days of the week to fully capture the life of a community. Be prepared to explain your presence to community residents if challenged—have your identification and a statement of your project with contact information available to hand out. And remember, use all five senses (and maybe also your sixth sense—intuition) as you observe (Box 13-1).

Key Informant Interview

There are people in the community who have much to offer an assessment team. They have perhaps lived there for a long time or are members of an aggregate of interest. Others may be in leadership positions (e.g., community association executive) or may serve the community in some capacity (e.g., police, fire, health and social services personnel, business people, school personnel). Their insights can be helpful in interpreting statistical findings or in offering information that other methods cannot capture. A variety of views and opinions can be obtained through key informant interviews that can be considered to reflect the views of the community at large (Conway, Hu, & Harrington, 1997).

TABLE 13-4 Windshield/Walking Survey		
I. COMMUNITY CORE	**OBSERVATIONS**	**DATA**
1. History—What can you glean by looking (e.g., old, established neighbourhoods; new subdivision)? Ask people willing to talk: How long have you lived here? Has the area changed? As you talk, ask if there is an "old-timer" who knows the history of the area.		
2. Demographics—What sorts of people do you see? Young? Old? Homeless? Alone? Families? Is the population homogeneous?		
3. Ethnicity—Do you note indicators of different ethnic groups (e.g., restaurants, festivals)? What signs do you see of different cultural groups?		
4. Values and beliefs—Are there churches, mosques, temples? Are there signs of diversity? Are the lawns cared for? With flowers? Gardens? Signs of art? Culture? Heritage? Historical markers?		
II. SUBSYSTEMS		
1. Physical environment—How does the community look? What do you note about air quality, flora, housing, zoning, space, green areas, animals, people, human-made structures, natural beauty, water, climate? Can you find or develop a map of the area? What is the size (e.g., square kilometers, blocks)?		
2. Health and social services—Evidence of acute or chronic conditions? Shelters? Alternative therapists/healers? Are there clinics, hospitals, practitioners' offices, public health services, home health agencies, emergency centres, nursing homes, social service facilities, mental health services? Are there resources outside the community but readily accessible to residents?		
3. Economy—Is it a "thriving" community, or does it feel "seedy"? Are there industries, stores, places for employment? Where do people shop? Are there signs that people can find employment (e.g., Help Wanted signs, classified ads)? Are there signs of thrift stores, pawn shops, and other services for people with money issues? How active is the food bank?		
4. Transportation and safety—How do people get around? What type of private and public transportation is available? Do you see buses, bicycles, taxis? Are there sidewalks, bike trails? Is getting around in the community possible for people with disabilities? What types of protective services are there (e.g., fire, police, sanitation)? Is air quality monitored? What types of crimes are committed? Do people feel safe? Are there signs of racism or intolerance?		
5. Politics and government—Are there signs of political activity (e.g., posters, meetings)? What party affiliation predominates? What is the governmental jurisdiction of the community (e.g., elected mayor, city council with single member districts)? Are people involved in decision-making in their local governmental unit?		

TABLE 13-4		
Windshield/Walking Survey (Continued)		
II. SUBSYSTEMS	**OBSERVATIONS**	**DATA**
6. Communication—Are there "common areas" where people gather? What newspapers do you see in the stands? Do people have TVs, mobile music devices, cell phones? What do they watch/listen to? What are the formal and informal means of communication?		
7. Education—Are there schools, universities, technical institutes, arts education in the area? How do they look? Are there libraries? Is there a local board of education? How does it function? What is the reputation of the school(s)? What are major educational issues? What are the dropout rates? Are extracurricular activities available? Are they used? Is there a school health service? A school nurse? Are there adult education and second-language programs readily available?		
8. Recreation—Where do children play? What are the major forms of recreation? Who participates? What facilities for recreation do you see? Are they in good order or disrepair? Are there signs that pets are welcome? What about the performing arts and social and other leisure activities (festivals, zoo, museums, sports teams, etc.)?		
III. PERCEPTIONS		
1. The residents—How do people feel about the community? What do they identify as its strengths? Problems? Ask several people from different groups (e.g., old, young, unskilled/skilled workers, service worker, professional, clergy, stay-at-home parent, lone parent), and keep track of who gives what answer.		
2. Your perceptions—General statements about the "health" of this community. What are its strengths? What community or population-level problems or potential problems can you identify? Who are the gatekeepers to the community and/or population of interest? Who are the champions that might support your work? Who in the community might become a partner in the process? Where will resistance be found?		

Note: Supplement your impressions with information from the census, police records, school statistics, Chamber of Commerce data, health department reports, and so forth to confirm or refute your conclusions. Tables, graphs, and maps are helpful and will aid in your analysis.

Adapted from Anderson, E. T., & McFarlane, J. M. (2006). *Community as partner: Theory and practice in nursing.* (5th ed., p. 220–221), Philadelphia: Lippincott Williams & Wilkins.

BOX 13-1

Using Your Senses to Collect Information About the Community

Sight—condition of streets, sidewalks, playgrounds; age, sex, racial distributions, clothing, general health condition of the people; housing and services (e.g., schools, businesses) visible

Hearing—noise levels and sources of noise

Taste—types of food supply stores, variety and prices of foods, water quality

Smell—pollutants, odours, sanitation levels

Touch—climate, psychological sense of safety, feeling of openness or oppression, friendliness

---

To prepare for interviews, the team should meet to:

1. Determine who are the key people/positions that should be included in interviews.
2. Outline the focus of each informant's potential contribution.
3. Determine the structure, timing, and recording methods.
4. Outline the questions and prepare the interview guide.
5. Create the invitation to participate and design the process.
6. Set the times and venues for interviews.
7. Invite the key informants to be interviewed.
8. Send out confirmation letters with the 'rules of engagement' clearly specified.
9. Send letters of thanks after the interviews.

It is helpful to send the questions to interviewees in advance so that they can prepare themselves. Be certain to outline the purpose of your assessment and the outcomes you hope to achieve. Send only the questions to which you want their specific responses, not the entire community assessment tool. Offer them something tangible in return for their participation (e.g., an Executive Summary of the final report, an invitation to a presentation). As with all inquiry methods that involve humans, you must be sensitive to ethical issues and ensure that no harm comes to your participants. Make sure they know in advance that the interview will be audiotaped or that you will be keeping notes or both.

Be certain to choose interview sites that are comfortable, confidential, and quiet. Make certain your equipment works and also take notes in the event of an equipment failure. Respect when your interviewee wants to go "off the record." Telephone interviews or the use of electronic surveys may be preferable in some instances, particularly if the questions are very structured or a key informant is not able to attend an interview in person.

Analysis of key informant interviews entails teasing out the main themes and patterns in the responses and capturing the essence of any discussion, debate, or differing opinion. If interviews are transcribed, software can help to identify themes, but in small samples, this may not be necessary.

Focus Groups

Focus groups are not intended to be group interviews in which new data are collected. Instead, they are best used when data themes have emerged from other sources and the team wants to add to the understanding of each theme and determine if they include a complete and accurate picture of community perspectives. Hence, focus group participants are limited to 8 to 12 homogeneous people (i.e., they share certain characteristics) with a variety of perspectives to facilitate in-depth discussion in an informal atmosphere where participants are encouraged to explore issues and express opinions freely. Focus group participants build on the comments of others and come to conclusions not considered individually. Additionally, it is possible to reach consensus about key issues and rank-order issues in terms of priority for action.

Focus group interviews need similar preparation as the key informant process. As well, skilled and unobtrusive facilitators are required to elicit the best information, ask open-ended questions, draw out reticent people, and keep the meeting on track with the stated objectives. Focus group interviews are usually audiotaped for later analysis, but a note-taker is important as well to assess interactions and keep track of points raised. It is important that results not be generalized to the whole population because the participants are not selected to be representative of the population.

There is more information on conducting focus groups in the literature that the team may find helpful (Hawe, Degeling, & Hall, 1990; Morgan & Kreuger, 1997).

Surveys and Questionnaires

Surveys can be used to collect information from people to supplement data from other sources, update information (e.g., demographic), solicit opinions (e.g., satisfaction, beliefs), assess risks (e.g., behaviours), and document exposure to various hazards (e.g., sexual harassment, pollutants). Information may be collected from people by questionnaires or surveys. Surveys can be in person (e.g., door-to-door, telephone) or in writing (e.g., mail-in). If administration methods are properly carried out and the instruments are valid, a survey can be relatively inexpensive in terms of the amount and quality of data collected for the expenditure of time and resources.

The following issues must be considered when planning to conduct a survey:

◆ *Purpose*. Knowing the goal of the survey will help to decide which format to use, the target for the survey, and how many people to include in the sample.
◆ *Resources*. Conducting a survey will use people, time, money, and support services to create the questionnaire, pilot test it, reproduce it, administer it, and do follow-up data entry, analyze, and report the data.
◆ *Information needed*. Instruments to collect data need to be sensitive (i.e., not intrusive), reliable, and valid. Developing or choosing a questionnaire that consistently measures what it is supposed to measure takes time and expertise.

◆ *Format*. Open-ended questions will provide richer data (e.g., unique perspectives) than fixed response questions (e.g., true–false, multiple choice, 1–5 scale), but they are more difficult to analyze.

◆ *Response rate*. In certain cases, a representative sample whose responses can be generalized to a wider population is desirable. At other times, the survey may need to reach everyone in a target group. Different methods to collect data and improve response rates may be used to ensure that the findings are not biased.

◆ *Training*. People who administer the survey need to be trained so that there is consistency among them. Data need to be recorded and input appropriately to facilitate analysis.

◆ *Analysis*. Responses to open-ended questions are analyzed thematically, seeking patterns and themes in the data. Results of fixed-response surveys are easily put into electronic form and analyzed statistically.

It is beyond the scope of this text to teach survey research, but excellent references are available to support the assessment team. As well, you may want to seek out the expertise of a statistician and appropriate software programs to support both qualitative and quantitative analysis.

Population Data

Several forms of data are collected in the course of everyday life: census, vital statistics, morbidity and mortality statistics, population health surveys, records of community services and schools, clinic records, screening records, environmental information (e.g., air and water quality), and the like. Many of these are in the public domain, but issues like confidentiality, data access, and quality of data must be assessed.

Population data can be used to establish baselines for the purposes of making comparisons, determining which indicators have enough support for their use, and setting benchmarks for measuring progress on goals and objectives, and when combined with critical reviews of the literature, they can be used to make program-related decisions.

Local data are often available from the municipality, health and social services departments, chamber of commerce, and similar groups in reports and on websites. As well, government ministries at both the provincial and national levels release population status reports that are available in local libraries or on the Internet. Health Canada regularly conducts a National Population Health Survey and makes reports available to the public. Statistics Canada also releases reports on population issues that may be of interest to the team for comparison purposes.

Other Assessment Strategies

The preceding is not an exhaustive list of mechanisms that can be used to collect information about a population or community. Other methods can be found described in the literature (for an example of photovoice technique, see Chapters 19 and 24). Additionally, the literature can be critically examined as issues arise and potential target populations surface. The team must meet frequently during data collection to share information and determine the scope and depth needed for analysis. Community members can be helpful in suggesting sources for further information (particularly regarding historical or recent events) and in providing evidence of community capacity and assets.

ELEMENTS OF A COMMUNITY ASSESSMENT

Begin by identifying your community. A system is a whole that functions because of the interdependence of its parts. A community, too, is a whole entity that functions because of the interdependence of its parts, or subsystems. The community assessment wheel (see Fig. 13-1) will be your overall framework. Five communities in downtown Calgary, Alberta, will be used to illustrate the use of the model in conducting a community assessment (as well as subsequent analysis, diagnosis, planning, intervention, and evaluation). Although we have chosen an urban community defined by census tracts, the guide can be used to assess *any* community, regardless of size, location, resources, or population characteristics. It can also be used to assess a "community within a community" such as a school, an industry, or a business. Examples of these communities are included in Part III of this book and in Appendices A and B. In addition, this guide can be used to assess a subpopulation, group, or aggregate (i.e., a defined group within the community [e.g., teenagers, lone parents, people of an ethnic group of interest, people living with a particular condition]) by providing the context in which this group is found. The *process* of assessment, regardless of where it is applied, always remains the same.

The use of a model to guide the assessment of a community, neighbourhood, population, or an aggregate assists with the organization of the process and of the data collected. This section will examine the data that describes the core, the eight subsystems, and the functions of the community according to the assessment wheel in Figure 13-1. The team may want to create its own process for data management or refer to Gerberich, Stearns, and Dowd (1995), who offer an assessment instrument with key questions for each subsystem that can be adapted to the community-as-partner model used here.

Take Note

Regarding information contained in tables throughout this chapter, our intention is to provide you with numbers, percentages, rates, and so on, along with their source. These figures, however, are for illustration only and do not necessarily reflect current data related to the areas where they are found. For your assessment, be sure to use the latest figures and include the date within the citation.

Community Core

The definition of *core* is "that which is essential, basic, and enduring." The core of a community is its people—their history, characteristics, values, and beliefs. The first stage of assessing a community, then, is to learn about its people to gain insight into their life experience. In fact, partnering with people in the community is an integral part of working with the community. Table 13-5 lists the major components of the community core along with suggested locations and sources of information about each component. Because every community is different, information sources available to one community may not be available to another.

The community core is described through information on sociodemographic, economic, and cultural variables and factors that describe social support. Lifestyle factors, employment patterns, resource production and consumption, and population-level personal health behaviours help to understand the people of the community and how their values influence the choices made. Indices of social cohesion or isolation, examples of stigma, prejudice or bullying, and predominant values and attitudes toward diversity are also signals of the health of the core/population of interest.

TABLE 13-5	
Community Core Data	
COMPONENTS	**SOURCES OF INFORMATION**
History	Library, historical society, museum, newpaper archives
	Interview "old-timers," town leaders
Demographics	Census of population and housing
Age and sex characteristics	Planning board (local, county, province)
Racial distribution	Chamber of Commerce
Ethnic distribution	City Hall, archives
	Observation
Household types by	Census (municipal, national)
Family	
Nonfamily	
Group	
Marital status by	Census (municipal, national)
Single	
Separated	
Widowed	
Divorced	
Vital statistics	Local and provincial departments of health (distributed through
Births	health department reports and websites)
Deaths by	
Age	
Leading causes	
Values and beliefs	Personal contact
	Observation ("Learning About the Community on Foot")
	(To protect against stereotyping, avoid the literature for this portion
	of the assessment.)
Religion	Observation
	Telephone book

To illustrate a community assessment, we will use examples from Calgary, Alberta. In the following sections of this chapter, data will be used to demonstrate what an assessment team might learn as it engages in the community-as-partner process.

In the summer of 1875, 50 members of the North West Mounted Police, sent to stop the whiskey trade and bring law and order to the West, arrived at the junction of the Bow and Elbow rivers to establish a new fort. Fort Calgary, named by Colonel MacLeod, became the Town of Calgary (pop. 1,000) in the Northwest Territories in 1884 and a city (pop. 3,900) in 1894, predating the creation of Alberta as a province in 1905. Situated at the gateway to the Rockies, Calgary was changed by the Canadian Pacific Railway from a frontier town to a major supply station. Although its beginnings were in fur trade, farming, and ranching, Calgary later became the hub of the petroleum industry and is famous for the Calgary Stampede "The Greatest Outdoor Show on Earth." Today, it is a thriving and vibrant city of nearly 1 million people.

Throughout its history, health and social services developed along with the city. Federal and provincial jurisdictions governed how human services were delivered, and municipalities filled complementary roles to protect the health and well-being of their residents. Over time, the organization of the systems of health and social services delivery became cumbersome, and in 1995, the province of Alberta restructured its health care delivery system and created 17 regional health authorities from over 200 separate boards that managed hospital, health units, and long-term care settings. Each health authority was responsible for amalgamating hospital, long-term care, emergency services, and community health and home care. Social services, children's services, mental health services, and other provincial services (e.g., tuberculosis and sexually transmitted infections) were also realigned over time to match health authority boundaries. In anticipation of this reorganization, a community needs assessment was carried out in 1994.

For the purposes of illustrating the process (from assessment to evaluation), 5 of 15 inner-city communities in Calgary, Alberta, will be described and used to demonstrate an application of the community-as-partner model. Fifteen communities were selected for the initial community assessment, representing approximately 51,380 residents (7.2% of the city's total population of 713, 610). An estimated 86,000 additional people come to the downtown area every day to work or to use services, and day care is provided to 2,500 children. The unique profile of each neighbourhood was obscured when the downtown area as a whole was considered. The five communities (of the original 15 in the study) that will be described and compared in this example are Bankview, Connaught, Victoria Park, Bridgeland, and Inglewood. Data from the most recent years from the following sources were used: Census Canada, City of Calgary, Alberta Environment, and Alberta Health. More complete and recent reports are available from the Calgary Health Region.

To begin the process, experienced community workers find it helpful to write thumbnail sketches that succinctly describe the community or communities of interest. In this case, we are assessing geopolitical communities (or neighbourhoods); their descriptions are found in Table 13-6.

TABLE 13-6
Community Descriptions

COMMUNITY	DESCRIPTION
Bankview (BNK)	In 1882, the land that became Bankview was purchased by an English immigrant for farming and ranching. In the early 1900s, the land was subdivided along a traditional grid pattern for housing development. Its character changed from low density in the 1950s to allow walk-up apartment buildings and now offers a diversity of housing units and an inner-city lifestyle. There are no schools in this community.
Connaught (CON)	In 1893, the city limits included the Connaught district that encompassed large estates of prominent citizens. By 1912, development had extended south and west with 2- and 3-story homes, treed boulevards, and large open spaces. Many of the city's first fine institutions (religious, educational, cultural) were located here. The character of the area has changed dramatically through the years, with the addition of many medium- and high-density commercial office buildings, apartments, and condominiums. There is one community elementary school (public).
Victoria Park (VIC)	This community predates Calgary's incorporation as a town. Named after Queen Victoria, the community prospered in its early days because of its proximity to Fort Calgary, the railroad station, and the developing downtown. By 1902, 83% of the existing structures had been built and by the 1950s and 1960s VIC found itself hemmed in by transportation corridors, so the community began to lose its appeal as a residential community. With the expansion of the Calgary Stampede and Exhibition in the 1970s, the construction of the Saddledome in the 1980s, and continuing rumours of further expansion, the community is under significant threat and even a neighbourhood improvement program has failed to revitalize the community. There is one public charter school.
Bridgeland (BRD)	This area, located across the Bow River, was enhanced in 1885 with the construction of the Langevin Bridge. It was annexed to the city in 1910. For many new Canadians, Bridgeland became their first home, originally Germans and Italians and more recently Vietnamese. There are two public schools (elementary and junior) and one separate school (elementary).
Inglewood (ING)	Calgary's oldest community, dating back to the late 1800s, located where the Bow and Elbow rivers join. People were attracted to the community by its industry (Burns Stockyards and Cross Brewery) and its proximity to the Fort. One environmentally sensitive industrial site (refinery) is located away from the residential area but could affect future development. Its residential community is low to medium density, and many projects are under way to restore its historical landmarks. It has one community elementary school.

Population Description

TOTAL POPULATION

Knowing the total number of people living in a neighbourhood or in a group of neighbourhoods allows the community worker to make certain judgements and comparisons between and among communities. Information that allows us to understand the elements of the community core is found in sociodemographic data that are often captured in the census. Table 13-7 provides an overview of the number of people residing in each of the communities that we are discussing.

TABLE 13-7	
Number of People Residing in Each Community	
NEIGHBOURHOOD	**POPULATION**
BNK	5,175
CON	11,115
VIC	4,755
BRD	4,685
ING	4,028

The five example communities have a population of 29,758, or 58% of the 15 downtown communities described in the initial study and 4.2% of the total population of the city. The communities are geographically arranged from west to east, with natural boundaries of the two rivers (Fig. 13-2). Description of the 5 communities will be compared with the "downtown" 15 (DT15) communities and to the city as a whole for the purposes of analysis (see Chapter 14).

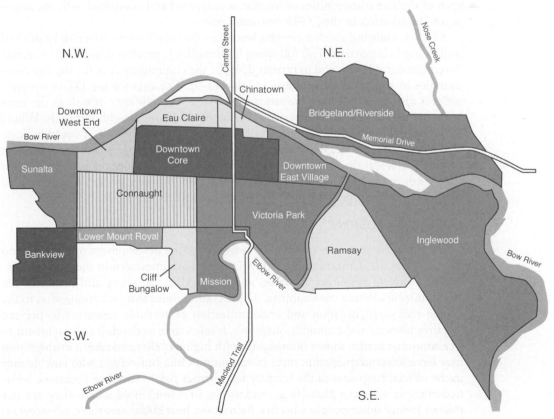

FIGURE 13-2 ◆ Map of 15 downtown Calgary communities.

TABLE 13-8

Percent of Community Population by Age Group

AGE	BNK	CON	VIC	BRD	ING	DT15
0–4 y	5.7	2.7	4.5	6.3	5.7	3.8
5–14 y	4.4	2.8	4.1	5.7	8.0	3.6
15–19 y	3.9	3.2	5.0	3.6	5.1	3.7
20–24 y	18.1	15.7	14.6	8.9	8.2	14.1
25–44 y	52.2	48.7	44.0	38.0	41.0	46.7
45–64 y	10.3	15.0	15.5	13.2	18.6	15.1
65+ y	5.4	11.8	12.3	24.3	13.3	13.6

AGE DISTRIBUTION

How a population is apportioned by age often provides important clues to potential issues that might be faced. For example, a neighbourhood with a high proportion of seniors will need different services and resources than a neighbourhood where young children predominate. In Table 13-8, the percent of age groups in each of the five communities of interest is presented and compared with the population distribution in the DT15 communities.

Further, knowing about some characteristics that can have an effect on health and well-being is important. The following information is presented to examine certain determinants of health and to further describe the community core for the five communities in which we are interested (Table 13-9). The data for the DT15 communities is also presented for comparison purposes. The raw data as well as the rates are provided to facilitate comparisons between and among neighbourhoods. Where rates are high, or higher in comparison to other neighbourhoods, it could indicate a concern; for instance, the youth unemployment rate in Inglewood is double that of the DT15 and three other communities. However, Bridgeland is markedly less (one tenth of the DT15 rate). Before taking action, however, more data are needed to analyze and interpret the meaning of these numbers.

SOCIAL INCLUSION

Geopolitical communities provide opportunity for the development of informal and formal social ties. Communities with people who are interested in their neighbourhoods, aware of resources available, and involved in the safety and health of the community are strong communities. Those communities that lack connection to the people risk social isolation and underutilization of available resources to prevent negative physical and economic outcomes. It takes time to develop an attachment to a community; hence, those communities with high mobility and recent in-migration may have lower participation rates in community life. Individuals who lack fluency in the official languages of the country face further risk of social or economic isolation. People who live alone (e.g., seniors) or in a household where they are not related to any other people who live there must bear social and financial stress on

TABLE 13-9						
Selected Sociodemographic Characteristics						
	BNK	**CON**	**VIC**	**BRD**	**ING**	**DT15**
Seniors living alone	125	685	365	285	125	3,435
(rate per 100 seniors)	(44.6)	(52.3)	(62.4)	(25.0)	(38.5)	(49.7)
Unemployed youth	110	190	115	70	85	930
(rate per 100 youth)	(9.7)	(9.2)	(11.4)	(1.3)	(22.7)	(11.5)
Unemployed adults (>25 y)	285	500	350	235	115	2,855
(rate per 100 adults 25+)	(8.0)	(6.0)	(10.5)	(7.9)	(6.5)	(7.4)
Lone-parent families	230	265	175	235	100	1,670
(rate per 100 families)	(49.5)	(45.2)	(44.9)	(45.6)	(32.8)	(45.5)
Persons in low-income households	1,750	3,870	2,365	1,595	840	19,020
(rate per 100 total population)	(34.0)	(35.6)	(51.6)	(39.6)	(43.4)	(40.6)
Home language not English	400	1,505	1,110	460	150	7,165
(rate per 100 total population)	(7.8)	(13.9)	(23.9)	(11.5)	(6.1)	(18.4)
Recent immigrants (past 5 y)	270	1,005	595	120	55	3,625
(rate per 100 immigrants)	(24.9)	(37.0)	(37.2)	(11.3)	(15.1)	(24.1)
Persons moved in past year	2,350	4,915	1,970	1,215	620	20,155
(rate per 100 population >1 y)	(45.9)	(45.3)	(43.1)	(30.7)	(25.5)	(37.0)
Persons moved in past 5 y	3,965	8,835	3,435	2,360	1,230	36,425
(rate per 100 population >5 y)	(76.5)	(79.5)	(72.1)	(50.4)	(50.1)	(70.9)
Education < secondary certificate (16+)	1,190	2,505	1,885	1,355	1,000	14,340
(rate per 100 population 16+)	(25.4)	(24.2)	(43.6)	(38.4)	(46.4)	(34.8)
Median household income	23,824	27,054	15,980	23,419	27,644	36,524

Note: Median household income for the city is $44,064

their own. Furthermore, they are more likely to have incomes below the low-income cut off (LICO). Seniors and those with disabilities may also face difficulties accessing services due to their frailty. In Table 13-10, the percent of people who live on their own in the five downtown communities of Calgary is presented, compared with the percent of people who live alone in the city as a whole.

SUBSYSTEMS

A review of a community's subsystems tell us about the context in which people live, work, play, pray, and go to school. It provides insights into factors that influence how people live, what choices they make, and why. A subsystems analysis

TABLE 13-10						
Percent of People Living Alone in the Downtown Area						
	BNK	**CON**	**VIC**	**BRD**	**ING**	**CITY**
Percent of unattached individuals	51.5	53.1	53.4	36.6	34.4	14.9

focuses on the external environment such as the sociopolitical and economic contexts and the infrastructures of the community and how these have an impact on the population. When we assess the subsystems, we are seeking to find if there are any stressors acting on them and what flexible lines of defence (temporary responses) and lines of resistance (strengths) are in place to protect the core.

Physical Environment

Just as the physical examination is a critical component of assessing an individual patient, so it is in the assessment of a community. And just as the five senses of the clinician are called into play in the physical examination of a patient, so, too, are they needed at the community level.

It is important to collect information about where and how the community/population is situated within the physical space to understand how the various elements have an impact on community life (e.g., weather, terrain, placement of services, population density, diversity). Such information allows us to assess availability, affordability, appropriateness, acceptability, adequacy and access to services, housing, green space, and so forth and associated issues of safety, utilization, and community capacity.

In Calgary, Centre Street is the major north–south thoroughfare, and Memorial Drive on the north side of the Bow River and 9th Avenue on the south side are the major east–west routes. The railway traverses the borders of Inglewood, Victoria Park, and Connaught. The Exhibition Grounds are located in Victoria Park, the Bird Sanctuary and Fort Calgary Historic Site in Inglewood, and the Zoo in Bridgeland. In all areas, there are businesses along main streets and a mix of housing options. Inglewood and Bridgeland have a lower population density than the others; Connaught, with its large number of high- and low-rise apartments, has the highest density. Victoria Park is in a state of decay as the Stampede and the City pursue urban renewal options. Connaught and Victoria Park amalgamated in 2003 to become the "Beltline." Inglewood is undergoing a renaissance, with an active main street revitalization program that is giving rise to quaint bistros, antique shops, art galleries, and specialty boutiques. Because parking is at a premium in the downtown, residential streets are crowded, and through streets are often jammed during rush hours.

The climate is mild, with sunny summer days and cool evenings. Chinooks (**http://www.mountainnature.com/Climate/Chinook.htm**) temper the winter chill, and the mountain playgrounds are nearby for hiking, skiing, high-country sports, and artistic pursuits. The Calgary climate is termed *moderate*; descriptive statistics are located in Box 13-2.

There are bike and jogging trails throughout the downtown and along the scenic riverbanks. Stately trees planted to remember the soldiers of the two world wars shade Memorial Drive; small parks dot the downtown with green space. The Alexandra Community Centre is a gathering place for the community of Inglewood. Connaught has a public pool. Downtown residents are served by churches

---

BOX 13-2

Climate Description for Calgary, Alberta

Moderate Climate
Mean rainfall per year: 30.1 cm (11.8″)
Mean snowfall per year: 152.5 cm (60.0″)
Days with measurable snowfall: 62

Seasonal Temperatures
Summer (June–August): 20°C (68°F)
Fall (September–November): 11°C (52°F)
Winter (December–February): −11°C (10°F)
Spring (March–May): 9°C (42°F)

---

of a variety of denominations, public and separate schools, museums, galleries, fire and police services, banks, supermarkets, and a large library. The downtown also contains services for the homeless (Drop-In Centre, Calgary Urban Projects Society [CUPS], Mustard Seed, EXIT Outreach for street youth, among others). In some areas, particularly the Beltline community of Victoria Park, yellow mailboxes are placed around the neighbourhoods to serve as receptacles for used needles. In this area, the sex trade has been an ongoing problem, accompanied by drug trafficking, crime, and alcohol abuse. Residents complain that because of the proximity to the light rail transit system, events at the Exhibition Grounds, and downtown bars, sex trade workers use the area to attract customers from other parts of the city, disrupting community life and making the community unsafe in the evenings. The condition of houses in a neighbourhood is a physical sign that indicates community well-being. If people are not putting effort into home maintenance, it may be a symptom of concern when considered with other information during the analysis process. The following information is available from the census.

Health and Social Services

A review of this subsystem allows an assessment of the "social safety net" infrastructure and provides insight as to how basic needs are met in the community. The focus is on need and utilization—how is it met (availability, access, affordability) by services within and outside the community. Various sectors that provide health and services are included in the assessment (e.g., formal [government] and informal [volunteer], publicly funded, and private).

One method of classifying health and social services is to differentiate between facilities located outside the community (extracommunity) versus those within the community (intracommunity). Once the health and social service facilities are identified, group them into categories, perhaps by type of service offered (e.g., hospitals,

TABLE 13-11	
Health and Social Services	
COMPONENT	SOURCES OF INFORMATION
Health Services	
Extracommunity or intracommunity facilities.	Chamber of Commerce
Once identified, group into categories (e.g., hospitals and clinics, home health care, extended care facilities, public health services, emergency care).	Planning board (district, county, city) Phone directory
For each facility, collect data on	Talk to residents
1. Services (fees, hours, and new services planned and those discontinued)	Interview administrator or someone on the staff Facility annual report and websites
2. Resources (personnel, space, budget, and record system)	
3. Characteristics of users (geographic distribution, demographic profile, and transportation source)	
4. Statistics (number of persons served daily, weekly, and monthly)	
5. Adequacy, accessibility, and acceptability of facility according to users and providers	
Social Services	
Extracommunity or intracommunity facilities.	Chamber of Commerce
Once identified, group into categories (e.g., counseling and support, clothing, food, shelter, and special needs).	United Way directory Phone directory
For each facility, collect data on 1–5 listed above.	Municipality Nongovernmental agencies and associations

clinics, extended care), by size, or by public versus private usage. Table 13-11 suggests a classification system as well as possible major components of each facility requiring assessment.

DOWNTOWN HEALTH FACILITIES AND SOCIAL SERVICES

At the time of the original community assessment, there were two acute care hospitals in the downtown area, two large long-term care facilities, and a veterans' facility. One hospital has since been demolished and one sold to private interests; the veteran's hospital has been moved out of the community. The Alexandra Health Centre is located in Inglewood; the Children's Hospital, once located in Scarboro (next to Bankview) has been moved out of the downtown to the University campus in the northwest of the city. The District Public Health serves the downtown from City Hall but is slated to move to the new building on the site of the former veteran's hospital in the Beltline community of Connaught. Home care is provided from the Central Office in the downtown area. Several general practice, walk-in clinics, and specialists have offices in the downtown communities. Pharmacies, laboratory and radiology services, dental offices, and vision care centres are located throughout the inner-city area. The food bank and a thrift store are situated in the downtown core near the housing shelters and other social services. The Victorian

Order of Nurses provides wellness services in seniors' housing apartments and a foot clinic out of the veterans' hospital.

Also located in the downtown are the Sexually Transmitted Disease Clinic, Southern Alberta Clinic (HIV/AIDS), Family Planning Clinic, Travel Clinic, Communicable Diseases Unit, Salvation Army Mission, YWCA, and Crisis Services (violence, mental health), along with churches and community schools that offer social outreach programs, "Inn from the Cold" emergency shelter, hot meals, and clothing programs. Vans roam the streets in the evenings to provide needle-exchange services, hot beverages and sandwiches, minor health care, and counselling services to street-involved people. In total, 54 health-related services are located in the downtown area (Fig. 13-3).

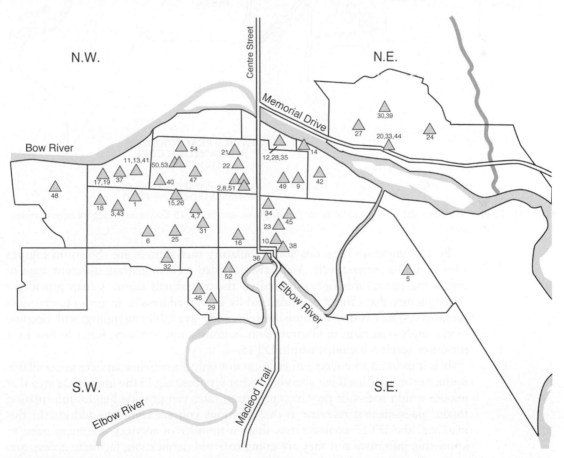

FIGURE 13-3   ◆   Map showing the location of health services in the 15 downtown Calgary communities.

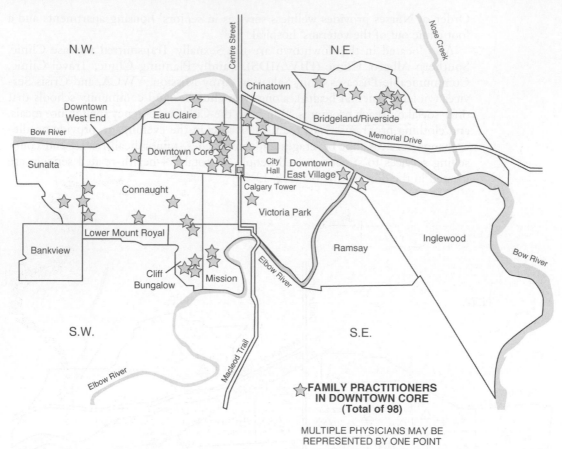

**FAMILY PRACTITIONERS
IN DOWNTOWN CORE
(Total of 98)**

MULTIPLE PHYSICIANS MAY BE
REPRESENTED BY ONE POINT

FIGURE 13-4 ◆ Map showing the location of family physicians in the 15 downtown Calgary communities.

Family physician locations and ambulatory care centres are shown on Figures 13-4 and 13-5, respectively. Maps are provided to demonstrate different ways of displaying the information gathered by the assessment team. A map provides a visual picture that cannot be illustrated by lists of addresses. As geographic information systems (GIS) become more readily available, mapping will become increasingly important to illustrate distributions across territory. Refer to Box 13-3 for other services included within DT15.

It is important to collect information not only about what services are available in the community itself but also about what services exist in the immediate area that people would access. If possible, utilization rates can provide helpful information to the assessment if relevant to the questions you are trying to address. In this instance, the DT15 communities share a number of services. Planners need to know this information if they are going to avoid duplication, facilitate access, and remove barriers or obstacles to utilization.

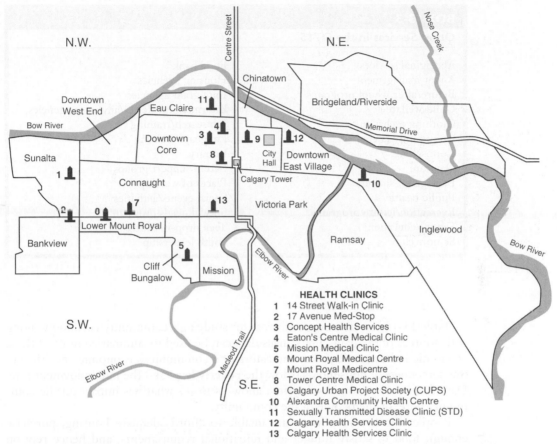

FIGURE 13-5 ◆ Ambulatory care centre locations in the 15 downtown communities.

HEALTH CLINICS
1   14 Street Walk-in Clinic
2   17 Avenue Med-Stop
3   Concept Health Services
4   Eaton's Centre Medical Clinic
5   Mission Medical Clinic
6   Mount Royal Medical Centre
7   Mount Royal Medicentre
8   Tower Centre Medical Clinic
9   Calgary Urban Project Society (CUPS)
10 Alexandra Community Health Centre
11 Sexually Transmitted Disease Clinic (STD)
12 Calgary Health Services Clinic
13 Calgary Health Services Clinic

Economics

The economic subsystem includes the "wealth" of a community—that is, the goods and services available to the community—as well as the costs and benefits of improving patterns of resource allocation. It should be evident that extra-community factors, such as the state of the national and world economies, affect in great measure the local economy. Nevertheless, intracommunity economic factors impinge on all other subsystems, so they must be included in the assessment.

The economy affects household finances through employment, business, and productivity, and measures that describe the labour force (e.g., employment rate, occupations) give insight into the "morale" of a population and the vitality of a community.

BOX 13-3

Other Services in the DT15

Aboriginal services	Food bank
Anger management	Housing agencies
Before/after school programs	Immigrant agencies
Child welfare	Information/referral/advocacy agencies
Clothing exchange	Job search/training
Community kitchen	Language training
Counselling	Library
Day care	Parent support groups
Emergency shelters	Places of worship
Public health	Social events/activities
Recreation/leisure programs	Special needs program
School/education	Teen drop-in centre
Seniors club	Youth leadership

Table 13-12 lists the suggested areas for studying a community's economy, along with sources of the data. The census data can be used to summarize most of these economic indicators. Two key indicators of a community's economic "health" are the percentage of households below the poverty level and the unemployment rate. Data from the economic subsystem allow us to see what has impact on the community core, or the people in the community.

People who live in poverty are unable to afford adequate housing, purchase enough food to satisfy hunger and nutritional requirements, and hence rely on social services for supplementary income, food banks for food, and thrift stores for clothing. When poverty becomes chronic, quality of life suffers, and in the long term, psychological consequences can have adverse effects on people, especially children and seniors. Seniors face a greater poverty risk because of their reliance on fixed incomes and the lack of employment opportunity. Seniors can receive a guaranteed income supplement (GIS), and families living in poverty may receive support for independence (SFI) (Table 13-13).

BUSINESS

Since the discovery of oil and gas in nearby Turner Valley in 1914, Calgary has become known as the energy capital of Canada. Building on that strength, the city's economy has diversified to include major activity in manufacturing, transportation, logistics, hi-tech, construction, tourism, and financial services. It is this diversity that has kept the city growing steadily and makes for a positive future of opportunity and prosperity. Calgary's traditional oil industry cycle of boom and bust has given way to the modern, international, technology-intensive operations of today.

TABLE 13-12	
Indicators and Sources of Information	
INDICATORS	**SOURCE**
Financial Characteristics	
Households	
Median household income	
% households below poverty level	
% households receiving public assistance	Census records
% households headed by females	
Monthly costs for owner-occupied households and	
renter-occupied households	
Individuals	
Per capita income	
% of persons who live in poverty	Census records
Labor Force Characteristics	
Employment Status	
General population (age 18+)	
% employed	Chamber of Commerce
% unemployed	Department of Labour
% not participating in employment	Census records
Special groups	
% women working with children under age 6	
Occupational Categories and Number (%) of Persons Employed	
Managerial	
Technical	
Service	Census records
Farming	
Production	
Operator/laborer	
Union Activity and Membership	Local union(s) office

The city has diversified its business to the point that in the late 1990s when the price of oil was low, Calgary's economy was still moving forward and growing. This stability prompted analysts to refer to Calgary's economy as "bullet-proof." The city is maintaining that reputation with forecasts, indicating Calgary will continue to lead the country in economic growth. In Figures 13-6 and 13-7, indicators of the economic subsystem are listed. These data will become important as teams analyze data (see Chapter 14) and plan interventions (see Chapter 15).

TABLE 13-13						
Economic Indicators for Five Communities and the Downtown						
	BNK	CON	VIC	BRD	ING	DT15
Percent of seniors receiving GIS	44.7	36.3	66.3	55.2	41.7	30.9
Percent of children living in SFI households	17.6	14.9	13.7	15.1	12.2	5.1

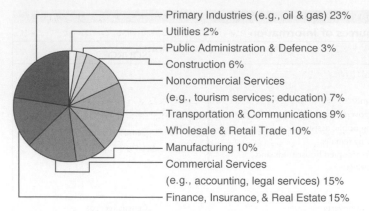

Primary Industries (e.g., oil & gas) 23%

Utilities 2%

Public Administration & Defence 3%

Construction 6%

Noncommercial Services
(e.g., tourism services; education) 7%

Transportation & Communications 9%

Wholesale & Retail Trade 10%

Manufacturing 10%

Commercial Services
(e.g., accounting, legal services) 15%

Finance, Insurance, & Real Estate 15%

FIGURE 13-6 ◆ Calgary gross domestic product by industry (% contribution to total, 2001). (Source: Conference Board of Canada.)

LABOUR FORCE

The labour force includes all persons over the age of 15 who were either employed or unemployed in the week prior to Census Day. Persons not in the labour force "refers to persons 15 years of age and over, excluding institutional residents, who . . . did not work for pay or in self-employment in the week prior to enumeration and (a) did not look for paid work in the four weeks prior to enumeration, (b) were not on temporary lay-off and (c) did not have a new job to start in four weeks or less. It also includes persons who looked for work during the last four weeks but were not available to start work in the week prior to enumeration." (Statistics Canada, 1997).

Work activity (number of hours and weeks worked per year) is related to income adequacy. People who work full time for less than a year, or part time, are almost three times as likely to have incomes below the low income cut-off (LICO) than full-time workers who worked for the full year. Particularly disadvantaged by earning inequality are women and youth workers.

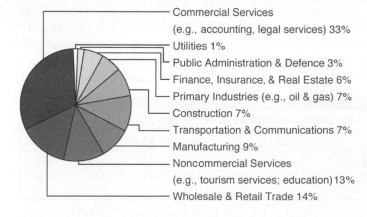

Commercial Services
(e.g., accounting, legal services) 33%

Utilities 1%

Public Administration & Defence 3%

Finance, Insurance, & Real Estate 6%

Primary Industries (e.g., oil & gas) 7%

Construction 7%

Transportation & Communications 7%

Manufacturing 9%

Noncommercial Services
(e.g., tourism services; education) 13%

Wholesale & Retail Trade 14%

FIGURE 13-7 ◆ Calgary employment by industry (% contribution to total, 2001). (Source: Conference Board of Canada.)

Educational attainment of the workforce tends to be related to income adequacy and employment opportunity. Rates of low income are highest for those workers with low education levels (i.e., less than high school certificate).

HOUSEHOLD STRUCTURE

The rate of lone-parent families in the downtown area is about twice that of the city average. In families headed by lone parents, one parent carries the full burden of finances and nurturing, increasing the risk of social and emotional stress and vulnerability. Of the 82% of lone-parent households in Canada headed by women, 57% were living in poverty.

SHELTER

The majority (83%) of people living in the DT15 communities live in apartments; in contrast, only 22% of Calgarians live in apartments. In Calgary, 53% of the population lives in single-family dwellings, but in the downtown area, only 7% reside in single-family dwellings. The ability to afford adequate housing contributes to the health of individuals, families, and communities. Families with low incomes may divert money from other necessities to cover shelter costs or may become homeless. The percentage of income devoted to shelter is a useful measure of housing affordability; this information is located in Tables 13-14 and 13-15 for the communities of interest and the downtown area.

Safety and Transportation

Without a safe and secure environment based on public order and respect for property, people will be fearful of participation in community events. Structures in this subsystem exist to reduce fear or anxiety and promote a sense of safety in a community or population. Hence, the availability of fire, police, sanitation, sewage, recycling, and solid waste services as well as those that protect air quality, monitor dangerous goods, and protect us from animals are assessed. Public and community services that offer health promotion, injury and disease prevention, and health protection services are important to the health and well-being of a community. Transportation safety measures (i.e., roads and road maintenance, private vehicle safety

---

TABLE 13-14

Percentage of Income Devoted to Shelter in Calgary and Downtown Communities

	BNK	CON	VIC	BRD	ING	CITY
Percent of renters spending >30% income on housing	42.7	36.8	43.1	42.0	50.9	37.8
Percent of families below the ownership affordability threshold	59.7	58.5	72.6	61.1	35.0	43.1

TABLE 13-15
Average Housing Values 2002 (in $100,000) According to Sales Records

	BNK	CON	VIC	BRD	ING	CITY
Condominium	140.6	165.9	169.8	118.3	138.6	150.0
Residential	274.1	288.5	165.0	202.5	263.0	196.0

regulations, public transit, air, and rail safety measures, lighting of public places and roads) protect the public from hazards. Community perceptions of safety are also important indicators for this subsystem—crime statistics give a picture of the community as do people's perceptions of racism, ageism, stigma, prejudice, and feelings of social isolation. For example, police calls for domestic situations, teacher reports of bullying, and racist graffiti in ethnic neighbourhoods are examples of communities in dysfunction. Crime statistics can usually be located on police services websites broken down by community (e.g., **www.calgarypolice.ca**), and often there are surveys that can be useful for assessment purposes. For instance, the 2005 Calgary Police Service Citizen Survey provides community perceptions on a number of points (**http://www.calgarypolice.ca/news/pdf/stats/2005-csurvey-pamru-final.pdf**) (Table 13-16).

To examine lines of defence (health status and temporary responses to stressors) and resistance (assets), consider what citizen protection mechanisms are in place: identification of children, seniors, and animals in case they wander from home, Amber Alert program, Block Watch programs, volunteer school safety patrols and crossing guards, school and mall security personnel, mall walk programs, and emergency call lines for children (Children's Help Phone), seniors, and people living with mental illness and experiencing domestic violence.

Table 13-17 lists the major components of safety and transportation that affect the community. Each of these will provide different types of data for the assessment process.

PROTECTION SERVICES

Fire, police, waste disposal, and sanitation services are provided by the City and paid for by property taxes. Crime rates are higher in the inner city than the Calgary average, ranging from 1.1 to 2.7 times the rate for the city as a whole (see Table 13-16). Police patrol the areas by car, on foot, and with bicycles. For the park areas, horse patrols are also used.

There are Neighbourhood Watch programs in the communities, and by-law enforcement officers pick up stray animals.

WATER AND SANITATION

Water supplies for the downtown area are from the Glenmore Reservoir; chlorine and fluoride are added at the source. There is no heavy industry in the area with

TABLE 13-16
2005 Calgary Police Services Citizen Survey

Perceptions of Safety

Question: How safe do you feel, or how safe would you feel, walking alone in your community after dark?

Data (expressed as percent of respondents):

Very safe	44
Reasonably safe	39
Somewhat unsafe	12
Very unsafe	5

Note: Respondents ages 65 or older are most likely to feel unsafe.

Question: How safe do you feel, or how safe would you feel around the light rail transit (LRT) areas such as the platforms or parking areas? In and around the downtown and city centre areas?

Data (expressed as percent of respondents):

	LRT AREAS	DOWNTOWN
Very safe	12	12
Reasonably safe	44	42
Somewhat unsafe	30	31
Very unsafe	14	15

Question: What do you consider to be the top city crime problems?

Data (expressed as percent of respondents):

1	Illegal gang activity/organized crime	43
2	Drug law enforcement	36
3	Traffic violations (speeding, unsafe driving)	31
4	House break-ins (break and enter)	14
5	Theft other than vehicles	9
6	Assault causing injury	8

From: Calgary Police Services. 2005 Calgary Police Service Citizen Survey. Retrieved June 30, 2007 from **http://www.calgarypolice.ca/news/pdf/2005-csurvey-sept-revisions.pdf**

Person and Property Crime Rates (per 1,000 population) for Selected Calgary Communities in 2006

	BNK		BELTLINE*		BRD		ING	
	2004	2005	2004	2005	2004	2005	2004	2005
Person crimes	9	9	39	36	12	11	12	9
Property crimes	53	64	146	144	82	77	74	68

*Combined Connaught and Victoria Park communities.
From Calgary Police Services Community Crime Statistics Reports. Created from materials from website at **www.calgarypolice.ca**.

the closure of the brewery and stockyards, so industrial pollution is minimal. Trains make some noise and traffic creates some air pollution. Occasionally, during the spring, people with respiratory disorders are advised to stay indoors because of the cottonwood pollen in the air.

TABLE 13-17	
Safety and Transportation	
INDICATORS	SOURCES OF INFORMATION
Safety	
Protection services	Planning office (municipality)
Fire	Fire department (local)
Police	Police department (municipality)
Sanitation	
Waste sources and treatment	Waste and water treatment plants
Solid waste	
Air quality	Environment department
Transportation	
Private	
Transportation sources	
Number of persons with a transportation disability	Census data: population and housing characteristics
Public	
Bus, subway, and light rail services (routes, schedules, and fares)	Local and city transportation authorities
Roads (number and condition; primary, secondary, and farm-to-market roads)	Provincial highway department
Interstate highways	
Freeway system	
Air service (private and publicly owned)	Local airports (Note: Local airports are frequently owned and operated by city government.)
Intercity rail service	CP Rail
	VIA Rail

TRANSPORTATION

Calgary is on the Trans Canada Highway and on the north–south truck route from Mexico to Alaska. An international airport in the northeast provides access to air travel. The Canadian Pacific Railway goes through the city, and Greyhound has a large terminal for passenger and freight service. Several smaller commercial airlines operate out of the airport in Calgary, and other bus services provide local access to the mountains and along the north–south corridor. There is a light rail transit system and regular bus service. A hazardous chemicals route goes through the city to the east of downtown. Traffic is heavy with people moving into and out of the downtown for employment and services. Parking is expensive, and people are encouraged to use "Park'n Ride." There are no special privileges for carpools on the many trails that move traffic around the city and few dedicated bike lanes on the major streets.

Politics and Government

The various forms and levels of government are responsible for public policymaking through legislation. We need to understand which government is responsible for the portfolios that influence healthy public policy, how special interest groups can influence policy, and how to gain access to these resources with the communities and population aggregates with which we are working. We must be aware of the influential people in positions of power to influence the health and well-being of people: mayor and alderpersons, school board and other trustees, provincial premier, key ministers in provincial government, leader of the provincial opposition, local medical officer of health, and heads of social and community agencies. On a national level, we must know who the persons of influence are with respect to issues of federal jurisdiction, including local members of parliament. Within the disciplines that are involved in community work, there are opportunities to bring issues and resolutions forward for action locally, provincially, and on the national scene. For instance, the Canadian Public Health Association (CPHA) has worked successfully with the various provincial branches and associations to influence public policy on gun control, home care, clean air, homelessness, and unemployment issues, among others.

The five example communities are situated within the downtown area of Calgary. Calgary has a mayor-council form of government with 14 aldermen elected every 2 years. City Council meets weekly and has several standing committees. The list of alderman is available on the City website (**http://calgary.ca**), and residents are encouraged to telephone, mail, or e-mail their representatives on a wide array of issues. There are seven trustees elected to both the public and separate school boards; the chairpersons are elected from among them (**www.cbe.ab.ca** and **www.cssd.ab.ca**). In 2001, nine elected and six appointed board members governed the local health region; the Alberta Minister of Health and Wellness appointed the chairperson. In 2003, the Province once again reorganized health regions, cutting the number of regions to nine and eliminating elected members to regional boards. Now, the health region has a chair and 13 members. Several members are from former rural boards now amalgamated into the expanded Calgary Health Region (**www.calgaryhealthregion.ca/board/board members/index.htm**). Twenty-one Members of the Legislative Assembly (MLAs) represent Calgary in the provincial government, and Calgary sends eight Members of Parliament to Ottawa. Each of these has an office in his or her home area, and residents are welcome to bring concerns to the staff. The Prime Minister at the time of writing, the Right Honourable Stephen Harper, represents a Calgary riding in Parliament.

Communication

This subsystem details how people communicate within the target population and the broad community on an everyday basis and also how emergency messages are conveyed. Access to communication links determines how well people are informed. Because information is key to awareness of goods and services, lack of a satisfactory means of gathering information can adversely affect access and utilization of needed services.

TABLE 13-18	
Communication	
COMPONENTS	SOURCES OF INFORMATION
Formal	
Newspaper (number, circulation, frequency, and scope of news)	Chamber of Commerce
Radio and television (number of stations, commercial versus educational, and audience)	Newspaper office
	Telephone company
Postal service	Yellow Pages
Telephone status (number of residents with service)	Telephone book
	Canada Post, courier services
Informal	
Sources: Bulletin boards; posters; hand-delivered flyers; and church, civic, and school newsletters	Windshield/walking survey
	Talking to residents
Dissemination (How do people receive information?)	Survey
Word of mouth	
Mail	
Radio, television	Reports, surveys

Communication may be formal or informal. Formal communication usually originates outside the community (extracommunity) as opposed to informal communication, which almost always originates and is disseminated within the community. Salient components of formal and informal communication, as well as sources of data, are presented in Table 13-18.

Two major papers serve Calgary, along with 7 AM and 13 FM radio stations and 8 television stations. Cable and satellite services are available. Every neighbourhood has a community association that is funded on a per capita basis by the city, and association executives are important routes of communication to aldermen. In the downtown, postal service is provided door-to-door, unlike in the suburbs where superboxes are the norm.

Education

Education is closely linked with employment and economic status of a community and population aggregate. The general educational status of a community can be summarized using census data. Census information lists the number of residents attending schools, years of schooling completed, and percentage of residents who speak English. This information describes the community core, but the infrastructure for learning—basic, specialized, literacy—is what comprises the subsystem.

To supplement this broad assessment, information is needed about major educational sources (e.g., schools, colleges, and libraries) located both inside and outside the community that people use for formal as well as continuing education and personal interest purposes. Table 13-19 is a suggested guide for assessing a community's educational sources.

TABLE 13-19	
Education	
COMPONENTS	**SOURCES OF INFORMATION**
Educational Status	
School enrollment by type of school	Census data
Dropout/completion rates	School board data.
Educational Sources	
Intracommunity or extracommunity (collect data for each facility)	Local board of education reports and websites
Services (educational, recreational, communication, and health)	School administrator (such as the principal or director) and school nurse
Resources (personnel, space, budget, and record system)	School administrator
Characteristics of users (geographic distribution and demographic profile)	Teachers and staff
Adequacy, accessibility, and acceptability of education to students and staff	Students and staff

It is sometimes difficult to decide which educational sources to include in the assessment. Community usage is probably the most important indicator. Primary and secondary schools attended by the majority of youngsters in a community, regardless of intra- or extracommunity location, are major educational sources and require a thorough assessment, whereas schools composed primarily of students from outside the community do not require such an extensive appraisal.

The Calgary Board of Education has elementary and junior high schools in the downtown communities that feed into the high school system. Similarly, the separate school system offers facilities throughout the downtown area. Children can take the bus to school if they live a certain distance away, and parents can opt into lunch programs if the children stay at school over the noon hour. Calgary also offers religious schools (Calgary Catholic Schools, Jewish and Christian schools), schools for special needs children, and charter schools in addition to an array of private schools. Public postsecondary education in Calgary is provided from several institutions: University of Calgary, Mount Royal College, Southern Alberta Institute of Technology, Alberta College of Art and Design, and Bow Valley College. All but Mount Royal College are accessible by light rail transit; public transportation is readily available at reduced rates for those who attend school in the city. Private postsecondary education can be accessed from DeVry Institute, Columbia Business College, and Rocky Mountain Bible College, among others.

Recreation

The recreation subsystem allows us to focus on assessing the degree of lifestyle support in the community. We will want to link recreation information with the data

TABLE 13-20	
Recreation	
Sports and fitness	City Parks and Recreation Services will list city-sponsored services; others will be listed under community associations or private business: arenas, playgrounds, bowling alleys, tennis courts, ball diamonds, soccer pitches, bike paths, walking paths, sport associations, fitness clubs, mall walk programs, outdoor skating rinks, water, mountain or forest activities. Professional and semiprofessional sports teams (e.g., hockey, baseball, football, basketball, soccer, lacrosse).
Social pursuits	Age-appropriate clubs (e.g., Brownies, Scouts), interest clubs (e.g., stamp collectors), community dances and celebrations, community courses for hobbyists. Library, faith, school-sponsored social events. Places people gather (e.g., coffee houses, restaurants, bars).
Leisure pursuits	Theatres, cinemas, dance, opera, music, artistic appreciation events and sites.
Other	Zoo and animal parks, museums, picnic areas.

on physical environment and safety subsystems for a complete picture, but collecting information on parks, sports facilities, jogging and bicycle paths as well as resources for social interaction (e.g., special interest clubs, seniors' centres, theatres, art galleries, restaurants, bars, festivals, zoo, museums, teams) offers insight into access, affordability, and use patterns that can suggest opportunities for community capacity-building and help to determine activity and social needs of the population (Table 13-20).

SUMMARY

A community assessment is never complete, because any community and the people who live in it are dynamic and ever evolving; however, we must pause at some point. Because we have addressed all parts of the model, this is where we will stop (see Appendix B and Chapter 18 for examples of completed profiles). A description of each community subsystem has been recorded. Note that at every step of the assessment, people in the community were included. Not only did we interview the "professionals" (e.g., school nurses, social workers, physicians, principals, police chief, alderman, and so on) but also individuals within the subsystems were included (e.g., parents, shoppers, patients, and people on the street). The assessment, like all steps in the process, is carried out in partnership with the community. The next step is analysis—a process that synthesizes the assessment information and derives from it statements specific to the community.

Crucial to community assessment is a model, or map, to direct and guide that process. The model (community assessment wheel) shown in Figure 13-1 provided a framework, and the tool "Windshield/Walking Survey" (see Table 13-4) guided the assessment of the neighbourhoods of the downtown area of Calgary,

Alberta. In the Suggested Readings list, several other approaches to community assessment are presented. As you are aware, there are other models that you may wish to consider as you continue your practice of community assessment. Workbooks to facilitate the process of community assessment are frequently available from local social planning departments. For instance, the Edmonton Social Planning Council (1988) offers "Doing it right! A needs assessment workbook" for sale ($5). See **www.edmspc.com** for information.

References

Barton, J. A., Smith, M. C., Brown, N. J., & Supples, J. M. (1993). Methodological issues in a team approach to community health needs assessment. *Nursing Outlook, 41*(6), 253–261.

Conway, T., Hu, T., & Harrington, T. (1997). Setting health priorities: Community boards accurately reflect the preferences of the community's residents. *Journal of Community Health, 22*(1), 57–68.

Diem, E. (2005). Team building. In E. Diem & A. Moyer, Community health nursing projects: Making a difference (pp. 26–54). Philadelphia, PA: Lippincott Williams & Wilkins.

Dimock. H. G., & Devine, I. (1994). *Making workgroups effective* (3rd ed.). North York, ON: Captus Press.

Edmonton Social Planning Council. (1988). *Doing it right! A needs assessment workbook*. Edmonton: Author.

Edwards, N. C., & Moyer, A. (2000). Community needs and capacity assessment: Critical components of program planning. In M. J. Stewart (Ed.), *Community nursing: Promoting Canadians' health* (pp. 420–442). Toronto: Saunders.

Gerberich, S. S., Stearns, S. J., & Dowd, T. (1995). A critical skill for the future: Community assessment. *Journal of Community Health Nursing, 12*(4), 239–250.

Gilmore, G. D., & Campbell, M. D. (1996). *Needs assessment strategies for health education and health promotion* (pp. 51–61, 73–87). Dubuque, IA: Brown & Benchmark.

Haglund, B., Weisbrod, R., & Bracht, N. (1990). Assessing the community: Its services, needs, leadership and readiness. In N. Bracht (Ed.), *Health promotion at the community level* (pp. 99–108). Newbury Park, CA: Sage.

Hancock, T., & Minkler, M. (1997). Community health assessment or healthy community assessment: Whose community? Whose health? Whose assessment? In M. Minkler (Ed.), *Community organizing and community building for health* (pp. 139–156). New Brunswick, NJ: Rutgers University Press.

Hawe, P., Degeling, D., & Hall, J. (1990). *Evaluating health promotion*. Sydney, Australia: MacLennan & Petty.

Kretzman, J. P., & McKnight, J. L. (1993). *Building communities from the inside out: A path toward finding and mobilizing a community's assets*. Chicago: ACTA Publications.

McDevitt, J., & Wilbur, J. E. (2002). Locating sources of data. In N. E. Ervin (Ed.), *Advanced community health nursing practice* (pp. 109–141). Upper Saddle River, NJ: Prentice Hall.

Morgan, D. L., & Kreuger, R. A. (1997). *The focus group kit.* (Vol. 1-6). Thousand Oaks, CA: Sage.

Parks, C. P., & Straker, H. O. (1996). Community assets mapping: Community health assessment with a different twist. *Journal of Health Education, 27*, 321–323.

Patton, M. Q. (1990). *Qualitative evaluation and research methods* (2nd ed.). Newbury Park, CA: Sage.

Statistics Canada. (1997). Guide to the Labour Force Survey. Catalogue no. 71-528-PB. Ottawa, ON: Author.

Suggested Readings

Bennett, E. J. (1993). Health needs assessment of a rural county: Impact evaluation of a student project. *Family and Community Health*, *16*(1), 28–35.

Beverly, C. J., McAtee, R., Costello, J., Chernoff, R., & Casteel, J. (2005). Needs assessment of rural communities: A focus on older adults. *Journal of Community Health*, *30*(3), 197–208.

Clark, N., & Buell, A. (2004). Community assessment: An innovative approach. *Nurse Educator*, *29*(5), 203–207.

Corso, L., Wiesner, P. J., & Lenihan, P. (2005). Developing the MAPP community health improvement tool. *Journal of Public Health Management and Practice*, *11*(5), 387–392.

Escoffery, C., Miner, K. R., & Trowbridge, J. (2004). Conducting small-scale community assessments. *American Journal of Health Education*, *35*(4), 237–241.

Gregor, S., & Galazka, S. S. (1990). The use of key informant networks in assessment of community health. *Family Medicine*, *22*(2), 118–121.

Keppel, K. G., & Freedman, M. A. (1995). What is assessment? *Journal of Public Health Management*, *1*(2), 1–7.

Lindell, D. H. (1997). Community assessment for the home health nurse. *Home Healthcare Nurse*, *15*(1), 618–626.

White, J. E., & Valentine, V. L. (1993). Computer assisted video instruction and community assessment. *Nursing and Health Care*, *14*(7), 349–353.

Williams, R., & Yanoshik, K. (2001). Can you do a community assessment without talking to the community? *Journal of Community Health*, *26*(3), 233–247.

Zahner, S. J., Kaiser, B., & Kapelke-Dale, J. (2005). Local partnerships for community assessment and planning. *Journal of Public Health Management and Practice*, *11*(5), 460–464.

Internet Resources

www.cchpr.org
Canadian Consortium of Health Promotion Research Centres

www.cich.ca
Canadian Institute of Child Health

www.cihi.ca
Canadian Institute for Health Information

www.cihr.ca
Canadian Institutes for Health Research

www.cpha.ca
Canadian Public Health Association

www.calgary.ca
City of Calgary Communities

www.hc-sc.gc.ca
Health Canada

www.sshrc.ca
Social Sciences and Humanities Research Council of Canada

www.statcan.ca
Statistics Canada

www.cdc.gov
U.S. Centers for Disease Control and Prevention

http://www.ctb.ku.edu/index.jsp
Community Tool Box

http://www.dph.sf.ca.us/Reports/Misc/4_01BosAsstRpt.pdf
International Institute of San Francisco

14

Community Analysis and Diagnosis

REVISED FROM THE ORIGINAL BY ARDENE ROBINSON VOLLMAN

Chapter Outline

Introduction

Community Analysis

Sample Community Analysis

Evaluation

Summary

Learning Objectives

This chapter is focused on the second phase of the community process, analysis, and the associated task of forming community diagnoses.

After studying the chapter, you should be able to:

❖ Practice within a team environment to critically analyze and synthesize data collected

❖ Classify community assessment data into the categories of the community-as-partner model

❖ Create summary statements and note aspects of incomplete or contradictory information

❖ Interpret summary statements in comparison with benchmark data and trends

❖ Generate inferences and formulate community diagnoses

❖ Validate information and inferences

Introduction

*A*nalysis is the study and examination of data by the processes of classification, summarization, interpretation, and validation of information in order to write community diagnoses and establish priorities (Helvie, 1998). These data may be quantitative (numerical) as well as qualitative. All aspects need to be considered. Analysis is necessary to determine community needs and community strengths as well as to identify patterns of responses and trends in service use. During analysis, any need for further data collection is revealed as gaps and incongruities in the community assessment data. The end point of analysis is the community diagnosis.

COMMUNITY ANALYSIS

Analysis, like so many procedures we perform, may be viewed as a process with multiple steps. The phases we will use to help in the analysis are classification, summarization, interpretation, and validation. Each is described and illustrated below.

Classification

To analyze community assessment data, it is helpful to first classify the data. Data can be classified into categories in a variety of ways. Traditional categories of community assessment data include:

◆ Demographic characteristics (family size, age, sex, and ethnic and racial groupings)
◆ Geographic characteristics (area boundaries; number and size of neighbourhoods, public spaces, and roads)
◆ Socioeconomic characteristics (occupation and income categories, educational attainment, and rental or home ownership patterns)
◆ Health and social resources and services (hospitals, clinics, mental health centres, welfare offices, etc.)

However, models are being used increasingly in the organization and analysis of community health data because they provide a framework for data collection and a map to guide analysis. Because the community assessment wheel (see Fig. 13-1) was used to direct the community assessment, that same model can be used to guide analysis. Each of the community subsystems will be analyzed, and the smaller components within each subsystem will help to describe the categories by which information is sorted.

Ultimately, we want to describe the community's normal line(s) of defence (NLD), that is, the health status of the population and/or the geographic community. We also want to locate sources of risk or hazard (stressors) and identify the flexible lines of defence (FLD) that are in place as well as the lines of resistance (LR) that represent the community's strengths and assets. The focus of analysis is the people (community core); the subsystems represent the context where people live, learn, love, work, play, and pray.

Summarization

Once a classification method has been selected, the next task is to summarize the data within each category. Both summary statements and summary measures, such as rates, charts, and graphs, are required.

> ### *Take Note*
>
> Many health care agencies and educational institutions have access to computerized information systems—a system through which formatted data can be retrieved in a variety of forms—including summary health statistics. For example, data entered into a computer system as census figures can be configured into population pyramids, and census and vital statistics information can be programmed to calculate birth, death, and fertility rates. Calculations that previously required hours to complete are now computed in seconds. In your practice, make it a point to inquire as to the availability of computer systems, and if possible, use computer processes to carry out quantitative data analysis. In addition, your local health department may be able to furnish the rates for you (e.g., the infant mortality rate [IMR]). Note, however, that the denominator used to calculate this rate may not be the community as you have defined it.

Interpretation

To interpret data often requires comparison to established standards or benchmarks, provincial and national statistics, and the community's own statistics for previous years (Helvie, 1998). Outcomes of data analysis include the identification of data gaps, inconsistencies, or omissions and the generation of inferences or hypotheses about the findings. Frequently, comparative data are needed to determine if a pattern or trend exists or if data do not seem correct and the need for revalidation of original information is required. Data gaps are inevitable, as are mistakes in recording data; the important task is to analyze data critically and be aware of the potential for gaps and omissions. It is helpful to have professional colleagues as well as community residents review the analysis. Every person has a unique perspective; it is only through the sharing of views that a whole and comprehensive picture of community assessment data can evolve.

Using the data from your community, compare them with other similar data to determine the size of the problem. For instance, you calculate (or discover) an IMR of 12/1,000 live births—how does this compare with other communities? The province? The nation? Is it for the entire infant population of your community, or are there differences among structural or demographic factors? Is the IMR different for different ethnic groups, ages and marital status of mothers, or geographic parts of the community? Have there been any changes for the better or worse in recent years or the past decade? (Note: This is a good time to review Chapter 3 to assist you with epidemiologic reasoning as you try to make sense of your data.)

Other resources for comparison are the documents produced as health report cards by regional health authorities, provinces, and Health Canada/Public Health Agency of Canada (and other federal departments such as Environment, Immigration and Citizenship, Human Resources Development). The Report on the Health of Canadians by Health Canada (2000) presents national figures, such as incidence and prevalence when available, for our major health concerns. Although Canada does not yet have a specific document regarding population health goals, Healthy People 2010 (U.S. Department of Health and Human Services, 1997), though not Canadian, can be invaluable to you because it contains goals and objectives that help in both data analysis and planning.

Having classified, summarized, and compared the data you have collected, the final phase is to draw logical conclusions from the evidence, that is, to draw inferences that will lead to the statement of a community diagnosis. An *inference* is a conclusion drawn from multiple observations. An inference synthesizes what you have learned about the community and the people—it states what the data *means*. These conclusions or inferences will identify stressors and strengths in succinct phrases; these phrases then form the basis for a community diagnosis. *Synthesis* is the linking of the summary statements from the classification process and formulating hypotheses about the connections among them.

Validation

It is a common complaint of communities that "experts" come in and collect data, make judgments, and then leave. It is important to validate the conclusions you reach and the hypotheses you generate to ensure that they are correct and reflect the community accurately. This requires the team to confirm their information and its interpretation by returning to sources for confirmation or additional data. Solicit feedback and check with key sources (e.g., community informants, external experts) to verify that your findings are appropriate. Validation can be carried out by town hall or focus group meetings, purposive surveys, or interviews.

Barton and coworkers (1993) discuss the issues that may face the team during its analytic process and offer suggestions to address them (Table 14-1).

The remainder of this chapter will walk you through analysis of the data that we collected in the community assessment of five downtown Calgary communities.

SAMPLE COMMUNITY ANALYSIS

After the analysis examples are presented, information on how to form community diagnoses is presented (see the Community Diagnosis section later in this chapter). The analysis of the five-community (DT5) assessment data, as in the assessment process, begins with the community core, because it is the core (the people and

TABLE 14-1	
Team Analysis Issues and Strategies for Solution	
ISSUES	**STRATEGIES**
Coordinating the sharing of volumes of data	Using electronic tools; sharing information during team meetings
Disagreement in interpretations of data	Ensuring the data are broadly representative of key community perspectives; if gaps exist, seeking to fill them with further information
Community-team disagreement on the meaning of data	Including community members in all aspects of analysis
Contradictory data from different sources	Seeking further data or clarification; reporting with recommendations for further exploration

their health) that is of interest to the community health professional. Recall that the core is affected by (and affects) all of the subsystems depicted in the model surrounding it. Some subsystems will influence certain problems more than others, but it is important to assess the subsystems because of their contribution to the causes and alleviation of problems in the core. As noted in Chapter 13, there may be three approaches to assessment—geographic community, issue, and aggregate—and this informs your analysis. In the example that follows, we use all three approaches at different times as illustration. You may need to return to Chapter 13 for data.

Community Core

An analysis of the core of the five communities (DT5) is presented in Table 14-2. Community core data include many sociodemographic measures, data that are especially amenable to graphs and charts. The adage "one picture is worth a thousand words" is particularly meaningful for demographic characteristics. The population (by age) of the five downtown communities in which we are interested is located in Table 14-3.

You will notice a data gap in Table 14-3; we cannot determine the sex composition of the population of these DT5 communities from this table. Perhaps the most representative illustration of the age and sex composition of a population is the population pyramid. In Table 14-4, the sex and age distribution of males and females are separately listed for the group of 15 downtown communities (DT15) and the city of Calgary. They are further illustrated as a population pyramid in Figure 14-1. Which of these best illustrates how the population of DT15 compares with the entire city on age and sex distribution?

The population pyramid is formed of bars; each bar represents an age group. Usually 5- or 10-year age groups are used, although adaptations can be made for smaller or larger age ranges. Bars are stacked horizontally, one on another, with bars for males on the left of a central axis and those for females on the right. The

TABLE 14-2
An Analysis of the Core of Five Downtown Communities

DATA CATEGORY	SUMMARY STATEMENTS	INFERENCES
History	• Inglewood is the historic site of Fort Calgary. Being revitalized. • Victoria Park grew around the Stampede grounds; very run down. • Bridgeland, originally called "Little Italy," now has a large immigrant population of Vietnamese. Borders the zoo. • Connaught has many high-rise apartment buildings. • Bankview is the newest of the five communities.	The downtown communities are not homogeneous; there is a great deal of variation in terms of neighbourhood history, pride, and attractions.

Demographics	• Connaught has the largest population of the five communities.
	• More than 43% of the residents over 1 year of age from Bankview, Connaught, and Victoria Park moved in the past year, above the downtown (DT15) average of 37%.
	• Inglewood and Bridgeland residents were less mobile than average downtown residents in the past year.
	• A similar pattern exists for 5-year mobility.
	• Immigrants comprise approximately 25% of the downtown population.
	• Connaught and Victoria Park have 37% new (past 3 years) immigrants among their residents; Bankview matches the downtown average, and Inglewood and Bridgeland are below the average at <15%.
	• Victoria Park has the highest proportion of people not speaking English as their first language at home (24%), compared with the average for downtown (10%).
	• Combined, the downtown communities (DT15) have a dependency ratio of 33. However, this obscures the differences among the five example communities:
	   Bankview 24
	   Connaught 26
	   Victoria Park 37
	   Bridgeland 67 (seniors)
	   Inglewood 47
		The five downtown communities have high mobility rates. A significant proportion of immigrants have settled in Victoria Park, accounting for the higher proportion of residents/households that speak a language other than English in the home.
		Bridgeland has the highest dependency ratio, due largely to the number of seniors living there. The other four communities are more evenly balanced between children and seniors.

Vital statistics	• Data gap: Unable to disaggregate the DT15 vital statistics data by neighbourhood. • In the period 1990–1992, there were 1,901 births in DT15. • Crude birth rate DT15: 12.3/1,000 population; Calgary: 15.6 • Proportion of births to women aged 15–19 in DT15: 11.3%; in Calgary: 5.1% • Teen birth rate DT15 is twice the Alberta rate; Calgary is half the Alberta rate. • DT15 low-birth-weight rate: 8.6%; Calgary: 6.1% • In the period 1990–1992, 688 DT15 residents died. The standardized mortality ratio = 0.9, not significantly different from the rest of the city.	DT15 women are at higher perinatal risk than other city women as a result of youth, immigration, mobility, and language.

(continued)

TABLE 14-2
An Analysis of the Core of Five Downtown Communities (Continued)

DATA CATEGORY	SUMMARY STATEMENTS	INFERENCES
Health status	• Causes of death: 　Cancer (28%) 　Ischemic heart disease (20%) 　Respiratory disease (20%) 　Cerebrovascular disease (8%) 　Injury (8%) • The most frequent reason for emergency room visits is injury (30%). Of these, falls account for the largest proportion. • DT15 accounts for 6.5% of the population of the health region but 8.5% of inpatient services, 6.7% of day procedures, and 10.5% of emergency room visits. • Bridgeland residents used all services more often than other communities. • DT15 patients aged 20–64 received 39.2% of home care service. In Alberta, patients aged 75 and older receive the largest percentage of care. • Infectious disease rates do not differ between DT15 and the city.	Bridgeland seniors are a risk group. Injuries (e.g., from falls) are a concern, particularly in Bridgeland where the senior population is high.

percentage of males and females in a particular age group is indicated by the length of the bars, as measured from the central axis. All age groups in a pyramid should be the same interval.

To construct a population pyramid, use Table 14-5 to calculate the percentage contribution of each age and sex group and Table 14-6 for actual pyramid construction. Note that parts of the population pyramids in Figure 14-1, those depicting people younger than 20 years and older than 65, are shaded; this was done to denote the dependent portions of the population. A dependency ratio (Table 14-7) can be calculated when we have this information.

TABLE 14-3
Age Distribution by Five Downtown Communities (DT5)

	BNK	CON	VIC	BRD	ING	DT15
0–4	295	300	214	295	230	1,952
5–14	228	311	195	267	322	1,850
15–19	202	356	238	169	205	1,901
20–24	937	1,745	694	417	330	7,245
25–44	2,701	5,413	2,092	1,780	1,651	23,994
45–64	533	1,667	737	618	749	7,758
65+	279	1,312	585	1,139	536	6,988

TABLE 14-4
Percent of Population by Sex and Age Group for 15 Downtown Communities (DT15) and City

AGES (YEARS)	MALES		FEMALES	
	DT15	City	DT15	City
<5	2.5	2.9	2.3	2.9
5–19	6.3	10.3	6.2	9.8
20–24	3.8	4.0	3.9	3.8
25–34	12.3	8.5	10.4	8.3
35–44	10.5	9.7	8.7	9.5
45–54	6.5	7.4	5.8	6.9
55–64	4.1	3.6	3.9	3.6
65–74	3.2	2.5	3.7	2.8
75+	2.2	1.4	3.9	2.3

The dependency ratio describes the potentially self-supporting portion of the population and the dependent portions at the extremes of age. It is usually calculated as follows:

$$DR = \frac{\text{population under 20 + population 65 and over}}{\text{population 20 to 64 years of age}} \times 100$$

The dependency ratio is interpreted as the number of persons under age 20 and over age 65 needing support (because of age) for every 100 persons aged 20 to 65 years.

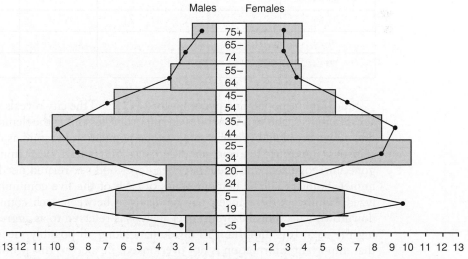

FIGURE 14-1 ◆ Population pyramid for DT15 (*bars*) with city superimposed (*lines*).

TABLE 14-5				
Calculations for a Population Pyramid				
Community Name, Census Tract, or Geographic Boundaries: _____				
Total Population: _____				
	MALES		**FEMALES**	
AGES (YEARS)	Number	Total Population (%)	Number	Total Population (%)
Total				
<5				
5–9				
10–14				
15–19				
20–24				
25–29				
30–34				
35–39				
40–44				
45–49				
50–54				
55–59				
60–64				
65–69				
70–74				
75+				

Studying the population pyramids for DT15 and the city reveals striking age and sex differences, and this illustrates an important lesson. If the demographics of the downtown area had been presented as one population pyramid as depicted by city statistics, important age and sex differences might have been minimized or have gone unrecognized, and their associated age- and sex-related needs would be left unmet. Similarly, if the demographics of each of the five communities were analyzed, significant differences may be detected between each community and the downtown data. This hazard in data analysis is referred to as aggregating or pooling the data. It is important to divide data along all possibly meaningful lines so that important information is not overlooked. Be alert to this problem as you proceed with your analysis.

TABLE 14-6
Constructing a Population Pyramid

Population Pyramid for _____ : Year _____

MALES								Age							FEMALES
								75+							
								70–74							
								65–69							
								60–64							
								55–59							
								50–54							
								45–49							
								40–44							
								35–39							
								30–34							
								25–29							
								20–24							
								15–19							
								10–14							
								5–9							
								<5							

8   6   4   2   0   2   4   6   8

Percentage of Population

TABLE 14-7
Data for Calculating the Dependency Ratios of DT5 and DT15

	BNK	CON	VIC	BRD	ING	DT15
Total population	5,175	11,115	4,755	4,685	4,028	51,380
Dependents	1,004	2,279	1,232	1,870	1,293	12,691
Working	4,171	8,825	3,523	2,815	2,730	38,897
Ratio	24	26	35	67	47	33

Studying the data presented in conjunction with the population pyramids, the following summary statements can be made about DT5's core.

◆ The DT5 population is more mobile than the general city population.
◆ Immigrants comprise one quarter of the DT5 population compared with 20% for the city.
◆ Compared with the city as a whole, DT5 has a higher proportion of recent immigrants.
◆ Young adults and seniors are in higher proportions in the downtown area than in the city.
◆ DT5 has a smaller proportion of school-age children than the city.
◆ The vast majority of DT5 residents live in apartments compared with 22% of city residents.
◆ In DT5, 62% of the senior population lives alone, more than double the proportion of seniors living alone in the city as a whole.

What inferences can we draw from these observations? We might infer that the built environment has an impact on the lifestyle of the population. We might wonder if the large proportion of seniors living alone presents any issues relating to health or social isolation. Does the large immigrant population represent a stressor with regard to employment, language, or cultural appropriateness of services in the downtown area? We will need to use other methods of data collection to test these inferences— perhaps by direct observation, key informant interviews, or group discussions with target populations; this is part of the iterative or cyclical nature of data collection, classification, summarization, and interpretation that makes up the analytic process.

Physical Environment

To study the physical components, data were collected by inspection (i.e., windshield surveys) and from written reports prepared by City Hall, Social Services, the Chamber of Commerce, and the regional health authority. Many of these reports are available on-line.

Rental accommodations in 2005 are scarce with less than 1.6% vacancy rate. There is a waiting list of 1,300 to 1,500 for public housing compared with 1,400 in 2001; no new public housing units are under construction. Average rent in Calgary, the highest of prairie cities, is $666 for one bedroom and $808 for two bedrooms (Box 14-1). For someone working full time at minimum wage (in Alberta, $7.00 per hour), affordable housing would have to be in the $350 per month range. New arrivals are at high risk of being homeless or inadequately housed because the first + last months' rent, damage deposits, and utility hook-up fees often cost up to $2,000. Homelessness is increasingly severe with 3,436 homeless persons enumerated on May 10, 2006 (32% more than in 2004), including 145 homeless families. Homelessness exists on a continuum, from "shelterless" individuals who sleep under bridges, in cars, or on the street (absolute homelessness) to the "hidden" homeless who are staying in inappropriate housing or are at risk of losing their homes (relative homelessness). The 51 facilities that were providing emergency and

---

BOX 14-1

Canada Mortgage and Housing Corporation Housing Report, 2005

According to the December 2005 Canada Mortgage and Housing Corporation (CMHC) Rental Market Report, vacancies have fallen dramatically, from 4.3% in 2004 to just 1.6%—the lowest level since 2001. The current inventory of rental apartments has once again decreased, from 42,335 units recorded in 2004 to 41,416 at the end of 2005. In real numbers, there were just 616 vacant apartment suites available in Calgary at December 2005 compared with 1,808 a year earlier.

The highest vacancies were recorded in three bedrooms at 3.5%, followed by bachelor units at 2.0% (down from 5.7% last year). Two-bedroom vacancies were recorded at 1.6% (down from 5.2% last year), and one bedrooms were at a low 1.4%, from 3.4% in December 2004. The Beltline saw a significant decrease in vacancy, from 4.1% in 2004 to 1.6% in 2005. Nationally, Calgary's overall vacancy rate of 1.6% was the sixth lowest in the country of 28 areas surveyed, compared with being tied with Toronto for 21st place or seventh highest in 2004. The lowest vacancies were found in Victoria at 0.5%, followed by Sherbrooke at 1.2%, and Quebec City and Vancouver at 1.4%.

Meanwhile, rents remained relatively unchanged, showing less than 1% average growth; the Beltline saw the highest average increases, of about 3%. The Beltline rents were in the range of $850 per month. As was the case in 2004, Toronto, Vancouver, and Ottawa once again recorded the highest average two-bedroom rental rates— Toronto unchanged at $1,052, Vancouver at $1,004 from $984 in 2004, and Ottawa at $920 in 2005. Trois-Rivières and Saguenay were once again the least expensive places to rent in Canada, where two bedrooms averaged $474 and $472, respectively.

Source: Canada Mortgage and Housing Corporation—Calgary Rental Market Report 2005. Retrieved July 10, 2007 from **www.cmhc-schl.gc.ca**. Document 64371: Calgary (enhanced).

---

transitional housing on May 10, 2006, have a capacity of 3,077 and operate at or above capacity (City of Calgary, 2006a; 2006b).

Summary statements include:

- DT5s are communities of contrast and diversity, both intracommunity and among them.
- There are many historical sites throughout the DT5 communities.
- Population density is the highest in the westernmost communities of Bankview and Connaught.
- There is little or no heavy industry in a DT5; commercial enterprises, professional offices, and small businesses are common along main thoroughfares and in strip malls.
- Housing values are higher in the westernmost communities, but Inglewood is undergoing significant revitalization. With the land available for development on the former Bow Valley Centre site, Bridgeland will soon experience a construction boom.
- Victoria Park is a community in decline with many abandoned buildings and property in disrepair. There is concern over homeless squatters, prostitution, and drug use in the area.

◆ Major transportation routes transect the DT5 communities, including trains that may carry hazardous materials.

◆ The proportion of good air quality samples for downtown DT15 is 95% compared with 87% in the industrial area and only slightly lower than suburban residential areas.

From this data, it can be inferred that the different communities will have different health and social needs and concerns, varying capacities to address issues, and different levels of motivation to develop a sense of community. Link this to the previous analysis of the community core to see what impact the physical environment (housing) exerts on the people in the downtown area. For instance, homeless people were found mostly in the inner city. Who are the homeless? On the night of the count, 82% of those enumerated were staying in facilities (49% of these in emergency beds), 5% were counted by service agencies, and 12% were staying on the streets. Male homeless persons accounted for 78% of the total. Forty-six percent of homeless individuals were between 25 and 44 years of age. Over two thirds are Caucasian; however, Aboriginal persons were disproportionately represented among the homeless compared with the city's population overall (City of Calgary, 2006a). A previous survey (City of Calgary, 1998) found that many homeless individuals were educated (20% with postsecondary education), and 45% were employed with average earnings of $7.40 per hour (when minimum wage was $5.90 per hour). Half had never been homeless before; the majority had been on the street for less than 3 months. One third reported mental health problems and addictions; 30% to 40% had serious mental health problems, and 34% were involved in substance abuse. We might infer from this that if there were adequate social housing, many members of this subpopulation would not be homeless. We might also infer that poverty is an important health determinant in this population and geographic area of the city.

Health and Social Services

Utilization of social services is primarily by people who require support for various reasons: low income, lack of shelter, need for support due to disability, and the like. Based on our analysis so far, we might want to focus on two key age groups: seniors and children. For example, seniors receiving old age security (OAS) pension will also receive the guaranteed income supplement (GIS) if they have no other source of retirement funds; this population might also receive other services from social agencies if they live alone and require assistance for activities of daily living. Another population group of concern to social service agencies are children, particularly those in low-income, lone parent families. Social safety net programs such as Supports for Independent Living (SFI, often referred to as "welfare") and Assured Income for the Severely Handicapped (AISH) allow people to live in the community rather than in group homes or shelters. However, when the benefits are compared with the costs for food and shelter, there is often a gap, indicated by people spending more than the recommended 30% of income on shelter (Table 14-8). To

TABLE 14-8

Social Characteristics by Percent of Population in 2001

	BNK	BRD	CON	ING	VIC	CITY
Persons living in low-income households	31.4	31.8	26.1	20.9	34.3	14.9
Children in SFI households of total population						
<20 years old	3.6	6.2	2.9	7.8	6.8	2.1
Lone parent families of total families with children	43.8	46.6	37.0	38.7	35.6	23.7
Seniors on GIS of total on OAS	47.5	58.8	31.9	38.2	65.8	28.8
Seniors living alone	61.9	52.8	56.9	25.0	80.8	26.3
Persons >15 without high school	14.8	22.1	13.4	18.0	25.1	20.1
Tenants spending >30% income on housing	38.1	45.5	31.6	40.2	36.8	36.4
Population receiving AISH	2.0	3.9	2.1	2.9	5.1	1.3

understand the capacity of this population, we examine unemployment rates and level of education because we understand the links between education, employment, and income. If we note low unemployment rates with high incomplete high school education rates, we might infer that those employed are not making high enough wages to accommodate rental costs. If these are lone parent heads of families, there might be opportunity for intervention.

We might also wonder what burden low income and inadequate housing places on the health care system—this is evident by hospital admissions and emergency room visits (Table 14-9).

Unfortunately, much utilization data are not easily available by community, and we have to rely on higher level information (Table 14-10) that might not provide the information that the team needs to draw inferences or make decisions.

In this instance, the best that can be done is to develop questions for further data collection: do lone parent mothers regularly receive mammograms? If not, why? What proportion of specific ethnic groups receives annual flu shots? Is there variation among men and women? What processes could be put into place to improve immunization rates?

Summary statements regarding the use of health and social services (using the data in the tables plus other reports) include:

♦ There is variation among the rates of day procedures by residents of DT5, with Bridgeland the highest at 108.4/1,000 population.

TABLE 14-9

Health Service Utilization by 1,000 Population, 2001

	BNK	BRD	CON	ING	VIC	CITY
Hospital in-patients	64	156	70	108	107	82
Emergency room visits	229	416	210	325	355	242

TABLE 14-10						
Percent of Population Reporting on Selected Health Indicators, 2005						
	CALGARY HEALTH REGION			ALBERTA		
	Total	Male	Female	Total	Male	Female
Positive self-rated health	65.2	64.8	65.7	62.2	61.6	62.8
Adult obesity	13.4	14.8	12.0	15.8	17.6	13.9
Self-rated positive mental health	76.2	78.2	74.3	73.4	73.7	73.1
Current smoker	19.8	22.1	17.5	22.7	25.5	20.0
Physical activity	56.6	56.1	57.2	53.5	52.4	54.7
Experiencing life stress	24.7	25.0	24.4	22.4	22.9	21.8
Sense of community belonging	59.4	58.2	60.6	62.8	60.9	64.8
Mammography			58.3			52.3
Influenza immunization	26.8	24.5	29.2	26.7	23.5	29.9
Has a regular medical doctor	84.3	79.0	89.5	82.4	76.3	88.6

- The top day procedure for Inglewood and Bridgeland is lens removal/replacement (for cataracts).
- Connaught and Bankview have higher rates of utilization for gynecologic services than the other communities.
- The utilization rates for in-patient services were higher for DT15 residents (152.9/1,000) than for the region (112.0/1,000). Bridgeland residents used all services more often than residents of other communities.
- Bridgeland's proportion of lone parent families is double the city's average.

Inferences we can draw are:

- Bridgeland residents account for a high use of health facilities because of the proportion and frailty of seniors in the community.
- Bankview and Connaught residents account for a significant use of reproductive health services, likely due to their youth and lifestyle.
- Many DT5 residents are at high risk for health-related problems due to low socioeconomic status.
- With high proportion of new immigrants, English as Second Language (ESL) services and translators will be needed.

Economics

The city has strong population growth with high net migration, a large proportion of which settle in the downtown area because of the proximity to resettlement and social services such as employment and second language training, and proximity to established communities of immigrants from their country of origin.

The Alberta economy led Canada in 2001 with 3% growth. The city had a low unemployment rate (4.5%) in 2002. There is a resurgence of construction because of the rising demand for office, warehouse, and residential space. Wages and prices

TABLE 14-11
Employment Characteristics by Percent of Population, 2001

	BNK	BRD	CON	ING	VIC	CITY
Unemployed persons over age 25 in labour force	4.3	4.3	4.7	5.2	8.6	4.0
Person aged 15–24 unemployed in labour force	3.5	5.1	5.6	4.9	10.0	10.1

are rising more quickly in Calgary than in the rest of Canada even though Alberta has the lowest minimum wage in the country at $7.00 per hour. Calgary's inflation rate as of April 2006 was 3.9% (highest in Canada), and the cost of living was 5.2% above the national average, driven largely by the cost of housing. Purchasing power has been eroded; price increases affect low-income budgets largely in food and shelter costs. The combined effect of inflation for basic needs and the level of Alberta's social assistance benefits amount to a significant decrease in purchasing power for single employable persons. With the aging demographic, the number of individuals leaving the labour market through retirements is expected to exceed the number entering it (City of Calgary, 2003).

The "low-income cut off" (LICO) is used in Canada as a measure of the "poverty line." A household is poor if it spends at least 20% more than the average household on the basic necessities (food, shelter, clothing). It has been determined that the average Canadian household spends 34.7% of its income on the basic necessities; therefore, a family is considered to be poor if it spends 54.7% of its income (or more) on food, shelter, and clothing (Statistics Canada, 1998).

The causes of poverty are many: prolonged periods of unemployment, employment that is part time or that provides inadequate wages for the household, and inability to work because of disability, lack of skill, or lack of opportunity. Youth, seniors, lone parents, single women, immigrants, persons who are visible minorities, Aboriginal people, and individuals with disabilities are more likely to experience unemployment (Table 14-11).

Households with low incomes tend to be more vulnerable to the fluctuating costs of goods and services and may not be able to afford basic needs (Box 14-2). This may be a threat to both the physical and mental well-being of those who live in low-income households.

Summary statements:

◆ The rate of people living in low-income households is 2.3 times higher in the downtown (DT5) than in the city as a whole. In Victoria Park, it is nearly three times higher.
◆ In Victoria Park, the median household income is one third that of the city; in the four remaining DT5 communities, the median income is half that of the city.
◆ Youth unemployment rate compares favourably with the city rate; Victoria Park is the highest but does not exceed the city average.

BOX 14-2

A Day in the Life of Poverty

Monthly family income: $1,666
Basic shelter, food, clothing: $1,596
Balance remaining: $70

A family of four with both parents working full-time (2,000 hours per year each) at minimum wage would have $13.69 available per family member per day. The daily cost of the bare essentials of shelter, food, and clothing are estimated to be $13.13 per day per family member, leaving only 56 cents a day per person to pay for child care, personal care items, household needs, furniture, telephone, transportation, school supplies, and health care. Because grocery money is more discretionary than other fixed expenses, poor families often run out of food before month's end. The impact of this is seen at food banks and in the nutritional health of families who are living in poverty.

◆ For adults over the age of 25, Victoria Park has the highest unemployment rate, at 8.6%.

What inferences can we draw from these observations? We certainly see that the economic "boom" has an effect on the price of housing and the amount of disposable income available for food and other basic needs. We can infer that people living without room in their budget for unexpected expenses will experience stress that will manifest in different ways: utilization of over-the-counter and prescription drugs and perhaps alcohol or substances, outdoor exercise in parts of the city that may be deemed unsafe, and/or seeking social support from local gathering places such as community or faith centres. Additional observation and data collection from service providers and community members about assets and challenges can help us to test and interpret inferences and suggest actions that can be considered in addressing issues of importance to the community.

Let us briefly present the summary statements for the remaining community subsystems with an issue (poverty) and a target population (lone parent families) in mind: Education, Safety and Transportation, Politics and Government, Communication, and Recreation.

There are many elementary and junior high schools in the inner city as well as one high school, but they suffer from age and declining enrolments as families have migrated to the suburbs. Further, the population is mobile and diverse, creating challenges for the teachers. On the other hand, couples who work downtown are seeking schooling and day care in the inner city close to where the parents work; this is creating some demand that is being met largely by private or charter schools. Public schools that remain in operation are suffering from major disrepair. The large proportion of lone parent families means that there is not a solid foundation for volunteers; there is some opportunity, however, to tap in to the senior population to

TABLE 14-12					
Fire Protection Service Statistics by 1,000 Population, 2001					
	BNK	BRD	CON	ING	VIC	CITY
House fires	2.7	3.6	5.0	4.5	8.9	1.9

provide support in the schools. With the ready access to the inner city by public transit, there are strong enrolments in day and evening English second language courses, educational upgrading and skilled worker programs at several post-secondary institutions (e.g., Bow Valley College), and nonprofit service providers (e.g., Calgary Immigrant Aid Society).

How safe is the inner city? In Chapter 13, data were presented on crime and perceived safety issues in the inner city. Table 14-12 provides information on residential fire incidence in the five inner city communities of interest. There is ample observational evidence of substance use, sex trade, and graffiti. Yet, members of the communities cite the vibrant nature of the art and entertainment scene as positive attributes that draw them to remain in the area notwithstanding its problems. Others cite the proximity to work as a benefit and appreciate the lifestyle offered by proximity to the river, jogging and biking paths, parks, and the like as attractions that allow them to maintain fitness. The evident problems of poverty are balanced by strong assets in the employed, well-educated population that has adequate disposable income and desires to invest in the health and sustainability of the communities in which they live.

There are formal and informal groups forming to address issues of environmental and personal protection (e.g., river cleanup, graffiti cleanup, community gardens, recycling programs, senior snow removal support for sidewalk safety, safewalk and school walk programs). Many of these are supported by local aldermen and faith institutions. As well, community spirit is supported by the local business associations. Downtown residents are vocal in political circles, advocating for (and against) the placement of certain social services through the four community associations. Political parties bring people out to vote by assisting with transportation. Homeless and poverty advocates volunteer at food banks, community kitchens, and in church basements that offer emergency shelter. City of Calgary provides ready access to social services in the inner city, and the health region operates or supports services to vulnerable populations in the downtown core.

On a walking survey, the community assessment team noticed active community bulletin boards in the supermarkets, health food stores, and coffee shops. Each community association publishes a newsletter delivered to its households on a regular basis. In these, community programs and services are advertised. Hydro poles also served as places to post notices of community events, lost pets, and the like. Schools and other gathering places celebrated a variety of festivals throughout the year that embraced the cultural diversity of the population and brought people out of their homes. For those without home computers, there is public access at cybercafés, public library, government offices, and some nonprofit agencies.

Recreational opportunities abound in the inner city—arts, entertainment, restaurants, the zoo, the library, the symphony, museums—and there are price subsidies for people of low income, youth, and seniors. Sports and fitness opportunities include several pools, skating rinks, skate-board parks, gardens, paths for walking, jogging and biking, curling rinks, professional and amateur sports facilities, and the like. Many of these can be enjoyed without cost or at low cost. Others are expensive (such as professional hockey games), but there are services that provide last-minute tickets to youth.

The overall well-being of a community is determined by both the volume (number of people in need) and risk (percentage of the population in need). One can infer the following about the downtown communities:

◆ All DT5 communities have social, economic, and health risks because of income, employment, and education deficiencies.
◆ Those who are young, elderly, immigrants, and women are at increased risk because of inequalities in employment, income, and independence.
◆ Because all communities have different risk factors, a single program will not serve all communities equally; Bridgeland is more in need of seniors' services, while Victoria Park is in more need of community safety services; single-parent families in several neighbourhoods may benefit from parenting programs to reduce their stress levels.
◆ The inner-city communities have many assets and strengths on which to build capacity.

Community Diagnosis

In the preceding pages, each subsystem of the DT5 has been analyzed in relation to its effect on the core (the people), the geographic community, and issues of importance. In each instance, inferences have been drawn and suggestions made for the collection of more data, comparative data, or data from different sources. The final task of analysis is the synthesis of the inference statements into community diagnoses (Neufeld & Harrison, 2000).

A diagnosis is a statement that synthesizes assessment data. A diagnosis is a label that both describes a situation (or state) and implies an etiology (reason) and gives evidence to support the inference.

A nursing diagnosis limits the diagnostic process to those diagnoses that represent human responses to actual or potential health problems nurses are licensed to treat. A medical diagnosis includes those issues a doctor is licensed to treat. A community diagnosis differs, however, in that it is focused on an aggregate or a community (rather than individuals), it requires multidisciplinary action to address (treat), multiple determinants must be considered when planning interventions, and outcomes of action may not be visible in the short term.

Although no standard format exists, most community diagnoses have four parts:

1. A description of the problem, response, or state
2. A statement indicating the aggregate, population, or community of focus

3. Identification of factors etiologically (causally) related to the problem
4. Signs and symptoms (manifestations) that are characteristic of the problem

A community diagnosis focuses the diagnosis on a *community*—usually defined as a group, population, or cluster of people with at least one common characteristic (such as geographic location, occupation, ethnicity, or housing condition). To derive a community diagnosis, community assessment data are analyzed and inferences are presented. Inference statements shape community diagnoses. Some inference statements form the descriptive part of the diagnosis; that is, they testify to a potential or actual community problem (risk, hazard, or concern) to a particular segment of the population (i.e., among).

For instance, health status data (NLD) may indicate that the low-birth-weight rate is higher than a comparison standard (stressor). Literature provides information regarding the causes of low birth weight, and these are compared with the data collected, the conclusions drawn about their applicability to the community of interest, and community resources available to address the issue (LR), and any FLDs (temporary responses to the situation) in place.

Finally, the signs and symptoms of the community diagnosis are the inference statements that document the duration or magnitude of the problem. Examples of documentation include data from record accounts, census reports, and vital statistics. This final piece of the community diagnosis establishes the relevant data and is linked to the first two parts with an "as manifested by" clause (Box 14-3). In Box 14-4, an example of a community diagnosis for an aggregate of adolescent pregnant women who reside in the downtown area is presented.

In comparison to taking a "problem" approach (Table 14-13/Box 14-4), there are many strengths exhibited by this community and the focus population that offer the opportunity to reframe the issue as a wellness or positive diagnosis. For instance, there is opportunity to improve the health status (issue description) of adolescent pregnant women in the downtown (focus) by maintaining attendance at school; receiving social assistance; enrolling in the Best Beginning program; and receiving support (manifestations) for effective parenting, stress reduction, and smoking cessation (etiology).

Although a single problem is stated, the causes and signs and symptoms may be multiple. Also notice that although the problem inferences are drawn from the analysis of one subsystem (such as the health and social services subsystem or the educational subsystem), the causation may be, and usually is, drawn from several subsystems. For example, regarding the issue of low birth weight, etiologic inferences

BOX 14-3

Template for a Community Diagnosis

| Issue description (risk, concern, issue, state, i.e., potential/actual) | Focus (boundaries of the population segment of interest) | Etiology/causal factors (signs and symptoms) | Manifestations (data in support of the etiologic inference) |

BOX 14-4

An Example of a Community Diagnosis

Issue Description	Focus	Etiology	Manifestations
Risk of low birth weight	*Among* teen pregnant women living in the downtown area	*Related to* (a) Inadequate income	*As manifested by:* Insecure housing, use of the food bank, unemployment rates
		(b) Use of tobacco	*As manifested by:* Smoking rates among pregnant teens

can be derived from four subsystems—educational, health and social services, safety and transportation, and economic.

This example sums up the most important lesson of community practice: All community factors (subsystems) join to determine the health status of a community. No one subsystem is more important or crucial than any other in determining a community's health. Every subsystem has a role in addressing community issues. Refer again to Table 14-13 for community diagnoses for the downtown communities.

The process of deriving community diagnoses always remains the same. First, assessment data are classified and studied for inferences that are descriptive of potential or actual problems (stressors that have penetrated the NLD or FLD); next, associated inferences are identified that explain the derivation or continuation of the problem and the community assets or strengths available to address the issue (LR); and last, documentation (data) is presented to support the inferences. Several community diagnoses may be stipulated; determining the order of priority among them is part of program planning and depends on existing community goals and resources. This important skill is discussed in the next chapter.

Deriving community diagnoses requires critical thinking, decision-making, and astute study; it is a challenging and vital task. The completeness and validity of the diagnoses that have been derived will be tested during the next stage of the community process and will form the foundation of that stage—the planning of a health program.

This is an excellent time to share your assessment data with colleagues and people in the community to solicit their analysis. Because we all have opinions and values that colour our perceptions, group critique and analysis of assessment data are ways to foster objectivity. Validating your community diagnoses with the community residents is an important step for establishing and maintaining the partnership. Equally important are the rights of community leaders, organizations, and residents to confidentiality of privileged information and to choose not to participate

TABLE 14-13

Community Diagnoses for the Downtown Communities

ISSUE	POPULATION	CAUSE	DATA
Lack of safety	For residents of Victoria Park	Due to crime after dark related to: • The sex trade, • Substance abuse, • Burglary • Vandalism	As manifested by Police Service crime statistics about: • Prostitution charges • Incidence of used needles and condoms found in vacant lots near school grounds and parks • Rate of break and enter crimes • Gang tagging graffiti on vacant buildings
Lack of adequate affordable housing	For the residents of the inner city	Related to single-parent families headed by women living in poverty	As manifested by: • The percent of single-parent families spending more than 30% on housing • The number of children living in homes receiving support for independence • The volume of inner-city single mothers using food banks, thrift stores, and other community services before month's end
Perceived stress	Of lone women heading families in inner-city communities	Related to lack of social support, isolation, and parenting stress	As manifested by: • Reports from Family Social Services
Capacity for instrumental support for community-living senior citizens in the inner city	By high school students	Related to the community service requirement at the local high school	As manifested by student-run programs for: • Snow shovelling program in winter • Grocery shopping and delivery • Daily telephone contact for at-risk seniors • Friendly visitor support
Poor nutritional status	Among female seniors in inner-city communities	Related to social isolation and inability to access affordable food	As manifested by: • Reports from home care nurses and parish-based social workers • Poor public transit access to the local supermarkets

in planning. Communities have the right to identify their own needs and to negotiate with the community assessment team with regard to interventions and specific programs. In turn, the community assessment team has the responsibility to provide or assist with the development of information needed for this process. This responsibility includes not using jargon when presenting data to community members—what words can you use besides "diagnosis"?

In the mid-1990s, Alberta was reorganizing its delivery of health, children's, and mental health services. As a result, Calgary service providers and concerned citizens met to discuss how they could best serve Calgary's inner-city communities and formally established itself in 1999 as the Inner City Family Resource Centre Network (ICFRN). The network was formed to coordinate resources and services to meet the needs of the residents (families and individuals) of Calgary's inner-city communities.

Its goal was to form one or more Community Coordinating Councils (CCCs) that would facilitate both community and service agency input into the planning and delivery of services (City of Calgary, 2005).

One of the network's first initiatives was to conduct a survey to confirm the findings of the community assessment report. The purpose of the "Inner City Survey" was to give community members a voice into services needed to address their concerns.

Before we continue, a few words are needed about composing questionnaires. Everyone is confronted daily with people who are asking questions. Questionnaires arrive in the mail, and people call on the phone. Frequently, the interviewees learn neither the purpose of the questionnaire nor how the information will be used. When you draft a questionnaire, begin with introductory information that states who you are and what the purpose of the questionnaire is. Emphasize that participation is voluntary and that the information given will be confidential. Sign your name, and if the questionnaire is to be mailed, include a phone number where you can be contacted. Write questions that can be answered quickly (the whole questionnaire should not take longer than 10 minutes to complete). Ideally, place all questions on one side of a standard 8-1/2-inch by 11-inch piece of paper that, if it is to be mailed, can be refolded so that a return address shows. Before sharing the questionnaire with agencies or community residents, administer it informally to friends and family; any comments made (such as "What do you mean by . . . ?" or "I don't understand . . .") signal the need for further rewriting and clarification. The same references used for the development of surveys in the assessment phase will be helpful as you plan a survey for this phase. Remember to check the reading level and language of the questions and allow for costs of translation as needed.

Take Note

How should the questionnaire be administered? Should the questionnaire be mailed to all households? Should the questionnaire be given to a specific group only? Or should the questionnaire be used as an interview guide and given to a selected number of participants at a specific site? (Recall from research that people who have been randomly selected can be considered representative of the total population.) What would you recommend? Before making a decision, list each option and consider the benefits and drawbacks of each. Here is some information for your decision-making: Mailed questionnaires have about a 50% return rate that can be increased somewhat with a reminder postcard or telephone call, whereas questionnaires administered as an interview potentially have a 100% return rate. However, interviews require trained people and about 5 minutes per person per page of the survey, whereas mailed questionnaires require less labour but have the financial cost of postage. Decisions . . . decisions . . . .

> **BOX 14-5**
>
> **Inner City Survey Content**
>
> Which community the respondent lives in and for how long
> Challenges faced and their importance
> Service utilization
> Service needs
> Reasons that prevent use of community programs
> Preferred location for services
> Demographic information

The Inner City Survey questionnaire consisted of 15 open- and close-ended questions and was produced in October 1999 in English and four other languages: Chinese, Serbo-Croatian, Tagalog (Filipino), and Polish. Convenience sampling procedures were used to obtain participants; the survey was distributed over 20 weeks through inner-city service agencies, schools, and recreational facilities in the downtown area. Three convenient downtown locations were designated as drop-off points for completed questionnaires. To encourage participation, those who submitted the survey were eligible to enter a contest. Two thousand forms were printed and distributed, with a return rate of 470 (23.5%); 43 responses were in languages other than English. It was recognized that limitations from the low response rate, the fact that respondents had to be literate, and the sampling process interfered with the ability to generalize across communities. Nevertheless, the findings were robust enough to be used to supplement the community diagnoses from the assessment phase and to begin the planning process. The details regarding the topics included in the survey are listed in Box 14-5.

Then, once the surveys were returned, the information was classified, analyzed, and summarized for the use of the steering committee. Next, the Health Department held meetings with the downtown community associations to set priorities among the issues identified and to begin the process of brainstorming ways of meeting the needs of downtown residents.

EVALUATION

At every stage in the community-as-partner process, individuals and teams should reflect on their performance—what went well, what did not, and what should be done differently as we move to the next phase. Did you participate honestly, fully, and respectfully? Did you engage others in the process? Did the team experience conflict, and how was it managed? Was the analysis process effective?

Think back on your analysis. Did you find yourself focusing on community or population deficiencies or its strengths? Did you identify ways people could contribute their talents to the community, or did you seek to find services for them? Did you impose your ideas on people, or did you foster participation and engagement in ways that empowered people? Sometimes, we are so overcome by community needs, challenging issues, or the vulnerability of groups of people that we forget their resilience and competence in the face of adversity. We need to remind ourselves that we are doing *with* people, not *to* or *for* them; that we seek to move people from being to belonging in a community.

At this point, teams that have been constructed to do an assessment and make recommendations for action will adjourn. Remember to file documents for future reference, prepare reports, and send letters of appreciation to your participants and the network of contacts you made. Goodwill is an important gift that you can give to future teams—the program planners, community developers, and evaluators will thank you for creating a supportive environment!! The assessment and analysis processes can be interventions in themselves—they raise awareness and expectations; they build capacity and empower people; they inform providers, politicians, and participants and ignite action that can be an important foundation for the next steps: program planning (Chapter 15), intervention (Chapter 16), and evaluation (Chapter 17). In the next chapter, the planning process will be detailed.

SUMMARY

Critical analysis of five downtown communities was completed using the community assessment wheel as a guide. Subsequently, community diagnoses were formulated based on the inferences gained from the analysis. Although community diagnoses are relatively new to practice, community workers have, since the inception of community development and advocacy work, derived inferences from assessment data and have acted on those data. However, the terminology and format that have surrounded these informally produced inferences (diagnoses) have been inconsistent. There is considerable discussion, and some controversy, regarding the structure and terminology that would be optimal for community-focused diagnoses. In your practice, you will be exposed to various formats for stating community issues and capacities—evaluate and test the usefulness of each. It is only through collaboration and vigorous testing that a standard format will evolve. In the Suggested Readings list, there are additional sources to help you as you develop community diagnoses.

References

Barton, J. A., Smith, M. C., Brown, N. J., & Supples, J. M. (1993). Methodological issues in a team approach to community health needs assessment. *Nursing Outlook*, *41*(6), 253–261.

City of Calgary. (1998). Count of homeless persons in downtown Calgary May 21, 1998. Community and Social Development Department, Social Research Unit.

City of Calgary. (2003). Socioeconomic profile Calgary 2003. Retrieved July 10, 2007 from **http://www.calgary.ca.**

City of Calgary. (2005). Calgary Centre City Social Plan (C3SP): Issues and opportunities in the Centre City: Research synthesis, 1999-2005. Community and Neighbourhood Services. Retrieved July 10, 2007 from **http://www.calgary.ca.**

City of Calgary. (2006a). Results of the 2006 count of homeless persons in Calgary homeless count, May 10, 2006. Retrieved July 10, 2007 from **http://www.calgary.ca.**

City of Calgary. (2006b). Community profiles. Community and Neighbourhood Services, Policy & Planning Division. Retrieved July 10, 2007 from **http://www.calgary.ca.**

Health Canada. (2000). *Second report on the health of Canadians*. Ottawa: Author.

Helvie, C. O. (1998). *Advanced practice nursing in the community*. Thousand Oaks, CA: Sage.

Neufeld, A., & Harrison, M. J. (2000). Nursing diagnosis for aggregates and groups. In M. J. Stewart (Ed.), *Community nursing: Promoting Canadians' health* (pp. 370–385). Toronto: Saunders.

Statistics Canada. (1998). *Low income cut-offs*. Ottawa: Author.

U.S. Department of Health and Human Services. Office of Disease Prevention and Health Promotion. (1997). *Developing objectives for Healthy People 2010*. Washington, DC. U.S. Government Printing Office.

Suggested Readings

Allor, M. T. (1983). The "community profile." *Journal of Nursing Education, 22*, 12–16.

Bjaras, G. (1993). The potential of community diagnosis as a tool in planning an intervention programme aimed at preventing injuries. *Accident Analysis and Prevention, 25*, 3–10.

Ervin, N. E. (2002). *Advanced community health nursing practice*. Upper Saddle River, NJ: Prentice Hall.

Stoner, M. H., Magilvy, J. K., & Schultz, P. R. (1992). Community analysis in community health nursing practice: The GENESIS Model. *Public Health Nursing, 9*, 223–227.

U.S. Department of Health and Human Services. Public Health Service. (1997). *Healthy People 2010: National health promotion and disease prevention objectives*. Washington, DC: U.S. Government Printing Office.

Internet Resources

www.cmhc-schl.gc.ca
Canada Mortgage Housing Corporation

Planning a Community Health Program

REVISED FROM THE ORIGINAL BY ARDENE ROBINSON VOLLMAN

Chapter Outline

Introduction
Planning in Partnership With the Community
Prioritizing Community Diagnoses

Planned Change
Developing a Program Logic Model
Summary

Learning Objectives

This chapter covers the planning of actions to promote the health of a community and its people.

After studying this chapter, you should be able to:

❖ Use principles of change theory to guide the planning process
❖ In partnership with the community, plan a community-focused health program that includes
  ❖ A process for validating community diagnoses with community partners
  ❖ A process for priority setting
  ❖ Development of a program logic model
  ❖ A sequence of actions and a time schedule for achieving goals
  ❖ Resources needed to accomplish the plan
  ❖ Potential obstacles to planned actions and revised actions
  ❖ Revisions to the plan as goals and objectives are achieved or changed
  ❖ Recording the plan in a concise, standardized, and retrievable form

Introduction

*O*nce a community has been assessed, the data analyzed, and community diagnoses derived, it is time to consider interventions that will promote the

306

community's health and development—to formulate a community-focused plan. Each of the three parts of the diagnosis statement—the descriptions of the actual or potential problem, its causes, and its signs and symptoms—directs planning efforts for the community team. All three provide equally important information from which to plan. Figure 15-1 displays the process for deriving a community diagnosis and summarizes how the parts of the diagnosis both describe the community assessment and give direction for program planning, intervention, and evaluation. Community-focused plans are based on the community diagnoses and contain specific goals and interventions for achieving desired outcomes. Planning, like assessment and analysis, is a systematic process completed in partnership with the community.

Take Note

Before proceeding, let us stop and consider the word *partnership* and its implications for community health. Recall that a community is a social group determined by geographic boundaries and common values and interests. Community members function and interact within a particular social structure that both creates and exhibits behaviours and values. The normative behaviours and value systems of individuals, families, groups, and the community that you have assessed may be very different from your own individual and family behaviours and values as well as the shared values of the community in which you reside. This creates a potential conflict. What may appear to you as a primary health problem of the community may not hold the same importance for the community's residents. They may be far more concerned about another possibility. Hence, there is a real need to prioritize community diagnoses with the community. There is one question to ask: Are the community diagnoses of importance to community residents? Methods of setting priorities among community diagnoses are presented in this chapter.

PLANNING IN PARTNERSHIP WITH THE COMMUNITY

It is important to validate community diagnoses with the residents and leadership of the community; it is their right to participate in decisions that affect them. The validation process can serve as an important trust-building activity in maintaining the partnership, and it is the role of the community worker to ensure they have all the information they need on which to base their choices.

In addition to forming a partnership with the community, the community worker must consider the influences of social, economic, ecological, and political issues. Larger policy issues directly and profoundly affect many (if not all) community issues. For instance, the number of injuries due to falls by seniors living in Bridgeland is related as much to the age and frailty of the people as it is to the condition of

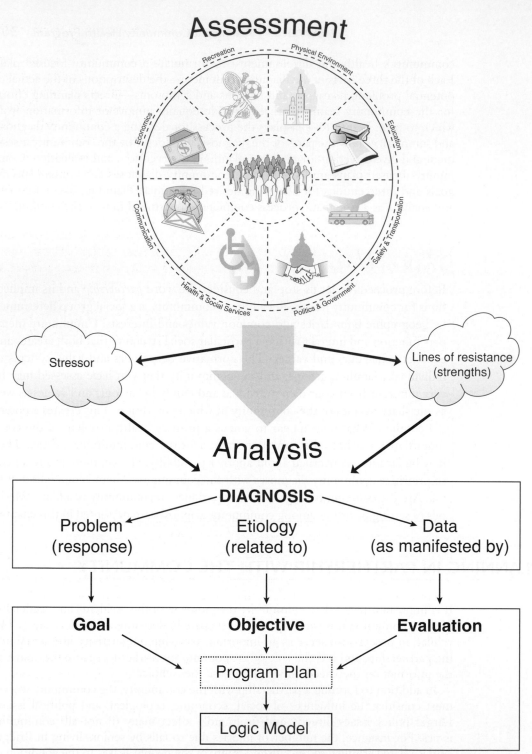

FIGURE 15-1 ◆ Relationship of assessment, analysis, and diagnosis with program planning.

the sidewalks, the knowledge of seniors about home safety, the lack of seniors' programs in the community, social isolation, and the nutrition levels of seniors and their access to adequate food. Each of these causes is related to municipal, provincial, and federal policies and legislation. Consider returning to the discussion of the Web of Causation in Chapter 3 for guidance. None of the diagnoses can be considered separate from others; all must be considered when doing community-focused planning.

The team involved in community-focused health planning must also consider the needs of populations at risk. Special at-risk groups reside in all communities—the homeless, the poor, new immigrants, pregnant women, infants, children, and the elderly are groups at increased risk. The health needs of at-risk groups must be considered as part of all community plans.

As is obvious from the assessment phase, resources exist within the downtown to serve the needs of residents. However, utilization was "spotty" at best—some services were appropriately and effectively utilized; others were underutilized or used by a population that was not its primary target, and others were overutilized because the demand for service was far greater than the resources available. The following reasons for not using available services were included on the Inner City Survey to assist in planning services that would be acceptable and accessible to the residents of the inner city:

- I don't have any way to get there.
- It is too far from home.
- It is not a convenient time.
- It is too expensive.
- I don't know what programs exist.
- Do not offer the programs I want.
- I don't know how to apply for the programs.
- Nobody to look after my children.
- Access issues for special needs.
- I have difficulties speaking/understanding English.
- The programs offered conflict with my cultural values.
- Other _____

The community's planning needs must be assessed when determining the membership of the planning team. It may be that the community team formed for assessment purposes and the team pulled together for the planning process will be somewhat different, depending on the nature and priority of the community diagnoses and the scope of the issues of concern. Smith and Maurer (2000) offer the following guidelines for those who should be represented on a planning team, keeping in mind that the team should be neither too large nor cumbersome to manage (p. 391):

- Broad segments of the community to provide wide base of support to the program
- Leaders with financial and legal authority for the problem

- Champions, people in a position to promote acceptance of the program (e.g., media, community leaders)
- Those who will implement the program
- Those who will be affected by the program (i.e., the target group)
- Those who will most likely offer resistance (i.e., the opposition)
- Specialists in the field who can contribute to understanding and offer alternative solutions

Last, community-focused planning involves an awareness and application of planned change—a process of well-thought-out actions to make something happen. Planned change is discussed in detail later in this chapter.

PRIORITIZING COMMUNITY DIAGNOSES

Not all issues can be addressed at the same time, so priorities must be determined. Many factors can influence the priority of an issue—a life-threatening emergency will take priority over everything else. Other factors are the seriousness of a concern, the desires of the community or aggregate, time, cost, and availability of resources. Five factors to consider are:

1. Magnitude of concern expressed by members of the community
2. Extent of existing resources to deal with the concern (e.g., knowledge, time, money, equipment, supplies, facilities, personnel)
3. Potential for success in solving the problem with existing resources
4. Need for special education or training
5. Extent of additional resources and policies needed for equitable, cost-effective, and efficient response

Several processes can be used to determine which issue or concern is the highest priority. For instance, each concern identified can be listed and posted around a meeting room at a community planning workshop. Members of the community and the team could be given a means to "vote" on their top three priorities (e.g., three coloured dots, three sticky notes), and those concerns that receive no "votes" are first removed from the list of priority issues.

In the next step, those issues that receive the most votes are assessed, one by one, according to a predetermined set of criteria, rated on a scale of 1 to 5, on which the team again "votes" or comes to consensus. The team may decide that community motivation is the most important criterion, and if that is not present to a high degree, action on the issue will fail. Or, the team may decide that quick success is most important, rating the speed criterion the highest. In any event, decisions about how to rate each criterion must be made in advance by the team, before the rating exercise begins.

- How aware is the community of the issue?
- How motivated is the community to resolve the issue?

TABLE 15-1

Ranking Each Issue by Criterion Weight

CRITERIA	CRITERION WEIGHT	AVERAGE RATING	RANKING (WEIGHT × RATING)	TOTAL POSSIBLE SCORE
Awareness	4	5	20	20
Motivation	5	2	10	25
Influence	3	4	12	15
Expertise	4	3	12	20
Severity	5	5	25	25
Speed	1	1	1	5
	Maximum (6 × 5) = 30	Maximum (6 × 5) = 30	Actual score = 80	Maximum score = 110

◆ How able is the team to influence the resolution of the issue?
◆ How available is the needed expertise to address the issue?
◆ How severe are the consequences if the issue remains unresolved?
◆ How quickly can the team achieve resolution?

As each participant rates each criterion for each issue, scores will indicate the order in which the community ranks its priorities. Discussions can then proceed regarding approaches to addressing the priority issue(s). So, for the first issue, compare the agreed-on issue weighting criteria with the average of the individual participants' ratings on each criterion by averaging the ratings, then multiplying them by the weighting. The sum of the ranking provides an overall assessment of the priority of the issue. This ranking process is detailed in Table 15-1.

In this way, issues can be examined and compared horizontally (across the row) to determine which criterion has the highest ranking overall and vertically (down the column) to determine which issue is the highest priority for action. As you continue to read this chapter, you will see in the example provided, the severity of the issue if left unresolved is clearly at a maximum. However, the speed with which the community can address it is at the minimum in the context of relatively low community motivation even though there is relatively high availability of expertise to address the concern. The community can discuss the meaning and interpretation of scores, and effective priorities can be set with efficiency.

The top issues in the five downtown Calgary communities in the example, as prioritized through the Inner City Survey and community meetings, are summarized in Table 15-2.

PLANNED CHANGE

We all experience change. As you read these words, your knowledge level is changing. Yet planned change differs from change in that actions occur in a definite sequence, with each one serving as preparation for the next. Planned change is a well-thought-out effort designed to make something happen; all efforts are

TABLE 15-2	
Priority of Community Issues	
THEME	RANK
Crime and safety	
In the neighbourhood	1
Break-ins/robberies	5
Vandalism	10
Prostitution	6
Teen gangs	9
Parenting issues	4
Access to services	7
Housing	
Cost	2
Homelessness	9
Having enough money	3
Literacy and training	
Cost of programs	11
Reading and writing skills	8
Job training	12

directed and targeted to produce change. (Many theorists have written about planned change; several works are listed at the end of this chapter.) Reinkemeyer's (1970) stages of planned change are presented in Box 15-1. The stages are like a recipe in that to produce the intended outcome, it is helpful to follow them strictly and completely to reach the intended outcomes.

BOX 15-1

Reinkemeyer's Stages of Planned Change

Stage 1	Development of a felt need and desire for the change
Stage 2	Development of a change relationship between the agent and the client system
Stage 3	Clarification or diagnosis of the client system's problem, need, or objective
Stage 4	Examination of alternative routes and tentative goals and intentions of actions
Stage 5	Transformation of intentions into actual change
Stage 6	Stabilization
Stage 7	Termination of the relationship between the change agent and the client system

Reinkemeyer, A. (1970). Nursing's need: Commitment to an ideology and change. *Nursing Forum*, 9(4), 340–355.

BOX 15-2

Lewin's Stages of Planned Change and Their Application to the Planning Process

Lewin's Stages of Planned Change	Application to the Planning Process
>> ◆ Unfreezing	◆ Unfreezing ● Identification of a need for change
>> >> ◆ Moving process	◆ Moving process ● Presence of a change agent ● Identification of problems ● Consideration of alternatives ● Adaptation of plan to circumstances
>> >> >> ◆ Refreezing	◆ Refreezing ● Implementation of the plan ● Stabilization of the situation

Lewin, K. (1958). Group decision and social change. In E. Maccoby (Ed.), *Readings in social psychology* (3rd ed.). New York: Holt, Rinehart and Winston.

One theorist, Kurt Lewin (1958), described three stages of planned change: unfreezing, moving, and refreezing, as shown in Box 15-2. It is during the unfreezing stage that the client system (in other words, the organization, community, or at-risk population) becomes aware of a problem and the need for change. Then the problem is diagnosed, and solutions to the problem are identified. From these alternative solutions, one is chosen that seems most appropriate for the situation. In the moving stage, the change actually occurs. The problem is clarified, and the program for solving the problem is planned in detail and begun. Finally, the refreezing stage consists of the accomplished changes becoming integrated into the values of the client system. In this stage, the idea is established and continues to be influential. Lewin also addressed forces that help or hinder change to occur, labelling them the *driving forces* and the *restraining forces*, respectively.

Theories of planned change are important because they can be used to guide and direct the planning process. Conceptual frameworks that suggest how individuals change their behaviour also inform the planning process. Table 15-3 details the key components of the transtheoretical (stages of change) model (Prochaska et al., 1995). The processes of change addressed by the transtheoretical model are located in Table 15-4 (Prochaska et al., 1995). Other models of change are described in the Suggested Readings section.

TABLE 15-3	
Stages of Change of the Transtheoretical Model	
STAGE OF CHANGE	CHARACTERISTICS
Precontemplation (PC)	Still engages in risky behaviour
	Has no intention of changing within the next 6 months
	May be uninformed, in denial, or demoralized from previous failures
	Defensive and resistant to change, avoids addressing risky behaviour
Contemplation (C)	Engages in the risky behaviour but is aware of problem
	Seriously considering change within 6 months but has not yet made a commitment to take action
	Indecisive, lacks commitment to enact significant change in high-risk behaviour
Preparation (P)	Still engages in high-risk behaviour but intends to take action within the next month
	Has typically taken some significant action in the past year
	Is on the verge of taking action and needs to set goals
Action (A)	Has modified behaviour, experiences, or environment within the last 6 months
	Involves overt behavioural changes and requires considerable commitment of time and energy
Maintenance (M)	Works to prevent relapse and consolidate the gains attained during action
	Is less tempted to relapse and has become increasingly more confident to continue changes
	A continuation, not an absence, of change
Termination (T)	Feels zero temptation and complete confidence
	New, healthier behaviour has become second nature
	Unlikely for most behaviours

Applying Change Theory to Community Planning

To validate the priorities and initiate the planning process, Reinkemeyer's stages of planned change (see Box 15-1) have been chosen as a guide.

STAGE 1: DEVELOPMENT OF A FELT NEED AND DESIRE FOR THE CHANGE

To initiate a felt need and desire for change within a community, those people and organizations involved in the assessment phase can be contacted and invited to a meeting to receive a report of the community assessment findings and proposed community diagnoses and to engage in an exercise to validate the findings and discuss priorities.

STAGE 2: DEVELOPMENT OF A CHANGE RELATIONSHIP BETWEEN THE AGENT AND THE CLIENT (PARTNER) SYSTEM

Both stages 1 and 2 are often completed during the assessment and analysis phases and the presentation of the report to the community and stakeholders because the team has entered the community and begun to establish connections with the people in it. At this point, community members (champions) and stakeholders express a

TABLE 15-4

Processes of Change of the Transtheoretical Model

PROCESS OF CHANGE	CHARACTERISTIC
Consciousness-raising	Individuals need to raise their awareness of the negative consequences of their behaviour.
Dramatic relief	Individuals need to release and express emotions related to their high-risk behaviour. Life events, such as the death of a close friend or family member, can move people into precontemplation emotionally, especially if the death was related to the high-risk behaviour.
Environmental re-evaluation	In precontemplation, individuals need to recognize how the presence or absence of a personal habit affects one's social environment.
Self-re-evaluation	This process is most important when the individual is moving from contemplation to preparation, when people assess how they feel and think about the behaviour. People may become aware of their guilt about a particular behaviour.
Self-liberation	While preparing for action, individuals need self-liberation, that is, the belief that they can change and the commitment to act on that belief.
Reinforcement management	During action, individuals need to provide consequences for taking steps in a particular direction, including the use of punishments for slips or rewards for making positive changes.
Helping relationships	Helping relationships can include those with health professionals who are actively involved in assisting the person to change or supportive members of a social network.
Counterconditioning	During the action and maintenance stages, individuals need to substitute healthier behaviours for the high-risk behaviours.
Stimulus control	People in action or maintenance need to remove stimuli that were associated with the unhealthy behaviour and add stimuli that signal the new behaviour.
Social liberation	Social liberation requires an increase in social opportunities or alternatives, especially for people who are relatively deprived or oppressed.

desire to become involved in the planning process to address the priority concerns. To preserve momentum and to expedite the planning processes, agencies/ groups often delegate a representative to the planning committee. At this point, a member of the community team is usually named to function as a change agent to guide and facilitate, but not to direct, the planning process. Sometimes a co-chair is elected from the community, the committee is given a mandate to plan, reporting measures are determined, and initial meetings are set. At this point, it is important to commit to build community participants' capacity in this process—remember to include the community co-chair in all meetings and decisions and to set meeting times that allow this to happen.

STAGE 3: CLARIFICATION OR DIAGNOSIS OF THE CLIENT SYSTEM'S PROBLEM, NEED, OR OBJECTIVE

Now the time has arrived for the planning team to confirm the community diagnoses and compare interpretations of the data with the perceptions of the selected target population. This process can be done by a questionnaire focused on a particular population or neighbourhood; it can be designed as a mail-out or completed as an interview. For instance, single parents who live in the target neighbourhoods and receive social assistance can be invited by social workers to provide information about the appropriateness of inferences drawn from the data about the need for parenting classes. Single parents can be approached by public health nurses when they bring their children for immunization to make suggestions about what services might meet their child-rearing needs. On the other hand, if you are planning to intervene at a community level with a community development project, you may choose to interview community leaders and civic groups (key informants) that are representative of the target population. The word *representative* is very important; the team needs to ensure that they are including the appropriate people in the validation process. For instance, if you are concerned about issues relevant to the well-being of a particular neighbourhood, people from a variety of walks of life, ethnic backgrounds, ages, religions, sex, marital status, family structure, and so forth should be included. Otherwise, a complete picture of life in the community will not be drawn. Validation from professionals and business owners, though informative, will not necessarily provide the most reliable perspective.

STAGE 4: EXAMINATION OF ALTERNATIVE ROUTES AND TENTATIVE GOALS AND INTENTION OF ACTIONS

At this stage, as the results are examined, planning committee members make suggestions about how to address the issues. Inventories of services, resources, and funding already available are compiled. Literature about successful programs in other jurisdictions is examined, program evaluation findings are analyzed, and decisions are made about a preferred approach to the issues.

As details emerge about how to address the issues, the planning committee must make decisions among suggested strategies based on the resources available, likelihood of success, acceptability to the community, and the time it will take to meet the goals.

We will return to stages 5 to 7 (transformation, stabilization, and termination) in Chapters 16 and 17.

Take Note

Each stakeholder will consider how information and suggested routes can be assimilated into existing or planned programs. All agencies have budgets and a set number of staff members to deliver services. Agencies must be as cost-efficient as possible and will want to consider how to include new services into an existing program or whether new funding will be needed. Community workers can facilitate this process by becoming familiar with the organizational structure and purpose of each stakeholder to learn as much as possible about their services and decision-making processes to facilitate the planned change interventions.

DEVELOPING A PROGRAM LOGIC MODEL

Now is the time to transform the ideas and proposals of each stakeholder into a community-focused goal and concrete intentions for action. A logic model is a diagrammatic representation of a program (Dwyer & Makin, 1997) that depicts the relationships among program goals, objectives, activities, indicators, and resources. It shows how different facets of a program are related and helps to integrate the program planning function with evaluation. The logic model also links back to the data collected in the community assessment phase and the diagnosis formulated in the analysis (see Fig. 15-1).

What is a program? It is an organized set of activities intended to meet specific goals and objectives (outcomes). A program may have a broad series of activities (e.g., a national tobacco reduction program), or it may be smaller and more specifically targeted (e.g., a prelunch hand-washing program for kindergarten students at a local school).

The program goal is a directional statement that specifies the desired outcome of the intervention. The target group is, as specified in the community diagnosis, the recipient of the program. This recipient group may be defined by age, sex, income level, ethnicity, health characteristics, or geographic location. Groups of activities that go together are called *components* and given a descriptive label. Then, for each component, outcome objectives are written using the SMART formula (i.e., specific, measurable, action-oriented, realistic, and time specific). Outcome objectives can be short term or long term and represent the desired end results of the intervention. Process objectives specify the activities that are needed to achieve the outcome objectives. Evaluation indicators based on the wording of the objectives need to be specified for each objective. Resources required to successfully carry out the intervention should be listed; they might include personnel, funding, materials, training, and promotional expenses (see Table 15-5 for a sample logic model).

Program Goals

A goal is stated as a long-term future condition, situation, or status (Ervin, 2002) of a particular population group that clearly identifies what outcome the intervention is designed to achieve or what change is expected in the target population.

From the setting of the goal, the target of an intervention becomes evident. The focus may be individuals, a group, or the community. When the focus is on individuals, their unique perspectives will govern the level of success attained. For instance, according to the Health Belief Model, the degree of behaviour change achieved may be related to the individual's perceived susceptibility to the condition, severity of the threat to personal health, benefits of acting, barriers to action, and cues to action (Rosenstock, Strecher, & Becker, 1988). Social support is a factor in how people adapt to situations, and other models (e.g., transtheoretical [stages of change] model [TTM]) define the stages people pass through as they go through the change process.

When the focus of an intervention is a group, we find that people in the group fall into five categories: innovators, early adopters, early majority adopters, late majority adopters, and laggards. The focus on a larger community requires different approaches such as those described by Lewin and Reikenmeyer (see Boxes 15-1 and 15-2). Understanding the processes of change is important for the team when making decisions about what activities to undertake to meet the stated goal.

Program Activities

Program activities map out the actions necessary to deliver the program and thereby reach the goal(s). Choosing an activity requires knowledge of a broad range of intervention strategies. Strategies can be classified as promotion, prevention, or protection and are aimed at education, engineering, or enforcement. Not all strategies are effective on all groups. For instance, an awareness program may be sufficient for action among innovators and early adopters, but personal contact may be needed for laggards. In many instances, a combination of education, policy change, and enforcement may be needed to help populations adopt healthy behaviours (e.g., seat belt campaigns).

In our Calgary example, the downtown Health and Social Services Department office had many pamphlets and resource materials for parents with advice about common parenting issues (e.g., toilet training, sibling rivalry, sleep patterns, nutrition, etc.) and also offered "Baby and You" classes to new parents. The recreation/pool centres offered "Parent and Me" swim and gym classes. The library had weekly story sessions for preschoolers. Yet, many parents still felt stressed and isolated. Based on this information, it was logical for community workers to suggest that "Nobody's Perfect" parenting classes be held in the downtown area. But in which neighbourhood? Where was the easiest access for the most people? Where was the highest need for this activity?

Calendar charts are an effective means of planning and documenting program activities. An example is shown in Figure 15-2. Note that the activities are sequenced in a stepwise manner, with start and completion months specified along with the initials of the person responsible to carry out the activity. Such charts are versatile and can show weekly or daily progress, depending on the needs of the program. They may be more or less detailed as required by funding agencies, administration, or working groups.

Program Objectives

Objectives are measurable and describe the behaviour expected in a specific time frame. They describe the step-by-step outcomes that are required to meet the long-term goal and specify who will perform the behaviour, under what conditions, how well they must perform (standard to be met), and how performance will be measured. The literature relevant to the health issue, population, group, and performance targets will need to be reviewed to ensure that the objectives are realistic in the time allotted.

	J	F	M	A	M	J	J	A	S	O	N	D
1. Invite partners to participate (AA)	0	X										
2. Create steering committee (AA)		0	X									
3. Develop logic model and work plans (ALL)				0	X							
4. Budget planning (CA)				0	X							
5. Protocols and policy development (DD)					0	X						
6. Develop program materials (CC)					0	→	X					
7. Hiring program staff (AA)						0	X					
8. Training staff (DD)						0	X					
9. Pilot test (CC)							0	X				
10. Evaluate pilot and revise (CC)									0X			
11. Set up demonstration site (DD)										0X		
12. Official launch (AA)											0X	
13. All sites participating (AA)												→

0= Begin task, X= End task (Initials of person responsible)

FIGURE 15-2 ◆ A calendar chart for coordinating and tracking planning activities.

Both process and outcome objectives can be written in sequential steps that are required to reach the goal, or each objective may have different aspects that, when combined, achieve the goal.

Take Note

The planning team must make every effort to involve community partners in the writing of outcome objectives if the program is to be acceptable to the target group. The team must also weigh the costs of intervention against the outcomes so that the most people can benefit at affordable cost.

Once program activities have been established, objectives are written. Outcome objectives focus on the client and are derived from a goal and describe the precise behaviour or changes that will be required to achieve the goal. Whereas process objectives map out the actions necessary to deliver the program, outcome objectives specify what changes in knowledge, behaviours, or attitudes are expected as a result of program activities.

If the activity chosen is health education, the objectives should detail the knowledge changes anticipated—for example, awareness, understanding, application, or evaluation. If the team is planning to engineer the environment to make the healthy choice the easy choice, it is the environment that must change. If the activity is to change policy, create new policy, or enhance the enforcement of policy, the objectives must reflect those elements that support this activity.

Objectives need to be stated in measurable terms. To make statements measurable, use precise words. Examples of precise terms and less precise terms are:

Less Precise Terms (Many Interpretations)
◆ To know
◆ To understand
◆ To realize
◆ To appreciate
◆ To be aware
◆ To lower

More Precise Terms (Fewer Interpretations)
◆ To identify
◆ To discuss
◆ To list
◆ To compare and contrast
◆ To state
◆ To decrease by 20%

In addition, strive for each objective to include:

◆ A time frame for attaining the change (e.g., "By June 15th. . . .")
◆ The direction and magnitude of the change (e.g., "Immunization levels at school entry will increase to 95%.")
◆ The method of measuring the change (e.g., "After the session, each participant will demonstrate. . . .")

Goals and objectives help to clarify a program and establish the expected changes that will result from the program. Although much has been written on the mechanics of writing goals and objectives (several such texts are listed at the conclusion of this chapter), little information exists on the collaborative relationship that must exist between the community team and community agencies before meaningful goals and objectives can result. Goals, objectives, and their indicators of success are absolutely crucial to the evaluability of your project. Clear and meaningful statements that articulate what measures will be used to assess achievement are necessary in the next steps of the community-as-partner process.

Interviews with single parents in the downtown area underscored the stress that they experienced, particularly with decisions about raising children. When asked about what could help, they suggested opportunities for parents to get together to learn from each other how to handle things, especially child (mis)behaviour; day programs to keep young children occupied while parents carried out activities such as food shopping or appointments with agencies; Adopt-a-Grandparent or Big Brother/Big Sister programs for positive role modelling; and so forth.

Action on access to day care was being led by a social service agency, and the Boys and Girls Clubs were sponsoring Big Brothers and Big Sisters, so the community planning team felt that the implementation of a Health Canada parenting support program called "Nobody's Perfect" would benefit the community in several ways. First, people in similar situations (lone parents of young children) would have the opportunity to meet in a central location with day care on site to learn effective parenting. Second, connecting in this way would serve to form connections and attachments that could provide social support and reduce isolation. Third, as parents became less stressed and more confident, they would have more energy to devote to the demands of being a lone parent and a community member. The logic model for the program is provided in Table 15-5.

Based on the logic model for the parenting program and with contributions from several service agencies, the planning team recommended that this program be implemented in the community of Bridgeland, where a high number and proportion (46.6%) of single parents resided (see Chapter 14). Data further revealed a high incidence of children living in households receiving social assistance (31.8%), and almost one third of the population living in low-income households. A program steering committee that consisted of the facilitator, partners, and community members (single parents) was formed and met regularly to carry out the details for implementation.

COLLABORATION

What is meant by a collaborative relationship? Could several community concerns be addressed in the same program? If they could, what would be the program goal? The objectives? This process is an example of collaborative planning and is the essence of community health practice. You may be wondering how to establish collaborative planning and inform agencies about the usefulness of goals and objectives. Although you may be convinced of the value of planned change, how do you convince others to agree, especially since planned change is not commonly practised in agencies? Role modeling is probably the best strategy. After reviewing the community diagnoses and validating data with an agency, propose goals and objectives that are congruent with the agency's purpose and organizational structure. Solicit input from the group, and continue to revise the goals and objectives until a group consensus is reached.

The advantages of collaboration include preventing duplication of effort, pooling resources for maximum impact, creating more publicity and credibility than

TABLE 15-5

"Nobody's Perfect" Program Logic Model

Overall goal: Parents will be capable of obtaining the support and information they need to maintain and promote the health of their children 0–5 years of age.
Target group: Parents who are young, single, socially or geographically isolated, or who have low income or limited formal education. Participation is voluntary and free of charge. The program is not intended for families in crisis.

PROGRAM COMPONENTS	SUPPORT	EDUCATION
Short-term objectives	Establish a group for mutual support development.	Increased knowledge and understanding of children's health, safety, and behaviour.
	Increased self-help knowledge and skill.	Increased coping skills.
Long-term objectives	Increased opportunities to offer aid to other parents in "Nobody's Perfect."	Positive change in parenting knowledge and actions regarding children's health, safety, and behaviour.
	Improved self-help, information, and assistance-seeking behaviour.	Improved self-image as a parent.
	Decreased sense of isolation in parenting.	Increased confidence in parenting skill and ability.
Short-term indicators	Referred parents will enroll in "Nobody's Perfect."	Able to demonstrate learning from each session.
	Parents will attend 75% of sessions.	Posttest scores greater than pretest scores.
	Parents will be engaged in session activities.	Appropriate responses to case study examples.
	Parents will be satisfied with group process.	Reported use of coping techniques at home.
	Parents will be able to articulate sources for self-help and mutual aid.	
Long-term indicators	Accepts assistance/advice from group members and facilitators.	Consistently displays positive responses regarding children's health, safety, and behaviour.
	Provides examples, ideas to group.	Views self as a good parent.
	Actively seeks and accepts support and information from community resources.	Is confident in ability to deal with new situations as children grow and develop.
	Feels more connected to the community.	
Program/facilitator activities	Recruitment of parents	Teach, using adult education principles.
	Facilitation of sessions	Facilitate session discussions and problem-solving.
	Encouragement of parents	
	Environmental support for learning	
Resources	Infrastructure for recruitment and registration	"Nobody's Perfect" materials
	Physical facility	Supplies
	Child care	Telephone and other contact resources
	Finances	
	Refreshments	
	"Nobody's Perfect" materials	

any stakeholder partner could accomplish alone, and increasing opportunities for sharing information.

To be effective, each objective needs to be supported by a clear work plan that details the specific steps to be taken in each facet of the planned program. What actions need to be done? How will they be accomplished? For instance, protocols and policies may need to be written to ensure that activities are carried out as designed by front-line workers. What resources are needed? A detailed purchasing or refurbishing plan may need to be developed, in-kind contributions tracked, and training programs developed and undertaken. Who is responsible for each action, when it is to begin, and by when is it to be completed can be detailed using a calendar chart such as in Figure 15-2. The work plan must consider communication methods to ensure that each working group is in concert with every other one. Coordination meetings must be held regularly with full attendance to ensure that the plan runs smoothly and the program is implemented on time. Be sure to keep stakeholder agencies and the community informed of progress along the way.

Resources, Constraints, and Revised Plans

Once goals and objectives are written, the next step is to identify available resources and any constraints to the plan. These are analogous to Lewin's (1958) driving and restraining forces. Last, revised plans are proposed to the planning group. Resources are all the available means for accomplishing a task, including staff and budget as well as physical space and equipment. Recall that part of your community assessment included the identification of strengths. As you consider resources, include those strengths that may facilitate meeting program goals and objectives. For program planning, it is important to identify the resources needed as well as the resources available. Constraints are obstacles that restrict or limit actions and can include a lack of staff, budget, physical space, and equipment. Constraints may be thought of as the difference between needs and resources. Revised plans are actions that are proposed based on the knowledge of resources and constraint.

Take Note

Universal constraints are staff and money—agencies never have enough. An additional constraint is resistance to change. All people are reluctant to change existing routines and patterns of behaviour. Initially, change is uncomfortable, and until new roles are learned, there is anxiety. Making people aware of the natural discomfort associated with change can build rapport and establish a collaborative relationship.

When each agency had shared its program goals, objectives, and activities, along with resources and constraints, several alternative actions became apparent. Therefore, the following revised plan was proposed.

Parenting classes will be held at a Bridgeland community school at 6:30 PM on Tuesdays because no early evenings were available at the community centre. Social workers, public health nurses, and teachers will place posters prominently in their offices, clinics, and classrooms. Professional partners also committed to inviting people to register. Registration will be done by the health clinic. The community police office will supply refreshments for three sessions; the seniors' group will alternate with them to provide refreshments for the remaining 3 weeks. The health department will supply the books and a nurse to facilitate the sessions. Grade 7 student volunteers will babysit in the child care room, and community volunteers from the steering committee will be present at the classes to welcome the participants and provide support to the sessions.

As word spread, the Vietnamese community in Bridgeland asked to be next on the schedule. To facilitate this, a Vietnamese-speaking community worker from Bridgeland was invited to attend the community sessions to learn the facilitation techniques with the mentorship of the nurse, social worker, teacher, and police officer involved. She also received advice and support from the community members on the steering committee about how to set up a similar process in the Vietnamese cultural centre. One woman even offered to go to the cultural centre business meeting with the facilitator to celebrate the parenting class success and encourage the Vietnamese community to get behind the project.

For each constraint identified, a revised plan was proposed, discussed, and adopted. This was a period of intense collaboration between the community team and community agencies, and only at the completion of this stage was the community ready for stage 5 of planned change—transformation of intentions into actual change behaviour. This transformation of intentions is the actual program implementation (which is covered in the next chapter). However, before the plan is implemented, costs must be calculated and the plan recorded.

BUDGETING

Several general areas require financing in any program. It is helpful to managers and funding agencies if you use a balance sheet format and specify sources of funds (e.g., new grants, in-kind contributions, funds already dedicated or earmarked for the intervention, donations) as well as the cost centres (e.g., personnel, supplies), staff expenses (e.g., travel, parking), operating costs (e.g., office administration, phone, fax, postage), and meeting expenses (e.g., refreshments, rent). Indicate how anticipated shortfalls or revenues will be managed. Budgets need not be overly detailed at this stage. As the plan progresses, financial expertise may need to be sought to prepare the accounting methods to ensure accountability.

RECORDING

Community plans must be recorded in standardized, systematic, and concise forms that clearly communicate to others the purpose and actions of the plan as well as the rationale for revisions and deletions of actions. Discuss with each agency its present recording system and decide on a format and system for recording the plan. The format need not be elaborate; a short written memorandum is a key component in the explicit agreement among people and agencies about what they agreed to do. The memo should include a background statement that details the key community assessment findings, the diagnosis, a description of the target population, and the model used for program planning. The components of the logic model should be clearly articulated (goals, objectives, indicators, etc.) along with a description of the program and its related activities. A separate section should present the proposed intervention itself and the details relevant to the delivery of the program. A statement of the available and needed resources, along with the current and anticipated constraints, will set the stage for the budget proposal. It is also a good idea to articulate the anticipated outcomes and impacts of the program without overstating your case and creating expectations that the program cannot be expected to achieve.

SUMMARY

The planning process begins with validation of the community diagnoses—a process that establishes the community's perception and value of community health needs. Next, using theories of planned change, the planning team and the community form a collaborative partnership to establish program goals, objectives, and the program logic model. Then, based on resources and constraints, intervention plans are proposed and revised, work plans and critical paths are recorded, and a final plan is adopted. Although only one example is offered here, the process of community planning is essentially the same for all programs that are developed. To create programs that are acceptable to the target population, the program planning and steering committees must encourage active participation by community representatives.

References

Dwyer, J. J. M., & Makin, S. (1997). Using a program logic model that focuses on performance measurement to develop a program. *Canadian Journal of Public Health, 88*(6), 421–425.

Ervin, N. E. (2002). *Advanced community health nursing practice*. Upper Saddle River, NJ: Prentice Hall.

Lewin, K. (1958). Group decision and social change. In E. Maccoby (Ed.), *Readings in social psychology* (3rd ed.). New York: Holt, Rinehart and Winston.

Prochaska, J., Norcross, J., & DiClemente, C. (1995). *Changing for good*. New York: Avon Books.

Reinkemeyer, A. (1970). Nursing's need: Commitment to an ideology & change. *Nursing Forum, 9*(4), 340–355.

Rosenstock, I. M., Strecher, V. J., & Becker, M. H. (1988). Social learning theory and the health belief model. *Health Education Quarterly, 15*(2);175–183.

Smith, C. M., & Maurer, F. A. (2000). Community diagnosis, planning and intervention. In C. M. Smith & F. A. Maurer (Eds.), *Community health nursing: Theory and practice* (pp. 381–406). Philadelphia: Saunders.

Suggested Readings

Bertera, R. L. (1990). Planning and implementing health promotion in the workplace: A case study of the DuPont Company experience. *Health Education Quarterly, 17*(3), 307–327.

deVries, H., Weijts, W., Dijkstra, M., & Kok, G. (1992). The utilization of qualitative and quantitative data for health education program planning, implementation, and evaluation: A spiral approach. *Health Education Quarterly, 19*(1), 101–115.

Dignan, M. B., & Carr, P. A. (1992). *Program planning for health education and promotion* (2nd ed.). Malvern, PA: Lea & Febiger.

Ervin, N. E., & Kuehnert, P. L. (1993). Application of a model for public health nursing program planning. *Public Health Nursing, 10*(1), 25–30.

Gold, R. S., Green, L. W., Kreuter, M. W. (1998). *EMPOWER: Enabling methods of planning and organizing within everyone's reach.* London, England: Jones & Bartlett. (Workbook with CD-ROM from **www.jbpub.com**.)

Green, L. W., & Kreuter, M. W. (2005). *Health program planning: An educational and ecological approach.* Mountain View, CA: Mayfield/McGraw-Hill.

Health Canada. (2000). *Second report on the health of Canadians.* Ottawa: Author.

Hedley, M. R., Keller, H. H., Vanderkooy, P. D., & Kirkpatrick, S. I. (2002). Evergreen Action nutrition: Lessons learned planning and implementing nutrition education for seniors using a community organization approach. *Journal of Nutrition for the Elderly, 21*(4), 61–73.

Helvie, C. O. (1998). *Advanced practice nursing in the community.* Thousand Oaks, CA: Sage.

Horacek, T., Koszewski, W., Young, L., Miller, K., Betts, N., & Schnepf, M. (2000). Development of a peer nutrition education program applying PRECEDE-PROCEED: A program planning model. *Topics in Clinical Nutrition, 15*(3), 19–27.

Hoyt, H. H., & Broom, B. L. (2002). School-based teen pregnancy prevention programs: A review of the literature. *Journal of School Nursing, 18*(1), 11–17.

Kelly, P. J. (2005). Practical suggestions for community interventions using participatory action research. *Public Health Nursing, 22*(1), 65–73.

Lippitt, G. (1973). *Visualizing change: Model building and the change process.* La Jolla, CA: University Associates.

Neiger, B. L., & Thackeray, R. (2002). CLIPS. Application of the SMART model in two successful social marketing projects. *Journal of Health Education, 33*(5), 301–303.

Patten, S., Vollman, A. R., & Thurston, W. E. (2000). The utility of the transtheoretical model of behavior change for HIV risk reduction in injection drug users. *Journal of the Association of Nurses in AIDS Care, 11*(1), 57–66.

Peterson, J., Atwood, J. R., & Yates, B. (2002). Key elements for church-based health promotion programs: Outcome-based literature review. *Public Health Nursing, 19*(6), 401–411.

Rew, L., Chambers, K. B., & Kulkarni, S. (2002). Planning a sexual health promotion intervention with homeless adolescents. *Nursing Research, 51*(3), 168–174.

Salazar, M. K. (1991). Comparison of four behavioral theories: A literature review. *AAOHN Journal, 39*(3), 128–135.

Shuster, G., & Goeppinger, J. (2000). Community as client: Using the nursing process to promote health. In M. Stanhope & J. Lancaster (Eds.), *Community and public health nursing* (pp. 306–329). St Louis, MO: Mosby.

Weist, M. D. (2001). Toward a public mental health promotion and intervention system for youth. *Journal of School Health, 71*(3), 101–104.

Wong-Rieger, D. (n.d.). *A hands-on guide to planning and evaluation.* Canadian Hemophilia Society: Ottawa. (Available from CPHA, **www.cpha.ca**.)

16

Implementing a Community Health Program

REVISED FROM THE ORIGINAL BY ARDENE ROBINSON VOLLMAN

Chapter Outline

Introduction

Promoting Community Ownership

Implementing a Unified Program

Setting Community and Population Health Goals

Community Health Focus

Community Interventions

Evaluation

Summary

Learning Objectives

Implementation is the action phase of the community process; it is carrying out the plan. Implementation is necessary to achieve goals and objectives, but more importantly, the implementation of interventions acts to promote, maintain, or restore population health and community well-being.

In this chapter, we discuss the process of implementing a community- or population-focused program. Intervention strategies are presented along with resources that are helpful in program implementation.

After studying this chapter, you should be able to:

❖ Suggest strategies to the community for implementation of health programs

❖ Working in partnership with the community:

   ❖ Implement planned programs

   ❖ Review and revise interventions based on community responses

   ❖ Use interventions to formulate and influence health and social policies that have an impact on the community

Introduction

O nce goals and objectives have been agreed on and recorded during the planning stage, all that remains for implementation is to actually carry out the activities to meet those objectives. This probably seems straightforward and simple. Indeed, at this point, you will have spent considerable time assessing, analyzing, and planning a program. You will be ready and eager to begin. But this very eagerness (and the associated impatience of the intervention stage) is a danger. You must take time to consider how you can promote community ownership, create a unified program that respects the overall goals of the community, and maintain a clear focus on your target population and the activities planned.

Take Note

This chapter focuses on the process of intervention and provides you with some general resources that may prove helpful in your community work. Many excellent examples of interventions in which community teams work as partners with the community are included in Part III.

PROMOTING COMMUNITY OWNERSHIP

Essential to achieving the desired outcomes of an intervention is the active participation of the community. The meaning of partnership and collaboration was discussed in the preceding chapter, but the present concern is ownership. The people of the community need to feel a sense of ownership of the program or event, which can only come with their full participation in the decisions regarding planning as well as their assuming some responsibility for implementation. Herein lies a potential conflict. The human service professions are dedicated to nurturing, sustaining, and caring for others. It is part of our professions to do for others what they would do for themselves if they were able. Indeed, many human service disciplines interact professionally with people during an altered state (crisis) that requires professionals to do for others; however, this is not true in community practice. Stepping into the community requires an attitude of doing *with* the people, not doing things *to* them or *for* them. When things are done to us or for us, our emotional commitment remains limited.

How might you ensure community ownership for a proposed program and planned interventions? How can you facilitate involvement? In Calgary, an inner-city network functioned to coordinate interagency planning for community-focused programming. When university students doing a course practicum completed the

Take Note

Recall Reinkemeyer's (1970) stages of Planned Change (Box 15–1). The goal of program implementation is to transform the plan into action so that the focus population, aggregate or community can achieve the changes desired (stage 5). Over time, as the program matures by going through several cycles, it will stabilize as part of ongoing community services (stage 6).

community assessment phase and submitted their report, community meetings had been held by the health department to determine priority issues, and planning was undertaken with community members on the various interagency planning teams. Once funding was located to support programming, the inner-city network directed its attention to the coordination of activities for implementation. The important point in this example is that a coordinating or "umbrella" group was already in place (the network). A separate working group within the network planned the "Nobody's Perfect" program and will be continuing to lead its implementation in the community.

The working group returned to the assessment data and learned that the United Way listed 14 agencies that served children and families in some capacity. The planning group decided to contact each of these agencies to inform them about the "Nobody's Perfect" program; enlist their support; inform them how parents were referred to the program; and invite them to provide speakers, audiovisual resources, and contributions for refreshments and babysitting costs.

Take Note

Do not panic at this point and feel that you must be knowledgeable about all agencies and their programs in the community that you have assessed. At the implementation stage, refer back to your initial assessment and consider logically which service agencies may have resources helpful to the planned program(s). Then, contact selected agencies, request information on their purpose and current programs, share with the agency your community-focused program plans, and solicit recommendations with regard to materials and resources. Many voluntary and NGOs have professional staff at the national and provincial levels and an affiliated or community linkage structure. These voluntary organizations have ongoing programs for a wide variety of issues, and most acknowledge health promotion as a vital part of their mission. The Internet is a good way to locate such resources in your community.

Health Canada (1999) and the Public Health Agency of Canada (PHAC) publish a tremendous amount of information that is designed to promote health among Canadians. Special attention is given to facilitating prevention activities. In addition, provincial health and social service ministries, Canadian Institutes for Health Research, the Canadian Consortium for Health Promotion Research, and other national and provincial departments (e.g., environment, education, justice, housing, transportation) and nongovernmental agencies (NGOs) have publications and initiatives that support population health. Several national or provincial libraries are designated as government repositories or information clearinghouses and, therefore, have many government publications. And do not ignore publications from other countries (such as the U.S. Centers for Disease Control and Prevention, World Health Organization).

Having discussed the importance of community participation and ownership of the program, the remaining issues to consider are a unified presentation of the program and an emphasis on community outcomes.

IMPLEMENTING A UNIFIED PROGRAM

Because of limited resources, staff constraints, and other situations beyond the control of the planners, many good programs are implemented in a piecemeal fashion that minimizes their impact. A unified program requires collaboration and coordination among the agency personnel who will implement the program, the program's recipients (the target population), and the community. Allowing plenty of time for publicizing the program (and how you perform the mechanics of publicity—the how, where, and to whom) can make a crucial difference in whether people attend and what the subsequent impact will be.

After a time and place have been selected (based on initial input from the survey questionnaires), how might you market a program? Public service announcements, notification in the newspapers, bulletin inserts for civic and religious associations, flyers sent home with school-age children, and posters and notices in community service buildings and local shopping centres are some of the methods to consider.

In the downtown communities, elementary school teachers placed articles in the school newsletter so that interested parents would know about the program, who was leading it, what costs were involved, that child care would be provided, and how to get a referral to participate. Community Associations put notices on their electronic bulletin boards and placed posters in grocery stores, arenas, pools, and other recreation centres. Social workers and public health nurses responded to requests from parents, suggestions from teachers and community workers, and registered parents into the program. A junior high teacher used the opportunity in a social studies course to offer class credits for those students who volunteered for the program in some capacity (e.g., child care).

SETTING COMMUNITY AND POPULATION HEALTH GOALS

The first *Report on the Health of Canadians* was released in 1996 and the second report *Towards a Healthy Future* in 1999. These reports summarize the current information available and comment on the state of the nation's health from a population health promotion perspective; they can be used as tools in identifying actions that can be taken to improve the health of Canadians, the residents of a province, city, or neighbourhood. The implicit goals of population health promotion is to reduce or eliminate disparities in health experienced by different groups of people, improve quality of life, and add years to life expectancy by strengthening communities and community action on the determinants of health. Provincial ministries of health and regional health authorities use these goals to establish performance objectives and determine funding priorities.

Many provinces and local health authorities have stated public health goals. At the present time, Canada is in the process of developing national public health goals that focus on:

◆ Opportunities for healthy development and learning throughout life
◆ Supportive communities and healthy working conditions
◆ Sustainable, diverse, and safe environments
◆ Vulnerable populations
◆ Supports for personal choices, skills, and capacities that enhance health
◆ An integrative, supportive public health system

(See **www.phac-aspc.gc.ca/hgc-osc/home.html**)

Take Note

Are the goals and objectives for your community realistic in terms of its past history, current context, and in relation to trends over time? Do the goals and objectives for your community-focused program further regional and provincial goals and objectives?

When the "Nobody's Perfect" working group examined its logic model and implementation plans, it was noted that its work was consistent with the overall purpose of the Network and the mandate of the Parent Advisory Committee and was congruent with the health ministry's children's initiative.

COMMUNITY HEALTH FOCUS

There is one remaining question to ask before initiating the program: Does it focus on community health? This may seem to be a strange question. You might wonder, do not all health programs focus on maintaining, restoring, or promoting health of the community? Frequently, the answer is no. Some community-based programs (i.e., located in the community, not in an acute care institution) focus on individuals and do not take the larger systems of family and community into context. Community-oriented and community-focused programs seek to improve the health of groups of people to benefit the quality of life and well-being of the community at large.

In the Inner City Project, the Network and designated staff had become very involved in planning specific activities and information modules associated with the various community projects. Several programs had been enlarged to include screening and health fairs (e.g., the seniors' health fair in Bridgeland and the community kitchen in Victoria Park), and additional activities were suggested at each meeting of the Network. The initial goal of promoting the health of downtown (DT15) residents had seemingly changed to providing lots of activities and information about health to individuals. Carrying out activities, going after every competitive funding opportunity announced, and being visibly "involved" had taken precedence over strategic planning, community participation, and collaborative coordination of activities to meet the needs of the community as expressed by the residents of that community and carried out in collaboration with community stakeholders. What had happened? Remember, we discussed the impatience and eagerness that are often associated with new programs. This situation is normal. Committees tend to overemphasize activities and knowledge and forget the initial reason for the program—to improve community health and quality of life. As activities were successful, more and more people approached the Network with more and more ideas and requests. In an effort to do as much as possible for as many people as possible, Network members found themselves in a state of burnout; community representatives felt burdened; and programs began, were carried out once, then fizzled.

It must be remembered that it is the sustained day-to-day use of knowledge and lifestyle practices that improve quality of life. Frequently, a program begins with enthusiastic momentum; media publicity attracts people to screening and information sessions—and then the program is over. Objectives are evaluated as having been achieved successfully, and another program is planned and implemented. But was there any real improvement in health? Was there any impact on participants' lifestyle practices? Will the changes be maintained and continued for a week? A month? A year? Most importantly, are the changed lifestyle or health practices supported by the surrounding environment and culture? Without sustained program activity and improvement over time, public policy that supports healthy choices and social support networks that create a positive environment, population behaviour change, and long-term impact on a community's health status will not be achieved.

Environmental and Cultural Support

Many parents in the downtown communities responded affirmatively to survey questions about child discipline. These parents believed that they or another person had hurt a child when the child was punished; parents wanted to learn ways to keep from hurting children when adults were angry. The Inner City Network responded with a series of programs on effective parenting that included information on various nonphysical strategies for disciplining youngsters as well as role-playing and open-discussion periods. However, as part of the community assessment, the school nurse recorded that the community school had a history of bullying and that no protocol for addressing it was in place because the Parent Advisory Committee had decided to focus instead on an antiracism initiative. Schoolchildren were experiencing harassment and bullying, but if it was not racial in nature, it often went unreported. The conflict between the effective parenting programs and the bullying at the school was obvious. What could be done? What would you suggest?

In Bridgeland, part of the planned "Nobody's Perfect" classes included discussion sessions on the difference between discipline and punishment and the importance of inquiring as to disciplinary techniques used by caregivers when parents left their children in someone else's care (e.g., at child care facilities, at schools, or with babysitters). During this discussion, parents with school-age children expressed their concerns about bullying on the school grounds. How, they wondered, could they deal with children who had to "fight back" at school and were acting the same way at home with younger siblings? Although some parents were unaware that the school board has an antibullying policy, most were aware of the reputation of the school as "tough" and believed that the environment could not be changed. Following a discussion of parental rights and responsibilities, one parent raised the issue with the community association president. A group of equally concerned parents subsequently came together to generate action against school violence; they made an appointment with the principal to discuss the situation. (After additional meetings with Parent Advisory Committee members and an open public meeting on school violence, the school changed its procedures regarding how it dealt with bullying, harassment, and racism. The process took 2 years, but resulted in a parent-supported peer antibullying program that created a positive school environment where children flourished in a context that valued diversity, leadership, and achievement.)

Take Note

Countless such incongruities exist between healthy lifestyles and environmental and cultural practices and policies. Here is one additional example: A school nurse taught hygiene to the elementary grades, emphasizing the importance of washing hands before meals and after using the toilet. However, the school did not provide soap in the washrooms, and for safety purposes, all taps ran with cold water. Additionally, those students who ate lunch at school were not allowed to go to the washroom to wash their hands before going to the lunch room. The reason? It was too disruptive, and students did not finish lunch soon enough. How would you approach this issue?

Identify the environmental and cultural practices and policies that are in conflict with the proposed community-focused health program that resulted from your community assessment. What can be done to increase community awareness of these conflicts, and how can change begin? To focus on health and the maintenance of healthy lifestyles, all of the community must be involved.

The best way to maintain a focus on health and not on the activities of the program is to use your practice model as a guide. The community practice model built and described in Chapter 12 (see Fig. 12-4) defines intervention as primary, secondary, and tertiary levels of prevention. Does the program that you propose address these three levels of prevention?

Levels of Prevention

Recall that *primary prevention* improves the health and well-being of the community, making it less vulnerable to stressors. Health promotion programs are primary prevention, as are programs that focus on protection from specific problems. Usually, health promotion is nonspecific and directed toward raising the general health of the total community (e.g., creating supportive environments for health by engaging community members in civic action, building healthy public policy through such actions as tobacco bylaws). Primary prevention can also be very specific, such as providing immunization against certain diseases, promoting the use of seat belts in vehicles, and purifying public water supplies. The Bridgeland peer leadership initiative that prevented school bullying by embracing diversity and teaching positive communication and conflict resolution strategies is an example of primary prevention.

Secondary prevention begins after a disease or condition is present (although there may be no symptoms). Emphasis is on screening, early diagnosis, and treatment of possible stressors that may adversely affect the community's health. The Mantoux test for tuberculosis, the Denver Developmental Screening Test for developmental delays, blood pressure assessments, and breast/testicular self-examinations are secondary prevention interventions to which we are accustomed. At a community level, Block Watch or Block Parent programs are often initiated after problems arise. Similarly, requests for services such as Boys and Girls Clubs escalate when local youth begin to get involved with vandalism and petty crime. A community kitchen or "Wheels to Meals" program might be offered as a remedy to poor nutritional status of certain populations (e.g., immigrants, seniors).

Tertiary prevention focuses on restoration and rehabilitation. Tertiary prevention programs act to return the community to an optimum level of functioning. Adequate shelters for battered women and counselling and therapy programs for sexually abused youngsters are examples of tertiary prevention. The Exit Outreach program is an example of a tertiary level preventive program intended to assist street youth. The Children's Cottage is another example, providing shelter for children when parents are experiencing a temporary crisis. The Calgary Drop-in Centre, Urban Projects Society, and Mustard Seed street ministry offer support for rehabilitation and recovery, advocacy for housing and employment, and assistance for street-involved people to gain access to treatment for financial, physical, and mental health issues.

The distinction between prevention levels is not always clear. Is a program on the assessment of fever in children (and the prevention of febrile convulsions and dehydration through use of tepid baths and extra fluids) secondary or tertiary prevention? How would you classify an effective parenting program? Support groups for lone parents? A crime prevention program? Workshops on stress reduction and physical fitness? Can some programs be primary, secondary, and tertiary depending on the needs of the persons who attend? Certainly, effective parenting classes for the parent with a child who has a behaviour problem will have a different purpose than classes designed for expectant parents of a first child. Likewise, the corporate executive who has been diagnosed with cardiovascular disease and placed on a low-cholesterol diet and activity program has very different learning needs from those of the senior citizen on a fixed income. Few programs are purely at one level of prevention. The important point is to assess your programs (the implementation phase of the community process) and ask if the interventions are consistent with the community practice model.

Levels of Practice

In addition to levels of prevention, we need to consider level of practice. This text promotes the community as partner; therefore, the level of practice is considered to be community, population, or systems focused. That is, while we may offer services and programs to individuals, (e.g., sexually transmitted infection (STI) screening, school lunches, bottled water to street-involved people) our primary purpose is to improve the conditions (health status, community core) of the population or community.

Specific criteria for population level community practice encompass:

- A focus on an entire population, subpopulation (aggregate), group, or community/ setting
- Reflection of community priorities and needs, as identified though participative processes
- Relationships with the community and its residents
- A philosophical foundation based on social justice, equity, respect, and appreciation of diversity
- The goal to improve health and reduce disparity among groups of people
- A broad definition of community and population health—mental, physical, emotional, social, spiritual, and environmental
- Evidence and research to support decision-making
- Collaboration and partnership in practice

COMMUNITY INTERVENTIONS

There are three types of interventions: education, engineering, and enforcement. In this section, we will briefly discuss each, with the focus of interventions being the group/aggregate or population.

Education

HEALTH EDUCATION

Learning can be defined as a measurable change in knowledge, attitude, or behaviour that persists over time. Learning occurs in three different domains: cognitive (memory, recognition, understanding, and application), affective (attitudes and values), and psychomotor (using the muscles and nervous system). For learning to be effective, learners must have the ability to perform and opportunities to practice. The environment needs to be supportive and the teaching format and communication process adapted to the needs of the group.

The health education literature is replete with helpful suggestions for teaching adults. For instance, Onega (2000) has adapted an acronym to describe the process of health education:

T—*Tune in*. Listen before you start teaching. Client needs should direct the content.
E—*Edit information*. Teach necessary information first. Be specific.
A—*Act on each teaching moment*. Teach whenever possible. Develop a good relationship.
C—*Clarify often*. Make sure your assumptions are correct. Seek feedback.
H—*Honour the clients as partners*. Build on clients' experiences. Share responsibility with the client group.

Knowles (1998), a scholar in adult education, offers six principles to guide adult learning:

Message—Send a clear message to the group. Avoid jargon. Select issues that are meaningful to the community.
Format—Select the most appropriate learning format. Begin where people are. Use learning aids judiciously.
Environment—Create the best possible learning environment, including physical space, interpersonal connections, and administrative aspects.
Experience—Organize positive and meaningful learning experiences—continuous, sequenced, integrated, and relevant to the group/community.
Participation—Engage learners in participatory learning. Encourage activity—discussion, role play—so that people learn by doing.
Evaluation—Evaluate and give objective feedback to learners, and receive feedback from them to modify the teaching process. (Meade, 1997, p. 168)

The educational process uses the same steps as the community process, making it straightforward for community educators to assess learner needs, plan and implement teaching interventions, and determine the effectiveness of the process.

Assessment	Identify the information needs and readiness, barriers to learning, and capacities of the target group.
Analysis and Diagnosis	State the educational goals and objectives.
Planning	Select methods, materials, site, time, and market the event.
Implementation	Carry out the sessions(s) as planned.
Evaluation	Assess the effectiveness of processes and achievement of outcomes.

Some formats for learning include brainstorming, demonstration, group discussion, lecture, role play, and panel discussion. Strategies to enhance learning may include printed material (bulletin boards, drawings, flash cards), audiovisual material (overhead transparencies, videotapes, photographs), computer-assisted software and on-line resources, guest speakers, peer presentations, and field trips. Care must be taken that materials are appropriate to the technology available, the culture, literacy and language levels of the participants, and the size of the group. Pretesting newly developed material is important, and critically assessing print resources for reading level, layout, type font and size, content (verbal and visual), and aesthetic quality is key to ensuring the resources are appropriate, culturally sensitive, and accurate.

SOCIAL MARKETING

In social marketing, mass media are used to "sell" health through particular behaviours or products. With its components of marketing and consumer research, advertising, and promotion, social marketing clearly has a central role to play in health promotion (Mintz, 1989). Mintz views the social marketing process as developing the right product, backed by the right promotion, and put in the right place at the right price. Although a social marketing campaign on its own cannot be expected to change the behaviour of large populations, it can be a potent component in a comprehensive health promotion program.

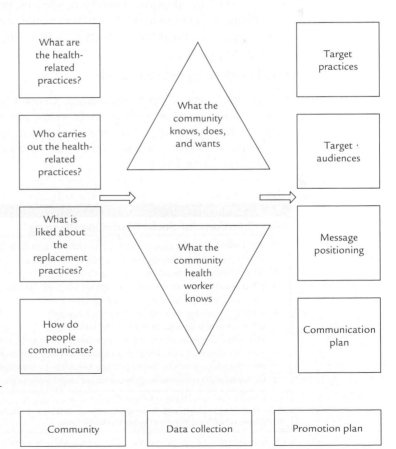

FIGURE 16-1 ◆ The process of social marketing.

Adapted from Department of International Development. (1998). *Guidance manual on water supply and sanitation programmes*. Loughborough University, Leicestershire, UK: Water and Environmental Health at London and Loughborough (WELL). Available at: **www.lboro.ac.uk/well/resources/Publications/guidance-manual/chapter_2-8.pdf**.

The *product* is the message and how it is presented. The price is not only the cost of producing and publishing the message but also the cost to the consumer of acting on it. *Promotion* is the means of persuasion or the communication function of marketing. *Place* respects adequate and suitable distribution as well as response channels or access to information. In other words, how can people who are motivated take follow-up action?

Social marketing is a systematic approach to public health problems. It offers a staged population-focused approach to convert community needs into demand and then provides the means to satisfy that demand (Figure 16-1). Social marketing is concerned with achieving a social objective. The key components of social marketing are:

- Systematically collecting data and analysing it to develop appropriate strategies
- Making products, services, or behaviours fit the felt needs of the consumers/users
- Using a strategic approach to promoting the products, services, or behaviours
- Incorporating methods for effective distribution of the message or product so that when demand is created, consumers know where and how to get the products, services, or behaviours
- Improving the adoption of products, services, or behaviours and increasing the willingness of consumers/users to contribute something in exchange
- Pricing so that the product or service is affordable to use or the behaviour is easy to perform

Social marketing processes include:

1. *Assessment, data collection, and analysis.* Consulting a sample of people from the target audience to assess their needs, wants, and aspirations (e.g., violence reduction in the community). Community members participate in the development of feasible, attractive solutions to the issues of concern (e.g., focus on schools and bullying) (Table 16-1).

TABLE 16-1

Ten Questions for Social Marketing Planning

1. What social or health issue does the community want to address?
2. What actions do community members believe will best address that issue?
3. Who is being asked to take action (target audience)?
4. What will the audience want in exchange for adopting this new practice/behaviour?
5. Why will the audience believe anything we say is true?
6. What is already out there about this issue/message?
7. What is the best time/place to reach the audience?
8. How often and from whom does the intervention need to be received in order to be effective?
9. How can the community integrate a variety of interventions over time in a coordinated fashion to influence the adoption of the desired practice/behaviour by the target group?
10. Do we have the resources to carry out this strategy? Who might be useful partners?

Adapted from Odor, R., & Franklin, R. (2005). Using social marketing for primary prevention of sexual violence in Virginia. From the Building Healthy Futures Prevention Conference, October 7, 2005. Available at: **http://www.vahealth.org/civp/sexualviolence/pubs.asp#pres**

2. *Market segmentation*. Based on an analysis of the initial data and the community, the target audience is divided into discrete units with common characteristics (e.g., parents, teachers, and children).
3. *Product and message development*. Products (e.g., posters, pamphlets, t-shirts) and messages (slogans, public service ads) are developed based on the preferences and characteristics of the relevant segments. These are tested among representative samples of target populations. Products and messages are modified, refined, and re-tested until they are acceptable.
4. *Launch*. The product or service is introduced.
5. *Evaluation*. The performance of the product or service is monitored and evaluated in the market and the strategy, marketing plan, or product itself revised accordingly.

Take Note

Primary target audiences are those people who are carrying out the risk practices.

Secondary target audiences are those who influence the primary audience and who are in their immediate society.

A third target audience leads and shapes public opinion (e.g. political leaders, religious leaders, traditional leaders, and elders) and exerts a major influence on the credibility and hence on the success or failure of a program.

Take Note

The community is made up of many different groups, or "segments." Each segment of the audience may need to be addressed separately. Programs are more effective if a small number of key messages are directed to specific target audiences. This concentrates resources and increases the chances that behaviour change will result.

For maximum efficiency of resource use and impact in the community, audiences and messages must be carefully targeted. Promotion must concentrate on the primary target audience and on those that influence them in their family circles or the wider community. The target messages must be those assessed as having the greatest adverse effects. Messages should bolster those aspects of the desired practice that users see as advantageous and not dwell on negative aspects of current practices. Odor and Franklin (2005) provide some ideas that you might find helpful.

No education or social marketing intervention is effective if the environment erects barriers to people taking action. In this instance, the community team must act to effect change by creating conditions that support making the healthy choice the easy choice.

Engineering

Engineering is the process of creating an environment that is supportive for change—that is, making the healthy choice the easy choice. For instance, in a context of rising obesity rates, Canadians value fitness and health and believe that healthy eating and activity are important, but they have trouble following through with their intentions to take action. People need support. Hence, the food industry has taken action in many ways: improved product choices are on the market; more nutrition information available to consumers on food packages; responsible marketing standards where children are concerned; and governments, media, food producers, and the public are working collaboratively to ensure that people have the information, the choices, and the environmental supports to make healthier choices.

MEDIA ADVOCACY

Media advocacy, based on the recognition that health is a result of the social and environmental conditions in which people live, uses the mass media to influence the development of healthy public policy through changing the nature of public debate on issues that affect health (Table 16-2). It is a political tool in that it exerts pressure to influence decision-makers and legislators.

There are several components of media advocacy. The first step of reframing the debate, or presenting the issue differently than it is usually discussed, results from setting the agenda, shaping the debate, and advancing policy. It involves capturing the attention of the media and demonstrating the newsworthiness of an issue. The

TABLE 16-2	
Program Communication Strategies	
Interpersonal communication training	Strengthen the ability of front-line workers to reach potential targets and to promote the message.
	Provide opportunities for front-line workers to develop communication skills.
	Ensure that quality support materials are available.
	Provide interpersonal support to front-line workers.
Mass media	Build on existing policies and strengthen government and private-sector capacity for creative presentation of standardized messages.
Print media	Promote the development and dissemination of a clearly defined program logo to build awareness and aid identification.
	Develop strategies using print media (e.g., billboards, posters, site-signs) and other learning materials, manuals, and program guidelines.
Community-based media	Use local media and employ traditional, community-based entertainment artists (e.g., popular folk singers, actors, and poets).

Adapted from Department of International Development. (1998). *Guidance manual on water supply and sanitation programmes.* Loughborough University, Leicestershire, UK: Water and Environmental Health at London and Loughborough (WELL). Available at: **www.lboro.ac.uk/well/resources/Publications/guidance-manual/chapter_2-8.pdf**.

second step is to tell the story from the perspective of the population, with emphasis on broad social issues rather than on individuals. The third step involves putting forward the policy solution that you are aiming to achieve (Wass, 2000). Community participation plays a key role in media advocacy. To be effective, media advocacy relies on the formation of coalitions that are sustained over a long period of time so that a grassroots movement can gain enough momentum to maintain the issue in the public eye for more than a short time.

Advocacy campaigns consist of providing newsworthy items to the media, writing letters to the editor, preparing media releases, releasing photographs or providing photo opportunities, and doing media interviews (Wass, 2000). Be certain to follow the protocols of your organization before contacting the media, and be prepared for questions that generate controversy!

POLICY FORMULATION

Healthy public policy is chiefly concerned with creating a healthy society (Glass & Hicks, 2000). Healthy public policy is multisectoral; it explicitly recognizes the contributions from other sectors that influence the determinants of health. It is founded on public involvement and principles of primary health care (Glass & Hicks, 2000): population health focus, equity, multidisciplinary approaches, intersectoral collaboration, participation, information systems, and health system reform.

Stages of policy formulation are:

Policy analysis	Identification of issues, analysis of options, and a choice of an optimal policy
Policy design	Communication with all sectors, problem identification, and definition
Policy development	Specification of goals and specific targets
Policy implementation	Deliberation on strategies and instruments that will incorporate policy into the system, funding models, legislation, and involvement of nongovernmental organizations
Policy evaluation	Monitoring the impact of policy on the population

Each stage is itself a political process (Helvie, 1998) and requires resource allocation, negotiation, conflict resolution, and compromise. Policy change takes a long time to occur, particularly because health and social policy are in provincial jurisdiction. Change challenges entrenched values and perceptions, requiring extensive consultation and development, and because of the complexity of the social situation, skill and patience are keys to eventual success. For examples of participative policy development, see the work of Smith (2002, 2003) that is available from the Government of Canada: **http://www.phac-aspc.gc.ca/canada/regions/atlantic/pdf/pub_policy_partic_e.pdf** and **http://www.atl.ec.gc.ca/community/pdf/public_policy_e.pdf**. Refer also to Chapter 7 and Figure 7-1 for more information.

Enforcement

When legislation is in place to require people to act in a certain way, and there is resistance or lack of compliance, protection services (e.g., police, fire, food inspectors) may enter the community to enforce the law. If community workers can combine education and engineering with this approach, then enforcement can be most effective. For instance, many health departments collaborate with the police and transportation officials during seat belt checkpoints. If children are unrestrained in a vehicle, or improperly restrained, professionals demonstrate proper restraint methods, provide information on purchasing appropriate restraints, and teach the parents the importance of restraints for child safety. The parents are given a "ticket" to attend a child safety workshop in their community, and when the parents attend, they receive a coupon for restraints at a local store. If, however, parents are found on check-stop to be repeat offenders, they are levied a fine that can be "paid" not only by money but also by attendance at the workshop. Notices regarding the check-stops are placed in community papers and school newsletters. If children are also taught car safety at school, they can be effective monitors of family vehicle safety, demonstrating the impact of multiple strategies on changing health behaviours.

What kinds of interventions support enforcement efforts? Letters to the editor, policy briefs, petitions, articles in community newsletters, town hall meetings, and knowledge exchange activities assist health workers to get the messages out to the community, opinion leaders, and policy-makers.

EVALUATION

At the conclusion of the planning and implementation phases of the community-as-partner process, it is important to assess team performance and reflect on individual contributions. Many teams disband at this point if external evaluators enter the process. Table 16-3 provides a framework for individual reflection; this can be used to begin a conversation about team function and the participatory process.

The program plan and its implementation need to be assessed at this time as well as throughout the process. Throughout, it is important to ensure that the program activities are congruent with its goals and objectives and that the activities target the appropriate audiences and practices. Did you honour the logic model (Chapter 15), or did you make adjustments along the way? Were those adjustments recorded and communicated? Did you collect data on the indicators? Did you collect additional information? Where is this data stored, and who has access to it for monitoring and evaluation purposes? At this time, assess what went well and why in program implementation—celebrate your successes. What did not go well? Try to explain why things went off track or did not turn out as well as expected. Were there aspects of the process for which you were unprepared? Did you have any surprises—good or bad? There are intended outcomes specified in any project plan; some unanticipated and unintended things happen as well.

TABLE 16-3
Participation Checklist

PERSONAL BEHAVIOUR	NEVER	OCCASIONALLY	OFTEN
I suggested a procedure for the group to follow or a method for organizing a task.			
I suggested a new idea, new activity, new problem, or a new course of action.			
I attempted to bring the group back to work when joking, personal stories, or irrelevant talk went on for too long.			
I suggested, when there was some confusion, that the group make an outline or otherwise organize a plan for completing the task.			
I initiated attempts to redefine goals, problems, or outcomes when things became hazy or confusing.			
I elaborated on ideas with concise examples or illustrations.			
I suggested resource people to contact and/or brought materials.			
I presented the reasons behind my opinions.			
I asked others for information and/or opinions.			
I asked for significance and/or implications of facts and opinions.			
I saw and pointed out relationships between facts and opinions.			
I asked a speaker to explain the reasoning that led him/her to a particular conclusion.			
I related my comments to previous contributions.			
I pulled together and summarized various ideas presented.			
I tested to see if everyone understood, and/or agreed with, the issue discussed or the decision made.			
I summarized the progress that the group had made.			
I encouraged other members to participate and tried to unobtrusively involve quiet members.			
I actively supported others when I thought their points of view were important.			
I tried to find areas of agreement in conflicting points of view and tried to address the source of the problem.			
I used appropriate humour to reduce tension in the group.			
I listened attentively to others' ideas and contributions.			

From Annis, R., Racher, F., & Beattie, M. (2004). *Rural community health and well-being: a guide to action* (p. 219). Brandon, MB: Rural Development Institute, Brandon University.

SUMMARY

Having considered the importance of community ownership of the program, the need to offer a unified program, and maintaining a focus on health and well-being, there remains one step in the process—evaluation. Before a program is implemented, the manner in which it is to be evaluated must be established, hence the importance of the logic model. The next chapter explains why this final stage of the community process is best considered before implementation begins.

References

Glass, H., & Hicks, S. (2000). Healthy public policy in health system reform. In M. J. Stewart (Ed.), *Community nursing: Promoting Canadians' health* (pp. 156–170). Toronto: Saunders.

Health Canada. (1999). *Toward a healthy future: Second report on the health of Canadians*. Ottawa: Health Canada. Available at: **www.hc-sc.gc.ca**.

Helvie, C. O. (1998). *Advanced practice nursing in the community* (pp. 287–313). Thousand Oaks, CA: Sage.

Knowles, M. (1998). *The adult learner: A neglected species*. Houston, TX: Gulf.

Meade, C. (1997). Community health education. In J. M. Swanson & M. A. Nies (Eds.), *Community health nursing: Promoting the health of aggregates* (pp. 155–192). Philadelphia: Saunders.

Mintz, J. (1989). Social marketing: New weapon in an old struggle. *Health Promotion, 28*(4), 6–12.

Mintz, J., & Steele, M. (1992). Marketing health information: The why and how of it. *Health Promotion, 31*(2), 2–5, 29.

Odor, R., & Franklin, R. (2005). Using social marketing for primary prevention of sexual violence in Virginia. From the Building Healthy Futures Prevention Conference, October 7, 2005. Available at: **http://www.vahealth.org/CIVP/sexualviolence/Social%Marketing%Handout%20of%20Slides.pdf**.

Onega, L. L. (2000). Educational theories, models and principles applied to community and public health nursing. In M. Stanhope & J. Lancaster (Eds.), *Community and public health nursing* (pp. 266–283). St. Louis, MO: Mosby.

Smith, Bruce L. (2002). Taking action through public policy: A focus on health and environment issues. A publication of the Community Animation Program, a joint Environment Canada & Health Canada program (Catalogue: En4-2/2002E ISBN: 0-662-32097-2). Available at: **http://www.atl.ec.gc.ca/community/pdf/public_policy_e.pdf**.

Smith, Bruce L. (2003). Public policy and public participation: Engaging citizens and community in the development of public policy. Population and Public Health Branch, Atlantic Regional Office, Health Canada. Available at: **http://www.phac-aspc.gc.ca/canada/regions/atlantic/pdf/pub_policy_partic_e.pdf**.

Wass, A. (2000). *Promoting health: The primary care approach*. Marrickville, AU: Harcourt.

Suggested Readings

Abraham, T., & Fallon, P. J. (1997). Caring for the community: Development of the advanced practice nurse role. *Clinical Nurse Specialist, 11*(5), 224–230.

Anderson, E. T., Gottschalk, J., & Martin, D. A. (1993). Contemporary issues in the community. In D. J. Mason, S. W. Talbott, & J. K. Leavitt (Eds.), *Policy and politics for nurses: Action and change in the workplace, government, organizations and community*. Philadelphia: Saunders.

Beddome, G., Clarke, H. F., & Whyte, N. B. (1993). Vision for the future of public health nursing: A case for primary health care. *Public Health Nursing, 1*(1), 13–18.

Chavis, D. M., & Florin, P. (1990). Nurturing grassroots initiatives for health and housing. *Bulletin of the New York Academy of Medicine, 66*(5), 558–572.

Courtney, R., Ballard, E., Fauver, S., Gariota, M., & Holland, L. (1996). The partnership model: Working with individuals, families, and communities toward a new vision of health. *Public Health Nursing, 13*(3), 17–186.

Dahl, S., Gustafson, C., & McCullagh, M. (1993). Collaborating to develop a community-based health service for rural homeless persons. *Journal of Nursing Administration, 23*(4), 41–45.

Duncan, S. M. (1996). Empowerment strategies in nursing education: A foundation for population-focused clinical studies. *Public Health Nursing, 13*(5), 311–317.

Durpa, K. C., Quick, M. M., Andrews, A., Engelke, M. K., & Vinvent, P. (1992). A collaborative health promotion effort: Nursing students and Wendy's team up. *Nurse Educator, 17*(6), 35–37.

El-Askari, G., Freestone, J., Irizarry, C., Mashiyama, S. T., Morgan, M. A., & Walton, S. (1998). The Healthy Neighborhoods Project: A local health department's role in catalyzing community development. *Health Education and Behavior, 25*(2), 146–159.

Farley, S. (1993). The community as partner in primary health care. *Nursing and Health Care, 14*(5), 244–249.

Flick, L. H., Reese, C., & Harris, A. (1996). Aggregate community-centered undergraduate community health nursing clinical experience. *Public Health Nursing, 13*(1), 36–41.

Flynn, B. C. (1997). Partnerships in healthy cities and communities: A social commitment for advanced practice nurses. *Advanced Practice Nursing Quarterly, 2*(4), 1–6.

Gamm, L. D. (1998). Advancing community health through community health partnerships. *Journal of Healthcare Management, 43*(1), 51–66.

Hawe, P., King, L., Noort, M., Gifford, S. M., & Lloyd, B. (1998). Working invisibly: Health workers talk about capacity-building in health promotion. *Health Promotion International, 13*(4), 285–295.

Heiss, G. L. (2000). Health teaching. In C. M. Smith & F. A. Maurer (Eds.), *Community health nursing: Theory and practice* (pp. 498–519). Philadelphia: Saunders.

Hollinger-Smith, L. (1998). Partners in collaboration: The Homan Square Project. *Journal of Professional Nursing, 14*(6), 344–349.

Jenkins, S. (1991). Community wellness: A group empowerment model for rural America. *Journal of Health Care for the Poor and Underserved, 1*(4), 388–404.

Kinne, A., Thompson, B., Chrisman, N. J., & Hanley, J. R. (1989). Community organization to enhance the delivery of preventive health services. *American Journal of Preventive Medicine, 5*(4), 225–229.

Labonte, R. (1993). Community development and partnerships. *Canadian Journal of Public Health, 84*(4), 237–240.

Murashima, S., Hatono, Y., Whyte, N., & Asahara, K. (1999). Public health nursing in Japan: New opportunities for health promotion. *Public Health Nursing, 16*(2), 133–139.

Perino, S. S. (1992). Nike-footed health workers deal with the problems of adolescent pregnancy. *Public Health Reports, 107*(2), 208–212.

Rutherford, G. S., & Campbell, D. (1993). Helping people help themselves. *Canadian Nurse, 89*(10), 25–28.

Scott, S. (1990). *Promoting healthy traditions workbook: A guide to the Healthy People Campaign.* St. Paul, MN: American Indian Health Care Association.

Wardrop, K. (1993). A framework for health promotion. *Canadian Journal of Public Health, 84*[Suppl l], S9–S13.

Woodard, G. R., & Edouard, L. (1992). Reaching out: A community initiative for disadvantaged pregnant women. *Canadian Journal of Public Health, 83*(3), 188–190.

17

Evaluating a Community Health Program

REVISED FROM THE ORIGINAL BY MARCIA HILLS AND SIMON CARROLL

Chapter Outline

Introduction

Evaluation Principles

The Evaluation Process

Components of Evaluation

Evaluation Strategies

Selected Methods of Data
  Collection

Summary

Learning Objectives

The cynic is a man who knows the price of everything, but the value of nothing. OSCAR WILDE

All evaluation should set as its primary task the avoidance of this pernicious cynicism. There is nothing more ruinous and disempowering than forcing good-willed communities into a 'gambit of compliance' with a set of reporting requirements that are mutually recognized as absurd, counterproductive, and energy-depleting travesties masquerading as rigorous evaluative technique. If anything, evaluation should be an empowering, supportive inquiry into how best to improve the everyday lives of our fellow human beings. In this mode, cynicism is the enemy that must be harried at every turn.

This may strike you as a strange beginning, one that is perhaps more appropriate for the conclusion to a much more comprehensive examination of evaluation, not as a comfortable and welcoming start to a benign introductory survey of community health program evaluation. Yet, we leave this here with you as a provocative application of the maxim that if you need to get one important point across, always be sure to put it at the beginning.

After studying this chapter, you should be able to act in partnership with the community to:

❖ Establish evaluation criteria that are timely and comprehensive

❖ Use baseline and current data to measure progress toward goals and objectives

❖ Validate observations, insights, and new data with colleagues and the community

❖ Revise priorities, goals, and interventions based on evaluation data

❖ Document and record evaluation results and revisions of the plan

❖ Participate in evaluation research with appropriate consultation

❖ Appreciate the complexity of program evaluation as well as the multiple paradigms that affect its implementation

Introduction

*P*rogram evaluation is the systematic collection of information about the activities, characteristics, and outcomes of programs to make judgments about the program, improve program effectiveness, and/or inform decisions about future programming (Patton, 1997, p. 23).

In addition to this generic perspective, in community health programming, evaluation *should* involve the community as a partner, meaning that all aspects of the evaluation process should be participatory, equitable, and empowering (Fetterman, Kaftarian, & Wandersman, 1996). Clearly, this definition places an explicit set of *values* up front as the basis of guiding principles that determine *how* and *why* community health program evaluations are conducted.

The most important decision to make before engaging with program evaluation is to determine what your working definition of *evaluation* is and to understand the implications of choosing a particular definition.

There are many different approaches to defining the concept and purpose of evaluation in community health programming. One of the broadest is that of Green and Kreuter (1991): "comparison of an object of interest against a standard of acceptability." However, as Rootman and colleagues (2001) point out, this leaves a lot to be determined. We do not know the nature of the 'object', nor the methods used to make the 'comparison', nor do we know *who* is setting the 'standard', nor *how* the standard is set. It is once we start to dig deeper into these questions that key ethical and political issues come to the fore.

Without listing all the possible definitions of *evaluation*, we can say that there are two primary dimensions, along which most approaches can be plotted. One dimension is about 'control'. Who controls the evaluation process? On this dimension, there is a continuum between external evaluator control on one end and total community control on the other. The second dimension is about knowledge and methods. This has a continuum with established social science methodologies on one end and pragmatic uses of the systematic collection and analysis of routinely produced data on the other.

While it is true that, at its very basis, evaluation is about the 'judgment' of, or the determination of, the 'worth or value' of something (Scriven, 1991), such a definition leaves aside just what is being judged and for what purpose (Patton, 1997). As we shall see, various components of program evaluation and various approaches to these components have different answers to these questions. Evaluations that are more community-controlled tend to be focused on pragmatic issues, concerning the ongoing assessment of how well a certain program is being implemented, and see the purpose of evaluation as the collection of evidence to support the immediate improvement of program processes; or at the extreme, the basis for completely changing the focus of the program or replacing it with a more relevant set of activities. Community practitioners and lay members tend to be less concerned about research and scientific rigour and more concerned that they utilize the information they already routinely collect to improve practice. On the other hand, external evaluations are often initiated by the requirements of large funding agencies and are focused on judging whether programs or projects they fund are meeting the overall policy objectives that form the basis on which the entire funding stream is constructed and the basis for its justification for continued existence. Often, with external evaluations of this kind, scientific rigour, based on established methodological approaches, is seen as a fundamental requirement for credible evaluations.

The community health team evaluates the responses of the community to a program to measure progress that is being made toward the program's goals and objectives. Evaluation data are also crucial for revision of the assessment database and the community diagnoses that were developed from analysis of the community assessment data.

Do you feel as if we are talking in circles? Evaluation is the "final" step of the community process, but it is linked to assessment, which is the first step. Professional practice is cyclic as well as dynamic, and for community-focused interventions to be timely and relevant, the community assessment database, community diagnoses, and program plans must be evaluated routinely. The effectiveness of community interventions depends on continuous reassessment of the community and on appropriate revisions of planned interventions. In fact, this has led some writers to argue that evaluation is a process that should take place throughout the life of the program; in other words, as soon as we begin, we should evaluate our progress so that we can use evidence to implement change immediately, rather than waiting until it is too late for that program, with that community. This principle is driven by the necessity of bringing benefit to each community we work with, as we work with them. Communities should always be better off having worked with you (Hills & Mullett, 2000).

Reflecting on the community-as-partner model (see Fig. 12-4), the purpose of evaluation is to determine if threats or challenges to health (stressors) have been repelled or minimized, if the health status of the population or community (normal lines of defence) is improved, and if the community's capacity (lines of resistance) or resilience (flexible line of defence) is strengthened as a result of the intervention.

Evaluation is important to community practice, but of equal importance is its crucial role in the functioning of human service agencies. Staffing and funding are frequently based on evaluation findings, and existing programs are subject to termination unless evaluation evidence can be produced that answers this question: What has been the program's impact on the community? Recent years have witnessed a growing focus on program evaluation; training programs on evaluation have become common, and evaluation has become big business. Unfortunately, evaluation is sometimes practised separately from program planning. It may even be tacked onto the end of a program just to satisfy funding sources or agency administration. The problems of such an approach are evident. Effective community practice requires an integrated approach to evaluation; it is a unique aspect of the field.

EVALUATION PRINCIPLES

Congruent with the theoretical foundations of working with the community as partner, we base our program evaluation on principles explicated by the W. K. Kellogg Foundation (1998). These principles are:

1. *Strengthen programs.* Our goal is health promotion and improving a community's self-reliance. Evaluation assists in attaining this goal by providing an ongoing and systematic process for assessing the program, its impact, and its outcomes.
2. *Use multiple approaches.* In addition to multidisciplinary approaches, evaluation methods may be numerous and varied. No single approach is favoured, but the methods chosen must be congruent with the purposes of the program.
3. *Design evaluation to address real issues.* Community-based and community-focused programs, rooted in the "real" community and based on an assessment of that community, must design an evaluation to measure those criteria of importance to the community.
4. *Create a participatory process.* Just as the community members were part of assessment, analysis, planning, and implementation, they also must be partners in evaluation. This can be a very difficult process, but not only is it more ethical, it creates enhanced validity for evaluation findings and builds commitment to change for community actors.
5. *Allow for flexibility.* "Evaluation approaches must not be rigid and prescriptive, or it will be difficult to document the incremental, complex, and often subtle changes that occur. . . ." (W. K. Kellogg Foundation, 1998, p. 3). The approach should be "able to respond changing circumstances, opportunities, challenges and priorities" (Rootman et al., 2001).
6. *Build capacity.* The process of evaluation, in addition to measuring outcomes, should enhance the skills, knowledge, and attitudes of those engaged in it. This includes both professionals and nonprofessionals alike.

THE EVALUATION PROCESS

There is a burgeoning literature on evaluation (see the References and Suggested Readings at the end of this chapter). Program or project evaluation has become a specialty with whole departments and consulting firms focused on measurement and evaluation.

There are many different models of the evaluation process, divided into various stages, phases, components, and the like (Table 17-1). For our purposes, there has been a developing consensus within the health promotion field that evaluation of community health programs can be broken down into the following steps:

1. Describing the program
2. Identifying the issues and questions
3. Designing the data collection process
4. Collecting the data
5. Analyzing and interpreting the data
6. Making recommendations
7. Dissemination
8. Taking action

TABLE 17-1

A Model for Program Evaluation

	PROCESS (FORMATIVE)	IMPACT (SUMMATIVE; SHORT-TERM OUTCOME)	OUTCOME (LONGER-TERM)
Information to collect	Program implementation, including • Site response • Recipient response • Practitioner response • Competencies of personnel	Immediate effects of program on, for example: • Knowledge • Attitudes • Perceptions • Skills • Beliefs • Access to resources • Social support	Incidence and prevalence of risk factors, morbidity, and mortality
When to apply	Initial implementation of a program or when changes are made in a developed program (e.g., moved to a new site, provided to a different population)	To determine if factors that affect health—both within the population and in the environment—have changed. For example did people's behavior change? Was the new policy implemented?	To measure if incidence and prevalence have been altered. For example, has the immunization rate of 2-year-olds increased? Did the rate of hospital admissions decrease? Did the industry filter its polluting smoke stack?

Process or formative evaluation is intended to improve the operation of an existing program. It answers the question: Are we doing what we said we would do? That is, did we deliver the program, provide a place to meet, include handouts at our meeting, and so forth? For example, when the pilot for the "Nobody's Perfect" program was offered in another Calgary community from 8 to 9 PM, very few parents attended regularly. They stated that the time was too late for them to return home and complete homework, family, and bedtime activities for their school-age children. As a result of this formative evaluation, the time chosen for the Bridgeland program was 6:30 to 8 PM to allow for refreshments and socializing; student volunteers provided babysitting on site. Participants were satisfied with this time frame, and there were few absences during the 6 weeks of the program. Some authors (Green & Lewis, 1986) make a distinction between formative and process evaluation by using *process* to denote evaluation conducted during the program and *formative* (as the name implies) at the program formation or preprogram stages.

Outcome (or summative) evaluation is concerned with the immediate impact of a program on a target group. It answers the question: Is our program effective? If your program is aimed at changing a group's knowledge and behaviour relating to sexually transmitted infection, for instance, you might build in a test to find out what they learned and what their intent is about modifying behaviour. In the case of the "Nobody's Perfect" program in Bridgeland, summative evaluation criteria might include parental self-reports that they have increased their knowledge about children's health, safety, and behaviour and that they have improved their coping skills with stressors related to child growth and developmental stages and needs. In addition, parents can provide feedback in terms of whether or not they feel they have had the opportunity to develop some supportive community connections.

It is in the long-term outcome evaluation, however, that you find out if the changes had a lasting and real effect. That is, did the incidence of child abuse drop in this population group? Because we are getting closer to the cause-and-effect question, careful evaluative research is needed to determine the actual contribution of the program to the outcome being measured.

Take Note

An in-depth review of evaluation research is beyond the scope of this text. There are several excellent texts that focus on evaluation research; these are included later in this chapter as Suggested Readings.

Before considering specific evaluation strategies, it is important to consider the "evaluability" of the program. To do this, review the program plan and ask yourself the following questions:

◆ Are program activities stated in precise words whose concepts can be measured?
◆ Is a time frame for attaining the change included?

- Are the direction and magnitude of the change included?
- Is a method of measuring the change included?
- Are the data that will be needed to measure the objectives available at a reasonable cost?
- Are the program activities that are designed to meet the objectives plausible?

If you find that any of these questions cannot be answered in the affirmative regarding your plan, review Chapter 15 and amend the plan and logic model to make them as concise and complete as possible. The plan for process and outcome evaluation should be built into your overall plan prior to its launch. Early planning ensures that you will be able to collect baseline data (how things were before you implemented your program) and collect the right data at the right time, from the right sources, using the appropriate methods. When these factors are considered, evaluation becomes a part of everyday program activities, not a burdensome add-on to program staff.

Take Note

A positive response to each of the "evaluability" questions would be an ideal state that few programs attain. Therefore, do not despair if your program is less than perfect but rather strive to increase your sensitivity to the issues that need to be considered in program planning to achieve optimum program evaluation.

COMPONENTS OF EVALUATION

Why collect evaluation data? To whom will the evaluation data be given, and for what purpose will it be used? What programs or activities will result from or be discontinued as a result of evaluation data? Before a strategy or method of evaluation can be selected, the reasons for and uses of the evaluation data must be established. An evaluation strategy appropriate for answering one type of evaluative question would not be useful for another. For example, if the Health Promotion Council wanted to know the relevancy to community needs of a program on crime prevention, then questions would be asked of the participants concerning the usefulness and adequacy of the information that was given. Possible questions would cover a range of topics:

- Did the information make a difference as to how residents protect themselves from crime?
- What protective behaviours do the residents practise now that were not practised before the program?
- Did the program answer the residents' questions?
- Did the program meet perceived needs?

However, if the Council wanted to know the outcome of the crime prevention program (such as if the program decreased the incidence of crime experienced by the participants), then self-reports and community crime statistics would be monitored. Usually, questions of evaluation focus on the areas of relevancy, progress, cost-efficiency, effectiveness, and outcome.

Relevancy

Is there a need for the program? Relevancy determines the reasons for having a program or set of activities. Questions of relevancy may be more important for existing programs than for new programs. Frequently, a program is planned, such as a blood pressure screening, to meet an expressed community need. Then, it is continued for years without an evaluation of relevancy. The question should be asked routinely—is the program still needed? Clearly, evaluation is not necessary just for new programs but for all programs. A common constraint to beginning a new program is inadequate staff or budget. A remedy to that constraint can be a relevancy evaluation of existing programs. Staff and budgets from a program that is no longer needed can be redirected to a new program.

Progress

Are program activities following the intended plan? Are appropriate staff and materials available in the right quantity and at the right time to implement the program activities? Are expected numbers of individuals participating in the scheduled program activities? Do the inputs and outputs meet some predetermined plan? Answers to these questions measure the progress of the program and are part of process or formative evaluation.

Cost-Efficiency

What are the costs of a program? What are its benefits? Are program benefits sufficient for the costs incurred? Cost-efficiency evaluation measures the relationship between the results (benefits) of a program and the costs of presenting the program (such as staff salary and materials). Cost-efficiency evaluates whether the results of a program could have been obtained less expensively through another approach. Cost-benefit analysis requires skills beyond the scope of this text, but references abound, particularly in economics and management literature.

Effectiveness (Impact)

Were program objectives met? Were the participants satisfied with the program? What behaviour changed as a result of the program? Were program providers satisfied with the activities and client involvement? Effectiveness focuses on formative evaluation as well as the immediate, short-term results.

Outcome

What are the long-term implications of the program? As a result of the program, what changes in quality of life or health can be expected in 6 months or 6 years? Effectiveness measures the immediate results, whereas outcome evaluation measures whether the program activities changed the initial reason for the program. The fundamental question is this: Did the program meet its goal? (Was health improved?)

EVALUATION STRATEGIES

Program evaluation can be defined as the consistent, ongoing collection and analysis of information for use in making decisions (W. K. Kellogg Foundation, 1998, p. 14). As such, the choice of approach or method to collect the information is an important decision in itself and needs to be agreed on by all parties involved in the program from the beginning. Realize that there is no one best approach to evaluation, but whichever approach is chosen needs to "fit" the questions you wish to answer.

SELECTED METHODS OF DATA COLLECTION

Four key points need to be considered as you decide which method to use:

1. What resources are available for the evaluation tasks?
2. Is the method sensitive to the respondents/participants of the program?
3. How credible will your evaluation be as a result of this method?
4. What is the importance of the data to be collected? To the overall program? To participants? (W. K. Kellogg Foundation, 1998)

Consider, too, that there are several frameworks or paradigms that may inform your choices. A summary of five such paradigms is included in Table 17-2.

Taking the key points and paradigms into consideration, let us review the various methods of data collection: case study, surveys, experimental design, process monitoring, and cost-benefit and cost-effectiveness analyses.

Case Study

A case study looks inside a program to determine its adequacy to meet stated needs. The case-study method provides insight into an entire program and, unlike many forms of evaluation, can be started at any time during the program. The data collected during a case study include observation of program activity, reports prepared by the program, unstructured conversations with program personnel, statistical summaries of program activities, structured or unstructured interview data, and

TABLE 17-2

Paradigms for Evaluation

	NATURAL SCIENCE RESEARCH MODEL	INTERPRETIVISM/ CONSTRUCTIVISM	FEMINIST METHODS	PARTICIPATORY EVALUATION	THEORY-BASED
Roots	Western "science"; European, white, male	Anthropology	Feminist research, power analysis	Education, community organization, public health, anthropology	Application in comprehensive community programs
Key points	Control of variables	Study through ongoing and in-depth contact with those involved	Women, girls, and minorities historically left out; conventional methods are seriously flawed	Create a more egalitarian process, make process more relevant to all, democratizing	Every social program is based on a theory—the key to understanding what is important is through identifying the theory
Approach	Hypothetico-deductive methodology, statistics	In-depth observations, interviewing	Contextual, inclusive, experiential, involved, socially relevant	Practical, useful, empowering	Developing a program logic model—or picture—to describe what works
Purpose	To explain what happened and show causal relationships between outcomes and "treatments"	To understand the targets of the program and the program's meaning to them	To include the feminine voice in all aspects of evaluation, being open to all voices	Actively engage all in process, capacity building	Revealing what works in comprehensive, community-based programs

information collected through questionnaires. Subjective data and objective data can both be collected. Subjective data include information collected primarily through observations of participants or program staff. Objective data are collected from organization or program documents or structured questionnaires and interviews. The distinction between subjective and objective is not readily perceptible. All questionnaires, regardless of how carefully written, have a subjective component, and, likewise, "objective" records or documents are all written by people and, therefore, introduce a subjective factor. It is optimum to have a mix of both objective and subjective data.

OBSERVATION

Observation is one method of collecting data for a case study. Observation can be participant or nonparticipant. The participant observer assumes a working role in the agency or organization and collects data about the program while working within the group. The nonparticipant observer remains an "outsider," does not assume a working role within the agency, and reviews and examines the program for designated periods.

The types of observations that are made are determined by the questions that have been asked about the program. For example, if the question is one of relevancy, the observer would concentrate on the "who, what, why, and when" of the program. Who is using the services? Record the demographics of age, ethnicity, geographic location, educational level, and employment status. What services are the participants receiving? (For example, what services are offered in the well-child clinic? Immunizations? Physicals? Health teaching? Screening? How often are the services offered, and what are the ages of the children who use the services?) Why is the population using the offered services? (Availability? Affordability? No other options?) Lastly, when are the services accessed? (Do people come at appointed times or only when they are ill? Or do people tend to cluster at opening and closing times?)

Some data can be collected from agency records; other information can be collected by informal conversations with the participants—both the professional health care providers and the clients. When interviewing, always have a checklist of topics that you want to consider, arranged in a logical sequence, along with the who, what, why, and when questions. Unstructured interviews in the form of informal conversations afford the opportunity to explore with the participants their perceptions of the program. The results of unstructured interviews provide specific areas from which a "structured" interview can be developed. Recall from Chapter 13 that an interviewer conducts the interview, whereas a questionnaire is self-administered. Observations and interviews share the criticisms of selective perception and interactiveness.

1. *Selective perception is the natural tendency of everyone to consciously classify into categories the behaviours or statements of others.* These categories have been established by our cultural values, learning, and life experiences. To a certain extent, this

process is desirable because it limits the number of observations that need conscious consideration and permits the rapid and effective handling of information. For example, if it were observed that a client waited 1 hour for a scheduled appointment, most people, based on the common orientation to time, would classify that observation as a negative aspect of the clinic's functioning.

Herein lays the major problem of selective perception. Statements and behaviours are classified according to the selective perception of the observer, which may be completely different from the selective perception of the client or provider. The most dangerous effect of selective perception in program evaluation is when the observer has a preconception that a program will be successful or unsuccessful. This can produce a self-fulfilling prophecy because the biased observer may unconsciously record only data that support the preconceived belief. Both selective perception and self-fulfilling prophecy are sources of subjective data. Perhaps the most important point is that you should be aware of the problem of selective perception and share your observation and interview data with a mixed group of clients and providers. Ask the group for categorization and summation implications.

2. *Interactiveness is an additional event to be aware of during all observations.* When an observer, whether participant or nonparticipant, observes and records program activities, the person's presence affects and shapes the activities observed. Productivity may increase because staff members are aware of being observed or because they are concerned about client satisfaction or dissatisfaction. All evaluation strategies can have an interactive component, but perhaps the interactive consideration is strongest in case studies because of the presence of an observer.

Two additional techniques of the case-study method are nominal group and Delphi technique. (References to both techniques and examples of their application are presented at the end of this chapter in the Suggested Readings.) Both techniques are based on the belief that the individuals in a program are the most knowledgeable sources on its relevancy.

NOMINAL GROUP

The nominal group technique uses a structured group meeting, during which all individuals are given a judgmental task, such as to list the functions of the program, problems of the program, or needed changes in the program. Each member is asked to write a response on paper and to not discuss it with other people. At the end of 5 to 10 minutes, all members present their ideas, and each idea is recorded (without discussion) so that everyone can see all of the suggestions. Once all ideas have been presented, a discussion is begun, during which ideas are clarified and evaluated. After the discussion, a vote is held to determine the order in which the group wants to address different areas. The nominal group technique allows all individuals to present their ideas before the entire group. Involving the entire group both decreases selective perception and promotes individual cooperation with the group's decisions because people believe that they have been involved in the decision-making process.

DELPHI TECHNIQUE

The Delphi technique tends to be used in large survey studies but is also useful as a case-study method. It involves a series of questionnaires and feedback reports to a designated panel of respondents. An initial questionnaire is distributed by mail to a preselected group (this could be all staff members, a group of clients, or program administrators). Independently, respondents express their thoughts through the questionnaire and return it. Based on the responses of the group, a feedback report and a revised version of the questionnaire are sent to the respondents. Using the feedback information, the respondents evaluate their first answers and complete the questionnaire again. The process continues for a predetermined number of feedback rounds.

USEFULNESS OF THE CASE-STUDY APPROACH TO EVALUATION

The case-study method of program evaluation can help to answer questions of relevance. Questioning clients and health care providers helps to explore perceptions of how well the program is meeting its defined goals as well as ascertaining problem areas and possible solutions. The case-study method would not point to any one solution but rather would offer several possible choices.

Questions of progress can also be addressed through the case-study method. The extent to which a program is meeting predetermined standards of service indicates progress. Because the case study provides an examination of the program, much can be learned if program activities are already in place.

Cost-efficiency of the program is difficult to evaluate using a case-study method. First, to evaluate if the program could have been offered more economically, a comparable program must exist, and second, the case-study method is designed to look at only one program. The method is not formatted to look at two programs and compare them. However, judgments can be made as to the operating efficiency of the program. These must be based on the experience and knowledge of the evaluator and cannot be based on comparisons with other operating programs.

Effectiveness determines if the program has produced what it intended to produce immediately after the program, as opposed to outcome, which measures long-term consequences. Although the case-study method may determine aspects of effectiveness, such as whether the aims of the program have been met in the short run, it is very difficult to measure long-term consequences unless the case-study method is conducted over a long period that allows a longitudinal or retrospective view of the program.

Surveys

A survey is a method of collecting information and can be used to collect evaluation information. Surveys are usually completed by self-administered questionnaires (the process used in DT5 to determine residents' perceptions of community health challenges) or by personal interviews. Surveys are formulated to describe (descriptive surveys) or to analyze relationships (analytic surveys), or both.

Surveys can be used to describe the need for a program, the actual operations of a program, or a program's effects. Along with the descriptive information, questions of analysis can be answered through a survey. For example, a survey could be used to describe the composition of the groups that attend crime prevention or weight reduction classes as well as to analyze the relationship between descriptive data of sex and weight reduction success.

Surveys are usually performed for summative (impact) evaluation. Did the program accomplish what it was proposed to do? Do clients perceive the program as successful? Program personnel? If the program was considered successful, what parts were most helpful? Least helpful? What should be changed? Left unchanged? The questions asked by the survey are determined by the initial list of questions about program evaluation.

Like the case-study method, the answers on surveys come from the perceptions, values, and belief systems of the respondents. The response given to questions of program usefulness by the team that planned and implemented the program may be very different from the answers of the participants. Awareness of perception bias can direct evaluation efforts to consider the perceptions of all people (providers, clients, and management) involved in program implementation.

Surveys that are used to measure program evaluation must be concerned with the reliability and validity of the information collected. Reliability deals with the repeatability, or reproducibility, of the data (i.e., if the same questions were asked of the same people 1 week later, would the same responses be recorded?). Validity is the correctness of the information. If questions are written to evaluate knowledge and the answers of the respondents reflect behaviours, then the questions are not valid because they do not measure what they claim to measure.

USEFULNESS OF SURVEYS TO EVALUATION

Surveys can be very valuable to answer questions of relevance, or the need for proposed or existing programs, especially if the perceptions of clients, providers, and management are solicited. In like fashion, progress can be measured. People critiquing surveys as an evaluation strategy may be concerned with the subjectivity of the survey—indeed, individual perception affects every response to every question. However, most decisions are based on subjective judgments, not objective reality. The important concern is to understand whose subjective impression is being used as a basis for judgment; it is imperative for community health workers to ensure that clients' perceptions are represented alongside those of health care providers and management.

Cost-efficiency, effectiveness, and outcome are difficult to measure by using a survey. Although a survey can measure the perceived efficiency of the program or the acceptability of ideas on alternative ways of operating to make the program more cost-efficient, these perceptions are formed only in the context of the existing program. There is no other comparison program against which recorded perceptions can be measured. A survey can provide information on the characteristics of program activities that are perceived by the respondents to have caused changes in their health status, but these impressions are reported in the absence of any comparison group. A comparison group is especially important with regard to effectiveness and impact because it is impossible to tell if an alternative program (or no program at all) might have been more or less effective in accomplishing the same objectives.

Take Note

You may be wondering—if a comparison group is so important and if perceptions cloud the evaluation with subjective impressions—why use surveys at all? Two pluses exist in surveys: A great deal of information for program evaluation can be obtained, especially about the activities of the program from the perception of several groups, and important evaluation data can be inferred if the instrument (questionnaire or interview schedule) is reliable and valid.

Experimental Design

Completed correctly, an experimental study can provide an answer to these crucial questions: Did the program make a difference? Are health behaviours, knowledge, and attitudes changed as a result of the program activities? *Is the community healthier because of the programs offered by the Inner City Health Promotion Council?* However, the problem with experimental studies in program evaluation is that they require selective implementation, meaning that people who participate are selected through a process such as random assignment to a control group and an experimental group. For many ethical, political, and community health reasons, selective implementation is difficult to complete and is sometimes impossible. Despite these problems, the experimental study remains one of the better methods to evaluate summative effects (outcomes) of a program and the only way to produce quantified information on whether the program made a difference.

Take Note

Reviewing the steps of the research process at this point may be of help to you in understanding the examples that follow. Indeed, each issue—such as a theoretical framework, sampling, reliability, and validity—must be addressed if an experimental design is proposed for evaluation.

The following designs are the most feasible and appropriate to health care settings. Apply the research process to each design.

PRETEST–POSTTEST ONE-GROUP DESIGN

The pretest–posttest design applied to one group is illustrated in Table 17-3. Two observations are made, the first at Time 1 and the second at Time 2. The observation can be the prevalence of a health state (e.g., the percentage of adults in the downtown area who exercise regularly, brush their teeth three times daily, or drink alcohol [beer, wine, liquor] more than five times a week; the teenage pregnancy rate; number of reported cases of domestic abuse, etc.), knowledge scores, or other important facts in the community. Between Time 1 and Time 2, an "experiment" is introduced. The experiment may be a planned program aimed at a target group, such as teen sexuality classes, or an intervention with a community-wide focus, like a crime prevention program. The evaluation of the program is measured by considering the difference between the health state at Time 1 and the health state after the program at Time 2.

If the experiment in Table 17-3 were teen sexuality classes for 10th-grade girls at Hampton High School, Time 1 was a teen pregnancy rate of 5/100, and Time 2 (1 year later) was a teen pregnancy rate of 3/100 among the girls taking the classes, then would you agree that the teen sexuality program was responsible for the decrease in teenage pregnancies? What other information do you need to know to decide? Are there other factors that could account for the decrease in the teen pregnancy rate? Perhaps family-planning programs have been focused on teenagers, or maybe local churches and social service agencies have sponsored teen sexuality programs. Teen access to and use of contraceptive methods may have increased, or laws regarding teen access to contraceptive methods may have changed. None of these factors can be eliminated on the grounds of not being associated with the decrease in the teen pregnancy rate. To eliminate other possible explanations for program effectiveness, a control group must be added.

PRETEST–POSTTEST TWO-GROUP DESIGN

A pretest–posttest with a control group design is illustrated in Table 17-4. The design has both an experimental group and a control group. At Time 1, an observation is made of both the experimental and control groups. Between Time 1 and Time 2, an experiment is introduced with the experimental group. At Time 2, second observations are made on both the experimental and control groups. Program

TABLE 17-3			
Pretest–Posttest One-Group Design			
	TIME 1		**TIME 2**
Experimental group	Observation 1	Experiment	Observation 2

TABLE 17-4			
Pretest–Posttest Two-Group Design			
TIME 1		TIME 2	
Experimental group	Observation 1	Experiment	Observation 2
Control group	Observation 1		Observation 2

evaluation is the difference between Observations 1 and 2 for the experimental group when compared with the comparison (control) group (which has been selected to be as similar as possible to the experimental group). Will the pretest–posttest with a control group design eliminate the effect of outside factors that occurred simultaneously with the experiment and that might account for the change between Observation 1 and Observation 2—the very problem that plagued the pretest–posttest one-group design? The answer is yes, if the experimental and control groups are similar.

To explain, let us return to the idea of a teen sexuality class for 10th-grade students at Hampton High School. If a group of 10th-grade students, similar in social, economic, and geographic characteristics, were randomly selected and then randomly assigned to the experimental or control group, then it could be assumed that any other factors that influenced the experimental group would also affect the control group. However, frequently, the decision is made that all students must be given the same program, thereby eliminating a comparison group. At the Health Promotion Council, when the information was received that all 10th graders must be given a teen sexuality program that had been proposed by the school nurse as a response to an increasing number of teen pregnancies, the suggestion was made that perhaps another high school could be used as a control group. How would you respond to that suggestion? Perhaps another high school class of 10th graders could be used, if the students were similar in social, economic, and geographic characteristics to the students at Hampton High (an unlikely situation).

Another possibility mentioned by the Health Promotion Council was to offer the program in one school year to one half of the Hampton High 10th graders (using the other half as a control) and then in the following year to offer the program to the remaining students. This method would ensure that all students would be given the program but would also allow for an experimental pretest–posttest design for evaluation.

A third method that was suggested to ensure an experimental design was to give the control group sexuality education and give the experimental group sexuality education plus assertiveness training. The assertiveness training would differentiate the groups and allow an experimental design. All of the suggestions were discussed with school officials, and it was decided to offer a traditional sex education class to half of the 10th-grade students (the control group); the remaining students (the experimental group) would get the traditional sex education material but would also receive classes on assertiveness training and values clarification. This design will not allow for evaluation of traditional sex education classes versus no information, but it will provide all students with the health information (an ethical compromise) and allow for evaluation of a traditional program on sexuality versus that traditional program plus assertiveness and values clarification information (an approach to reduce teenage pregnancies that is supported in the literature).

Take Note

Notice that the decision to offer information on assertiveness and values clarification as part of teen sexuality classes was based on documentation from the literature. Hampton High School is not the first school to offer health promotion programs. Many schools and communities have assessed the status and perceived needs of their publics and have followed up by planning and implementing programs that have been evaluated and have reported their findings and results in the literature. One contribution that the community health team can make is to do a literature review about the ways in which other communities have addressed and evaluated similar programs, critically review and synthesize the results of these programs, and present this information to the community to use when making choices and decisions.

USEFULNESS OF THE EXPERIMENTAL DESIGN TO EVALUATION

An experimental design can yield data on whether a program has produced the desired outcomes when compared with the absence of such a program or, alternatively, whether one program strategy has produced better results with regard to the desired outcomes than some other strategy. However, the experimental design is not useful for evaluation of program progress or program cost-efficiency.

Monitoring (Process)

Monitoring measures the difference between the program plan and what has actually happened. Monitoring focuses on the sequence of activities of the program—specifically, how the program is to be implemented (the activities), by whom (the personnel and other resources), and when (the timing of activities). Monitoring is usually done with a chart, and although there are several different styles of charts, all arrange activities in a sequence and specify the time allotted to complete each task. In Chapter 15, Figure 15-2 illustrated one form of calendar chart for planning purposes. Figure 17-1 provides another example of a calendar chart that illustrates the sequencing of events in a program.

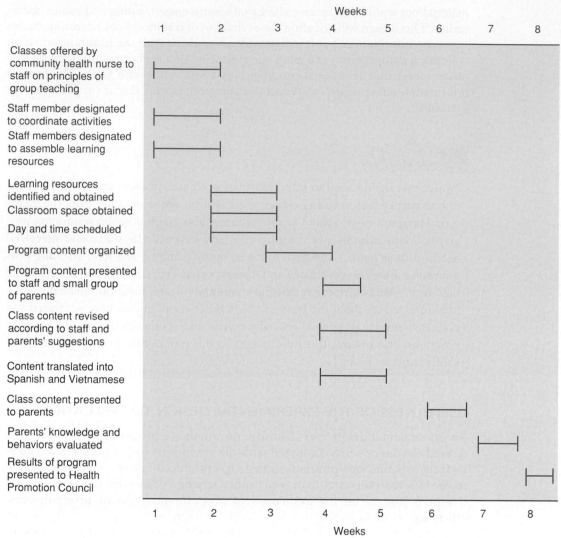

FIGURE 17-1 ◆ Sequence of events for program: Common health problems of children.

MONITORING CHARTS

To construct a monitoring chart for your program plan, information is needed on the inputs (resources necessary to carry out the program such as personnel, equipment, and finances), the process (the program activities, their sequencing, and timing) and outputs (the expected results of the program, including immediate and long-term health effects). It is helpful to make a list of inputs, processes, and outputs.

Take Note

You have already recorded this information as part of your program plan and logic model. Resources are the same as inputs, program activities correspond to processes, and objectives describe expected outputs or outcomes. You may have also made calendar charts of the detailed processes for each program component in the planning process. So, all that remains is to plot implementation information (i.e., what actually happened) onto the existing calendar chart for monitoring purposes—to see if activities happened on time, by the people who were assigned, and what effects (if any) the context had on the schedule.

It is difficult to decide on the amount of time that will be needed to complete any task. After assessing the organizational structure and management methods of the agency, you determined the approximate amounts of time that would be needed to complete the activities of the program. Do not be surprised if you made errors in your estimates. With experience, you will begin to be more accurate in gauging time requirements for specific activities. Evaluation data will be valuable to future estimates. The Suggested Readings list at the end of this chapter includes references to several other types of monitoring charts, including the Gantt, Program Evaluation and Review Technique (PERT), and Critical Path Method (CPM). These provide a slightly different variation of the basic time-sequencing, activities-monitoring charts that appear in Figures 15-2 and 17-1.

USEFULNESS OF PROCESS MONITORING TO EVALUATION

A monitoring chart measures progress and can be used to evaluate whether a program is on schedule and within budget. Perhaps no other evaluation method is as perfectly suited to process evaluation as the monitoring chart. In addition, monitoring can provide information on the cost-efficiency of the program by measuring the average cost of the resources required per client served. The effectiveness of the program can be measured by monitoring if the chart records outputs achieved. Monitoring charts cannot determine program relevance or the long-term impact of a program, however.

Cost-Benefit and Cost-Effectiveness Analyses

Much has been written and discussed about the escalating cost of health care services and on ways that cost can be reduced. The turmoil over health care reform in Canadian provinces and the intense debate regarding the pros and cons of various alternative approaches to health care delivery are testimony to the need to contain cost and yet increase access and maintain quality. Every program has a dollar price both in terms of the resources needed to offer the program (e.g., personnel and equipment) and the dollar benefits to be gained from improved health (e.g., increased worker productivity).

Two of the most common methods of analyzing the economic costs and benefits of a program are cost-benefit analysis (CBA) and cost-effectiveness analysis (CEA). Both CBA and CEA are formal analytic techniques that list all costs (direct and indirect) and consequences (negative and positive) of a particular program. The distinction between CBA and CEA is based on the value that is placed on the consequences of a program. In CBA, consequences or benefits of a program are valued in dollar terms; this makes it possible to compare different projects because all measurement is made in dollars. Therefore, the worth of a project can be judged by asking if dollar benefits exceed dollar costs and, if so, by how much. In contrast, CEA does not place a dollar value on either the consequences or the costs of a project. Another outcome is used for programs whose benefits or costs are difficult to measure. (For example, how could a dollar value be placed on each suicide prevented by a primary prevention program to decrease teenage suicide?) Therefore, CEA, unlike CBA, does not determine if total benefits exceed total costs.

However, CEA can be used to compare programs with similar goals and objectives. (For example, two different primary prevention approaches to decrease the incidence of teenage suicide share the same benefits, so only costs need to be compared—a CEA.) A CEA can also be used if the costs of alternative programs are the same or if only a given amount of money exists and the objective is to select the program with the greatest benefits (not measured in dollar terms). The decision is obvious—select the program that produces the most effectiveness; that is, the most benefits per dollar spent or the least cost for each unit (individual, family, or community) benefited.

The choice between CBA and CEA depends on the type of questions and programs considered. Neither technique is superior to the other. Both techniques can be used in planning for future programs or as an evaluation strategy of present or past programs. The actual procedures for completing a CBA or CEA are beyond the scope of this book; however, several references that include the procedural steps are listed in the Suggested Readings list. Obviously, both CBA and CEA are strategies for measuring program cost-efficiency and do not address the issues of relevancy, progress, effectiveness, or impact.

SUMMARY

Several methods of evaluation have been presented and discussed. No one method will evaluate components of relevancy, progress, cost-efficiency, effectiveness, and outcome equally well. It is important to be knowledgeable about different methods of program evaluation and to discuss the benefits and limitations of each with the community as the program is being planned and before program implementation occurs. Table 17-5 presents a summary table of appropriate evaluation methods for program components. Once evaluation methods are selected, then the methods (case study, experimental design, or process monitoring) become part of the program plan.

TABLE 17-5				
Examination of the Appropriateness of Different Evaluation Methods for Program Components				
	METHOD			
COMPONENTS	Case Study	Survey	Experimental	Monitoring
Relevancy	Yes	Yes	No	No
Progress	Yes	Yes	No	Yes
Cost-efficiency	No	No	Yes	Yes
Cost-effectiveness	Some	No	Yes	Some
Impact	No	No	Yes	No

You may be wondering which evaluation methods were used to evaluate health promotion programs in downtown Calgary. A variety of strategies were used. To evaluate the relevancy of the crime prevention program, nominal group meetings were scheduled, and both human service providers (e.g., police service, public health, social services, community outreach agencies) and residents of the community attended. In addition, the utilization rates and demographics of the participants in the various crime prevention activities were assessed, as were the participants' perceptions of the value of the information. Crime reports and arrest and conviction data are being logged to determine if crime rates reveal a downward trend over time for the neighbourhoods in the program.

For the "Nobody's Perfect" program in Bridgeland, program progress was evaluated with monitoring charts; the effectiveness and impact of the program on individuals were evaluated with knowledge, attitude, and behavioural intent surveys (e.g., questionnaires) given to participants before the program began, immediately after the program ended, and at predetermined follow-up times (6 weeks and 3 months). As well, satisfaction was measured to make decisions about program adaptations that could be made before the next session was planned.

In both instances, costs were calculated, both real and in-kind, to determine the ongoing budget that would be needed to sustain the programs and perhaps expand to other communities as needs warranted. To assess impact, further data are required to measure and interpret the consequences (benefit and effectiveness) of the programs on the communities involved and the health of families and individuals residing there.

When providing a final report of your evaluation to the community, you will inevitably be asked to make recommendations for future action. This must be done with caution and in consultation with the key stakeholders in community action—politicians, funders, informal leaders, local businesses, and the residents themselves. To help prevent people from taking offence, refer to community diagnoses and problems from a positive or wellness perspective, acknowledge the limitations as well as the strengths of the data collection processes, and defer to the wisdom of those who live in the community when suggesting future interventions.

Take Note

Presenting an evaluation report is often the stage in the process where the program is handed over from the team to an agency or to the community itself for ongoing action. This completes Reinkemeyer's (1970) Stages of Planned Change (see Box 15-1); stage 7 is where the change agent (community team) and the client part ways and the relationship changes so that the community leads future program action. All steps in the process have been leading to this outcome through the participation of community in each stage of the community-as-partner process.

One approach many evaluators find useful is to do a SWOT (strengths, weaknesses, opportunities, threats) analysis and use this to frame recommendations. For instance, the fact that residents were willing to bear the costs of leaving outdoor lights on all night (strength) could be used to overcome the darkness in the back alleys (weakness) that allowed drug deals and prostitution to occur. The risk of parental stress and consequent child abuse in a community with a high number of single-parent families (threat) was balanced by the opportunity for the community to come together to create healthy environments for child development and family support—a school providing space for a parenting program, students volunteering for child care, and service agencies and businesses in the area supporting the initiative in many ways. Community action teams and external evaluators can take community strengths and opportunities into account when making recommendations for action against perceived weaknesses in and threats to the community.

You are ready now for program implementation and the reinitiation of the community process, namely, assessment of the program's effects. As you implement the planned program, data will be added to the community assessment profile, which will demand addition, deletion, and revision of the community diagnoses and the associated program plans and interventions. Let us take a final look at the community-as-partner model (see Fig. 12-4) and ask, Will the planned programs assist the community to attain, regain, maintain, and promote health? Strengthen the community's ability to resist stressors? Enhance the community's competence and self-reliance?

Take Note

It is fitting that the final chapter of this section on the application of the community process in practice ends with questions. Community practice is the constant questioning, prodding, probing, and pondering of the health status of a population. Although individual and family health statuses are always important, the uniqueness of our field is the application of multidisciplinary professional practice techniques to the health and well-being of a community. Each community is unique and special. There is no other community quite like the one in which you are practising!

References

Fetterman, D. M., Kaftarian, S. J., & Wandersman, A. (Eds.). (1996). *Empowerment evaluation: Knowledge and tools for self-assessment and accountability*. Thousand Oaks, CA: Sage.

Green, L. W., & Lewis, F. M. (1986). *Measurement and evaluation in health education and health promotion*. Palo Alto, CA: Mayfield.

Green, L. W., & Kreuter, M. W. (1991). *Health promotion planning* (2nd ed.). Mountain View, CA: Mayfield Publishing Company

Hills, M. & Mullett, J. (2000). *Methodologies and methods for community-based research and evaluation*. Victoria, BC: University of Victoria Community Health Promotion Coalition.

Patton, Q. M. (1997). *Utilization focused evaluation: The new century text* (3rd ed.). London: Sage Publications.

Rootman, I., Goodstadt, M., Potvin, L., & Springett, J. (2001). A framework for health promotion evaluation. In I. Rootman, M. Goodstadt, B. Hyndman, D. McQueen, L. Potvin, J. Springett, et al. (Eds.), *Evaluation in health promotion: Principles and perspectives*. Copenhagen, Denmark: World Health Organization.

Scriven, M. (1991). *Evaluation thesaurus* (4th ed.). Newbury Park, CA: Sage Publications.

W. K. Kellogg Foundation. (1998). *Evaluation handbook*. Battle Creek, MI: Author.

Suggested Readings

Allen, J. (1993). Impact of the cholesterol education program for nurses: A pilot program evaluation. *Cardiovascular Nursing, 29*(1), 1–5.

Birch, S. (1990). The relative cost effectiveness of water fluoridation across communities: Analysis of variations according to underlying caries levels. *Community Dental Health, 7*(1), 3–10.

Ervin, N. (2002). *Advanced community health nursing practice*. Upper Saddle River, NJ: Prentice Hall.

Finnegan, J. R., Murray, D. M., Kurth, C., & McCarthy, P. (1989). Measuring and tracking education program implementation: The Minnesota Heart Health Program experience. *Health Education Quarterly, 16*(1), 77–90.

Helvie, C. O. (1998). *Advanced practice nursing in the community*. Thousand Oaks, CA: Sage.

Horne, T. E. (1995). *Making a difference: Program evaluation for health promotion*. Edmonton: WellQuest Consulting. Available at: **tamhorne@web.net.**

Kohler, C. L., Dolce, J. J., Manzella, B. A., Higgins, D., & Brooks, C. M. (1993). Use of focus group methodology to develop an asthma self-management program useful for community-based medical practices. *Health Education Quarterly, 20*(3), 421–429.

Minkler, M. (Ed.). (1997). *Community organizing and community building for health*. New Brunswick, NJ: Rutgers University Press.

Nas, T. F. (1996). *Cost-benefit analysis: Theory and application*. Thousand Oaks, CA: Sage.

O'Brien, K. (1993). Using focus groups to develop health surveys: An example from research on social relationships and AIDS-preventive behavior. *Health Education Quarterly, 20*(3), 361–372.

Porteous, N. L., Sheldrick, B. J., & Stewart, P. J. (1997). *Program evaluation tool kit: A blueprint for public health management*. Ottawa: Public Health Research, Education and Development Program, Ottawa-Carleton Health Department. Available from: Public Health Agency of Canada **www.phac-aspc.gc.ca/php-psp/toolkit.html.**

Rossi, P. H., Freeman, H. E., & Lipsey, M. W. (1998). *Evaluation: A systematic approach* (6th ed.). Thousand Oaks, CA: Sage.

Smith, C. M. (2000). Evaluation of nursing care with communities. In C. M. Smith & F. A. Maurer (Eds.), *Community health nursing: Theory and practice* (pp. 407–423). Philadelphia: Saunders.

Thompson, J. C. (1992). Program evaluation within a health promotion framework. Canadian *Journal of Public Health*, *83*[Suppl 1], S67–S71.

Tonglet, R., Sorogane, M., Lembo, M., WaMukalay, M., Dramaix, M., & Hennart, P. (1993). Evaluation of immunization coverage at local level. *World Health Forum*, *14*(3), 275–281.

Wheeler, F. C., Lackland, D. T., Mace, M. L., Reddick, A., Hogelin, G., & Remington, P. L. (1991). Evaluating South Carolina's community cardiovascular disease prevention project. *Public Health Reports*, *106*(5), 536–543.

Part 3

Community as Partner
in Practice

Chapter 18
Community Profile: Exemplar Health District / 373

Chapter 19
Assessing the Health of Communities in Northern
Canada / 397

Chapter 20
Promoting the Health of Pregnant Women / 414

Chapter 21
Promoting the Health of Schoolchildren / 432

Chapter 22
Youth Engagement in Health Promotion / 449

Chapter 23
Workplace Health Promotion / 470

Chapter 24
Promoting the Health of Vulnerable Populations / 493

Chapter 25
Using Technology to Promote the Health of Homebound Seniors / 508

This section is intended to serve two purposes: to offer an opportunity to share success stories and to provide educators and students with case stories to study. Each author has presented a different story—of one community issue, with one target population, in one particular setting. The stories have been written with the community-as-partner model in mind, but different components of the process have been emphasized. These stories can be used to apply the model components. For instance, you can ask of each:

◆ What data represent the *community core*? Embedded within the stories are the social, economic, and demographic data relevant to the population of interest.
◆ What is the *normal line of defence*? Health status data are also contained within each story. Recall that the normal line of defence can be drawn around the core to represent population health status or around the assessment wheel to incorporate the subsystems and represent the community's health.
◆ What *stressors* are acting on the population, and what *lines of resistance* are preventing them from invading the community core? What are the community's strengths and assets?
◆ What *flexible lines of defence* have been erected to preserve the integrity of the core when stressors have affected the health of the community? What indicates that the community or population is resilient?

Additionally, you can observe, vicariously, the processes undertaken in each of the stories. In each instance, assessment and analysis information is presented. Can you suggest community diagnoses from this information? Can you present them as problem statements and as positive statements? If you were involved in this project, how would you have presented diagnostic statements to the community or to funding agencies?

As you read about the interventions, are you able to discern the logic models inherent in the approach and activities? Are the indicators and evaluation processes coherent?

Throughout each of the stories presented in this section, you will see aspects of the community health worker using the strategies of the Ottawa Charter (1986) and the principles of the Declaration of Alma-Ata (1978) as described in Chapter 1. Can you also discern the issues of culture, diversity, ethics, and advocacy that the professionals faced while working in and with those communities?

Critical reflection is an important component of learning. Reflection demands that we use various lenses to critique what we hear, see, and read. Using lenses of population health promotion (Chapter 1) and epidemiology and demography (Chapter 3), the authors have presented narratives of community practice that represent advocacy and ethical practice (Chapter 2) based on principles of public participation, partnerships, and accountability through evaluation.

There are many additional settings and population groups of interest to the Canadian community health worker. This section presents a small number of contributions for the reader to consider. It is my hope that it will inspire you to do three things: try new strategies in your community practice, share your stories (successes and challenges) with others, and be inspired to contribute to the next edition of this Canadian publication.

18

Community Profile: Exemplar Health District

ARDENE ROBINSON VOLLMAN

Chapter Outline

Introduction
Demographic Data
Health Determinants
Health Status

Observations and Recommendations
Regional Health Indicators
Summary

Learning Objectives

After studying this chapter, you should be able to:

❖ Appreciate how large amounts of community assessment data can be displayed

❖ Understand how summary statements and inferences can be incorporated into text

❖ Recognize the utility of local, regional, and national data for comparison purposes

Introduction

This is a fictional case example that makes use of data available from various sources: Statistics Canada, Health Canada, Human Resources Development Canada, and others. No citations are given because the data have been adapted for presentation in this example, and no provincial or local identifiers are used.

The current environment for the health professional, community board, citizen, and elected official in deciding health policy and expenditures is a challenging one. The cost of health care in the Province has been rising more rapidly than income and the cost of living. Public policy, at both the national and provincial levels, is clearly aimed at managing the debt and deficit.

These and other forces, such as reconceptualization of health from sickness care to wellness and health, the interest in coordinated local / regional decision-making, a more knowledgeable consumer, and so forth are causing health districts to initiate processes that will assess and improve the health of its citizens. One component of the process is the gathering of information on the health of residents. The purpose of this report is to gather data as it pertains to the health of residents in the geographic area of the Exemplar Health District (EHD).

The first issue that arises is, "What is an appropriate definition of health?" Increasingly, the trend is to a broader definition such as the one noted herein: health is a state of physical, mental, emotional, social, and spiritual well-being.

In deciding on the measures one might use to describe the health of a region and the categories is which data should be grouped, a review of similar studies and of health indicator literature was undertaken. The framework chosen for this project is a simple one with four categories of which only the first three are covered in this report:

◆ Demographic profile: a description of the population of the Health District, including data on birth rates, age, family characteristics, and so forth
◆ Determinants of health: socioeconomic, environmental, and lifestyle indicators such as measures of income, employment, social supports, and alcohol consumption
◆ Health status indicators: objective and subjective measures of well-being such as causes of death, dental health, communicable diseases, and mental health
◆ Health care system: descriptors of the health system, policies, use and cost—for example, inventory of health care facilities, medical services offered, actual services provided, patient days, and cost-effectiveness

Where possible, we have sought to obtain 10-year data and compare the information for the Health District geographic area with data for the Province. As might be expected, the desired information was not always available. Sometimes, there was a problem in obtaining data for this length of time for the geographic area of the EHD, or the most recent data from the 2001 Canada Census were not published. This is not an unusual situation with which community workers must contend; census surveys are undertaken in different years and on different cycles for municipal, federal, or other purposes. Then, there is a time lag between the collection of information and its publication. During this time, the data are entered and statisticians prepare it for release, ensuring the accuracy of the data, the appropriateness of the display methods, and the relevance of the interpretations of the data.

DEMOGRAPHIC DATA

Population

The population in the EHD geographic area has decreased from 29,305 in 1991 to 27,525 in 2001. The Health District contributed 1.3% of the Province's total population in 1991 but decreased to 1.08% in 2001. The population growth is detailed in Figure 18-1; you will notice that the bars go below zero, indicating

FIGURE 18-1 ◆ Population growth for the Exemplar Health District geographical area and Province, 1991–1996 and 1996–2001.

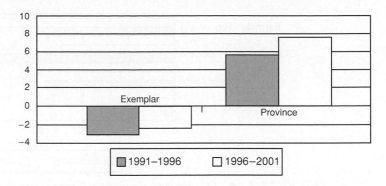

net population loss in Exemplar. Comparatively, the Province had a net population gain.

Age Distribution

In comparison to the Province, the Health District area's population has a much higher concentration of seniors (Fig. 18-2). However, the percentage of people in the Health District geographic area over 65 years of age has declined over the last 10 years from approximately 24% to 19% of the total population.

Birth and Death Rates

Because of the preponderance of seniors, the death rate in the Health District area has been higher than the provincial average. The death rate in the Health District geographic area has been increasing over the 10-year period (1991–2001), while the rate in the Province is remaining fairly constant.

The birth rate per thousand population has been correspondingly lower in EHD than in the Province. In 2001, the birth rate per thousand population was 13.70 in the Health District and 16.64 in the Province. However, women in the Health District geographic area are giving birth at the same rates as women in other regions of the Province. In 2001, there were approximately 54 babies born

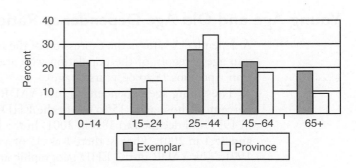

FIGURE 18-2 ◆ Population distribution by age category for the Exemplar Health District geographical area and Province, 2001.

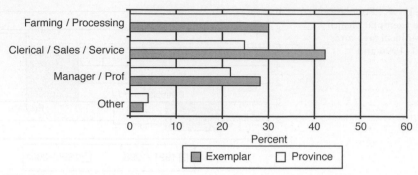

FIGURE 18-3 ◆ Occupational distribution for the Exemplar Health District geographical area and Province, 1996.

per thousand girls/women aged 10 to 49 in both the Province and the EHD geographic area.

Occupational Distribution

Generally, in 1996, approximately half of the EHD geographic area work force is employed in farming or processing occupations compared with about 30% in the Province (Fig. 18-3). The number of persons employed in the professional/managerial-type occupations increased from 1991 to 1996 (the most current information available). There are more women than men in the clerical/sales/service professions in both the Province and the Health District geographic area, although there are more people in those professions in the Exemplar area than in the Province.

Single-Parent Families

The number of lone-parent families in the EHD geographic area as a percentage of all families is lower than in the Province: 7.65% for the Health District in 2001 compared with 12.4% for the Province. Female-led lone-parent families represent approximately 75% of all lone-parent families in the EHD geographic area as compared with 82% for the Province.

Young Age and Old Age Dependency Ratios

A dependency ratio is the expression of the number of persons belonging to a certain age category of the population who are dependent on the "working population" (persons 15 to 64 years of age).

The young age dependency ratio (YADR) is those aged 0 to 14 expressed as a percent of those aged 15 to 64. In the EHD geographic area, the YADR was 39.4 in 1991 and declined to 38.5 in 2001. In the Province, the YADR was 35.3 in 1991 and 35.1 in 2001. That is, there was .35 of a child for each adult (aged 15 to 64) in 1991. The YADR in the EHD geographic area was only moderately higher.

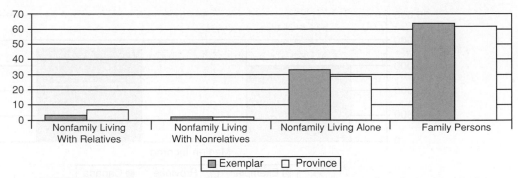

FIGURE 18-4 ◆ Living status of persons 65+ as a percentage of total persons 65+ for the Exemplar Health District geographical area and the Province, 2001.

The old age dependency ratio (OADR) is those aged 65+ expressed as a percentage of those aged 15 to 64. The OADR for the EHD geographic area in 1991 was 25 and rose to 28.8 in 1996 and to 32.4 in 2001. The Province OADR was 10.7 in 1991, 11.9 in 1996, and 13.5 in 2001. This means that the working population in the Health District geographic area "supported" about 2.5 times more seniors than the number supported by 15 to 64 year olds in the Province as a whole.

Living Status of Persons 65 and Older

The biggest difference between the living status of those persons 65 and older in the EHD geographic area and the Province is the number of nonfamily persons living alone. As illustrated in Figure 18-4, 32% of those persons aged 65 and older in the Health District are living alone compared with 29% in the Province. This suggests that more seniors are living without family or companion support in the Health District area than in the Province.

HEALTH DETERMINANTS

Income

The EHD geographic area had the lowest average private household income of all the Health Districts in the Province as of 1996. The average private household income for provincial Health Districts in 1996 was $36,800 in contrast to $28,784 in Exemplar.

The median income per tax filer in 1996 was lower in Exemplar ($14,943) than in both the Province ($19,900) and Canada ($19,200), as illustrated in Figure 18-5.

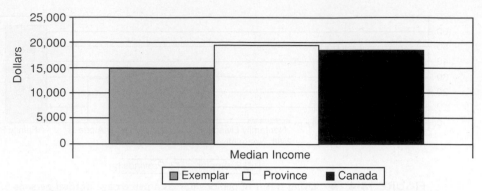

FIGURE 18-5 ◆ Median income in dollars for the Exemplar Health District geographical area, the Province, and Canada, 1996.

Levels of Education

In the EHD geographic area in 1991, 25.8% of the population 15 years of age and over had less than a grade 9 education (12.7% for the Province), and 9.1% had university education (18.4% for the Province). These figures are illustrated graphically in Figure 18-6.

The percentage of people with some university education increased from 8.1% in 1991 to 11% in 1996. The percentage of people with less than a grade 9 education declined from 25.8% in 1991 to 22% in 1996, a change that is possibly related to a reduction in the number of older, less educated citizens. The proportion of people with more than a grade 9 education but no university education also increased slightly from 65.1% in 1991 to 67.1% in 1996.

Labour Force

The EHD experiences a higher unemployment rate than the Province or the nation, with similar participation and employment rates as the national average. However, in comparison to the Province, these rates are somewhat depressed.

The *unemployment rate* is the percentage of the labour force that actively seeks work but is unable to find work at a given time. Discouraged workers—persons

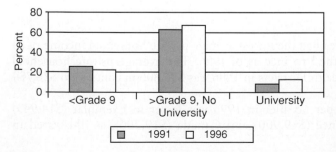

FIGURE 18-6 ◆ Levels of education for the Exemplar Health District geographical area, 1991 and 1996.

who are not seeking work because they believe the prospects of finding it are extremely poor—are not counted as unemployed or as part of the labour force.

$$\text{Unemployment rate} = \frac{\text{Number of unemployed people}}{\text{Number of people in the labour force}} \times 100$$

The number of persons unemployed is not the same thing as the number of people receiving employment insurance (EI, formerly unemployment insurance) benefits, because not all unemployed people are eligible for those benefits and some people receiving EI benefits for things like maternity leave and fishing benefits may not be considered unemployed.

The labour force *participation rate* is a measure of the extent of an economy's working-age population that is economically active; it provides an indication of the relative size of the supply of labour available for the production of goods and services. The labour force participation rate is calculated by expressing the number of persons in the labour force as a percentage of the working-age population. The labour force is the sum of the number of persons employed and the number unemployed. The working-age population is the population above age 15.

The *employment rate*—also called the *employment-to-population ratio*—is the percentage of working-age people who have jobs. For example, in 2001, there were 24.6 million Canadians of working age (aged 15 years and over). Of those, 15.1 million were employed full-time or part-time. The employment rate was therefore 61.2%.

The employment rate denominator is the source population, not the labour force. The source population includes all working-age people not in the military or institutions, but the labour force includes only those persons who either have a job or are looking for one. In 2001, the latter number was 16 million people. Whereas the source population grows fairly steadily from one year to the next, the labour force tends to fluctuate as persons become encouraged or discouraged by prevailing economic conditions. The employment rate shows a country's ability to put its population to work and thereby generate income for its citizens. Countries with higher employment rates are likely to have higher standards of living, other things being equal. As you can see from Table 18-1, Exemplar's unemployment rate is nearly double that of the Province and higher than the national rate.

TABLE 18-1			
Unemployment, Participation, and Employment Rates Percent for EHD, the Province, and Canada, 2001			
	EHD	**PROVINCE**	**CANADA**
Unemployment rate	8.0	4.6	7.2
Participation rate	66.3	72.3	66.0
Employment rate	61.0	69.0	61.2

At present, the number of active EI claimants in the Province is 130,000 people, a number typical of the last several years. The two largest cities each have about 40,000 to 50,000 claimants, with the remainder scattered throughout other regions of the Province.

In both the Exemplar sample area and the nearest large city region, approximately 67% of all claimants are men and 33% are women. By age, in both the Exemplar sample area and the nearest large city region, about 20% are in the 15- to 24-year age category. About 58% are in the 25- to 44-year age category, and 22% are in the 45 and older category. The average length of time on EI is currently 10 to 12 weeks.

Female claimants are concentrated in the clerical, service, and health areas, whereas male claimants are most likely to be in the construction trades, transportation, and resource operations. The unemployment rate by age and sex for the province indicates that unemployment for men is higher than for women. Table 18-2 compares the rate of EI claimants in Exemplar with that of the Province in several employment categories.

TABLE 18-2

Percent of Regular[a] Active Claimants by Occupation in EHD Geographic Area and Province, Various Dates, 2001

TITLE	EHD	PROVINCE
Managerial and professional	2.6	4.7
Natural sciences, English, and math	2.1	3.4
Social sciences	1.8	1.2
Religion	—	—
Teaching and related	0.3	2.0
Medicine and health	4.2	1.8
Artistic, literary, and performing arts	0.3	0.8
Sport and recreation	0.3	0.4
Clerical	15.1	15.7
Sales	5.7	6.3
Service	5.6	11.1
Farming and related	2.6	2.3
Fishing, hunting, and trapping	—	—
Forestry and logging	—	0.4
Mining, oil, and gas	3.7	2.4
Processing	2.1	2.0
Machining and related	3.7	3.5
Production fabric, assembly, and repair	4.4	6.3
Construction trades	32.8	25.4
Transport equipment operation	6.3	5.5
Material handling	3.5	1.5
Other crafts and equipment operating	0.8	0.7
Occupations not elsewhere classified	1.6	2.1
ALL OCCUPATIONS	100.3	99.9

[a]Excludes claimants on maternity or sick leave or receiving other special benefits.

TABLE 18-3			
Social Allowance Cases Exemplar (Region 3) Regional Office[a] by Month, FY[b] 1997–1999			
	1997–1998	1998–1999	1999–2001
April	331	351	452
May	307	353	419
June	318	352	421
July	300	351	427
August	301	349	437
September	307	367	456
October	320	375	466
November	327	396	486
December	334	415	500
January	357	449	529
February	360	474	504
March	326	458	513
Yearly Average	324	391	468

[a]Approximately equals the EHD excluding an estimated 750 people in Township 4 that are covered by the Region 2 Office of Social Services.
[b]Fiscal year runs from April of one year to March 31 of the next year. For example, the 1997 fiscal year runs from April 1997 to March 31, 1998.

Social Allowance

Social Allowance (SA) benefits are to be used for shelter, food, clothing, and household goods. The SA program encourages independence and encourages the individual's responsibility to work toward self-sufficiency.

The SA caseload in the Province increased substantially throughout the 1990s and reached historically high rates in early 1993. There is an average of 1.8 people per case. The caseload for the Exemplar Regional Office of Social Services has again shown growth in the 3 years from 1998 to 2001, as is shown in Table 18-3. There is some difficulty in interpreting these data because the social services regions are not contiguous with the health regions.

Take Note

This is a situation that often arises in community assessment; for instance, data may be available for electoral wards, but not by neighbourhood, which may include parts of several wards.

Those receiving assistance through the SA program are placed into one of five categories: the Aged (60+), Single Parent, Physical Illness or Disability, Mental Illness or Disability, and Employable. This breakdown is graphically illustrated in Figure 18-7.

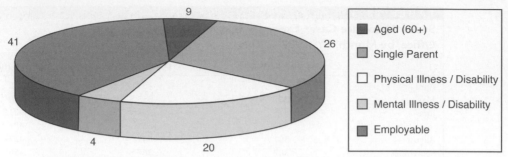

FIGURE 18-7 ♦ Active cases for Social Allowance program for the Exemplar regional office as of March 31, 2001.

Child Protection Cases

The number of child protection cases in the Province as of March 31, 2001, was 8,000, whereas the number of cases being administered on that date by the Exemplar Regional Office of Social Services was 88.

Over the last decade, there have been changes to the legislation as well as to the methods by which the child protection caseload is determined. The most significant legislative change was the introduction of a new Child Welfare Act. One of the aspects of the new law was the view that the families of origin are generally best able to provide the child the warmth and stability it requires. This led to a drop in the number of cases in this period.

Further, the transfer of 3,500 Disabled Children's Service Agreements from the Child Protection Services caseload in 1996 further reduced the size of the Child Protection Services caseload. Hence, as of March 31, 1997, the number of Child Protection cases stood at 7,684, down from 11,263 the previous year. The data prior to 1995 are not comparable to that of following years because of the changes in legislation and also because of the reorganization of health, children's, and social service regions in the Province. Table 18-4 details the number of children in protection by the legal authority that governs them.

For the first 4 years of the period (1995–2001) being covered, the Exemplar area had less than 1% of all child protection cases in the Province. However, during the last 3 years, the Exemplar area has exceeded the 1% rate and hence rose above the provincial average based on population. (With the provincial population growing and the Exemplar population declining, the rate of cases in the Exemplar area is somewhat greater than these percentages would suggest.)

Over the 6-year period, the number of provincial cases varied by as much as 9% from the base of 1995, with the number of cases in 2001 being about 4% higher than 1995. The number of cases in the Exemplar Regional Office declined by 32% between 1995 and 1996 but has been climbing every year since and presently stands at 33% higher than the number of cases in 1995.

TABLE 18-4

Provincial Child Welfare Child Protection Cases by Legal Authority, Exemplar Regional Office,[a] Cases Active as of March 31, 1995–2001

	1995	1996	1997	1998	1999	2000	2001
Custody agreement	6	3	4	13	6	1	3
Support agreement	27	14	22	23	45	28	35
Apprehension	0	0	4	0	0	0	0
Permanent guardianship order	31	20	21	17	16	17	18
Supervision	0	0	3	4	0	0	3
Temporary guardianship order	5	6	5	7	8	4	5
Extend custody to 3 yr	—	—	—	—	0	0	0
Extend care past age 18	—	—	—	—	0	3	3
Interim custody order	—	—	—	—	0	1	2
Other	6	2	1	2	0	4	2
No legal authority in effect	1	0	4	1	0	28	17
TOTAL	55	45	64	67	75	86	88
Province total	7,584	7,712	8,247	7,855	7,520	7,109	7,998
Exemplar Office as % of Province	0.9	0.6	0.8	0.9	1.0	1.2	1.1

[a]Approximately equals the EHD excluding an estimated 750 people in Township 4 covered by the Region 2 Office of Social Services.

Alcohol Sales

Excessive use of alcoholic beverages can be detrimental to the heart, primarily by increasing blood pressure, raising serum cholesterol levels, and increasing the ability to gain weight and fat. Excessive consumption is also closely linked to cirrhosis of the liver, poisoning, falls, domestic abuse, violence, psychosis, vehicle collisions, and problems in the workplace.

The preferred indicator relating to alcohol would be one based on consumption of ounces of alcohol. The published data by the Provincial Alcohol Office uses very large regions, and the EHD geographic area is combined within a larger rural-urban region. An alternative indicator using sales data of 11 liquor stores within the EHD geographic area was chosen; these data are presented in Table 18-5.

TABLE 18-5

Alcohol Sales in Dollars, by Stores in EHD Geographic Area, 1996–2001

	1996	1997	1998	1999	2000	2001
Area sales	8,367,038	8,523,988	8,525,213	8,690,137	8,436,464	8,514,585
EHD sales per capita	297.07	304.37	306.27	313.89	306.50	Not available
Province sales	942,061,103	994,895,681	1,003,436,423	1,044,804,522	1,019,915,078	1,004,989,345
Province sales per capita	395.76	410.60	413.07	423.03	400.67	392.97

Alcohol sales per capita within the EHD geographic area appear to be three quarters the level of sales in the Province. Sales per capita in these 11 stores increased between 1996 and 2001, peaking in 1999 at $314 per capita. A similar trend is noted for the Province with a peak of $423 per capita that year.

As noted, the data presented relate to sales. When converted into quantity, there has been a steady decline in consumption in the Province during the 1990s (there was a slight increase in beer consumption in the 1990s). The consumption pattern in Canada has been similar to that experienced in the Province.

Alcohol consumption is quite strongly correlated to age and sex, with high consumption by young people in their late teens and twenties. With the EHD area consisting of a generally older population, lower sales per capita would be expected. More specific information is needed to confirm the extent to which patterns of consumption are of concern. Finally, notwithstanding that recent research notes that moderate alcohol consumption can provide a degree of protection against coronary heart disease, the impact on overall mortality is not clear. However, as a local physician noted, alcohol consumption should not be promoted if it involves "trading a couple of months of extra life in a nursing home, in the case of an older person who benefited from alcohol consumption, for decades of lost life in the case of a 20-year-old who dies on the road." Such minor health benefits cannot be compared with the tremendous social costs of alcohol use by young people and those who are addicted.

HEALTH STATUS

No report on the health status of a community would be complete without a discussion of physical indicators of health. The following discussion summarizes the physical indicator findings presented in the main report. The physical indicators presented here include the leading causes of death, injury deaths and hospitalization, potential years of life lost (PYLL), the incidence of low-birth-weight births, congenital anomalies, teenage pregnancy, communicable diseases, sexually transmitted infections (STIs), and dental health.

Causes of Death

Table 18-6 gives the actual frequencies of the seven leading causes of death in the EHD geographic area between 1991 and 2000. Diseases of the heart and cancer claimed more lives than any other cause. This was true for both the EHD geographic area and for the Province overall throughout the entire time period. In the EHD geographic area and in the Province, suicide was the least frequent major cause of death.

From 1995 to 2000, the annual number of suicides in the EHD geographic area fluctuated between 2 and 10. In four of the five remaining years during this time

TABLE 18-6

Incidence of Seven Leading Causes of Death in EHD Geographic Area, 1995–2000

	1995	1996	1997	1998	1999	2000
Diseases of the heart	98	89	103	96	105	100
Malignant neoplasm (cancer)	73	73	73	70	84	89
Cerebrovascular disease (strokes)	18	22	22	23	21	34
Accidents / adverse effects	14	15	19	19	16	19
Chronic obstructive lung disease	4	10	12	7	14	18
Pneumonia / influenza	6	12	13	9	16	11
Suicide	2	4	3	4	4	10
Other	47	38	50	69	55	63
TOTAL	262	263	295	297	315	344

period, the number of suicides was four or fewer. However, in 2000, the number of suicides in the EHD area increased to 10 (7 men and 3 women). The predominance of male suicides over female suicides was consistent for every year from 1995 to 2000. The suicide rate in the EHD geographic area did not differ significantly from the provincial suicide rate during the 5-year period from 1995 to 2000.

The number of deaths from accidents and adverse effects in the EHD geographic area showed no apparent trend. On the other hand, the number of accidental deaths in the Province as a whole decreased between 1995 and 2000, although there are considerable fluctuations from year to year.

In comparison with provincial data, the rate of death from heart disease increased slightly more in the Province as a whole than it did in the EHD geographic area between 1995 and 2000 (32% and 26%, respectively).

Table 18-7 presents the rates per 100,000 of the seven leading causes of death in the EHD geographic area and in the Province in 1996 and 2001.

Generally, the rates of death from the seven major causes were higher in the EHD geographic area than in the corresponding provincial rates. However, it

TABLE 18-7

Mortality Rates Per 100,000 of the Seven Leading Causes of Death in EHD Geographic Area and Province, 1996 and 2001

	1996		2001	
	EHD	Province	EHD	Province
Diseases of the heart	310	157	382	149
Malignant neoplasms (cancer)	240	135	305	145
Cerebrovascular disease (strokes)	71	44	76	41
Accidents/adverse effects	64	43	76	41
Chronic obstructive lung disease	18	21	51	23
Pneumonia/influenza	35	20	58	22
Suicide	18	18	14	18
Other	208	124	200	128
TOTAL	964	562	1,144	559

should be kept in mind that in both 1996 and 2001, the EHD geographic area had more than twice as many persons over the age of 65 as the provincial average. Elderly persons tend to die from all causes at higher rates than the general population, and this can inflate the overall death rates. The specific trends and differences between the EHD geographic area and the Province are described in Table 18-7.

The overall death rate in the EHD geographic area rose between 1996 and 2001. Of the specific causes of death, chronic obstructive lung disease had the sharpest jump. In the EHD geographic area, the rate of death from cancer and pneumonia/influenza also increased substantially. The rate of death from heart disease also rose, but the rate of death from other (miscellaneous) causes dropped between 1996 and 2001.

Injury Deaths and Hospitalization

A more detailed examination of injury deaths indicates that in the 6-year period from 1995 to 2000, there were three times as many male as female fatalities from injuries. Figure 18-8 notes the three most significant causes of injury death for the EHD geographic area and the Province.

The number of persons hospitalized due to injuries increased from 572 in 1999 to 653 in 2000. The average length of stay remained constant at 8 days. Falls and motor vehicle crashes were the two leading causes of hospitalization due to injuries. The rate of hospitalization due to motor vehicle crashes was, as with deaths from motor vehicle crashes, significantly higher than the provincial rate.

Motor vehicle crash data obtained from Provincial Transportation indicates that four of five of motor vehicle crashes in the EHD area resulted only in property damage.

Potential Years of Life Lost

The number of PYLL is a measure of premature death. It is based on the assumption that all people have the potential to live up to an average life expectancy of 75 years of age. Table 18-8 compares the total number of PYLL in both the EHD area and in the Province in 2000 broken down by the leading causes of death.

When considering these data, it is useful to keep in mind that the population of the EHD area represents approximately 1% of the total population of the

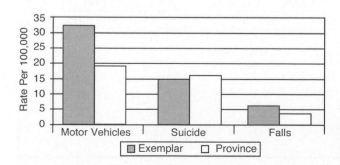

FIGURE 18-8   ◆   Injury death rate for the Exemplar Health District area and Province, 1995–2000.

TABLE 18-8			
Total Number of Potential Years of Life Lost in EHD Geographic Area and Province, 2000			
	EHD	PROVINCE	EHD (% OF PROVINCE)
Cancer (malignant neoplasms)	473	35,688	1.3
Ischemic diseases of the heart	294	17,128	1.7
Strokes (cerebrovascular disease)	66	3,818	1.7
Chronic obstructive lung disease	40	1,854	2.2
Suicide	237	16,764	1.4
Pneumonia/influenza	13	1,531	0.8
Accidents	313	24,882	1.3
Other	635	72,310	0.9
TOTAL	2,081	173,975	1.2

Province. Using this rough estimation, it is clear that the number of PYLL in the EHD area in 2000 was higher than 1% of the provincial figure for all of the leading causes of death, with the exception of pneumonia/influenza and miscellaneous causes. In these two cases, the figure for the Health District area was slightly less than 1% of the provincial rate.

Also note that when ranking causes of death in the EHD geographic area with PYLL, accidents move from fourth to second and suicide from seventh to fourth.

The PYLL for men in the EHD in 2000 exceeded the PYLL for women for ischemic heart disease, suicide, and accidents. On the other hand, women exceeded men in the total number of PYLL for strokes, chronic obstructive lung disease, and miscellaneous causes of death during 2000.

Low-Birth-Weight Babies

In the EHD area, the number of low-birth-weight babies born from 1991 to 2002 fluctuated between a high of 29 in 1991 and a low of 13 in 2002. The rates also fluctuated throughout this time period between approximately 3 and 7 low-birth-weight babies per 100 live births.

During the same time period, the number of low-birth-weight babies in the Province varied between 2,699 and 2,286. However, the rate of low-birth-weight babies per 100 live births in the Province remained fairly constant throughout this time period at approximately 5.7. The data for the EHD and the Province are located in Figure 18-9.

Congenital Anomalies

Figure 18-10 presents the rate of congenital anomalies per 1,000 births in both the EHD geographic area and in the Province between 1990 and 2000. Through the entire time period, the rate of congenital anomalies in the EHD geographic area was lower than the provincial rate. The rate for the EHD geographic area fluctuated

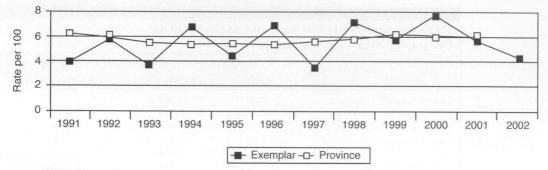

FIGURE 18-9 ◆ Rate of babies born weighing less than 2,500 grams per 100 live births, Exemplar Health District and Province, 1991–2002.

between a low of 12.6 in 1993 and a high of 42.7 in 1999. Between 1990 and 2000, the Health District area rate rose by a net 3.2%. In comparison, the provincial rate fluctuated between 35.9 congenital anomalies per 1,000 births in 1990 and 47.8 in 2000, and increased by 33% during the same time period.

Adolescent Pregnancy

Table 18-9 shows the number of live births to all girls under the age of 19 in the EHD area and in the Province. In the EHD geographic area, there was a total of 48 live births to girls 19 years and under in 1991. By 1998, the number of live births had dropped to 21, less than half of the 1991 figure. Although the total number of live births to girls aged 19 years and under also dropped in the Province during the same time period, the drop was less dramatic.

In Figure 18-11, the rates of live births per 1,000 girls aged 15 to 19 years in the EHD geographic area and in the Province during the years from 1998 to 2001 are

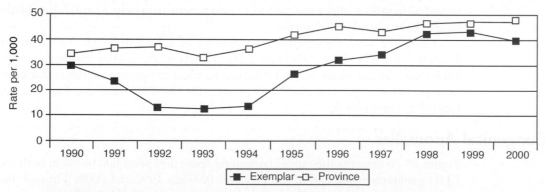

FIGURE 18-10 ◆ Rate of congenital anomalies per 1,000 births, Exemplar Health District geographical area and Province, 1990–2000.

TABLE 18-9		
Total Number of Live Births to Girls Aged 19 Years and Under in EHD Geographic Area and Province, 1991–2001		
YEAR	EHD	PROVINCE
1991	48	4,255
1992	27	4,188
1993	26	4,515
1994	25	3,303
1995	23	3,120
1996	23	3,155
1997	22	3,064
1998	21	3,032
1999	37	3,189
2000	25	3,339
2001	16	3,477

shown. In the EHD geographic area, the rate of live births per 1,000 girls aged 16 to 19 years decreased 47% between 1991 and 1997 (from 45.1 in 1991 to 23.9 in 1997). This trend continued during 1998 through 2001, with a further 9% drop in the rate of live births per 1,000 girls between the ages of 15 and 19 occurring during this time period.

The provincial live birth rate for girls aged 16 to 19 years also decreased between 1991 and 1997 (214%). However, between 1998 and 2001, there was a 22% increase in the number of live births to girls aged 15 to 19 years in the Province.

In Table 18-10, the percentage of teen mothers in both the EHD geographic area and in the Province in 1991 and 2001 who were not married at the time of their child's birth is illustrated. The proportion of single teen mothers more than doubled in the EHD geographic area during this time period (from 40% to 94%). In the Province, the trend was similar but not quite as pronounced (a rise from 53% to 84%).

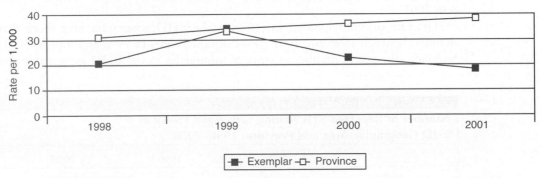

FIGURE 18-11 ◆ Live birth rates per 1,000 females aged 15 to 19 years, Exemplar Health District geographical area and Province, 1998–2001.

TABLE 18-10

Proportion of Adolescent Women Unmarried at Time of Birth in EHD Geographic Area and Province, 1991 and 2001

	1991	2001
EHD	40%	94%
Province	53%	84%

The acquisition of sexually transmitted infections (STIs) is a health risk of sexual activity. Table 18-11 gives the number of reportable STIs among young women aged 15 to 19 years in the EHD geographic area and in the Province from 1998 to 2000. In 2000, there were seven reported cases of STIs in the EHD geographic area among young women aged 15 to 19 years, resulting in a rate of 6.84 per 1,000. By comparison, the provincial rate was 30.3 in 2000.

Communicable Diseases

Tables 18-12 and 18-13 give the rates per 100,000 of vaccine-preventable and enteric communicable diseases in both the EHD geographic area and in the Province in 1996 and 2002. Enteric communicable diseases are infections that occur within the digestive tract or intestines.

An outbreak of pertussis (whooping cough), which began in 1999, is undoubtedly responsible for the large jump in the rates of pertussis in both the EHD geographic area and the Province between 1996 and 2001.

The number of diagnosed cases of measles in both the EHD geographic area and the Province dropped considerably between 1996 and 2001, with the rates also showing corresponding decreases.

There were no reported cases of either tetanus or poliomyelitis in the EHD geographic area between 1996 and 2002.

The number of diagnosed cases of giardiasis in the EHD geographic area fluctuated somewhat but showed an overall downward trend, from 20 cases in 1996 to 6 in 2001.

The rate of campylobacter infection in the EHD geographic area more than doubled between 1996 and 2001 (two diagnosed cases in 1996 and four in 2001). Similarly, the yearly number of cases of salmonella in the EHD geographic area

TABLE 18-11

Number of Reported STIs Among Girls Aged 15–19 in EHD Geographic Area and Province, 1998–2000

	1998	1999	2000
EHD	18	117	
Province	2,708	2,896	2,676

TABLE 18-12

Rate per 100,000 of Selected Vaccine-Preventable Communicable Diseases in EHD Geographic Area and Province, 1996 and 2001

	1996		2001	
	EHD	Province	EHD	Province
Diphtheria	–	–	–	–
Mumps	14.1	9.8	3.6	3.7
Rubella	45.9	48.9	14.5	2.4
Haemophilus influenzae type b	3.5	6.1	3.6	1.9
Pertussis	7.1	7.8	32.7	42.0
Tetanus	–	–	–	0.1
Poliomyelitis	–	–	–	–
Measles	74.1	34.3	–	0.3

peaked at 23 (1998). In comparison to the Province as a whole, the rates of salmonella infection in the EHD geographic area were lower than the provincial figures in both 1996 and 2001.

There were no diagnosed cases of *Escherichia coli* in the EHD geographic area in either 1996 or 2001; however, there was one reported case in 1997 and another three in 1999.

Sexually Transmitted Infections

Table 18-14 shows the rates per 100,000 of the three most common STIs (gonorrhea, nongonococcal urethritis/mucopurulent cervicitis [NGU/MPC], and chlamydia) for the EHD geographic area and for the Province in 2001. The EHD geographic area had substantially lower rates of all three STIs than the provincial average. In the EHD geographic area, the rate per 100,000 of chlamydia, the most frequently occurring STI, was approximately one quarter of the provincial rate in 2001 (72.7 and 272.5, respectively). The rates of gonorrhea and NGU/MPC in the EHD geographic area in 2001 were close to one seventh of the provincial figures. The positive diagnosis of an STI is a highly sensitive and confidential matter; thus,

TABLE 18-13

Rate per 100,000 of Enteric Diseases in EHD Geographic Area and Province, 1996 and 2001

	1996		2001	
	EHD	Province	EHD	Province
Giardiasis	70.6	68.0	21.8	61.2
Salmonella	21.2	32.0	18.2	35.8
Shigellosis	45.9	36.8	29.1	40.8
Campylobacter	7.1	7.6	14.5	7.8
Escherichia coli	–	6.2	–	4.1

TABLE 18-14

Incidence Rates per 100,000 of Selected STIs in EHD Geographic Area and Province, 2001

	EHD	PROVINCE
	Rate	Rate
Gonorrhea	7.3	54.7
NGU/MPC	18.2	133.0
Chlamydia	72.7	272.5

NGU, nongonococcal urethritis; MPC, mucopurulent cervicitis.

the following data need to be interpreted in light of the possibility that the number of reported cases may be less than the actual number of cases, particularly because infections such as chlamydia often exhibit few symptoms.

Dental Health

Figure 18-12 shows the average number of decayed, missing, and filled teeth (DMF) among school-age children in the EHD geographic area between 1992–1993 and 2001–2002. During this time period, the average number of DMF teeth decreased by almost half (47%).

OBSERVATIONS AND RECOMMENDATIONS

Frameworks and Understanding Health

It is clear that our concept of health is becoming broader. This is evident in both the reflections of local citizens and professionals. In a recent report of residents of five communities in the Province that were exploring concepts of health, health

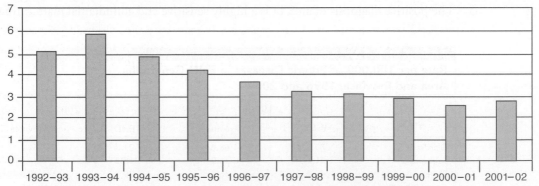

FIGURE 18-12 ◆ Average number of decayed, missing, or filled teeth among school-age children, Exemplar Health District geographical area, 1992–1993 to 2001–2002.

issues, and making health information available in the community, it was noted that rather than seeing health as something to work toward (i.e., dedication to a rigid regime) focus group participants tended to favour a balance of activities and interests where enjoyment was the goal. The societal framework, the focus groups suggested, should be one that allows for individual differences in needs, tastes, capabilities, personal histories, and lifestyles.

A senior researcher in mental health of the Provincial Health Ministry has been examining data on mental illness and social problems and concluded physical health, mental vulnerability, social problems, and social structure are interconnected and interdependent. Further, although we still need to know more about the way in which these connections operate and how to deal with them, the evidence of their existence is clear enough to warrant, and in fact demand, a change in direction.

As our understanding of health and wellness grows and broadens, we will undoubtedly revise the frameworks used for data collection in similar health indicator studies so as to more clearly draw conclusions and develop useful strategies for improving the population's health.

Data

The limited availability of certain useful data, such as the lack of information about a condition in the desired geographic region, for enough years to discern possible trends, and so on, is generally acknowledged. Although the provincial Health Ministry has organized a committee to look at health indicator information, it is suggested that much more energy and attention need to be given to this area.

There is concern that the provincial government decisions to reduce expenditures will inhibit the availability of data on a timely basis. The regional office of Statistics Canada is a source for some data, but cost and turnaround time need to be factored into the data collection process if different breakdowns of data are needed.

Data Interpretation

Statistical information by itself would not normally be the sole basis for decision-making in a Health District or community. For example, low income has been closely correlated with poor health. Hence, one might conclude that because average income is high, good health should be expected. However, additional exploration might point to continuing concerns—for example, although the average family income in Canada rose during the 1990s, there was also an increasing disparity between those with lowest income and those in the uppermost income categories.

With respect to "hard" data, one needs to be open to interpretations other than those initially considered. Qualitative data and measures that reflect health-promoting processes must also be given serious consideration in analysis of complex situations.

Additional Measures

Future health indicator studies that should be considered include data on:

◆ Prescription and over-the-counter drugs
◆ Mental health
◆ Spiritual health

Decision-Making Structure

In the development of a comprehensive community health plan, the community infrastructure and decision-making process must be considered. That is, health in the first instance is individual—it is based on each person's physical, mental, emotional, and spiritual condition. However, one could be in a healthy caring society or in a sick society, in one that promotes health and wellness of all or one that limits access or freedoms unnecessarily, or in one which ensures that legislation and decision processes reflect current issues and needs or one that neglects to change laws that are no longer current.

REGIONAL HEALTH INDICATORS

The core list of health indicators is presented in Table 18-15, within the Statistics Canada and Canadian Institute of Health Information (CIHI) indicators framework. Data for the indicators included in this framework are available at the health region level and include subsets for each indicator. Subsequent releases will add indicators and time series as these data are developed at the regional level and new health data are collected. Reports are available from the Canadian Institute for Health Information (www.cihi.ca).

SUMMARY

In this chapter, the report of the EHD was presented to illustrate how an assessment and analysis of a geopolitical district might be consolidated in a form that could be taken to decision-makers for planning purposes. In the real world, this report would include a series of community diagnoses with recommendations for action. However, the report stops short to allow you, the reader, to take it further. You can contemplate the data, drawing on what you view as salient to generate community diagnoses, both risk-related and wellness-oriented, and postulate hypotheses for action. From this, an intervention plan, logic model, and evaluation guides can be created and used as templates to guide action. As you become familiar with the process by using this chapter as a case study, you will develop skills that are transferable to the community practice setting.

TABLE 18-15

Health Indicator Framework

HEALTH STATUS

How healthy are Canadians?
Health status can be measured in a variety of ways,
including well-being, health conditions, disability or death.

Well-being	Health conditions	Human function	Death

NON-MEDICAL DETERMINANTS OF HEALTH

Non-medical determinants of health are known to affect
our health and, in some cases, when and how we use
health care.

Health behaviours	Living and working conditions	Personal resources	Environmental factors

HEALTH SYSTEM PERFORMANCE

How healthy is the health system?
These indicators measure various aspects
of the quality of health.

Acceptability	Accessibility	Appropriateness	Competence
Continuity	Effectiveness	Efficiency	Safety

COMMUNITY AND HEALTH SYSTEM CHARACTERISTICS

These measures provide useful contextual
information, but are not direct measures of
health status or the quality of health care.

Community	Health system	Resources

EQUITY

Canadian Institute
for Health Information

Institut canadien
d'information sur la santé

Statistics
Canada

Statistique
Canada

Canadian Institute for Health Information (2007). Health Indicators 2007. Ottawa: Author, p. 15. Available: www.cihi.ca

395

Internet Resources

http://secure.cihi.ca/indicators/en/tables.shtml

http://www.statcan.ca/english/freepub/82-221-XIE/free.htm

http://www.cich.ca/

http://library.usask.ca:9003/data/health/2002.comparable.tables.html

http://www.canadian-health-network.ca/customtools/homee.html

http://www.ainc-inac.gc.ca/gs/soci_e.html

http://www.camh.net/

http://www.brandonu.ca/rdi/

http://www.sustreport.org/issues/sust_comm2.html

http://www.smartcommunities.ncat.org/

http://www.ccsa.ca/ccsa/

http://www.cewh-cesf.ca/

http://www.spheru.ca/

http://www1.oecd.org

19

Assessing the Health of Communities in Northern Canada

GWEN K. HEALEY

FRANCES E. RACHER

Chapter Outline

Introduction

Inuit Women's Health

Promoting Youth Participation in Community
Development Through Photovoice

Summary

Learning Objectives

After studying this chapter, you should be able to:

❖ Discuss stressors for the health of Inuit women

❖ Detail the benefits of qualitative inquiry in community assessment

❖ Identify challenges to implementing programs in Nunavut

❖ Discuss the Community Health Action Model

❖ Identify ethical challenges of using photovoice in community practice

Introduction

*I*n this chapter, we present two stories of working in and with remote northern Canadian communities to assess the assets, capacities, and stressors facing them. In each, qualitative methods of inquiry are used to generate stories of life in these communities from the points of view of two groups that tend to be vulnerable in society—women and youth.

Community development has been defined as a philosophy, a process, a project, or an outcome, and perhaps all four at once (English, 2000). As a philosophy, community development entails the fundamental belief that people can identify and solve their problems. As a process, it supports citizens as they find their power to effect change. As a project or an outcome, it involves work with citizens to bring about change in their community. The community development process involves engagement, assessment, planning, implementation, and evaluation. While this circular process may become convoluted at times, it remains continuous. Throughout community development processes, products for communication and mobilization are generated and disseminated first within the community and eventually beyond the community for research, practice, and policy purposes (Racher & Annis, 2005). The work of one community becomes a case study with tools and outcomes to be shared with others, translated for their purposes, and adapted for their use.

The first story by Healey, *Inuit Women's Health*, focuses on the assessment and community diagnosis (priority-identification) aspects of the Canadian community-as-partner model. After reading this case study, the reader will have gained some insight into the use of qualitative, face-to-face interview methods as a part of community assessment and identification of issues and priorities for both health promotion and health research in the population.

The second story by Racher, *Promoting Youth Participation in Community Development Through Photovoice*, describes a project undertaken in Leaf Rapids, Manitoba, when the community reached a point of crisis and sought to engage community members and to rebuild a sense of community. In an effort to regenerate their community, engaging youth through a photovoice project became a valuable and useful strategy to meet that goal and assess the community from the eyes on one subpopulation.

INUIT WOMEN'S HEALTH

Inuit women's health is a crucial part of the health of their communities, and in recent years, several aspects of life in the North have had a negative contribution to the health of Inuit women. For example, Inuit women face serious health issues related to reproductive and sexual health, such as high rates of sexually transmitted infections and medical evacuation for childbirth. Wellness, suicide, and stress are more significant issues for Inuit women compared with non-Inuit women. Food security and accessibility is an issue for all northerners; however, it is a particular concern for Inuit women, as they often have sole responsibility for children and, therefore, have many mouths to feed. Alcohol and substance abuse as well as exposure to violent situations endanger both the health and safety of Inuit women in Nunavut.

The challenging circumstances facing Inuit women and their health are numerous; however, literature examining these contexts and the processes through which health is affected is virtually nonexistent. Additionally, no research to date has been conducted that examines women's perspectives about how the determinants of health affect Inuit women's day-to-day well-being. Published research that explores the relationship between social determinants of health and disease conditions in First Nations women is sparse. For Inuit women, it is virtually nonexistent. This case story will examine a qualitative assessment process that explored the determinants of health for Inuit women in Nunavut Territory, Canada, from the perspective of women living in a Nunavut community.

Background

The Inuit are the indigenous inhabitants of the North American Arctic, from the Bering Strait to eastern Greenland, a distance of over 6,000 kilometres. The Inuit live in Alaska, Greenland, and the Canadian Arctic and share a common cultural heritage, language, and genetic ancestry. Of the approximately 150,000 Inuit living in the Circumpolar region, 45,000 live in Canada's North (Morrison, 2005). There are four regions within Canada that are traditionally inhabited by the Inuit. Those regions are the Inuvialuit region of the Northwest Territories, Nunavut Territory, the Nunavik region of northern Quebec, and the northern regions of Labrador.

Nearly three centuries ago, the arrival of European whalers and explorers to the Arctic marked a significant turning point in the health of the Inuit. Interaction with European visitors through trade and gift exchange resulted in the introduction of alcohol, infectious diseases, and unhealthy lifestyles to Inuit communities (Morrison, 2005; Inuit Tapiriit Kanatami [ITK], 2005). Since then, the Canadian Inuit have undergone a tremendous cultural shift from a nomadic, subsistence lifestyle to working and living in communities year-round. The Inuit of northern Canada, as with other indigenous groups in Canada, have experienced and are continuing to experience a shift in their way of living and their traditional practices over the last several decades. What makes the experience unique to the Inuit is that this transition has been extremely rapid compared with the centuries-long process among other Canadian indigenous peoples, taking place in the last five to seven decades.

Nunavut, Canada's newest territory, came into being on April 1, 1999, when the Northwest Territories was partitioned (Fig. 19-1). *Nunavut* means "our land" in

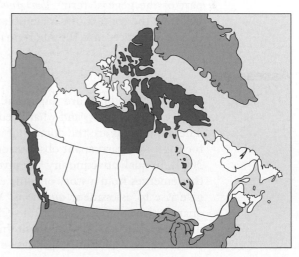

FIGURE 19-1 ◆ Map of Nunavut.

Inuktitut, the most common local indigenous language, and its boundaries were created based on knowledge of traditional Inuit hunting grounds.

In 2003, Statistics Canada estimated Nunavut's population to be 29,357 (Statistics Canada, 2003), of whom approximately 22,000 are Inuit. Compared with the rest of Canada, Nunavut residents are less likely to obtain a high school diploma or attend postsecondary studies, less likely to hold a job, likely to have lower income and be less likely to own their dwellings, more likely to live in overcrowded conditions, and are less likely to eat fruits and vegetables (Nunavut Department of Health and Social Services [NDH&SS], 2005). These factors play a role in determining the health of Nunavut's population.

In a workshop held in Nunavut in March 2005, representatives from a variety of fields related to health, well-being, policy, and Inuit culture met to discuss the determinants of health for the Nunavut population. They identified the following as factors influencing health in Nunavut: acculturation / self-determination, education, quality of early life, productivity, income and its distribution, food security, health care services, social safety net, housing, and environment (NDH&SS, 2005).

The current state of health of the Canadian Inuit is under investigation by researchers, government departments, and Inuit organizations in Canada. In a review of health research conducted with indigenous populations in Canada about their health needs, Young (2003) reviewed 254 articles pertaining to the First Nations, Inuit, and Métis populations in Canada. Of the articles reviewed, 122 (48%) were relevant to Canada's Inuit population, which constitutes a significant over-representation of Inuit studies in the literature given their relative proportion in the indigenous population in Canada (Young, 2003). This body of research also highlights that indigenous women's health in general is under-researched and that little, if any, literature (published or otherwise) exists that is specific to the determinants of Inuit women's health. In addition, the Inuit do not see themselves as part of the general term *Aboriginal*; therefore, it is important to examine their health in the context of Circumpolar Inuit and the Arctic region and not subsume their experiences into the Aboriginal health literature in Canada.

Assessment

Qualitative methods are important for determining what is important and why, what variations exist, and what lived experiences mean to individuals and groups. These questions are the domain of qualitative methods, which include interviews, focus groups, participant observation, and document analysis (Crabtree & Miller, 2004). In qualitative inquiry, the investigators usually start with a problem or issue that emerges from a story or some experiential context; these problems and issues give rise to assessment questions. What distinguishes qualitative research from quantitative approaches is that it seeks to search inductively for understanding and meaning. Little is known about Inuit women's health in the Canadian Arctic; therefore, an exploratory qualitative design was appropriate for this assessment.

A Participatory Action Research (PAR) approach was used in this study (Macaulay et al., 1999). One of the most important aspects of qualitative research is that it can be participatory in nature (Creswell, 2003), marked by the fact that individuals are afforded the opportunity to participate directly in the study by sharing their knowledge and providing their perspectives on the research question. Participatory research attempts to negotiate a balance between developing valid generalizable knowledge and benefiting the community that is being researched and to improve research protocols by incorporating the knowledge and expertise of community members. Collaboration, education, and action are the three key elements of participatory research. Historically, northern researchers and anthropologists were viewed by some communities to be disrespectful of the Inuit and Inuit *Qaujimajatuqangit* (traditional knowledge), often documenting aspects of Inuit lifestyle and traditional knowledge, or even conducting experiments on the Inuit, and then leaving the community never to be heard from again. This has left many communities with a negative view of health research and researchers in general. Berg (1999) states that the lack of participation in projects by understudied cultural groups has been attributed to language barriers, distrust of the inquiry process, and criticism that past research has done little to benefit the community. One of the benefits of using a PAR approach in this population is that it stresses the relationship between researcher and community, the direct benefit to the community of the potential outcome of the research, and the community's involvement itself as beneficial (Macaulay et al., 1999). A goal is that research subjects should 'own' the research process and use its results to improve their quality of life.

For this work, individual face-to-face interviews were used to gather data from a sample of nine Inuit women living in Iqaluit, Nunavut, Canada. Interviews were audio recorded with permission and transcribed verbatim. Data were analyzed using a process of immersion and crystallization (Borkan, 1999). All nine women participants, currently living in Iqaluit, Nunavut, identified themselves as Inuit, and each had at least one Inuk parent. Women were born in a variety of Nunavut communities and had moved to Iqaluit for school, work opportunities, or with family. Women in the project were given the option of conducting the interviews in English or Inuktitut; they universally chose to conduct the interviews in English. Women ranged in age from 27 to 51 years and came from a variety of family and educational backgrounds.

Participants were asked to comment on the contexts and issues that affect their health—for example, the broad determinants of health. In particular, they were asked to comment on how these issues contribute to their well-being and impact their daily lives. The women were then asked to comment on what aspects of their health they believe could be improved and how this might be achieved as well as to comment on these issues for women in the community in general.

Issue Identification

Participants discussed their health in terms of mental, emotional, spiritual, and physical aspects, illustrating both positive and negative influences on health. They talked about the strains that they, and other women in their community, experience as mothers, grandmothers, spouses, students and career women and the physical and emotional burdens that these issues can bring. In all of the interviews, women discussed their health concerns in terms of gender roles, traditional beliefs and values, and education and knowledge. Participants used stories that illustrated their issues or their own experiences or those of others they knew, to share their perspectives on the determinants of health and well-being of Nunavut women.

Three themes were identified from the data: (1) tradition and culture, (2) knowing, and (3) wellness. The first two themes were discussed by women in the context of relationships, reproductive and sexual health, and food accessibility. The third theme, wellness, was universally identified by participants as the desired health outcome for women in Nunavut. Participants used stories and examples of teenage pregnancy and parenting issues to illustrate points about the importance of traditional practices related to childbirth and child-rearing in Nunavut communities. Women described the importance of having learned Inuktitut, the indigenous language of the Eastern Arctic, and teaching it to their children. They associated the ability to speak Inuktitut with their ties to cultural tradition—for example, sharing stories and history—and felt that without it, many young people are left with a sense of not belonging to the community. Women talked about the grief that is experienced from loss of culture that can cause significant problems related to identity, social inclusion, wellness, and suicide.

Knowledge, as discussed by the participants, moved beyond simply receiving information and came from many sources, including formal education, parents, life experience, traditional teachings, and community sharing. It is the collection of knowledge from these different sources that helps contribute to the health and well-being of Inuit women.

Women who shared their insight in this project clearly illustrated the importance of culture in their lives and in their community, yet also illustrate the tension between traditional and nontraditional (or southern) influences on their health. At the same time, women identified and recognized their knowledge deficits as sources of harm to their health. In turn, they viewed knowledge as a resource for health and made suggestions for how knowledge can be gained. Well-being was described holistically, yet, in their words, women illustrate how it is undermined in personal and cultural interactions and injuries. Women shared health experiences through stories and used examples to illustrate points about underlying health-related issues, such as knowledge and education.

Insight

While this project was not designed to examine specifically how Inuit women communicate their health experiences, it became apparent in the analysis process that participants used stories to explain community health issues conceptually. For example, they used the stories to describe situations or events that illustrated underlying issues in the community. Although some cultural practices may be disappearing, the use of these stories to communicate information remains part of the culture. The Inuit have a very strong oral history and oral culture. The telling of stories is a millennia-old tradition used not only for entertainment but also for the sharing of information; it is an essential aspect of the Inuit culture (Bennet & Rowley, 2004). This tradition was reflected in the way that women in the study talked about health issues. Participants drew on examples from the community and used stories to illustrate points about important health issues, which illustrated aspects of the broader health context involving the community and society relating to education and cultural practice. Understanding this mechanism for sharing information allowed more insight into the data and the meaning of the stories and brought a different lens to the understanding of issues in the community.

This project has highlighted the importance of several key issues in Inuit women's health, including the role of culture and traditional knowledge, the need for health information, and the mental and emotional strains women experience due to family and personal relationships as well as the role of wellness and community support. Participants reinforced the notion that women's health is only one part of community health and that efforts must be made to approach health holistically and inclusively in Nunavut communities. We learned about the value women place on Inuit traditions and values; that important resources for community health include formal, informal, and public health education; and that the strategies used by communities for communicating information include the sharing of stories, examples, and personal experiences. These local practices are important to recognize and encourage.

The knowledge generated by this project will make an important contribution to policy and programming initiatives in Nunavut and add to the growing body of knowledge about the health of Inuit communities in Canada. It will also help decision-makers, health professionals, and caregivers to further understand Inuit women's health issues and help to identify priorities for policy and program development that will target their specific needs. Furthermore, the insight into the health perspectives of Inuit women in Nunavut has the potential to carry over into other Arctic regions both in Canada and in the Circumpolar community. The information gained may also inform questions related to the health of northern First Nations and Métis Canadians.

PROMOTING YOUTH PARTICIPATION IN COMMUNITY DEVELOPMENT THROUGH PHOTOVOICE

A Community in Crisis

In July 2002, the Ruttan Mine, located near the community of Leaf Rapids in northern Manitoba, closed. The copper and zinc mine owned and operated by Hudson Bay Mining and Smelting had been the impetus for building the town in the mid 1970s. With the closing of the mine, the Leaf Rapids Advisory Committee reported that the population declined from 1,309 in 2001 to an estimated 391 by 2005. As many of those employed at the mine and their families left the community, others from nearby Aboriginal communities and other locations moved into the town. The composition of the population shifted, and those now living in the town struggled to build a sense of community.

In 2004, representatives of the Town Council and Community Labour Adjustment Committee approached the Rural Development Institute (RDI) of Brandon University to seek its assistance in bringing the residents of the community together, undertaking a community assessment, and engaging the community members in setting goals and developing plans for the future of the community. Earlier work of the RDI, including *Rural Community Health and Well-Being: A Guide to Action* (Annis, Racher, & Beattie, 2004) and the *Community Health Action Model*, provided tools and strategies to support the process and work to be undertaken.

The Community Health Action Model

The Community Health Action Model evolved through collaboration and consultation among rural and northern community residents, organizations, and researchers. Literature on community development processes and documentation of community assessment models with quality-of-life indicators (including the community-as-partner model) informed the process (Racher & Annis, 2006).

The Community Health Action Model is unique in its ability to merge the community development process with a compatible community assessment, planning, implementation, and evaluation framework (Fig. 19-2). By using this model as a guide, the community takes ownership, gives direction, and assumes responsibility for its activities and the resulting outcomes. Through public participation, community members come together and interact as a collective unit. They express and demonstrate a sense of community before moving into action to gather information, determine goals, implement plans, and evaluate outcomes. This community development process is sequential (but not necessarily linear) and is often iterative. The Community Health Action Model supports community participation leading to community-engaged assessment and change.

Interaction as a Collective Unit

Through discussions with various groups and organizations in the community, the Town Council, Labour Adjustment Committee, and RDI undertook a collaborative project directed by the newly formed Leaf Rapids Advisory Committee. Two goals were addressed simultaneously: (1) to bring members of the community together and foster their participation in community planning and development and (2) to begin gathering data for a community assessment to provide information to be used for future planning. In addition to the broad community representation

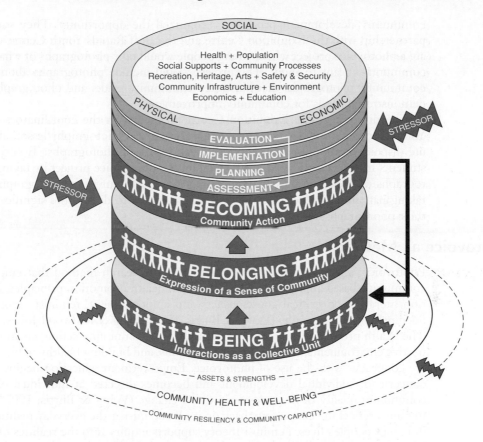

Used with permission. © Rural Development Institute, Brandon University, 2005

FIGURE 19-2 ◆ Community Health Action Model.

on the advisory committee, a series of community meetings were scheduled to encourage and support participation by community members.

Engaging Youth in Expressing a Sense of Community

Although youth representatives participated on the advisory council, young people in the community were not well engaged in the community development processes and activities. At this critical time in the community, a display of photography by local residents happened to be on exhibit at the Leaf Rapids National Exhibition Centre. While researchers from the RDI were viewing the exhibit, the director of the Exhibition Centre mentioned her plan to provide tours to schoolchildren and her desire to make an opportunity available to the students to engage in photography as an art form. The researchers, looking for ways to engage youth in the community development processes recognized the opportunity. They sought a partnership with the Exhibition Centre and the Leaf Rapids Youth Centre to create a photovoice project where young people would take photographs of what their community meant to them. The project would include photographs about their community, photographs that illustrated community pride, and photographs that demonstrated needs for community improvement.

The director of the Exhibition Centre worked with the coordinators of the Youth Centre to involve the young people, organize a photography lesson, distribute disposable cameras, and plan for a local display of photographs. Twenty-eight students from grades 5 to 12 participated in the photovoice project by taking photographs of their community, completing journals about their photographs, and taking part in individual interviews with researchers to discuss the significance of their photographs.

Photovoice as Method

Photovoice is an innovative participatory action research method that employs a community-based approach and is founded on health promotion principles, education literature on critical consciousness and empowerment, feminist theory, and documentary photography (Wang & Burris, 1994; Wang & Redwood-Jones, 2001). The health promotion principles of strengthening community action, creating supportive environments, developing personal skills, and building healthy public policy are congruent with the use of photovoice. Empowerment education begins with a concern for individual development and becomes directed at individual change, community quality of life, and institutional change (Wang & Burris, 1997). Photographs reflect the community back on itself and mirror the everyday realities that influence people's lives. Feminist theory supports inquiry into the realities of those who live with limited power, by and with those individuals instead of on them, in ways that empower them, honour their intelligence, and value their knowledge that is grounded in their experience. Documentary photography has used visual images to portray the social realities and quality of life of its subjects and the societies to which they belong. Photovoice places the cameras in the hands of community members, encouraging them to be the recorders and engaging them in sharing their images and thoughts of the communities in which they live.

Overall, photovoice is a tool for communication, using visual artefacts and a grass roots approach for community development and social action. Photovoice is an effective mechanism for sharing the perspectives of those who may be marginalized or not often heard. According to Wang (2006), photovoice is a method that enables people to define for themselves and others what is worth remembering and what needs to be changed.

BENEFITS OF PHOTOVOICE

Photovoice employs cameras as motivating tools. Participants become interested in the artistic aspects of photography and its potential for self-expression. The resulting photographs and the opportunities for sharing creativity and thoughts are reinforcement for participation. Photographs are used as tools for communication, and the old adage "a picture is worth a thousand words" rings true and is extended to "a picture is a way of gaining insight into the humanness that surrounds us" (Moffitt & Vollman, 2004, p. 189). The visual artefacts are works of art, visual stories, enduring records, and mechanisms for conversation and reflection. Photovoice enables people to record and reflect on topics or issues of importance. Discussion of the photographs raises awareness and promotes dialogue regarding perspectives and related concerns. Through the use of photovoice, individual residents become agents of change as they use their expertise, mobilize for change, and influence policy.

LOGISTICS IN UNDERTAKING PHOTOVOICE

The logistics in undertaking a photovoice project are multiple and must be identified and addressed to ensure the success of the project and its outcomes. Issues include seeking and securing funding to pay for cameras, developing, and printing of photographs; management and decision making prior to, during, and after the project; organization and project coordination; communication with participants, project partners, and the community at large; education on the use of the cameras and photography techniques; consent to participate in the project, to have one's photo taken and to use the photographs; ownership of materials, photographs, and research findings; and recognition of photographers and those who are the images in the photographs. In addition, research components of data management, data analysis, and dissemination of the findings are challenges to be considered largely by the researchers but are also of concern for other project participants and partners. Literature on the findings of photovoice research is becoming more available; however, information to guide the application of this method is less accessible. In this case study, the benefits and the logistics will be discussed as they applied to the youth photovoice project.

Leaf Rapids Though the Eyes of Youth

An informal partnership between the leaders at the Leaf Rapids Youth Centre, the director and staff of the Exhibition Centre, and researchers from the RDI directed and organized the project. The partners worked together to plan and implement the project and pay attention to ethical considerations (Box 19-1).

Initiating the Project

The director of the Exhibition Centre placed posters about the town centre announcing the photovoice project. Young people in grades 5 to 12 were invited to attend an educational session to learn about the project and hear tips on camera use and photography techniques. A local teacher who had been a professional photographer generously offered to teach students the basics of camera use,

---

BOX 19-1

Consent

Three carefully constructed consent forms were developed: (1) for permission for students to participate in the project signed by parent or guardian, (2) for the use of their photographs to be signed by students, and (3) for individuals in the photographs agreeing to use of their images. Consents were distributed with cameras; students did not receive copies of photos of people that were not accompanied by consents. The project had to discard those photos as well.

---

photographic composition and style, lighting, and image-building. Thirty disposable cameras each with 24 exposures were purchased for the project. Pairs of younger students shared cameras, with each student taking 12 photographs. Each high school student received a camera and took 24 photographs. In all, 31 students chose to participate in the project; that is, about half of children in grades 5 to 12 in school in Leaf Rapids. Students were asked to take photographs of their community, to demonstrate through their images what was important to them, what they wanted to stay the same, and what they believed needed to change in their community (Box 19-2).

Students had two weeks to take their photographs and return their cameras.

DISTRIBUTING AND DISCUSSING THE PHOTOGRAPHS

When researchers returned to the community with the photographs, participating students eagerly signed up for interviews to share their photo logs and the opportunity to see their photographs. When sharing their photo logs, students discussed the contents of their photographs in more detail, with researchers making notes of their comments. Once students had provided their photo logs and the necessary consent

---

BOX 19-2

Cameras

Cameras were labelled and numbered so that careful documentation of the distribution of the cameras could be maintained. All cameras were sent for development of the images; duplicate photographs were ordered (one set for the photographer), and images were placed on CDs. In a file created for each camera, numbered photographs, corresponding photo logs, and photograph consent forms were organized. The back of each photograph retained by the project contained both the camera number and the related image number; these numbers were placed also on the photo logs provided.

BOX 19-3

Photo Logs

Photo logs or journals were distributed, and students were asked to record the completion of three statements for each photograph. When students had not written journals, they were allowed to tell the stories into an audio recorder or to a researcher:

This photograph is of. . . .
I took this photograph because. . . .
This photograph is important to me because. . . .

---

forms for use of the photographs, they were given a set of their prints and chose a photograph from their prints for enlargement and display (Box 19-3).

LEARNING FROM THE PHOTOGRAPHS AND PHOTO LOGS

The youth photographers provided a wonderful array of creative photographs that demonstrated their appreciation for the people in their community and the environment in which they lived. In their photographs, the youth illustrated their perspectives on the importance of people and place, people in relation to place, and their connection to the northern environment (Box 19-4).

Through the analysis of the photographs and photo logs, six themes emerged.

1. *People*. First and foremost, youth took pictures of family members and friends. "These are my brothers and sisters, and aunties and cousins." Often, the pictures demonstrated the roles of people in their community. "My mom is an ambulance attendant." "This is my teacher; he is also a volunteer fireman." "The Churchill River is where everyone fishes, and people work at the fish plant."

BOX 19-4

Analysis

All data were managed by hand. Researchers reviewed all photographs and corresponding photo logs to identify themes and categorize the images by these themes. The importance of the words of the photographers in relation to the photographs facilitated clearer understanding of the images and proved to be vital in the data analysis. For larger data sets, the use of qualitative software is recommended.

In an ideal world, participant photographers would be involved in the analysis, interpretation, and display of data; this is not always possible, so project staff must be critically reflective in their analysis.

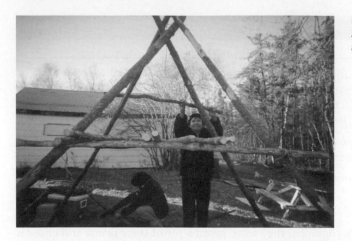

FIGURE 19-3 ◆ My Mom and Auntie are building a smoke house. Shannon, age 11.

2. *Community structure.* Youth took photographs of their unique town centre. In this industrial Northern community built in the mid 1970s, the Town Centre under one roof includes the business sector, school, hospital, post office, bus depot, and recreation centre. Residential bays loop out from the town centre. Students took photographs of community services, including the fire and ambulance departments and Royal Canadian Mounted Police (RCMP) offices. Transportation emerged as a subtheme. Many youth took photographs of the Greyhound Bus. This primary mode of transportation connects Leaf Rapids to the City of Thompson via a three-hour bus trip over rough weather-dependent gravel roads. Youth also took pictures of semi-trucks, the local taxi, the conservation officer's truck, and the medical evacuation airplane landing on the gravelled runway.

3. *The "big back yard" of trails, bush, lakes, and the rock gardens.* Central to their photography was the maze of trails that connect the residential areas to the town centre. Youth took pictures of "the trail leading from my house to the town centre" and "the trail my sister and I take to go to school." One young girl stated, "This is the trail to the rock gardens. It is a passage that everyone follows. I have walked here many times." Through their photos and conversations, young people demonstrated the time that they spend in their "big back yard."

4. *The culture and history of the community.* Culture and history came to the foreground in several of the photographs. "My family is from Newfoundland and these musical instruments are part of our culture." Several students took pictures of the Canadian flag located at the entrance to the town centre. One student stated, "It's the flag of our country. I like being Canadian" (Figs. 19-3, 19-4).

5. *Appreciation for the natural environment.* One of the strongest messages shared by the youth of Leaf Rapids was their love of and appreciation for the natural environment in which they lived. Their numerous photographs of nature and the surrounding beauty demonstrated their connection to the land; these photographs were some of the most influential, as they reminded the community of the vast magnificence of the surrounding environment.

FIGURE 19-4 ◆ Some of our friends are Inuit, and they showed us how to build an Inukshuk. Hugh, age 14.

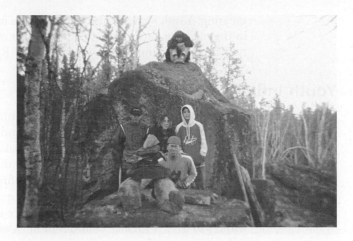

6. *A sense of loss of friends and neighbours, community activities, and the way life used to be*. Photographs of residential areas demonstrated the loss of friends and neighbours. "It is so sad to see these vacant houses in Leaf Rapids." "My dad and one of his buddies built that cabin. When we have to move that is one of the biggest things I'll miss, that cabin." "We have lost a lot of businesses; even the hotel has closed." "We don't use the arena any more because it costs too much to put in the artificial ice."

The vast majority of photographs demonstrated the pride that youth felt about their community. They focused on the positives: the people, the place, the natural environment. Some pictures were also taken of vacant businesses and homes, some of vandalism, and some of graffiti.

What is missing from the photographs also contributes to the analysis. Photographs of community activities centred on children playing in the "big back yard" and near the school. No photographs were taken of the traditional winter activities of skating, hockey, or curling, as the community could no longer fund the maintenance of the expensive community facilities and they sat dormant. Few photographs were taken of community events, for few events were taking place and few attended the activities. Could the students' photographs contribute to the efforts to bring people together and rebuild a sense of community?

SHARING THE PHOTOGRAPHS WITH THE COMMUNITY

The students' enlargements were placed on display at the Exhibition Centre for a month. Image after image, complete with quotes and names of the photographers, lined the walls of the Exhibition Centre. Young people took great pride in their talent to capture images that represented their community. Researchers were asked to build a composite presentation of the photographs to be shared at a community meeting. Youth were invited to participate in the presentation and stay to take part in the meeting, setting the stage for youth to attend community meetings and participate in planning for the future of Leaf Rapids.

Youth Influence Community Action

The Leaf Rapids Advisory Committee wanted to utilize short-term planning activities as a means to bring people together and generate a sense of community. When the youth were asked what short-term goal was their greatest community priority, they responded with the request for an outdoor rink. Maintaining the existing indoor community arena was beyond the financial capacity of the town, so it stood empty. Some community members were quick to reject this idea due to concerns about injury, insurance costs, and future ice surface maintenance; others were more willing to give it further consideration. A volunteer fireman suggested that it was time to "test the hoses on the fire truck"; another resident suggested a good location "for the testing." Several community members offered to build a border to contain the water. Youth offered to keep the ice surface cleaned. A supply of worn skates lingering in the arena would be moved to the school for students to use. The community buzzed with plans as the enthusiasm for the project grew; people were coming together, young and old alike. A common vision was being created as a sense of community began to evolve.

Lessons Learned

The potential of youth participation in community planning is increasingly being recognized (Frank, 2006). The photovoice project engaged community youth in a meaningful and creative way. Photographs provided a means for their perspectives to be heard and their opinions and views to gain respect. Their pride and enthusiasm were contagious; photographs reminded community members of their connection to the land and the benefits they had grown to know through living in the North. Community members began to feel a rekindled sense of belonging and to share the desire to work together for the enrichment of their community.

SUMMARY

In this chapter, the authors illustrated two methods of acquiring assessment data from subpopulations of interest—key informant interviews and photovoice. Each of these methods requires skill in person-to-person and person-to-community interaction and in qualitative data analysis. Often, these methods are introduced after a more broad assessment has been completed and issues or populations in need have been identified.

References

Annis, R., Racher, F., & Beattie, M. (2004). *Rural community health and well-being: A guide to action*. Brandon, MB: Rural Development Institute, University Press.

Bennet, J., & Rowley, S. (Eds.). (2004). *Uqalurait: An Oral History of Nunavut* (pp. xxv–xxiv). City, Province-Québec Montreal, QC: McGill Queen's University Press.

Berg, J. A. (1999). Gaining access to under-researched populations in women's health research. *Health Care for Women International, 20*, 237–243.

Borkan, J. (1999). Immersion/Crystallization. In B. F. Crabtree & W. L. Miller (Eds.), *Doing qualitative research* (pp. 169–193). Thousand Oaks, CA: Sage Publications.

Crabtree, B., & Miller, W. (2004). Research methods: Qualitative. In R. Jones, N. Britten, L. Culpepper, D. A. Gass, R. Grol, D. Maut, et al. (Eds.), *Oxford textbook of primary medical care* (pp. 507–511). Oxford, UK: Oxford University Press.

Creswell, J. W. (2003). *Research design: Quantitative, qualitative, and mixed methods approaches* (pp. 179–182). Thousand Oaks, CA: Sage Publications.

English, J. (2000). Community development. In M. Stewart (Ed.), *Community nursing: Promoting Canadians' health* (pp. 403–419). Toronto, ON: WB Saunders Canada.

Frank, K. I. (2006). The potential of youth participation in planning. *Journal of Planning Literature, 20*(4), 351–371.

Inuit Tapiriit Kanatami (ITK). (2005). Meeting of two worlds. Retrieved January 27, 2005, from **http://www.itk.ca**.

Macaulay, A. C., Commanda, L. E., Freeman, W. L., Gibson, N., McCabe, M. L., Robbins, C. M., et al. (1999). Participatory research maximizes community and lay involvement. *British Medical Journal, 319*, 774–778.

Moffitt, P., & Vollman, A. R. (2004). Photovoice: Picturing the health of Aboriginal women in a remote northern community. *Canadian Journal of Nursing Research, 36*(4), 189–201.

Morrison, D. (2005). Canadian Inuit history: A thousand year odyssey. Canadian Museum of Civilization Online Resource. Retrieved January 29, 2005, from **www.civilization.ca**.

Nunavut Department of Health and Social Services (NDH&SS). (2005). *Social determinants of health in Nunavut*. Workshop report March 8–10 (pp. 1–27). Iqaluit, NU: Government of Nunavut.

Racher, F., & Annis, R. (2005). Community partnerships: Translating research for community development. *Canadian Journal of Nursing Research, 37*(1), 169–175.

Racher, F., & Annis, R. (2006). *The Community Health Action Model: Health promotion by the community*. Unpublished paper.

Statistics Canada. (2003). The Daily, Thursday, December 18, 2003. Retrieved January 27, 2007, from **http://www.statcan.ca/Daily/English/031218/d031218c.htm#tab3 ftnotepp.**

Wang, C. (2006). Photovoice: Social change through photography. Retrieved August 6, 2006, from **www.photovoice.com**.

Wang, C., & Burris, M. (1994). Empowerment through photo novella: Portraits of participation. *Health Education Quarterly, 21*(2), 171–186.

Wang, C., & Burris, M. (1997). Photovoice: Concept, methodology and use for participatory needs assessment. *Health Education and Behavior, 24*(3), 369–387.

Wang, C., & Redwood-Jones, Y. A. (2001). Photovoice ethics: Perspectives from Flint photovoice. *Health Education and Behavior, 28*(5), 560–572.

Young, T. K. (2003). Review of research on aboriginal populations in Canada: Relevance to their health needs. *British Medical Journal, 327*, 419–422.

20

Promoting the Health of Pregnant Women

TRUC HUYNH

DOROTHY NICOLAOU

ALIYAH MAWJI

Give light and people will find their own way.   ANONYMOUS

Chapter Outline

Introduction

Empowering Immigrant Women
 in Canada

The Silk Road: Health
 Promotion in Northern Pakistan

Summary

Learning Objectives

After studying this chapter, you should be able to:

❖ Describe the Empowering Community conceptual model

❖ Discuss the challenges that face pregnant immigrant women

❖ Describe health promotion and prevention strategies at the individual,
 group, and community levels

❖ Outline some challenges of promoting health in developing countries

❖ Describe the role of culture in provision of health services

❖ Describe the Capacity Building Framework

Introduction

*I*n this chapter, three authors share two stories of working with pregnant and parenting women. In both instances, empowering techniques were used to build the capacity of women to care for themselves and their families. Huynh and Nicolaou tell a story of empowering immigrant women in Canada, while

Mawji illustrates the plight of women in Pakistan. As you read, you will notice how women were involved in the empowerment processes in each instance and how lay providers and peer supporters facilitated the development of these communities.

Friere (1993) describes *empowerment* as the process of putting power back into the hands of lay individuals in matters concerning their life and health (Laverack, 2006). *Power* can be viewed as "power over" when a person has the authority to influence and determine social events affecting his or her life and "power within" when the individual's self esteem is enhanced as a result of his or her actions of self-determination in life and self-control over his or her health. *Community empowerment* occurs when a population works together to change the social environment so that collective social and health needs are met.

EMPOWERING IMMIGRANT WOMEN IN CANADA

In community health programs, empowerment can illuminate the interaction process between health professionals and community members to co-create opportunities whereby both gain decision-making authority in some areas of their life. The key processes of this empowerment model are extensive collaboration on an equal footing and reciprocal health education among health professionals and community members (Lewis et al., 2003). The outcome of these processes is the increased sense of "power-over," "power-within," and of connection at the individual and community level. Figure 20-1 depicts the LOV Parc-Ex conceptual model of empowering community.

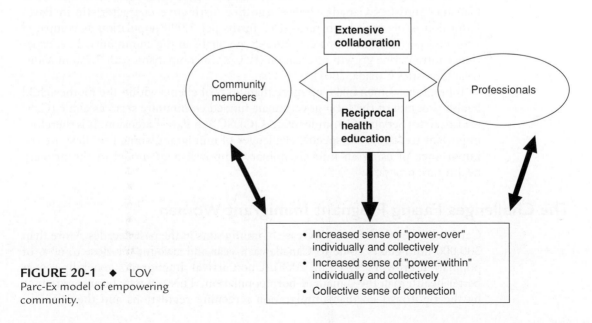

FIGURE 20-1 ◆ LOV Parc-Ex model of empowering community.

In this section, we illustrate a community health empowerment project in a small neighbourhood of Montréal (Parc-Extension). First, a brief community analysis was done by looking at the community's sociodemographic characteristics. Then, we planned an intervention that used an interdisciplinary empowerment model to demonstrate immigrant women's work and health professionals' efforts in primary prevention (i.e., to prevent low-birth-weight infants) and in health promotion (i.e., to empower immigrant women and enhance their sense of well-being). This section tells the story of our intervention.

Community Analysis: Sociodemographic Characteristics of Parc-Extension

The neighbourhood of Parc-Extension has been identified as one of the poorest and most densely populated communities in Canada. Of its 31,365 residents, 52.1% have an annual income below the Canadian poverty line, and 25% of the population is on public financial assistance (Statistics Canada, 2001). The average household income in Parc-Extension is $28,876, compared with the greater Montréal average of $49,429 (Statistics Canada, 2001).

The community has one of the most ethnically diverse populations in Montréal, with 62% of the population being immigrants (Statistics Canada, 2001). There also exists a linguistic barrier; in 12% of total households, neither French nor English is spoken at home, as compared with 2.3% in Montréal. More dramatically, 41% of the women who gave birth between the years 2000 and 2002 spoke neither French nor English, and 90% of the women who gave birth came from outside of Canada (Statistics Canada, 2001). Another distinctive characteristic in Parc-Extension is the high birth rate—16.7 births per 1,000 population as compared with 11.3 per 1,000 in Montréal. Among the births in the community, 12% experience intrauterine growth retardation (IUGR) in comparison with 7.7% in Montréal (Statistics Canada, 2001).

Immigrant women make up more than 90% of clients within the mother-child health program of the local government-funded community services clinic (Centre Local des Services Communautaires [CLSC]) in Parc-Extension. It is therefore important to discuss the specific challenges of immigrant women to illustrate the importance of using an interdisciplinary empowerment model in the primary health care program.

The Challenges Facing Pregnant Immigrant Women

Canada has seen a dramatic increase of immigrants in the past decades. More than 200,000 immigrants come to Canada each year and account for close to 60% of population growth (Ng et al., 2005). Upon arrival, immigrants generally report better health than the Canadian-born population. This fact may be accounted for by the rigorous Canadian immigration screening regulations and the selection process. Most immigrants are found to have the necessary stamina to undertake the tremendously stressful migration process. However, immigrant health declines significantly as their stay in Canada increases. This fact may be associated with the adoption of unhealthy lifestyles by the immigrants as a process of adapting to a new culture (Ng et al., 2005). Research has also established that immigration entails extensive stress and a period of adjustment, particularly in the area of social relations (Hyman et al., 2004). Stressors that have potentially negative consequences on immigrant health have been identified: feeling of loss of social status, loneliness, poverty, social exclusion due to prejudice, discrimination, lack of knowledge of existing services, and barriers to accessing the health system (Thurston & Vissandjée, 2005). Immigrants' feelings of being discriminated against based on their racial origin by members of the dominant society have been voiced frequently in the academic literature (Thurston & Vissandjée, 2005) and the mass media.

Social isolation of immigrant women is found to be rooted in linguistic barriers. Loneliness and social isolation is amplified by the loss of their premigration social system and predispose them to depression (Ahmad et al., 2004). In addition, their cultural adherence to gender hierarchy often leads them to ignore or deny their ailments (Ahmad et al., 2004) and to put the needs of loved ones before their own (Itzhaky, 2003).

For Canadian women, pregnancy and the process of becoming a mother are stressful events. They rely on their social support (e.g., partner, extended family members, friends, and coworkers) to buffer stress that comes with this transitional and transformative period of life. For pregnant immigrant women, however, there is little or no social support system, and many also face financial hardship. Most of their husbands work as unskilled workers earning minimum wage, and a large portion of their salary is spent on the high-cost city housing. In Parc-Extension, 41% of the households pay 30% or more of their earnings on rent (Statistics Canada, 2001). As a result, immigrant women often neglect their nutritional intake during pregnancy, which can have consequences for foetal health. Evidence shows that moderate (and even mild) foetal malnutrition impacts negatively on the foetal cognitive development (Global Health Watch, 2005).

It is therefore vitally important for immigrant, non-French and non-English–speaking, economically disadvantaged, pregnant women to have access to comprehensive and effective prenatal care. Furthermore, empowering immigrant women is essential to promote a shared sense of accountability of foetal health outcomes.

The provincial nutritional supplement program OLO (Oeuf [egg], Lait [milk], Orange [orange]) intended for the francophone and anglophone "native" pregnant women was found to be ineffective, as it could not adequately and linguistically reach out to immigrant women. To address this gap, health professionals at the Parc-Extension CLSC conceptualized the LOV (Lait [milk], Oeuf [egg], Vitamin [vitamin]) Parc-Ex program in 2000 (Nicolaou et al., 2003). Later, the program was modified and owned jointly by the immigrant women and the community professionals.

The LOV Parc-Ex program illustrates how a community, as composed of its people and health professionals, collectively built the flexible line of defence to buffer the identified stressors: absence of social support system, poverty, and inaccessibility to health services.

LOV Parc-Ex Program

NEED TO ADAPT THE PROVINCIAL PROGRAM

In 1992, a multidisciplinary team composed of a social worker, a nurse, and a community organizer implemented the provincial OLO program targeting the pregnant immigrant women of the community of Parc-Extension. The objectives of this provincial program are to: (1) identify high-risk pregnancies, (2) reduce the incidence of low-birth-weight infants, and (3) improve the overall health of new mothers.

At the local level, an objective was added to form a self-help group among the women identified as carrying "high-risk pregnancies." This last objective had never been crystallized because clients who received their nutritional supplement in the form of coupons were only seen on an individual basis. They were referred to prenatal meetings, which were conducted in either English or French. The non-French and non-English–speaking pregnant immigrant women could not understand what was going on during prenatal meetings; they rarely spoke up to ask any questions and generally kept silent. They were merely responding to what the CLSC professionals had asked them to do—attend the meetings! A few immigrant women communicated their sense of being disempowered in feeling obligated to attend prenatal meetings without being able to participate meaningfully.

EMPOWERING INTERDISCIPLINARY WORK

Nurses and social workers historically worked separately and occasionally worked together on cases; each discipline sought to guard its professional boundary as if respective practices were mutually exclusive. Unfortunately, this practise contributes to fragmentation of services for pregnant immigrant women. For example, women were expected to talk to the nurses about their physical health and to see the social workers about their feelings of sadness and grief due to migration.

After years of debate, nurses and social workers came together to use the strengths of their respective fields. Discussions ensued to find alternate ways of responding to pregnant immigrant women that would be more effective. In grouping their professional strengths, they were empowered to bring a collective voice to CLSC administrators. The administrators agreed to transform traditional teaching at prenatal groups.

TABLE 20-1
LOV Parc-Ex Logic Model

PROGRAM OBJECTIVES	PROGRAM ACTIVITIES	OUTCOMES
a. To reduce social isolation b. To increase the pregnant immigrant women's sense of self-esteem and control of their lives c. To increase the pregnant immigrant women's level of involvement in community activities d. To reduce the number of low-birth-weight babies due to poor maternal nutritional intake in the community	a. Individual meeting between the pregnant immigrant woman and the nurse b. Biweekly group meetings of pregnant immigrant women to exchange information on pregnancy and child care and to create different ethnic networks for social support c. Biweekly meetings between professionals and group leaders d. Distribution of food coupons	a. Increased knowledge for pregnant immigrant women regarding pregnancy, child care, and associated subjects b. Establishment of formal and informal network of social support according to ethnic origins and language c. Improved nutritional intake of immigrant women

Program Activities

INDIVIDUAL MEETINGS

The first contact of pregnant immigrant women with the CLSC is an individual meeting with the nurse. During this meeting, the pregnant immigrant woman talks about her life experiences in her homeland and Canada and discusses her health needs with the nurse. Then, together, they decide a plan of health services. The pregnant immigrant woman is invited to join the biweekly group meetings (Table 20-1).

GROUP MEETINGS

At the group meetings, the pregnant immigrant women are greeted by CLSC professional staff—two nurses and one social worker. The women are weighed and can ask any questions that they have about their pregnancies. While waiting for everyone to arrive, the women are invited to an adjacent room where they exercise and practice relaxation techniques. Once all of the women have arrived, they are divided into small groups. They are free to make their own groups; when the women have met and have gotten to know each other slightly (usually by the third or fourth meeting), they often form natural clusters made up of the different languages (Urdu, Tamil, Punjabi, Creole, Arab, French, or English).

The professionals facilitate discussion in the groups by identifying a leader within each group. The subjects discuss nutrition, baby care, labour and delivery, changes during pregnancy, postpartum life, baby safety, and dental care. The group leader and professionals further facilitate the discussion and the exchange of information by identifying veteran mothers who can act as mentors to new mothers. They are asked to recount their personal experiences on a particular topic (e.g., delivery), how they coped, and what they learned. Professionals will intervene to add (if need be) their North American scientific perspective and their personal experiences. Participants compare their experiences back home and in Canada. They often talk about the difficulties that the older immigrant women faced and how they coped in Canada. The exchanges not only serve to inform women about vital health information but also serve to create a supportive and open environment where women feel free to discuss whatever issues they are experiencing. The professionals do not offer advice but are constantly redirecting discussion so that the younger, newly arrived and immigrant women look for answers from women who are veteran mothers and who have been in Canada for many years.

PROFESSIONAL AND LEADER MEETINGS

Once the group leaders are comfortable in their roles, the professional staff asks them to join in planning subsequent prenatal subjects. This group work evolves as individual perceptions among professionals and leaders change. Professionals perceive leaders not as poor and vulnerable immigrants but as capable women whose strength lies in their self-belief and their own cultural knowledge about childbearing and child-rearing. Community members view health professionals not as authoritative experts but as women whose life experiences are similar to theirs and have insider knowledge about the health services.

Together, they explore what the group members need and how they can respond to those needs. These biweekly planning sessions help this small number of women to discover (or rediscover) the strengths and assets that they have and what they may have thought that they left behind in the immigration process. In essence, the immigrant women and professionals become partners in the LOV Parc-Ex experience by planning the content and the process of the prenatal meetings.

CIRCLE OF EMPOWERMENT

In 2004, the professional staff and group leaders decided collectively to approach a nongovernmental organization (NGO) in the neighbourhood to ascertain the possibility of organizing prenatal group meetings at this NGO to increase the accessibility of health services for pregnant immigrant women and to promote community ownership of the program.

Evaluation

In a small phone survey conducted by one of the nurses of the project, 50% of the women in the group kept in touch with other women they met in the program. In fact, some reported that they call each other first when they have questions about baby care, since they often speak the same language and these women are

BOX 20-1

What LOV Parc-Ex Gave Me

1. Confidence, knowledge & enthusiasm.
2. Conviction that I could make a difference.
3. The very best friends that I could ask for.
4. The final push that set the ball rolling for me.
5. Something that looks good on my resume.
6. Memories to last a lifetime.

Memories . . . the fall of 2001, I had just given birth the second time in the last 14 months. . . . I was reading self-help and mothering books, articles, brochures and product labels trying to learn the "natural" art of being a mother.

I had immigrated to Canada in 1999 to join my husband; I was on my own without my immediate family. . . . The next 2 years brought 1 miscarriage, 2 babies and many challenges. When I was pregnant a nurse at my doctor's clinic said I should take pre-natal classes at a CLSC. Though convinced at the time that I could not learn anything new, I signed up for classes. The nurses led us through those classroom style classes where we watched scary birthing videos, took in lectures about anatomy, did sensible pre-natal exercises and had nice, healthy snacks. We were given hand-outs and had brief discussions. The next year I was pregnant with my daughter, I participated in the LOV program. I was given vitamins, and coupons for free milk and eggs. There were 2 groups, French & English, on separate days.

So, that brings me to the time after my second child was born when I was learning the "natural" art of being a mother. Truc asked me to demonstrate infant massage to a group of new moms. I had learned the techniques of infant massage by magazine and had months of practice doing it on my 2 babies, who loved it. I described my actions in English with Dorothy translating in French. I supplemented various times in Urdu and Punjabi when needed because many moms did not understand much of either of the official languages. Moms did not feel shy asking me questions because they feel I am one of them.

Thereafter, I was asked if I would be interested in helping out with the revolutionary LOV Parc-Ex prenatal groups. I loved the idea of helping pregnant immigrant women because I knew their challenges.

We learned pre-natal exercise routines and led women in these exercises each session while the nurses did weight, blood pressure, etc. The groups were divided into smaller groups on the basis of languages and each group had an animator to facilitate discussions according to each week's theme. There was lots of discussion and many questions now that there was almost no language barrier.

The ladies were curious to know about us and our roles as facilitators. They actually started to look up to us and the whole exchange was empowering to both of us at our ends. We were happy to be so important to someone and the participants regained confidence because we were immigrant women like them who were doing an "important" job. We told them they could also help out later like us. Many of them agreed and were actually part of the team.

I have since moved to another city but will forever cherish my one year working with LOV Parc-Ex. Apart from all the fun & friends, the big confidence booster was the way we were treated as one of the team. Our opinions were heard & valued. We had a great learning experience in our planning and evaluation meetings, about how things were actually done. The meetings were so satisfying in terms of exchange of wisdom and energy—an energy so strong that you could almost hear and see the sparks, if you believed enough.

For me, it was this energy that fuelled me to accomplish various milestone feats, for which I thank LOV Parc-Ex.

also available after 5:00 PM and weekends—times when professionals are not available. Informal networks of social support according to each ethnic group were constantly being developed and enhanced.

Since the project began in 2000, nine women have become project leaders. Of the nine women, three went back to school to complete a trade or degree, three found jobs, and three went to work in the community on specific projects. The same nine women also acted as leaders in creating a women's group, Extension Liberty, in Parc-Extension. They recruited other women in the community, and other CLSC professionals involved their clients in the process. Together, they organize a Christmas party for the community every winter, and they also organize Women's Week activities every year. In 2003, they produced the *Vagina Monologues* (a play to sensitize communities to stop violence against women) in an effort to raise funds for their group.

Box 20-1 shows written testimony from one of the leaders.

In summary, the LOV Parc-Ex program originated from the perceived gap between existing health services and the needs of pregnant immigrant women in the community. Professional staff learned to redirect and reframe traditional intervention strategies that often excluded the very individuals that they set out to help in the first place. LOV Parc-Ex maximized the potential of individual immigrant women who are often seen as poor and with few resources. It also maximized the potential of the multidisciplinary team—instead of acting individually within one's own profession, the professionals merged their respective strengths. The process formed a bridge over tradition, experience, and professional knowledge; crossing this bridge makes individuals more knowledgeable, empowered, and with more possibilities to create a hopeful future.

THE SILK ROAD: HEALTH PROMOTION IN NORTHERN PAKISTAN

Introduction: Pakistan's Magic Mountains

Unique challenges face the communities of northern Pakistan, which is one of the most remote and resource-poor areas of the world. Northern Pakistan borders with Afghanistan, China, and India and is home to some of the world's highest mountain ranges: the Western Himalaya, Karakoram, Hindu Kush, and Pamir. Its centuries-old Silk Road is the most historically important trade route between China, Central Asia, and the West. Alpine farming and grazing livestock are the main sources of income—often amounting to less than one Canadian dollar a day. Amid numerous villages scattered throughout the mountain pastures, much diversity exists in terms of language, religion, and culture. Harsh winters coupled with extremely difficult terrain makes this area impossible to access in the winter months, even by helicopter.

Travel by Jeep in the summer months is challenging at best. The information for this case story is presented in terms of geographic landmarks in northern Pakistan. First, the various stakeholder groups are likened to the famous Silk Road. With every route travelled, "The Silk Road" is often visible and appears to accompany the various paths taken from village to village. This represents the constant guidance through interactions with local stakeholders, a few of which were "constants" and had existing relationships with several villages. Second, information was gathered through interactions with various stakeholders. This exercise is equated to "Navigating the Silk Road," as it was necessary to determine which information would be best obtained from the diverse groups. The Rakaposhi Viewing Point (Fig. 20-2), a landmark between valleys, symbolizes the analysis. From this viewing point, one is able to obtain a bird's eye view of the varying factors, and their relationships, that affect "life" in the region. The Rakaposhi Viewing Point represents taking the pieces of information gathered and "putting the puzzle together." Third, building the capacity of the various stakeholder groups (the Silk Road) is likened to construction that is often required to maintain roads and generate resilience. This corresponds to the strengthening of work currently taking place at various levels with respect to the Health Promotion Program.

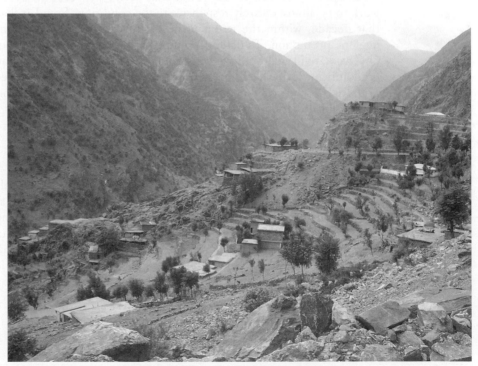

FIGURE 20-2 ◆ Rakaposhi Viewing Point.

Background: Suraj Health Network

Suraj Health Network (SHN), an NGO, began its work in northern Pakistan in the 1970s. It works in four districts and serves a program population of approximately 600,000 people. SHN provides services though two tiers. The first tier consists of village level volunteers: community health workers (CHWs) and skilled birth attendants (SBAs). Their roles include providing prenatal and postpartum care, assisting women at low risk for complications through the birthing process, and engaging in health promotion and disease prevention activities. The second tier includes 45 mother and child health (MCH) centres, 18 family health centres (FHCs), and 6 secondary health care facilities. The MCH centres will be the focus of this case story. Each MCH centre is staffed with two lady health providers (LHPs) who serve, exclusively, women and children in the community 24 hours a day, 7 days a week. They treat minor illnesses, ensure safe deliveries, and carry out health promotion and illness prevention activities including health education for schoolchildren and information sharing through home visits.

Assessment: Suraj Health Network Health Promotion Program

Since the 1970s, much of SHN's work has been reactive, as it was necessary for the work to be almost entirely responsive to the conditions found at that time. During that decade, within the realm of health promotion, there was much need for hygiene promotion. To date, the culture of providing care in response to what is observed at village level has been maintained. Since providing curative care is the predominant focus, health promotion messages are those that were put into place in the 1970s and are, therefore, few and far between. As a result, the SHN Health Promotion Program was called for review. At present, SHN views its health promotion activities only as disseminating messages.

Method: The Silk Road

The descriptive information about the population and the Health Promotion Program was collected during meetings, field visit observations, and group discussions in various villages with staff members of SHN (including senior managers, middle managers, and LHPs); CHWs (SHN-trained volunteers); SBAs (SHN-trained volunteers); community members, community leaders (including heads of mosques); and school teachers. Broad open-ended questions were used to guide the group discussions; local translators fluent in the Chitrali, Burushuski, Wakhi, Shina, and Urdu languages were employed.

Results: Navigating the Silk Road

After an initial review of morbidity and mortality patterns in the region, the most significant findings were the alarmingly high rates of pneumonia in the winter months and water-borne illnesses (e.g., diarrhea) in the summer months. Children

---

BOX 20-2

Appropriate Hygiene to Prevent Illness

Personal Hygiene
Hand-washing with soap after latrine use and after taking children to the toilet.
Hand-washing with soap before eating and before feeding children.
Hand-washing with soap after working in the fields.
Regular bathing (e.g., once daily during summer and twice weekly during winter).

Domestic Hygiene
Keeping boiled water covered (to prevent insect breeding sites).
Encouraging mothers to provide bottled water (that has been boiled) to their
    school-going children in villages that do not have clean drinking water.
Washing fruits and vegetables before consuming.
Covering food, cooked and uncooked, to prevent insect infestation.
Washing dishes and kitchen utensils with soap.
Appropriate garbage disposal.

Environmental Hygiene
Promoting latrine use and appropriate disposal of human excreta.
Garbage disposal techniques at village level.

---

carry the majority of the illness burden. The main sources of drinking water are free-flowing open water channels. Many villages lack basic sanitation infrastructure. Discussions revealed that deworming initiatives are nonexistent in the region. The evaluation of the Health Promotion Program was strongly influenced by these initial findings and largely focused on health promotion messages related to water-borne illnesses and pneumonia prevention. Message transmission during pregnancy and the postpartum period was also reviewed.

MESSAGES RELATING TO PREVENTION OF ILLNESS

Messages regarding the prevention of water-borne illnesses fall within three distinct categories: personal hygiene, domestic hygiene, and environmental hygiene (Box 20-2).

The messages pertaining to pneumonia prevention were focused on obtaining adequate nutrition in the winter months. As wasting due to inadequate nutrition and a resulting decrease in immunity levels is common in the winter, much effort during the agricultural season is put into drying adequate amounts of food for the difficult winter months. In addition, initiatives aimed at improving ventilation in typical traditional houses are promoted. At present, wood-burning stoves are used inside the small, windowless, one-room houses to prepare simple meals and to keep families warm. The lack of adequate ventilation in combination with the confined space provides an ideal opportunity for bacteria and viruses to transmit from person to person.

Health Promotion During Pregnancy and the Postpartum Period

Some prevention messages are delivered to pregnant mothers during antenatal care visits. Most mothers are given messages regarding:

♦ Adequate nutritional intake
♦ Vitamin and micronutrient supplementation
♦ Importance of clean and safe deliveries
♦ Danger signs of pregnancy, such as vaginal bleeding and severe headaches
♦ Malaria prevention

In addition, when observing mothers breast-feeding during group discussions, and those waiting their turn in the MCH centers, it was clear that little attention was given to coaching them on appropriate breast-feeding techniques. For example, many latches observed were poor, and breast-feeding positioning was not conducive to effective feeding. Furthermore, it was difficult to determine whether the nursing mothers were aware of the importance of monitoring the amount of breast milk consumed and whether or not the infant is feeding well.

AN INTERESTING ISSUE IDENTIFIED

In a few districts, plagiocephaly (parallelogram head shape and a persistent flat spot on the back of one side of the head) and brachycephaly (disproportionately wide head with a flat area on the back) were widely observed. After discussion with people from different valleys, it was identified that from a cultural perspective, flat heads are perceived to be beautiful. As a result, family members deliberately flatten the heads of their babies either by continuously laying the child down in the same position or using a flat stone and rubbing the back of the infant's head in efforts to make it as flat as possible!

Analysis and Diagnosis: Rakaposhi Viewing Point

During the beginning of the analysis phase, it was evident that staff members working at various levels in the network have different working definitions of health promotion. Therefore, it was essential to review the comprehensive definition of health promotion as outlined in the Ottawa Charter for Health Promotion with them to ensure a common understanding (WHO, 1986).

Before initiating discussion on which way to steer the SHN Health Promotion Program with respect to its water-borne illness prevention, pneumonia prevention, and maternal and child health components, it was important to triangulate information from various sources to gain a comprehensive understanding of significant gaps that need to be filled. This was accomplished by looking at published literature as well as comparing the program with what is recommended by global leaders in health such as the World Health Organization. This information was then linked to the context in northern Pakistan.

In efforts to curb the pneumonia disease burden, it was appropriate to study the causes of pneumonia and how it could be prevented in children ages 5 years and younger. Available literature suggests that the *Haemophilus influenzae* bacteria is a common cause of childhood pneumonia and usually strikes children between the ages of 3 months and 5 years (WHO, 2003). With the awareness of this fact, it was necessary to review the available morbidity and mortality data more thoroughly and determine the pathogens responsible for causing pneumonia in northern Pakistan. It was found that 40% of pneumonia cases in infants and children were attributed to the *H. influenzae* type B.

Group B streptococcus (GBS) is another causative agent of infant pneumonia. GBS, a common pathogen in the vaginal tract of many women, can be transmitted vertically to newborn infants. As no data is available on prevalence rates of GBS in northern Pakistan, it was necessary to find an estimate. According to the World Health Organization, 10% to 30% of pregnant women in Pakistan are colonized with GBS in the genital tract and 50% to 75% of their infants become infected, usually during labour or birth (Arab & Mashouf, 2006; WHO, 2006). After this information was presented, SHN estimated that 20% or more of its infant and child pneumonia mortality can be attributed to this pathogen. Babies who do survive can be left with speech, hearing, and vision problems. It was also noted that most cases of GBS in infants can be prevented by giving pregnant women antibiotics during labour. At present, screening for GBS is not common practice in northern Pakistan.

As there is no research available on the incidence of parasitic infections in northern Pakistan, it was important to look for research that could be generalized to the region in question. For example, a recent study conducted in Abbottabad, Pakistan, demonstrated significant parasite infestation (81%) of children ages 5 to 12 (Ahmed et al., 2003). It is well known that the Abbottabad area has better water and sanitation conditions than northern Pakistan. Therefore, it is reasonable to hypothesize that one would find similar, if not poorer, results if such a study were conducted in northern Pakistan.

Clear evidence exists suggesting the effectiveness of professional support during the breast-feeding period, even in areas where breast-feeding has always been part of the culture. Research has shown that certain attitudes create barriers to breast-feeding promotion. These include the assumption that health workers know enough already, the reluctance to allocate staff time to breast-feeding support, and the failure to recognize the impact of inconsistent or inaccurate information, all of which are apparent in northern Pakistan (OlaOlorun & Lawoyin, 2006). Although babies delivered by trained practitioners are brought to the breast during the first hour after delivery, it is unclear if indicators of effective breast-feeding (rooting, latching, suckling, and swallowing) are assessed (Riordan, Gill-Hopple, & Angeron, 2005).

As SHN has no experience in deworming, it was necessary to look for guidance to others with insight. WHO recommends *routine* deworming during antenatal care. There is also evidence that anthelminthic treatment of women during pregnancy (and lactation) improves maternal health, increases infant birth weight, and reduces infant mortality (WHO, 2004). Deworming as part of routine antenatal care is proven to be a cost-effective strategy for reducing maternal anaemia that in turn has broader health benefits related to birth outcomes. Furthermore, anthelminthics are also now recommended for children as young as 12 months of age. The impacts of such deworming initiatives are immeasurable and include increased growth rates of children and increased school attendance and school performance, including an increase in short-term memory, long-term memory, language, problem solving, and attention span (WHO, 2004).

After information was gathered from a variety of sources, a broad diagnosis was formulated: There is an opportunity to improve the health status of children in various communities in northern Pakistan by exploring changes to the immunization schedule, implementing deworming initiatives, and improving the quality of antenatal and postpartum care, which will likely result in decreased morbidity and mortality rates of pneumonia and water-borne illnesses and, more broadly, healthy growth and development of infants and children.

Before planning could begin, it was necessary to submit recommendations for changes to the Health Promotion Program to the SHN Board of Directors. The recommendations in Table 20-2 relate to the diagnosis presented previously. After

TABLE 20-2

Recommendations for Changes to the Health Promotion Program

RECOMMENDATION	ACTIONS
Determine immunization coverage, particularly for diphtheria, measles, hepatitis B, pertussis, and oral poliomyelitis to compare with literature regarding coverage needed to attain herd immunity.	SHN could then discuss steps needed to meet these target percentages *at minimum*. After this, the management team could consider the introduction of the *Haemophilus influenzae* type B vaccine into its immunization schedule to assist with decreasing the pneumonia disease burden.
Assess the potential to incorporate deworming initiatives with the routine immunization schedule in regions with no access to safe drinking water.	It would also be beneficial to introduce concurrent vitamin A and iron supplementation, as these micronutrient deficiencies are common consequences of worm infestation.
Incorporate screening for GBS infection into routine antenatal care to prevent a portion of newborn pneumonia morbidity and mortality attributed to this particular pathogen.	Screening data could then be used to validate the estimate received from the World Health Organization on the prevalence of GBS infection in pregnant women in Pakistan.
Revisit the SBA training program to support efforts to promote effective breast-feeding.	SBAs could be trained to inform mothers about the length of time an average breast-feeding session takes, indicators of effective breast-feeding, and signs and symptoms of infant dehydration.
Train LHPs, CHWs and SBAs in behaviour change and communication (BCC) techniques as part of efforts to promote healthy child growth and development.	Armed with these skills, various cadres of health workers could implement initiatives that focus on minimizing practices that lead to conditions like plagiocephaly and brachycephaly, which have implications for early child development.

approval from the Board, these recommendations will be prioritized, and the active planning phase will begin.

Building Capacity: Silk Road for Construction

It is evident that before SHN can put plans into place to implement the outlined recommendations, capacity would need to be built at various levels of the organization. It is with this understanding that a capacity-building framework was introduced. The Capacity Building Framework was most comprehensive, easily understood, and similar in structure to SHN (McKinsey & Company, 2001). It defines *nonprofit capacity* in a pyramid of seven essential elements: three higher-level elements—target, strategy, and organizational skills; three foundational elements—human resources, systems and infrastructure, and organizational structure; and one cultural element that serves to connect all the others (Fig. 20-3).

These elements are defined as:

◆ **Target:** an organization's mission, vision, and overarching goals, which collectively articulate its common sense of purpose and direction

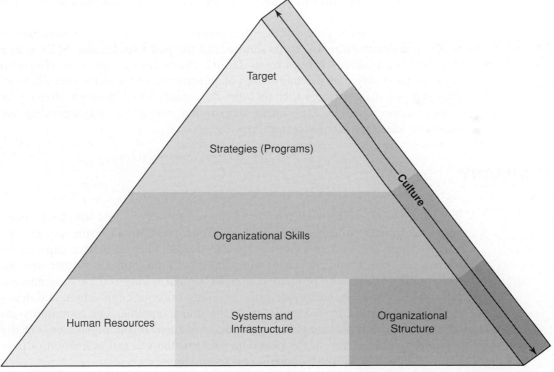

FIGURE 20-3 ◆ The Capacity Building Framework (adapted from McKinsey's 2001 Capacity Framework).

- **Strategy:** the coherent set of actions and programs aimed at fulfilling the organization's overarching goals
- **Organizational skills:** the sum of the organization's capabilities, including such things as performance measurement, planning, resource management, and external relationship building
- **Human resources:** the collective capabilities, experiences, potential, and commitment of the organization's management team, staff, and volunteers
- **Systems and infrastructure:** the organization's planning, decision making, knowledge management, and administrative systems as well as the physical and technological assets that support the organization
- **Organizational structure:** the combination of governance, organizational design, interfunctional coordination, and individual job descriptions that shapes the organization's legal and management structure
- **Culture:** the connective tissue that binds together the organization, including shared values and practices, behavioural norms, and the organization's orientation toward performance

By combining the different elements of organizational capacity in a single, coherent diagram, the pyramid emphasizes the importance of examining each element both individually and also in relation to the other elements as well in context of the entire SHN. The Health Promotion Program is one of the strategies for building capacity.

In summary, SHN provides essential primary care to many communities in northern Pakistan. Building on its successes of the past two decades, SHN is in a position to introduce changes to its Health Promotion Program in efforts to improve morbidity and mortality rates of pneumonia and water-borne illnesses. The analysis demonstrates that this can be accomplished through altering its immunization schedule, introducing deworming initiatives, and improving the quality of antenatal and postpartum care.

SUMMARY

Pregnant and parenting women in developing countries or those who have immigrated to Canada from less developed countries have distinct challenges in supporting their personal and families' health needs. They also have capacity to address these needs and challenges when linked with programs and other women. Community-based health programs can assist women as long as these programs are culturally appropriate; congruent with prevailing traditions and values; and delivered in manners that are accessible, affordable and acceptable. The community-as-partner model can provide guidance to the assessment of the population and the community context and to the planning, implementation, and evaluation of programs designed to address population needs and interests.

References

Ahmed, A. K., Malik, B., Shaheen, B., et al. (2003). Frequency of intestinal parasitic infestation in children of 5–12 years of age in Abbottabad. *Journal of Ayub Medical College, 15*(2), 28–30.

Ahmad, F., Shik, A., Vanza, R., et al. (2004). Popular health promotion strategies among Chinese and East Indian immigrant women. *Women and Health, 40*(1), 21–40.

Anonymous. (n.d.). Retrieved July 17, 2007, from **www.quotationsbook.com/subject/ giving/page-12.**

Arab, S. R. M., & Mashouf, R. Y. (2006). Epidemiologic pattern of vaginal colonization by Group B streptococcus in pregnant women in Hamadan, Central West of Iran. *Iran J Med Sci, 31*(2), 106–108.

Friere, P. (1993). *Pedagogy of the oppressed.* New York: Continuum.

Global Health Watch. (2005). *An alternative world health report.* London: Zed Books.

Hyman, I., Guruge, S. Mason, R., et al. (2004). Post-migration changes in gender relations among Ethiopian couples living in Canada. *Canadian Journal of Nursing Research, 36*(4), 74–89.

Itzhaky, H. (2003). Developing empowerment and leadership: The case of immigrant women in Israel. *Affilia Journal of Women and Social Work, 18*(3), 289–301.

Laverack, G. (2006). Improving health outcomes thru community empowerment: A review of literature. *Journal of Health, Population and Nutrition, 24*(1), 113–120.

Lewis, W., Labonté, R., & O'Brien, M. (2003). Empowering social action through narratives of identity and culture. *Health Promotion International, 8*(1), 33.

McKinsey & Company. (2001). *Effective capacity building in nonprofit organizations.* Report prepared for Venture Philanthropy Partners. Retrieved July 17, 2007, from **http://vppartners.org/learning/reports/capacity/capacity.html.**

Ng, E., Wilkins, R., Gendron, F., et al. (2005). *Healthy today, healthy tomorrow? Findings from the National Population Health Survey.* Retrieved July 17, 2007, from **http://www. statcan.ca/bsolc/engish/bsol?catno=82-618-M.**

Nicolaou, D., Huynh, T., Quirion, M., Ahmed, A., & Imran, A. (2003). *The LOV Parc-Ex program.* Document presented to the Quebec Ministry of Cultural Communities.

OlaOlorun, F. M., & Lawoyin, T. O. (2006). Health workers' support for breastfeeding in Ibadan, Nigeria. *Journal of Human Lactation, 22*(2), 188–194.

Riordan, J., Gill-Hopple, K., & Angeron, J. (2005). Indicators of effective breastfeeding and estimates of breast milk intake. *Journal of Human Lactation, 21*(4), 406–412.

Statistics Canada. (2001). *Statistics on population characteristics of CLSC Parc Extension.* Retrieved January 6, 2006, from **http://www.santepub-mtl.qc.ca.**

Thurston, W. E., & Vissandjée, B. (2005). An ecological model for understanding culture as a determinant of women's health. *Critical Public Health, 15*(3), 229–242.

WHO. (1986). *Ottawa Charter for Health Promotion.* Geneva: Author Retrieved July 17, 2007 from **http://www.who.int/healthpromotion/conferences/previous/ottawa/en/ index.html.**

WHO. (2003). *Immunization, vaccines and biologicals:* Haemophilus influenzae *type B (Hib).* Retrieved July 17, 2007, from **http://www.who.int/immunization/topics/hib/ en/index.html.**

WHO. (2004). *Deworming for health and development.* Report of the Third Global Meeting of the Partners for Parasite Control, Geneva, November 29–30. Retrieved July 17, 2007, from **http://whqlibdoc.who.int/hq/2005/WHO_CDS_CPE_PVC_2005.14.pdf.**

WHO. (2006). *Initiative for Vaccine Research (IVR): Group B* Streptococcus. Retrieved July 17, 2007, from **http://www.who.int/vaccine_research/diseases/soa_bacterial/en/index6. html.**

21

Promoting the Health of Schoolchildren

JENEAN JOHNSON

HEATHER McELROY

CANDACE LIND

Chapter Outline

Introduction

Oral Health Programming—Getting
to the Evidence

Promoting School Health Through a
Partnership Model

Summary

Learning Objectives

After studying this chapter, you should be able to:

❖ Discuss oral health challenges in Canada

❖ Detail the components of a dental health survey

❖ Discuss best practices in survey methodology

❖ Articulate two approaches to oral health promotion in schools

❖ Describe how labelling and stigma influence health

❖ Discuss wellness diagnoses in capacity-building

Introduction

R ural Canada occupies 9.5 million square kilometres, or around 99%, of Canada's territory. Towns with fewer than ten thousand residents account for 22% of the Canadian population, about 6.4 million people. Rural Canadians are served by about 10% of Canada's physicians; Canadians in some rural communities have life expectancies of less than 75 years, four years less than Canada's average (Health Canada, 2001).

In this chapter, the authors present two different ways of intervening for health promotion and capacity-building in rural Canadian schools. In the first story, *Oral Health Programming—Getting to the Evidence*, Johnson and McElroy offer a traditional epidemiologic survey approach to public health practice. In the second story, *Promoting School Health Through a Partnership Model*, Lind describes a more participatory approach. Regardless of the approach used, the implications of socioeconomic status and disadvantage on ill health are evident. Additionally, the risk-based and capacity-building approaches to health promotion are detailed by the authors so that readers can discern the relative strengths of each as they are applied in rural school settings.

Communities are located in different sites—for example, the school—and can be targets of intervention as well as locations for groups. Elementary schools were the target for the first section, and an alternative high school was the setting for the second. The community-as-partner model allowed the community health team (in this chapter, a team of dental health professionals and a team of nursing students) to work through a process of assessment and analysis to plan and implement a program that addresses the needs of the community of interest.

When we speak of being "at risk," we assume that there is a potential for harm or some danger to health and well-being. This hazard may be imminent, or its consequences may occur long after the exposure to the risk. In the first section, the authors assess the actual harm to the oral health of school children and act to prevent further harm by applying preventive measures. In the second section, the harm is less of a physical nature than it is psychosocial—loss of self-esteem and identity—that can have long-lasting implications for school achievement, eventual employment, and income. In both cases, the population level consequences of harm are evident.

ORAL HEALTH PROGRAMMING—GETTING TO THE EVIDENCE

In 2003, a reorganization of Alberta health regions resulted in the expansion of the David Thompson Health Region (DTHR) from the British Columbia border to the Saskatchewan border across the centre of the province. The DTHR covers an area of over 60,000 square kilometers and serves a population of 290,000 people, making it the third largest health region in Alberta. Similar to other health regions in Alberta, the DTHR includes programs and facilities such as hospitals, continuing care, public health, mental health, rehabilitation, and community care. With regionalization came the amalgamation of four previous health regions and the necessity to combine four distinct dental programs. The newly formed dental program found itself facing the question: "How do we plan evidence-based school oral health programs for such a large and diverse region?"

Oral Health and Quality of Life

Dental caries (cavities or decay) is one of the most common diseases globally, affecting 60% to 90% of schoolchildren and the vast majority of adults (Sheiham,

2005). It is a ubiquitous disease found in all age groups, social strata, and countries. However, the distribution of the disease is not equitable—the greatest burden of disease is experienced by people who are disadvantaged and / or living in poverty.

Dental caries is a multifaceted disease comprising several factors, including host biological resistance, oral environment; causative microbial agents (e.g., *Streptococcus mutans*), substrate, and time before initiation of disease. These factors are linked to and affected by many of the social determinants of health (Chapter 1). The significant role of sociobehavioural and environmental factors in oral disease is well demonstrated in a large number of epidemiological surveys (Petersen et al., 2005). Cavitation of tooth surfaces is more complex than what the public believes; it is not as simple as "brush + floss + see your dentist = good oral health." Hence, dental caries remains a prevalent and significant problem even in developed nations.

Dental caries represents a huge financial burden on the health care system. The cost of dental care in Canada in 1989 was $3.1 billion, with only 14% of these costs covered by public funds. It is estimated that those costs doubled by 2000, making the treatment of dental disorders the third highest health expenditure after cardiovascular diseases and mental disorders (Locker & Matear, 2001). In Canada, with its privatized dental industry, parents of children with oral disease personally incur high treatment expenses. Children are viewed as a disadvantaged segment of the population when considering oral health.

The personal toll of oral disease is great because poor oral health detracts from quality of life. Advanced dental caries cause pain, discomfort, disfigurement, acute and chronic infections, eating and sleeping disturbances, higher risk of hospitalization, and loss of school/work days with the consequently diminished ability to learn/earn (Sheiham, 2005). In addition to the oral impact of dental disease, there is direct impact of oral health on systemic conditions such as diabetes, cardiovascular disease, cerebral incidents, and respiratory health (Locker & Matear, 2000).

Approaches to Oral Health Promotion

There are essentially two public health approaches to the prevention and reduction of disease: population and high risk. The population approach uses public health measures to reduce the level of risk for the entire population (e.g., fluoridation of the water supply). The high risk approach focuses attention on individuals within a population who have been identified as most likely to succumb to or currently have a specific disease. These individuals then receive an intervention to mitigate the disease. Health professionals often utilize this approach, as it is a good fit within the clinical model to disease prevention and management. There are benefits and shortcomings to each method, depending on the intervention implemented. The population approach assumes that an intervention applied to an entire population will decrease disease levels in those most at risk; however, this is not always the case, as benefits may be unevenly distributed across socioeconomic status (SES) groups, with higher SES populations responding better to interventions than those groups with lower SES (WHO, 2006). From a public health perspective, the high risk approach can present two key pitfalls (Sheiham, 2005): it does not address the underlying cause of the disease, which invariably results in new cases; and it relies on screening tools that may not be sensitive, specific, or predictive (Watt, 2005). In the recent past, prevention of oral disease has been dominated by the high risk approach. It is now accepted as best practice that a combination of high risk and population based approaches is the best option to limit the shortcomings of each (Beaglehole & Bonita, 1998; Petersen et al., 2005; Rose, 1992).

With this in mind, the DTHR Dental Program defined its high risk target schools based on epidemiological data and then offered oral health services to the entire school population. This targeted approach to disease prevention is appealing as it focuses action on higher risk subgroups (i.e., target schools), resulting in more efficient use of health resources than would be the case if a prevention program were applied to the entire population (i.e., all schools in the health region) (Tickle et al., 2003). In addition, the application of effective preventive measures and health promotion strategies is more effective than treating the dental disease after it occurs (Wright et al., 2000).

Community Assessment

In order to implement this approach, school populations in the greatest need of oral health services had to be identified. Since Canada is one of the only developed countries without a national oral health plan or recent oral health data on its citizens, we needed to look elsewhere for oral health epidemiological data. Similarly, the province of Alberta does not have a mandated oral health program, dental public health standards, or provincial data on the oral health status of its children. Thus, the first step in program planning was to acquire the epidemiological data on the region's school populations through a comprehensive school-based dental health survey.

While dental health surveys had previously been conducted in many parts of the region, the data did not reflect the newly formed regional boundaries. The Dental Program developed a set of criteria and protocols for a region-wide school oral health survey with a sample population of every student (with parental consent) in grades 2 and 6 in all 179 schools within its catchment area, for a potential total of over 8,300 students.

Why were these age groups targeted for assessment? Our goal was to acquire data on age groups where oral health interventions would be most effective. Eruption of the 6- and 12-year molars is most likely to happen by grades 2 and 6, and the placement of dental sealants is recommended shortly after tooth eruption. Information on these age groups also allows approximate comparisons to the minimal oral health goals established by the World Health Organization (WHO) and World Dental Federation (FDI) in 1981 (Table 21-1).

With an average of 67% consents returned, the data collection teams surveyed 5,786 students, representing an oral exam completion rate of >95% of the students

<table>
<tr><td colspan="2">TABLE 21-1</td></tr>
<tr><td colspan="2">Oral Health Goals for Children by Year 2000</td></tr>
<tr><td colspan="2">World Health Organization and World Dental Federation Oral Health Goals</td></tr>
<tr><td>Goal 1</td><td>50% of 5 to 6 year olds (grade 2) will be caries free.</td></tr>
<tr><td>Goal 2</td><td>The global average to be no more than three decayed/missing/filled teeth at 12 years of age (grade 6).</td></tr>
<tr><td colspan="2">From World Health Organization. Oral health information systems. Retrieved July 20, 2007, from www.who.int/oral_health/action/information/surveillance/en/print.html.</td></tr>
</table>

with parental consent. Seven dental hygienists and nine dental assistants collected data on oral health indices including:

◆ deft—decayed, extracted, and filled primary teeth (grade 2 only)
◆ DMFT—decayed, missing (due to disease), and filled permanent teeth
◆ Students with no decay experience
◆ Students with untreated dental disease
◆ Students who required sealants
◆ Students who required a professional dental cleaning
◆ Students who required urgent dental treatment (e.g., abscessed teeth, student was in pain, or more than half the tooth was missing due to decay)
◆ Students who were considered to be high risk (i.e., two or more untreated dental caries lesions)

The results for each index were aggregated by grade and then for each school, providing complete comparative data for each school and regional averages for each index. When comparing these results with the Oral Health Goals established by WHO (Table 20-1), it is important to note that the standards established by WHO are inclusive of both developed and developing nations. High-risk students in the DTHR are just barely meeting this standard.

Some significant results to be noted in terms of level of disease were that among grade 2 students surveyed, there was an average of 2.47 deft. If we looked only at those students with disease, the rate rose to 4.26 deft per student. The results for grade 6 were more encouraging at an average of 0.68 DMFT per student. Again, however, when we focused only on those students with disease, that number more than tripled to 2.25 DMFT. Other important information provided by the survey was the percentage of untreated dental caries: 25% of grade 2 students and 14% of grade 6 students needed treatment on their permanent teeth. Of greater concern was that 4% of grade 2 students and 2% of grade 6 students were in urgent need of treatment. Overall, 15% of grade 2 students and 5% of grade 6 students were considered to be at high risk for dental disease. On the positive side, over 40% of grade 2 students had never had any decay in either their primary or permanent teeth, and 70% of grade 6 students had not experienced decay in their permanent dentition (Patterson, 2004).

Determining the Target Schools

Further analysis involved examining each of the risk indicators and determining how many and to what degree they existed for each school. The schools were then ranked from worst to best according to their oral health status. From the original pool of 179 schools, 47 of the highest risk schools (representing about 26% of the total school population) were identified as potential participants in the Target School Oral Health Program.

Planning the Program

In the tabulation and statistical analysis of the dental survey, the data from the small schools that had the potential to greatly skew the statistical outcome had been omitted. By excluding these schools from the data aggregation, they were effectively eliminated from the potential target school list, creating cognitive dissonance for many dental team members, as it meant that they would no longer be working with and offering services to schools that their intuition told them were in the high risk category. How can this issue be reconciled? We recognized further that another limitation of the targeting process is the resultant lack of school-based oral health interventions for high risk students attending low risk schools. How can these students receive needed services given the resource limitations?

An unexpected outcome of the oral health survey came about as a direct result of efforts made to use best practices in survey methodology, wherein the premise is that all surveyors are calibrated to the same standard of data collection. For the DTHR school oral health survey, data collection standards were set by the regional Dental Officer of Health (DOH) and a colleague at the University of Alberta. Our DOH then calibrated the DTHR dental team surveyors to these set standards. Subsequently, as dental programs from other regions have undertaken oral health surveys, they used the same set of standards, resulting in valid comparative oral health data for Alberta.

Implementing an Oral Health Promotion Intervention

Guided by the epidemiological data, dental public health personnel began a school-based program that was responsive to individual schools' identified oral health risk indicators and the school-community context. Interventions selected to be the foundation of target school services are the "gold standard" for the prevention of dental caries, particularly in high risk populations: screening and referral (Wright, Satur, & Morgan, 2000), fluoride varnish application (Patterson, 2002a), and applying pit and fissure sealants (Patterson, 2002b). The empirical evidence for these interventions is conclusive, especially when applied in high risk populations (Simonsen, 2002).

In addition to clinical services, dental public health professionals respond to requests from school staff for oral health presentations with the understanding that knowledge and awareness are first steps toward behaviour change. Building capacity around oral health and creating a positive oral health environment within the school

TABLE 21-2	
Activities for Promoting Oral Health in Schools	
ORAL HEALTH STRATEGIES	**EXAMPLES OF ACTIVITIES TO SUPPORT ORAL HEALTH IN SCHOOLS**
Healthy school environment	• Safe playgrounds to prevent oral injuries • No smoking on school premises • Smoking cessation services and counselling • Restricted sale of unhealthy foods and substances
Healthy eating	• Healthy foods made available in the school canteen, tuck shop, and kiosks • Nutritious meals served in the school cafeteria • Education for cooks and food providers regarding dentally acceptable foods • Restriction of sugary foods and drinks on the school premises
Oral health education	• Oral health education as part of all subjects in the school curriculum • Parent education regarding good oral health and encouragement to take part in health promotion activities at school • School staff education on oral health issues
Oral health services	• Working closely with local oral health service providers • Encouraging teacher role in identification of oral health issues • Applying dental sealants • Providing oral health screenings and fluoride varnish services
Oral injury	• Education on accident prevention • Protocol of actions for oral injury • Information and protocol on the use of mouth guards in sports
Policy development	• Encouragement for and participation in development of policies and action plans for oral health • Involvement of students, school staff, families, and community members in policy development
Other	• Commitment to an integrated school community for optimal oral health

Adapted from Kwan, S. Y. L., Petersen, P. E., Pine, C. M., & Borutta, A. (2005). Health promoting schools: An opportunity for oral health promotion. *Bulletin of the World Health Organization, 83*(9), 677–685.

comprise the desired next steps in the journey to improved oral health in the DTHR. Some of the potential activities within schools that would help to achieve this long-term goal are highlighted in Table 21-2.

Discovering how a program can weave into the fabric of a school and become an integral part of the school community is key to its acceptance and ultimately to its success in building school capacity. Experience taught the personnel in the DTHR Dental Program several lessons about working in and with the school community (Table 21-3).

Evaluating the Intervention

Program success is established by evaluation; the DTHR Target School Oral Health Program will be evaluated based on changes in oral health status of

TABLE 21-3

Lessons Learned From the Dental Health Promotion Program

Search out a champion within the school community.	Allies who are familiar with the school culture can facilitate the process. The most important ally is the principal.
Be flexible.	Ensure that your own agenda does not interfere with your ability to affect positive change with regard to oral health.
Be patient.	Both capacity building and the process to bring about measurable change take time. Take the time to get to know your schools, and encourage the school community stakeholders in the process. Elicit school buy-in and engagement.
Determine priorities identified by the school; look for integration points for your program.	Provide data on status of children's health. Determine priorities for oral health integration with school input.
Acknowledge small successes. Celebrate baby steps.	Realize that not all components of a recommended program will be adopted by all schools.
Understand that it is difficult to build capacity when you cannot provide ongoing funding, support, and resources within the school.	Sustainability is the key to success; without continued support, it is difficult to achieve. Recognize that it is more difficult to obtain school and staff commitment, as they are required to add additional subjects to an already burgeoning agenda.
Take the opportunity to critically reflect on what activities are working and where change is needed.	Monitor health indices, and adjust programs to provide appropriately targeted services.

students in these schools after the next survey. While it is acknowledged that changes in oral health status during the 5-year cycle cannot be directly attributed solely to school interventions, it is important to bear in mind that process is also an important part of evaluation. The dental team screens students' oral health on an annual basis, and these data are used to monitor change. Program activities are constantly adjusted as a result of school input and the oral health data. Lessons learned are also documented and shared with other dental team members in order to extrapolate an approach that is successful in one school and apply it to others.

Evaluating how school oral health activities impact change within the culture of the school is important. To do this, it is necessary to describe changes that occur, document the precipitating factors, detail how changes were implemented (e.g., parent, student, and staff involvement), and the outcome of such interventions. Examples of change might include integration of dental health into the school curriculum, adoption of a mouth guard policy for school sports, or the removal of school vending machines.

The journey to improving the health status of a population can be slow and challenging yet, when successful, extremely rewarding. The school years are the most influential stage of children's lives; health messages that are reinforced throughout these years will help students to develop the lifelong beliefs, attitudes, and skills needed for good oral health.

PROMOTING SCHOOL HEALTH THROUGH A PARTNERSHIP MODEL

An alternative high school in a rural Alberta town provided clinical placements over an academic year for two groups of community health students from the University of Calgary, Faculty of Nursing. This alternative high school was different from most of the student nurses' high school experiences; the school's population comprised adolescents who were not able, for a variety of reasons, to complete their education in a mainstream school. Curriculum was delivered using a personalized, student-directed approach. At first glance, the school appeared to be unstructured, with students talking amongst themselves and teachers helping individual students as needed. Expecting to see a traditional classroom setting with a teacher lecturing from the front, it took time for some students to discover that there was structure beneath what appeared to be chaos.

In addition to its primary focus on education, this alternative high school also assisted students in obtaining food, clothing, shelter, and medicine. Fifteen percent of the school's student population lived in foster families, group homes, or elsewhere under the care of the Public Guardian. Many were lone parents; the school offered a program for parenting students who were able to bring their children to school with them. More than half of the students had jobs to support themselves while they struggled to obtain a high school diploma. Traumatic life situations were common, and many students had experienced or were considered to be at risk for a variety of health and social problems, including violence, crime, drug and alcohol use, mental health issues, poverty, early pregnancy, sexually transmitted infections (STI), tobacco use, and poor nutrition.

Many alternative school students are well aware that they have been labelled "at risk," and many feel stigmatized by this label. Adolescents are often stereotyped by the media as impulsive, unreliable, immature, incapable, hormonally driven, untrustworthy, criminals, or drug abusers (Brendtro, Brokenleg, & Van Bockern, 1998; Lesko, 2001), and students attending alternative schools may be even more likely to be portrayed negatively. Feelings of low self-worth and ability were evident among many of the students at this school. Staff who were dedicated to helping these adolescents provided a sense of family. Offering a safe, relationship-based environment for learning was therefore a mainstay of the school; the school mission was to help students find strength, acceptance, and hope and to connect them with the community.

Compared with students attending regular high schools, students attending alternative high schools have been described in the research literature as "high risk," experiencing a substantially higher prevalence of violence and other behavioural issues, truancy, learning disabilities, homelessness, family problems, substance use, and risky sexual behaviours (Grunbaum et al., 2000; Knutson, 1999; NW Regional Educational Laboratory, 1997). Alternative school adolescents report approximately twice the rate of attempted suicide compared with regular school adolescents (Grunbaum et al., 2000; Kann et al., 2000). Adolescents attending alternative high schools are often considered to be at higher risk for engaging in behaviours that lead to early mortality (i.e., injury, suicide) or morbidity (i.e., sexually transmitted infections, mental illness), resulting in a decreased ability to be fully contributing members of society.

In contrast, it is difficult to locate explorations in the literature from the perspective of the majority of "high risk" adolescents (approximately 80%) who do not contemplate suicide, even though they too may experience difficult life situations. What personal strengths or situational contexts might enhance resiliency? Research has shown that adolescents who are active participants in society become adults with fewer health issues (Health Canada, 2001). It is important for health professionals to look beyond the labels attached to students and move past interventions that focus on telling students what to do. Education about risk behaviours does not by itself reduce risk behaviours for adolescents; we know that knowledge is insufficient for behaviour change. Partnerships, relationship-building, the development of trust, environmental actions, and addressing multiple interventions at multiple times and with multiple targets are ways to act within a community-as-partner model to fulfil the goals of population health promotion and promote the health of communities and aggregates. Strengthened public participation is health promoting. How did students work with this population? This section is an example of the community-as-partner approach in action.

Assessment and Analysis

What might be considered a natural starting point when entering a new setting, the first group of nursing students (fall term) focused mainly on gathering health assessment data about the school and the adolescents from both internal and external sources, while the next group of students (winter term) directed their energies to validating and furthering the assessment, analysis, and diagnosis process within the school environment. External sources of information included the local police, public health nursing staff, local family services, town hall staff, school board personnel, pamphlet information from local community agencies, and Internet sources such as Statistics Canada.

The assessment process began with a review of the literature on alternative high schools and then a windshield survey in order to understand the context and environment of the school and the community. For one group of nursing students, this included entering a local diner to ask staff about the school and how it fit within the community. A variety of reactions was received—some of which were very supportive of the school and its good work with and for students, and other reactions were consistent with the stigmatization of adolescents that has been reported in the literature and are commonly portrayed by the media.

Nursing students spent time in the school, talking with students, helping them with their homework, answering questions about their presence, and generally "hanging out." They discovered that it took time to develop a relationship and trust for some of the students to talk to them. One group found that participating in an art class by making pottery alongside the students was a fun activity that helped to break down some of the communication barriers that arose when the student nurses appeared to be on site for their own purposes, which was perceived by the high school students as an attempt to "find out what is wrong with them." Many of the high school students had been "assessed" by the child welfare system, for psychological purposes or for educational testing, and it is understandable that the students held negative perceptions of the process, expecting that they would be found somehow inadequate.

In the fall term, student nurses conducted a written survey to determine the health needs and interests of staff and students. A survey was a nonintrusive means of collecting information that helped to refine the assessment process and narrow down areas for further exploration by key informant interview and focus group methods. Participant-observation strategies were also used to collect impressions, with field notes capturing the data. Student nurses found that including a variety of methods of data collection afforded a holistic, in-depth assessment of the context and the people. However, assessment was a time-consuming process, resulting in a large amount of data to sift through and analyze. Many issues that required further exploration were identified, including risky health behaviours (e.g., drug and alcohol use, smoking, unsafe sexual practices), poor dietary habits, poor sleeping patterns, and low levels of physical activity. Also identified were issues of racism and high levels of stress experienced by school staff. On the positive side, high school students expressed willingness to accept and/or seek out external supports. It was evident to the nursing students that the issues uncovered were very complex; many factors influenced student behaviour choices, including poverty, history of violence/abuse, lack of support, transient lifestyle, lack of acceptance by the larger society, and paucity of positive role models.

In the winter term, the second group of nursing students concurred with the assessment and themes identified by their colleagues. They suggested some options for potential intervention: hygiene, nutrition, and sense of community. The school community's strengths were resiliency; recreation; art; creativity; and peer, staff, and community support. Both groups of nursing students focused not on the deficits or concerns that their assessment and analysis had uncovered but on the numerous strengths that they found in the school environment and within the students themselves. With this insight, the process of partnering for diagnosis and planning activities became an important health promoting strategy. By focusing on process, student nurses believed that change might occur in the environment and in behaviour. This approach to working with communities would build individual and community capacity, promote health, and build relationships consistent with the Ottawa Charter definition of *health promotion*—"the process of enabling people to increase control over, and to improve, their health" (WHO, 1986)—and with the Canadian Community Health Nursing Standards of Practice (Community Health Nurses Association of Canada, 2003).

Diagnosis

Wellness diagnoses are congruent with the asset building, strengths based approach taken by nursing students in this practicum. Wellness diagnoses support the participatory capacity of communities by inviting members into a strengths enhancing process that is empowering. Empowering strategies increase people's participation in health activities (Wallerstein, 1992); citizens gaining control through empowering processes is a strategy for promoting health (Wallerstein & Bernstein, 1988). Strategies used to empower staff and students result in personal efficacy and competence and a sense of mastery and control, and the process of participation and action influences institutions and policy decisions (Falk-Rafael, 2001; Israel et al., 1994; Labonté, 1994) (Table 21-4).

Three wellness diagnoses were verified and prioritized through a rank-ordering process with staff and students of the school (see Table 21-4). The focus of attention was chosen to be on the diagnosis proposed by the high school students: "The school community has the potential to enhance the nutritional status of its students *related to* the school's current food bank donations, breakfast program and home economic studies *as manifested by* data from participant observation, focus group and key informant interviews." This community health diagnosis was viewed as an area with excellent potential for growth, as resources and community connections were already in place. The nursing students noted that enhanced nutritional health has been linked in the literature to improved stress management and better academic performance. Undernutrition in children results in reduced immune status, poorer cognitive functioning, and poorer educational outcomes (Nelson, 2000). Further, students could create an intervention project that would be tailored to student interest and could engage them in partnering to promote their own health.

The school had strong connections to a number of community agencies that provided donations of food, baby care items, clothing, and other necessities on a regular basis (e.g., local grocers, food banks, and the community at large). Concerns

TABLE 21-4	
Community Health Diagnoses	
RANK	**WELLNESS DIAGNOSIS**
#1	The school community has the potential to enhance the nutritional status of its students *related to* the school's current food bank donations, breakfast program, and home economic studies *as manifested by* data from participant observations, focus group, and key informant interviews.
#2	The school community has the potential to enhance the coping mechanisms of its students *related to* the availability of community resources, including peer support, community connections, and academic flexibility *as manifested by* data from participant observations, focus groups, windshield surveys, and key informant interviews.
#3	The school community has the potential to enhance its community relations *related to* recreational opportunities, volunteer work placements, and corporate sponsors *as manifested by* data from key informant interviews, focus groups, and participant observations.

arose from participant observation that foods donated regularly included pies, cakes, and other items of low nutritional quality (i.e., high salt, fat, and/or sugar content). Perhaps some donors did not have other foods to donate. It was also possible that each organization providing food was unaware there were others donating such "treats" that, when combined, were the predominant source of food choice and thus formed a substantial contribution to the students' diets. Food donors were "killing them with kindness," since students' main caloric consumption during the week often occurred at school.

Planning

Strategies were developed to improve student nutrition by capitalizing on existing strengths in partnership with school staff and students. Three main areas of focus were community connections, nutrition education, and a home economics course. Student nurses suggested meetings between the school and community food donors to discuss the nutritional needs of the students. Guest speakers were suggested for health education, accompanied by a food fair to provide students with access to a variety of healthy, simple, tasty, low-cost, and multicultural foods that could be prepared at home. Student nurses recommended that high school students bring recipes from their own cultural backgrounds to the home economics class for teaching, cooking, and sharing. Many meals prepared in the home economics course were offered to the school population at lunch, further extending an impact to the whole school. For their part, nursing students incorporated the Canada Food Guide into discussions with students and staff, making the Guide a living document. They felt that it was important to include staff in these discussions, as teachers are role models as well as educators and sources of information for adolescents. The food fair idea was discussed at length with the principal who, in turn, led efforts to implement a food fair after the school's involvement with the student nurses ended.

An Unexpected Outcome

Through the development of relationships and the creation of a partnership with a rural alternative high school using the community-as-partner model, an unexpected positive outcome was achieved. As part of a final class presentation, the nursing students from the winter term created a short video about the school, weaving music and captions into a variety of photos that they had taken of the school, which captured the essence of the school's mission in a very powerful manner. For example, their pictures of the art room included the captions such as "using paint brushes to promote healing" and "what sculpture is to a block of marble, education is to the soul." Pictures of the bowling alley included "breaking down barriers." The school principal attended the farewell presentation and was teary-eyed by the end. The nursing students had left behind a legacy of their work—a valuable tool for the school to use to introduce itself to others, thus supporting its continuing emphasis to form community connections to benefit its students.

Lessons Learned

Partnering with members of a school community to conduct an assessment or plan an intervention is time-consuming and difficult to complete within the dual constraints of an academic school year (with competing priorities for adolescents' attention), in addition to the constraints of a 13-week clinical nursing course.

A sense of participatory competence was fostered in adolescents (Gibson, 1991) in order to engage them in a health-promoting process. One way that this sense of competency was fostered was by engaging high school students in the needs assessment and planning processes. However, this takes time. Trust is built through trustful interactions—engaging in activities together. Adolescent participatory roles led to increasing the likelihood of intervention programs being perceived as empowering, holistic, relevant, and sustainable by the students.

Student nurses recognized the importance of working interdependently with the community to gain a sense of having accomplished something of mutual value. Thanking the community was also important for closure. One group of nursing students thanked the school community by hosting a healthy school lunch for staff and students on their last day. For the second group of students, the semester ended with an afternoon of socializing and a bowling outing with the students.

Nursing students felt that their semester at the alternative high school provided them with an excellent opportunity to experience the connection between theory and practice by applying the community-as-partner process. They applied the theoretical principles that they had learned in class directly, witnessing firsthand how they functioned within a real community setting. In addition, the opportunity allowed them to determine which strategies were effective or ineffective, and they learned how to quickly adapt to changing circumstances. For example, what do you do when your plans to interview a teacher fall apart because she suddenly has to deal with a student crisis and is no longer available? What do you do when you have a plan set in place to conduct a focus group with students and then discover on your arrival that they have all gone on a field trip that day? What do you do when you are ready to interview a staff person with preselected questions and she suddenly asks you if the four or five students in the room can be a part of it? The student nurses discovered that crucial components of community health work include flexible planning—always having a back-up plan in mind, openness to changing plans at the last minute, and an eye for seeing opportunities as they arise. Working with community partners is also a challenge, as it means that the plans you have made ahead of time may not be the direction in which a project goes—sharing control in a partnership also means relinquishing control at times.

In conclusion, participatory learning has benefits for the learners and the recipients of the community process. The community-as-partner model, the theory learned from population health promotion researchers, and the practical elements of community work contribute to effective preparation for students in a nursing program. Similar experiences and results can be achieved by learners in other disciplines. Ideally, a mixed (interprofessional or interdisciplinary) learning group will better model desirable community practice for the future.

SUMMARY

In this chapter, there are two levels at issue: rural health and youth. Canada has developed a rural health strategy to address the health needs and concerns of rural and remote populations. Many of these concerns relate to access and availability of services—hence, a population risk-based analysis is helpful in targeting subpopulations most at need, as, for instance, Johnson and McElroy discussed with regard to the oral health of schoolchildren in targeted schools in a rural health region. But school health services are not only delivered at a setting level (i.e., schools) but also at the school-community intersection to benefit vulnerable groups within the school population. As Lind points out, the school exists as a community within a neighbourhood or town, and interventions can incorporate a wider array of people and activities that address an identified need and encourage people to help people in a reciprocal manner.

ACKNOWLEDGMENTS

Gratitude and acknowledgement of their important contribution is extended to the following student nurses: Ashley Blakeman, Jacquelyn Comeau, Kelsie Guagliano, Nancy Guillen, Jessica Hardwicke, Dianna Hong, Navpreet Kang, Carolyn Kathol, Jana Kurilova, Ashley MacKenzie, Michelle Madamesila, Kaitlin McHenry, Karen McIsaac, Hendrik Schipper, Tyler Smith, Minghui Katherine Wang, and Leona Wright.

References

Beaglehole, R., & Bonita, R. (1998). Public health at the crossroads: Which way forward? *Lancet, 351*(9102), 590–592.

Brendtro, L. K., Brokenleg, M., & Van Bockern, S. (1998). *Reclaiming youth at risk: Our hope for the future*. Bloomington, IN: National Educational Service.

Community Health Nurses Association of Canada. (2003). Canadian community health nursing standards of practice. Retrieved July 20, 2007, from **www.chnac.ca**.

Falk-Rafael, A. R. (2001). Empowerment as a process of evolving consciousness: A model of empowered caring. *Advances in Nursing Science, 24*(1), 1–16.

Gibson, C. H. (1991). A concept analysis of empowerment. *Journal of Advanced Nursing, 16*, 354–361.

Grunbaum, J. A., Kann, L., Kinchen, S. A., Ross, J. G., Gowda, V. R., Collins, J. L., et al. (2000). Youth risk behaviour surveillance national alternative high school youth risk behaviour survey, United States, 1998. *Journal of School Health, 70*, 5–17.

Health Canada. (2001). Canada's Rural Health Strategy: A one-year review (Cat. H39-579/2001). Ottawa: Author.

Israel, B. A., Checkoway, B., Schultz, A., & Zimmerman, M. (1994). Health education and community empowerment: Conceptualizing and measuring perceptions of individual, organizational, and community control. *Health Education Quarterly, 21,* 149–170.

Kann, L., Kinchen, S. A., Williams, B. I., Ross, J. G., Lowry, R., Grunbaum, J. A., et al. (2000). Youth risk behavior surveillance—United States, 1999. *Journal of School Health, 70,* 271–285.

Knutson, G. G. (1999). Alternative high schools: Models for the future? Retrieved November 25, 2002, from **http://horizon.unc.edu/projects/HSJ/Knutson.asp**.

Labonté, R. (1994). Health promotion and empowerment: Reflections on professional practice. *Health Education Quarterly, 21,* 253–268.

Lesko, N. (2001). *Act your age! A cultural construction of adolescence.* New York: Routledge Falmer.

Locker, D., & Matear, D. (2001). Oral disorders, systemic health, well-being and the quality of life: A summary of recent research evidence. Health Measurement and Epidemiology, No. 17; Community Health Services Research Unit, Faculty of Dentistry, University of Toronto: Toronto, ON. Available at: **http://www.utoronto.ca/dentistry/faculty/research/dri/CDHSRY-reports.html**.

Nelson, M. (2000). Childhood nutrition and poverty. *Proceedings of the Nutrition Society, 59,* 307–315.

NW Regional Educational Laboratory. (1997). Alternative schools: Approaches for students at risk. Retrieved November 25, 2002, from **http://www.nwrel.org/request/sept97/article2.html**.

Patterson, S. (2002a). *Fluoride varnish: Effectiveness, patient assessment, protocols for appropriate use.* Dental Public Health Centre: University of Alberta.

Patterson, S. (2002b). *Pit and fissure sealants: Effectiveness, decision making, protocols for appropriate use.* Dental Public Health Centre: University of Alberta.

Patterson, S. K. (2004). *Children's Oral Health Survey 2003-2005.* Red Deer, AB: David Thompson Health Region Dental Program.

Petersen, P. E., Bourgeois, D., Ogawa, H., Estupinan-Day, S., & Ndiaye, C. (2005). Policy and practice: The global burden of oral diseases and risks to oral health. *Bulletin of the World Health Organization, 83*(9), 661–669. Available at **http://www.who.int/bulletin/volumes/83/9/661.pdf**.

Rose, G. (Ed.). (1992). *The strategy of preventive medicine.* Oxford: Oxford University Press.

Sheiham, A. (2005). Editorial: Oral health, general health and quality of life. *Bulletin of the World Health Organization, 83*(9), 644–645. Available at **http://www.who.int/bulletin/volumes/83/9/644.pdf**.

Simonsen, R. J. (2002). Pit and fissure sealant: Review of the literature. *Pediatric Dentistry, 24*(5), 393–414.

Tickle, M., Milsom, K. M., Jenner, T. M., & Blinkhorn, A. S. (2003). The geodemographic distribution of caries experience in neighboring fluoridated and nonfluoridated populations [Abstract]. *Journal of Public Health Dentistry, 63*(2), 92–98.

Wallerstein, N. (1992). Powerlessness, empowerment, and health: Implications for health promotion programs. *American Journal of Health Promotion, 6,* 197–205.

Wallerstein, N., & Bernstein, E. (1988). Empowerment education: Freire's ideas adapted to health education. *Health Education Quarterly, 15,* 379–394.

Watt, R. G. (2005). Public Health Reviews: Strategies and approaches in oral disease prevention and health promotion. *Bulletin of the World Health Organization, 83*(9), 711–718. Available at **http://www.who.int/bulletin/volumes/83/9/711.pdf**.

World Health Organization (WHO). (1986). *Ottawa charter for health promotion.* Geneva: Author.

World Health Organization (WHO) European Office. (2006). Largely preventable chronic diseases cause 86% of deaths in Europe: 53 European Member States map a strategy to curb the epidemic. Press release EURO/05/06: September 11, 2006. Copenhagen, DK.

Wright, F. A. C., Satur, J., & Morgan, M. V. (2000). Evidence-based health promotion resources for planning: No.1—Oral health. Health Development Section, Public Health Division Department of Human Services. Victoria, Australia: Dental Health Services. Available at **http://www.health.vic.gov.au/healthpromotion/quality/oral_health.htm**.

Internet Resources

http://www.hc-sc.gc.ca/ahc-asc/alt_formats/cmcd-dcmc/pdf/media/releases-communiques/ 2001/2001_76ebk1.pdf
Canada's Rural Health Strategy

www.phac-aspc.gc.ca/rh-sr/index.html
Office of Rural Health

www.who.int/oral_health/action/information/surveillance/en/print.html
WHO Oral Health Reports

http://www.engagementcentre.ca
Centre of Excellence for Youth Engagement

22

Youth Engagement in Health Promotion

MICHELLE SULLIVAN

NANCY SULLIVAN

DONNA HARDY-COX

ANNETTE JOHNS

SHARON M. YANICKI

KAROLINE PHILIPP

Chapter Outline

Introduction
Way Out There: Youth Engagement in Social Policy Action Planning
Community Partnerships for Postsecondary Tobacco Reduction
Summary

Learning Objectives

After studying this chapter, you should be able to:

❖ Discuss social exclusion as a health issue

❖ Discuss the health effects of tobacco

❖ Describe the use of the community-as-partner process to plan a community-based project

❖ Describe community health worker roles in supporting community mobilization, coalition development, and project evaluation

❖ Describe the assessment of multiple policy contexts

❖ Describe the process of selecting multiple interventions in a community-based project

❖ Appreciate how multilevel community partnerships strengthen project effects

Introduction

*Y*outh engagement is central to social inclusion and social policy development. Research reviewed by the Centre of Excellence for Youth Engagement (2003) demonstrates a link between youth engagement and greater well-being and positive health outcomes. Social inclusion, including connection to one's peer group, family, and community, is linked to healthy child development and greater life opportunities (Canadian Council on Social Development, 2006a; Hanvey, 2003; Hertzman, 2002). Therefore, youth engagement in social policy is important to community development and strategic planning. Operating from a strengths perspective and community capacity building framework recognizes the developmental assets that young people bring to their communities, including their life experiences and a keen sense of understanding or wisdom of the issues that impact on their lives. Importantly, youth engagement in social policy is an opportunity for young people to have their voices heard in relation to the issues that are important and relevant to them. This opportunity is particularly important for those who experience social exclusion. Involving youth in social policy can provide the mechanism for young people to build relationships, gain a sense of active citizenship, and make a contribution in their communities in the short- and potentially long-term.

In this chapter, two stories of youth engagement are described with respect to the development of healthy public policy. In the first story, *Way Out There: Youth Engagement in Social Policy Action Planning*, Sullivan, Sullivan, Hardy Cox, and Johns detail a process that engaged socially excluded youth in Newfoundland and Labrador (NL) in a project designed to enhance their participation in NL in social policy development through education and skill development. The process that they describe is one of participatory democracy and action research. In the second story, *Community Partnerships for Postsecondary Tobacco Reduction*, this time from the province of Alberta, Yanicki and Philipp describe the development of a coalition to promote tobacco reduction that used multiple interventions and multilevel partnerships to create awareness of an important public health issue and develop support for policy change. In both examples, the processes used demonstrate how participatory action-oriented interventions can affect social policy.

WAY OUT THERE: YOUTH ENGAGEMENT IN SOCIAL POLICY ACTION PLANNING

This section of the chapter will describe a project in which young people throughout the province of NL were invited to develop, implement, and participate in a workshop focused on social policy action planning and skill development. The project was funded by Health Canada, Atlantic Region, Population Health Fund, and conducted by Memorial University's School of Social Work in collaboration with the provincial Community Youth Network (CYN).

Background and Context

This project was designed to enhance the participation of socially excluded youth in NL in social policy development through education and skill development. It was set within the context of a broader Community-University Research Alliance (Community Services Council, 2002) and was based on the premise that the depth and breadth of the social capital among the youth population in rural and remote communities involved in the project could be improved by an increased appreciation of the implications of social policy at the local, regional, provincial, and national levels.

The project's target group was youth (ages 12 to 18 years) who were engaged in the CYN hub sites in St. John's, Harbour Grace, Harbour Breton, and Happy Valley–Goose Bay. The CYN, funded by the National Child Benefit Reinvestment Plan, is an organization of youth centres throughout the province whose mandate is to provide outreach and support for youth at risk. The organization's four primary business lines include employment, learning, support services, and community building (CYN, 1998).

The majority of youth involved in this project faced multiple barriers to their general well-being and future life chances. These included limited education, literacy difficulties, drug and alcohol use, poverty, learning disabilities, and absence of positive role models and supports. These barriers relate to the social determinants of health as outlined by Public Health Agency of Canada (2002) (Table 22-1).

Description of the Project: Planning and Methodology

The project as a whole and the development and delivery of the workshop in particular were based on principles of empowerment and participatory democracy. Prior to developing the project proposal, initial contact was made with several CYN coordinators to discuss the potential project and to develop collaborative partnerships (pre-engagement activities). CYN hub sites at St. John's, Harbour Grace, Harbour Breton, and Happy Valley–Goose Bay collectively represented urban, rural, and remote areas of the province (Fig. 22-1) and also incorporated the voices and experiences of Aboriginal youth.

The CYN hubs in each of these regions embraced the project, and the local coordinators took leadership roles in recruiting youth participants in St. John's for establishing a reference group and at the other sites for attending the policy workshop. An additional project site was chosen in the St. John's region as part of a collaborative partnership with the Brother T.I. Murphy Learning Resource Centre, an alternative school for youth.

TABLE 22-1

Determinants of Health Impacting on Newfoundland and Labrador Youth

DETERMINANT OF HEALTH	SUMMARY STATEMENT	INFERENCE
Income and social status	According to Campaign 2000 (2005), Newfoundland and Labrador (NL) continues to have one of the highest rates of youth poverty in the country (21.8%).	Poverty is an issue facing communities in rural NL with many areas falling below the low-income cut-off levels (Government of NL, 2005a).
Social support networks	NL continues to face issues such as youth outmigration, a declining birth rate, and changing demographics (declining population) in rural areas of the province (Government of NL, 2005b).	These changes continue to have an impact on traditional patterns of extended family and community support.
Education	Research completed by the Canadian Council on Social Development (2006b) on school enrolment in elementary and secondary schools throughout Canada reported that NL had the largest decrease in full-time school enrolment (6.6%).	Educational opportunities for youth in NL are compromised by a marked decrease of the school-age population and declining birth rate. This reduction will have an impact on educational programming and resources, particularly in the more rural and remote parts of the province.
Employment	In June 2006, the youth unemployment rate was 23.5%, compared with 21.4% in 2005 (Statistics Canada, 2006).	The unemployment rate for youth in NL remains very high in comparison to historical trends and in relation to rates for other parts of Canada.
Social environments	In NL, the level of social cohesion and patterns of citizen inclusion traditionally have been perceived as very positive. According to the Canadian Council on Social Development (2006a), there has been an increase in youth participation in volunteering.	A focus on increasing the social capital of communities is consistent with the current literature, which links social capital to general economic performance, reduced levels of crime and general civil unrest, immigrant employment, and health trends (Schuller, 2001). This demonstrates the importance of youth engagement in civic activities.

PHASE I: PARTICIPATORY DEVELOPMENT OF SOCIAL POLICY TRAINING AND ACTION PLAN WORKSHOPS

The first task was to hire a project coordinator based in St. John's, whose work initially was to develop a youth reference group for the project. Staff at the St. John's CYN worked collaboratively with the project team to form this group, which was drawn from 15 young people who participated in a 10-day peer mentoring outreach

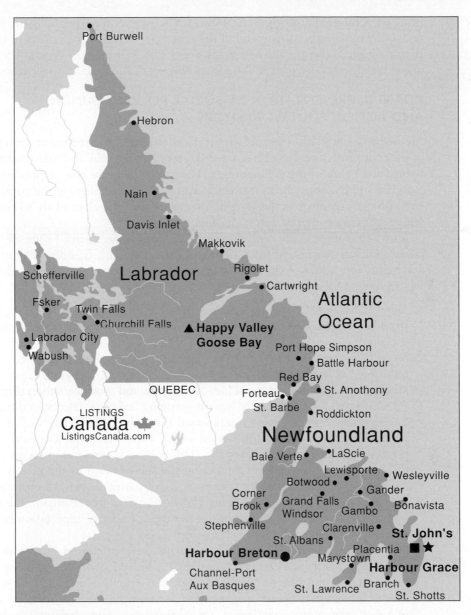

Key: Symbols represent project sites.

■ = Harbour Grace
★ = St. John's
● = Harbour Breton
▲ = Happy Valley–Goose Bay

FIGURE 22-1   ◆   Map of Newfoundland and Labrador.

program conducted through the St. John's CYN over a 5-week period in the summer of 2002. These youth were typical of the provincewide CYN population in terms of their multiple challenges and barriers to health and well-being. The youth reference group consisted of five girls and two boys ranging in age from 15 to 19 years.

PHASE II: PRESENTATION OF SOCIAL POLICY TRAINING AND ACTION PLAN WORKSHOPS

Members of the youth reference group travelled as part of the project team to each of the four project sites to deliver the 2-day workshops, held on Friday evening and Saturday, in each of the communities. They took an active role in presenting the material and engaging the participants. Although the members of the youth reference group were seen as the leaders, they were able to relate easily to the other youth participants involved in each of the project sites.

The workshop was the central means for youth engagement. From site to site, it was generally consistent in content and format—youth friendly, activity based, and highly interactive. Following is a brief outline of the various activities that were incorporated in the workshop design.

1. *Social Policy Definition*. Youth participants were asked for their ideas and definitions of social policy to provide a baseline for participants' understanding of social policy.
2. *Social Policy Spheres*. The youth reference group created and presented a model outlining five levels of society where social policies exist, including the self, living arrangements, school and social life, community, and province/nation (Fig. 22-2).
3. *Person-Mapping Activities*. Five person-mapping activities, corresponding to the Social Policy Spheres, were interspersed throughout the 2-day workshop and provided a tiered framework within which youth participants could identify polices that impact them personally. This was an incremental process moving through the five levels, from a focus on the self outward to the provincial and national levels. Operationally, groups of youth participants were provided with life-sized outlines of a human figure and were invited to personalize the outline by contributing written indications of the type of activity/expectation or policy that they experienced in each sphere (Fig. 22-3).
4. *Survivor Island Activities*. Youth participants were organized into "tribes" for seven "Survivor Island" activities, designed as if suddenly they had found themselves on an island with no pre-existing societal structures or policies. The activities facilitated participants' engagement in navigating toward the development of a new community, identifying community needs, and working in collaboration to develop useful social policy. For example, an "Island Tribe" would receive a message indicating that a member of its community had developed a severe physical disability and there was now a need to re-examine how the community operated in order to accommodate this new circumstance.
5. *Kitchen Kaper*. This activity was designed to illustrate the unique capacity of different tribes working together from a problem-solving framework. Each tribe

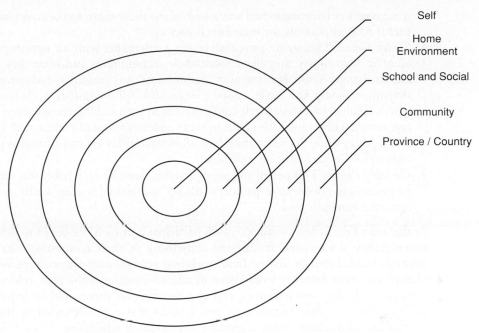

FIGURE 22-2 ◆ Five levels of society depicted by youth.

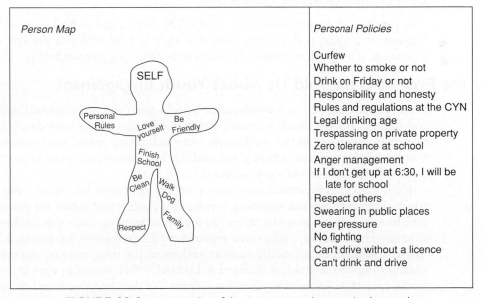

FIGURE 22-3 ◆ Results of the person-mapping exercise by youth.

was given five basic items and was asked to use these them to construct as many useful tools as possible for their Island society.

6. *Spider Game*. This game provided youth participants with an opportunity to identify what things they liked about their communities and what they would like to change. A visual portrayal of "community" was created as each youth participant, standing in a circle, tossed a large yarn ball to another while speaking, which resulted in a spider web configuration of yarn linking the whole group as one entity. This helped the youth in their understanding of community life and social policy while demonstrating how all communities are constituted as groups of interwoven participating individuals.

7. *Guessing Puzzle*. This pencil and paper activity, done by each tribe, was intended to encourage cooperative problem-solving and model a community working toward a common goal.

At the end of the 2-day workshop, youth participants at each site began to develop a social policy action plan, identifying something in their community that they believed needed change. As the final workshop activity, participants were asked to identify the steps that they would need to take to implement the plan, relevant key community leaders and resources, and specific activities that would be required to proceed with the plan. Examples of policy issues that were identified by the local groups included school policy regarding discretionary scheduling ("Fast Fridays"), the need for additional recreation and support programming in local communities, and the need for environmental initiatives focused on cleaning up the land and water.

PHASE III: DEVELOPMENT AND MONITORING OF SOCIAL POLICY ACTION PLAN

The youth, with support from their local CYN, were asked to further develop and implement a social policy action plan that they had identified at the end of the workshop. This work continued in the months following the workshop.

What the Project Data Told Us About Youth Engagement

Project data consisted of a combination of logs from the meetings of the project coordinator and the youth reference group, videotapes of the workshops, written materials generated in the workshops, team debriefing notes, workshop evaluations, workshop groups' action plans, and the logs generated by the project coordinator following each of the workshops.

Each workshop generated many opportunities for insight into factors that facilitate and interfere with engagement, serving as a context and means for young people's learning related to social policy. To maximize learning from this extraordinary volume of information, a structured approach to data reduction was essential. Qualitative data methods, primarily content analysis of the data, were conducted using standard stepwise techniques (Lofland & Lofland, 1995). Raw data were transcribed by the project coordinator to allow for reduction of data into significant themes, for comparison on a multidimensional basis. Themes became evident on analysing the data from each of the project sites. The conceptual framework for this project sought to identify factors that focused on what facilitated and what impeded youth engagement in the process of social policy development within and across CYN sites.

Highlights From Project Analysis

From the perspective of the project as a research study, analysis of the data demonstrated that youth who are socially excluded have a vital role to play in social policy development. Notable success indicators are:

◆ The youth were able to identify the issues that had an impact on their overall health and well-being.
◆ The youth were able to identify the various contexts (i.e., local, regional, provincial, and/or national) in which social policies are developed and implemented.
◆ The youth expanded their basic understanding of the nature and role of social policy in their lives through skill development and capacity building.
◆ The youth were able to apply a preliminary understanding of policy development around issues in their own communities.
◆ The youth were able to apply and hone their abilities to build social connections and networks through collaboration and teamwork.

Themes that focused on what worked in the engagement of youth in social policy development include:

◆ *Workshop design*. The workshop was designed by the youth reference group in a way that allowed the complex issue of social policy to be understood within the context of youth development and relevance.
◆ *Involvement of youth with pre-existing relationships with the CYN*. The project team was able to tap into existing community resources that helped to engage youth in the workshop.
◆ *Underlying principles*. The overall project was built on principles that were empowering and youth centred and fostered skill development by promoting capacity-building from a strengths perspective.
◆ *Practical supports*. Food, transportation, and personal encouragement were essential to engaging youth in the workshops.
◆ *Previous or current involvement with youth organizations or groups*. Youth who were involved with other youth organizations brought a greater understanding of social policy issues.

Themes that focused on what did not work (barriers) in the youth engagement process are:

◆ *Preplanning activities and pre-engagement activities*. Although the researchers had met with the CYN coordinators at the beginning of the project, the full team had not met with any of the sites prior to the workshops.
◆ *Distraction from the youth reference group*. There were some challenges with respect to youth reference group members who were disruptive during the

workshops, particularly during the first workshop when their own comfort level was low.

◆ *Limited exposure to social policy issues*. Many of the youth engaged in the workshops, including reference group members, had limited exposure to social policy and limited knowledge prior to being involved in the project.

◆ *Lack of clarity around changes in the roles of adult team members.*

Accomplishments and Reflections

The major objectives of the project were completed beyond expectations. As planned, the youth reference group successfully participated with project team members in:

◆ Crafting the design, content, and methodology of the interactive 2-day workshop intended to increase youths' information and skill base regarding social policy

◆ Reviewing and revising the workshop format following each site visit in preparation for the next one

◆ Participating in the delivery of the workshops at the selected sites

The seven youth reference group members from the St. John's CYN hub provided continuous engagement in the project (relationship development and/or on-task work) over a 15-month period, for a total of 120 days of meaningful youth engagement.

In addition to the youth members of the reference group, 36 youth (ages 12 to 18) participated in the workshops, designed to increase their understanding of social policy, the impact of policy on their lives, and the social capital that exists in their communities for addressing community issues and concerns. The workshops served as a significant vehicle for engaging and informing youth about social policy as it relates to the multiple spheres of society.

It had been anticipated that each of the workshop groups would continue with its implementation of a social policy action plan. However, this may have been unrealistic to expect as an immediate project outcome. From the outset, the project team was aware that time would be a significant variable as to the youths' ability to embrace this opportunity to engage with one another on a local policy issue and that in such a short time frame, it would be unlikely that major shifts in policy could occur. These considerations were monitored, and adjustment to the expectations related to action plans proved necessary. While full action plan development and implementation was beyond the scope of this project, the workshop served the function of making concrete some strategies that could enable youth to have a voice in influencing policies that affect them.

Although there were challenges throughout the project, most of these were addressed through a process of participatory democracy as they arose. The workshop was developed and refined. The youth participants experienced a sense of pride and ownership of the project. One of the reference group members stated at the conclusion of the project, in a tone of heartfelt sincerity, "I feel proud."

Evaluation

Evaluation of the project focussed on both process and outcome. It was important to view youth engagement as a dynamic rather than static process. This feature made the project rich and meaningful to the youth participants. There are a number of lessons or recommendations, however, that would be helpful to incorporate in future projects. For purposes of this chapter, we will highlight three of the key recommendations.

1. To enhance the effectiveness of youth engagement in the project, it may have been beneficial to increase the level of pre-engagement activities with the youth and the CYN project sites prior to the delivery of the workshops. This may have allowed the participants to take a greater leadership role in moving forward with the social policy action plans. More pre-engagement activities could have been undertaken with community partners to introduce the project and discuss how they might have become involved in the implementation of the action plans developed by the youth. It would have been important for the youth to take a leadership role, as able, in creating these networks and collaborative relationships with community stakeholders.

2. The short-term nature of project funding made it necessary to strike a balance between operating within the parameters of the funding organization and being sufficiently flexible with time to facilitate a deepening of youth engagement in the social policy work. Such a process requires a realistic understanding of the developmental needs of youth in terms of their understanding of social policy and how to build a sustainable momentum.

3. Once the workshop groups had proposed their social policy actions plans, it may have been useful for the project team to maintain a collaborative and supportive relationship with each site to facilitate ongoing leadership and participation and to encourage and assist site groups to seek opportunities to showcase their work and to involve adult policy-makers at various stages of development.

In summary, this project highlights the critical dynamic of youth engagement in community-based social policy work and provides a greater understanding of factors that may impede or facilitate its development. The social policy workshop is a tool that will be used in an additional follow-up research project. This project was built on the principles of genuineness, respect, social justice, appreciation of diversity, recognition of the developmental needs of youth, and a belief that engaging marginalized youth in social policy can have meaningful outcomes.

COMMUNITY PARTNERSHIPS FOR POSTSECONDARY TOBACCO REDUCTION

Students for Tobacco Reduction, a student-led coalition at the University of Lethbridge (UL), was formed in 2003 in response to the Students' Union accepting tobacco industry sponsorship for a concert.

On September 28, 2003, tobacco giant Benson & Hedges sponsored a David Usher concert in The Zoo (the campus restaurant and pub) at the University of Lethbridge. Benson & Hedges displayed their logo at the concert and circulated cigarette vendors on the concert floor. The UL Students' Union had signed a contract with Benson & Hedges on September 16, only twelve days before the concert . . . [and] exposed 500 students to the negative press of tobacco advertising. (Students for Tobacco Reduction, 2004, as cited in Yanicki, 2005)

This event can be considered the community 'stressor' that acted as an impetus for a group of students to take action.

In the fall of 2003, grant funding became available from the Alberta Alcohol and Drug Abuse Commission (AADAC) (2006) Young Adult Tobacco Reduction Strategy (YTRS), and AADAC held an information session at the UL campus on October 7, 2003. A small group of students attended the session to voice their concerns regarding recent tobacco industry tactics on campus and the lack of student awareness of the issue. The Chinook Health Tobacco Reduction Coordinator was in attendance at this information session and offered to assist the student group. The combination of student passion to take action on an issue of concern, available funding, health promotion expertise, and administrative support assisted this group of young adults in rapidly mobilizing to form a coalition and receiving funding to take action.

Take Note

- ◆ Community development ideally starts from issues identified by community members.
- ◆ Taking action on an issue that coincides with available funding opportunities can lead to a more rapid community mobilization process and implementation of interventions.
- ◆ Self-identified community leaders (local champions) bring knowledge of the local context critical to understanding the issue and selecting appropriate interventions.

Mobilization

A small group of first-year university students formed Students for Tobacco Reduction (STR), a coalition (a small action group) that quickly moved through group formation steps and mobilized for action. Two students emerged as natural group leaders and became the co-chairs of the coalition. The co-chairs had known each other for a number of years, were both political science students, and had a shared interest in policy issues; they quickly mobilized a group of acquaintances to take action on a policy concern, with a secondary interest in changing smoking behaviour. The co-chairs played a key role in setting direction for the project and in bringing suggestions to the coalition members for decisions. The coalition remained a small, fluid group of students and did not expand to include faculty or community members. Partnerships with external agencies and coalitions were developed to support specific project activities. The co-chairs changed in the second year of the project, creating a shift in some of the project's priorities. This project concluded after reaching several key policy changes during a two and a half year period.

Take Note

♦ Coalition-building usually begins with gathering a group of people who have shared interests and expands to include a large group of stakeholders.

♦ Most groups take considerable time to build trust, develop consensus on the issues, and determine options for action.

♦ A small action-oriented group can mobilize quickly on an issue of shared local concern.

♦ Sustainability of a small action-oriented group requires maintaining leaders to sustain the focus and energies of the group.

Assessment

TOBACCO USE IN YOUNG ADULTS

Baseline information on tobacco use at UL was available from an on-line student survey, based on a convenience sample of 419 respondents; 73% of respondents were 18 to 24 years of age (Meyer & Weber, 2003). Of the respondents, 10% reported being current smokers and 90% nonsmokers; this suggested lower smoking rates at UL than the provincial and national averages; however, this was a nonrepresentative sample. In another local survey conducted in 2003, the rate of reported tobacco use among 18 to 24 year olds in Lethbridge was 24% (Meyer, 2004). Tobacco use trends in Canada have been monitored in the Canadian Tobacco Use Monitoring Survey (CTUMS) since 1999. While tobacco use trends showed a general decline through the years, 30% of Canadian and 31% of Albertan young adults aged 20 to 24 years reported being current smokers in 2003, representing the highest rate of smoking by age group (Health Canada, 2006). Recent trends in young adult tobacco use and differences in smoking rates by level of education are described in Box 22-1.

AWARENESS OF TOBACCO INDUSTRY TACTICS

The co-chairs were very concerned that UL students were either unaware of or unconcerned with the tobacco industry sponsorship of a Students' Union event on campus. A group interview was conducted with a convenience group of students in

---

BOX 22-1

Key Facts About Tobacco and Young Adults

Young adults remain an important target group for tobacco reduction interventions.

◆ Young adults aged 20 to 24 years reported the highest rates of being current smokers—27% for Alberta and 26% for Canada (both sexes combined) in 2005.

The prevalence of smoking declined in Canada across all age groups, including young adults.

◆ Tobacco use in young adults aged 20 to 24 years dropped by 13 percentage points between 1985 and 2003.

Rates of tobacco use vary by province.

◆ In 1999, Alberta reported the highest rate of smoking among 20 to 24 year olds in the county—40% compared with the national average of 35%.

Smoking rates differed by sex.

◆ In 2005, males aged 20 to 24 years reported higher rates of current smoking (32%) than did females (21%).

Smoking rates differed by education.

◆ In 2005, daily smoking rates for Canadians 15 years of age and older were lowest among university graduates (11%), higher among college graduates (20%), and highest among those with grade 12 (22%) or less than grade 12 (21%) educations.

From Canadian Tobacco Use Monitoring Survey (CTUMS), Health Canada, 2006.

---

early January 2004, prior to launching educational sessions for National Non-Smoking Week. Participating students expressed varied attitudes toward tobacco industry tactics and sales at the sponsored event (Yanicki, 2005). One student noted that tobacco was already available at The Zoo in vending machines and saw little difference with cigarettes being sold by people who circulated at the event. In contrast, another student was concerned that their Students' Union was giving the tobacco industry direct access to students. An AADAC-sponsored report in 2003 suggested that young adults in Alberta were unaware of many forms of tobacco industry marketing and were ambivalent about many aspects of tobacco industry sponsorship of social, cultural, and sporting events (Malatest & Lavack, 2003).

THE POLICY CONTEXT

Tobacco policies can be viewed from multiple levels. The initial focus of the coalition was on the policy decisions of the Students' Union and the smoking policy of the UL Board of Governors. The broader community policy context (City of Lethbridge), regional policies (Chinook Health), and provincial legislation (Alberta) also needed to be considered. The co-chairs had a keen interest in influencing policy decisions, and other policy targets were added as the project progressed. The Tobacco Reduction Coordinator shared her knowledge of tobacco policies at multiple policy levels.

The Students' Union decision to accept tobacco industry sponsorship and the signing of a 5-year contract allowing the sale of tobacco products at The Zoo in the Students' Union building were key policy issues. The UL banned smoking indoors on campus in 2001; this policy was intended to prevent exposure to environmental tobacco smoke. However, students were allowed to smoke on the third floor of the Students' Union building. A policy change in June 2003 completely banned indoor smoking (University of Lethbridge, 2003), making The Zoo one of the first smokefree pubs in Lethbridge. The co-chairs were interested in further strengthening the existing policy, as it still allowed students to smoke outside of entranceways, and nonsmokers entering and leaving buildings were forced to pass through the cloud of smoke created by the many smokers gathered around doorways.

Take Note

◆ Health care providers can share their knowledge of public policies in supporting community coalitions.
◆ Policies can be viewed from *multiple levels:*
  Organizational context
  Institutional context
  Government contexts (municipal, provincial, and federal)
  International corporate context
  International agreements between governments
◆ A review of policy contexts is helpful prior to selecting policy targets for intervention.
◆ Policies can be viewed as *lines of resistance or strengths* extending from community subsystems. These lines of resistance can help to defend the community core from stressors.
◆ Policies can also help to reset the *normal lines of defence* in a community by:
  Restricting some behaviours (smoking bans)
  Reducing exposure to toxins (smokefree public places)
  Making healthy choices easier (supporting smoking cessation)

Analysis and Diagnosis

The community diagnosis in Table 22-2 provides a compilation of the concerns identified by the co-chairs, the issues based on demographic data, and opportunities for policy intervention.

TABLE 22-2
Community Diagnosis

ISSUE DESCRIPTION	FOCUS	ETIOLOGY	MANIFESTATIONS
Targeting of young adults to recruit new smokers	Postsecondary students	Tobacco industry marketing	Industry sponsoring a concert Contract with the Students' Union for tobacco sales and marketing
Knowledge deficit regarding tobacco marketing	Students, postsecondary governance bodies, and the public	Lack of awareness of tobacco industry marketing tactics	Students' Union accepting sponsorship Lack of university policies on sponsorship

Project Development, Roles, and Responsibilities

HOW DID THE TOBACCO REDUCTION COORDINATOR SUPPORT MOBILIZATION?

The coalition formed with a purpose in mind. Time lines for developing a proposal for funding were short. The coordinator helped to focus the group, called meetings for proposal writing, provided her knowledge and expertise on tobacco reduction as a population health issue, and identified options for project activities and outcomes as well as the community resources available to support action. A project proposal was developed and submitted on November 23, 2003, by the co-chairs with the support of Chinook Health and the coalition. By December 16, 2003, the coalition identified a small group of students who accepted voluntary board positions. The Tobacco Reduction Coordinator assumed the role of secretary/treasurer on behalf of Chinook Health. The project received a $37,750 YTRS grant in early 2004.

HOW DID THE PROJECT EVALUATOR SUPPORT THE PROJECT?

The project evaluator (a health promotion consultant) was identified early in the planning process (December 2003). A participatory evaluation process was used and included the evaluator in coalition meetings. The evaluator facilitated a discussion to clarify how the selected project activities would result in the intended actions and outcomes of the project. This process led to the development of a project logic model early in January 2004 (Fig. 22-4). The logic model helped to focus the group's efforts and identified the types of data required to evaluate the project outcomes and processes.

Partnerships With a Purpose

Developing partnerships was essential to gather the resources needed to implement a wide range of project strategies during the two main university school terms (fall and winter sessions). The support of the Tobacco Reduction Coordinator was

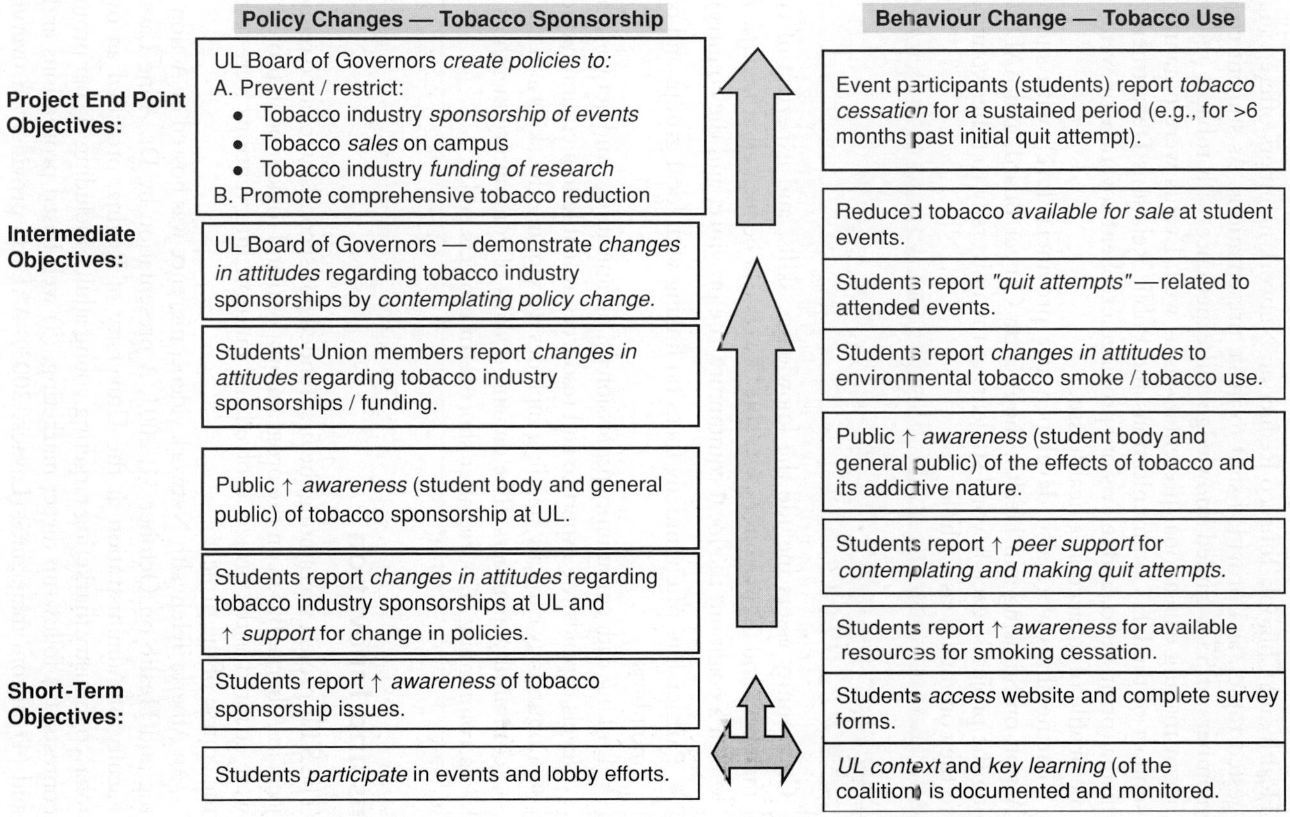

FIGURE 22-4 ◆ Program Logic Model—Students for Tobacco Reduction.

Behaviour Change — Tobacco Use

Event participants (students) report *tobacco cessation* for a sustained period (e.g., for >6 months past initial quit attempt).

Reduced tobacco *available for sale* at student events.

Students report *"quit attempts"*—related to attended events.

Students report *changes in attitudes* to environmental tobacco smoke / tobacco use.

Public ↑ *awareness* (student body and general public) of the effects of tobacco and its addictive nature.

Students report ↑ *peer support* for *contemplating and making quit attempts*.

Students report ↑ *awareness* for available resources for smoking cessation.

Students *access website* and complete survey forms.

UL context and *key learning* (of the coalition) is documented and monitored.

Policy Changes — Tobacco Sponsorship

Project End Point Objectives:

UL Board of Governors *create policies to:*
A. Prevent / restrict:
- Tobacco industry *sponsorship of events*
- Tobacco *sales* on campus
- Tobacco industry *funding of research*
B. Promote comprehensive tobacco reduction

Intermediate Objectives:

UL Board of Governors — demonstrate *changes in attitudes* regarding tobacco industry sponsorships by *contemplating policy change.*

Students' Union members report *changes in attitudes* regarding tobacco industry sponsorships / funding.

Public ↑ *awareness* (student body and general public) of tobacco sponsorship at UL.

Students report *changes in attitudes* regarding tobacco industry sponsorships at UL and ↑ *support* for change in policies.

Students report ↑ *awareness* of tobacco sponsorship issues.

Short-Term Objectives:

Students *participate* in events and lobby efforts.

important to maintaining momentum throughout the project. A series of education sessions were held during National Non-Smoking Week each year. Chinook Health and Chinook Tobacco Reduction Network members offered support, suggested topics, and provided staff to make presentations. As student co-chairs and members of STR gained knowledge and experience with tobacco reduction, they began making educational presentations as well. Events were organized with the support of the UL Communications and Public Relations Department. The local media (print, radio, and television) provided excellent coverage of events and raised the profile of tobacco as a health issue.

Partnerships were also developed at a provincial level, with such groups as Action on Smoking and Health, the Alberta Cancer Board, and AADAC, extending the project's reach beyond students at the university to other young adults and to the community as a whole.

Take Note

Community assets include the knowledge, skills, and expertise of community members and the resources available. Assets can be located at *multiple levels* (e.g., within a coalition, the local community, the province, and the country).

◆ Partnerships often initially focus on linking with local groups and community members.

◆ Linking with community professionals, organizations, and networks at multiple levels expands the expertise and resources available to a community coalition.

◆ Community capacity building includes developing the skills and confidence of community members. The enhanced skills of community members remain as a community resource after short-term projects end.

Interventions and Innovation

The STR project was among the first funded postsecondary tobacco reduction projects in Alberta. Based on the program proposal and logic model, project strategies were adapted as the project evolved and multiple interventions were tested during the course of the project.

An Alberta Telehealth Network videoconference was hosted by Action on Smoking and Health on October 31, 2003. A presentation by Dr. Anne Lavack, of the Faculty of Administration at the University of Regina, provided an overview of tobacco industry marketing targeting young adults, including (1) bar promotion and contests, (2) follow-up direct marketing, (3) web-based promotions and contests, and (4) custom magazines (Lavack, 2003). AADAC provided an overview of the YTRS grants and principles of tobacco reduction with young adults to (1) develop tobacco policies, (2) increase awareness of tobacco marketing and advertising,

(3) prevent initiation of tobacco use, (4) support smoking cessation, and (5) protect nonsmokers from environmental tobacco smoke (Freeman, 2003).

In 2003, little evidence was available on tobacco reduction at the postsecondary level, so creativity and evaluation were encouraged to test innovative approaches. STR began to forge new ground in implementing creative tobacco reduction strategies:

◆ Incentives (food, prize draws, and a scholarship draw) to promote educational events (Lunch N Learn) and completion of evaluation surveys
◆ Lobbying (e.g., Students' Union elections and the Lethbridge bylaw amendment)
◆ Social marketing (Licensed to Kill[1], Drop Dead events,[2] and UR the Target campaign[3])
◆ Countermarketing/denormalization (Smoke-Free Concerts and Smoke-Free Night Life)
◆ Linking to external resources to bring in high-profile speakers (Heather Crowe and Georgina Lovelle).

Evaluation

AADAC acted as a support to the projects funded under the YTRS by bringing project leaders and evaluators together each year for an evaluation workshop and providing project leaders an opportunity to showcase progress on their projects and share their innovations. Combined evaluation paradigms and data collection approaches were used to monitor and evaluate project processes, the relevance and perceived effects of project strategies, and project outcomes.

Overall, there was excellent implementation of a broad range of activities to address the project outcomes of interest. The use of multiple strategies provided good target group exposure to information. Several key policy changes occurred over a two and a half year period, meeting key policy objectives of the project (University of Lethbridge, 2004). While it is not possible to document that the STR project caused the resulting policy changes, it is clear that the intended effects were largely achieved for the policy targets. The project model moved away from the initial plan of offering smoking cessation support due to a lack of student interest; thus, the project had no direct measures of smoking cessation, although there was regular use of the website and regular uptake of cessation information.

In summary, we have described the development of a postsecondary, student-led coalition promoting tobacco reduction. Assessment of policy contexts and of community focussed the issues to be addressed in the project. A program logic model mapped the intended actions of the project in tobacco policy change and individual level change. A participatory evaluation process monitored project processes

---

[1] UL drama students acted the part of a tobacco company, informing students of their strategies.
[2] Action on Smoking and Health sponsored events to dramatize annual deaths due to tobacco.
[3] Alberta Cancer Board social marketing materials pilot tested by STR.

and outcomes. Partnerships extended the expertise and reach and expanded the resources available to the project. Use of multiple interventions created broader impacts on young adults in university and community settings. The success of the coalition was built on the strength of these factors.

SUMMARY

In this chapter, the authors described two examples wherein youth were involved in health promotion. In both instances participation, engagement, and the use of democratic process developed participats' skills and helped them to become empowered in their respective contexts. Further, the use of multiple interventions and partners created as environment that fostered success.

References

Alberta Alcohol and Drug Abuse Commission. (2006). Young Adult Tobacco Reduction Strategy (YTRS). Edmonton, AB: Author.

Campaign 2000. (2005). Decision time for Canada: Let's make poverty history. Retrieved July 20, 2007, from **http://www.campaign2000.ca/rc/rc05/index.html**.

Canadian Council on Social Development. (2006a). The progress of Canada's children & youth. Retrieved July 20, 2007, from **http://www.ccsd.ca/pccy/2006/tools.htm**.

Canadian Council on Social Development. (2006b). Stats & facts: A profile of education in Canada. Retrieved July 20, 2007, from **http://www.ccsd.ca/factsheets/education/index.htm**.

Centre of Excellence for Youth Engagement. (2003). Youth engagement and health outcomes: Is there a link? Toronto ON: Author.

Community Services Council Newfoundland and Labrador. (2002). Values Added Community University Research Alliance. Retrieved July 20, 2007, from **http://www.envision.ca/templates/cura.asp?ID=3667**.

Community Youth Network. (1998). *Framework document*. St. John's: Author.

Freeman, B. (2003). Young adult tobacco reduction strategy grants (YTRS): Community presentation. Videoconference on Alberta TeleHealth Network, hosted by Action on Smoking and Health, October 31, 2003.

Government of NL. (2005). *Reducing poverty in Newfoundland and Labrador: Working towards a solution*. St. John's: Queen's Printer.

Government of NL, Department of Finance. (2005). Demographic change: Newfoundland & Labrador issues & implications. Retrieved July 20, 2007, from **http://www.economics.gov.nl.ca/pdf2003/demography.pdf**.

Hanvey, L. (2003). Social inclusion research in Canada: Children and youth. Retrieved July 20, 2007, from **http://www.ccsd.ca/events/inclusion/papers/hanvey.pdf**.

Health Canada. (2006). Canadian Tobacco Use Monitoring Survey (CTUMS). Retrieved July 20, 2007, from **http://www.hc-sc.gc.ca/hl-vs/tobac-tabac/research-recherche/stat/ctums-esutc/index_e.html**.

Hertzman, C. (2002). *Leave no child behind! Social exclusion and child development*. Toronto: The Laidlaw Foundation. Available at **http://www.cccabc.bc.ca/res/pdf/hertzman.pdf**.

Lavack, A. M. (2003). Tobacco marketing to young adults. Videoconference on Alberta Tele-Health Network, hosted by Action on Smoking and Health, October 31, 2003.

Lofland, J., & Lofland, L. (1995). *Analyzing social settings: A guide to qualitative observation and analysis* (3rd ed.). California: Wadsworth Publishing Company.

Malatest, R. A., & Lavack, A. (2003). Framework for developing tobacco reduction strategies for young adults. Report for Alberta Alcohol and Drug Abuse Commission. Edmonton AB: AADAC.

Meyer, C. (2004). *Tobacco use in the city of Lethbridge 2003: Preliminary report*. Lethbridge: Chinook Health Region and City of Lethbridge.

Meyer, C., & Weber, L. (2003). *2002 University of Lethbridge Student Health Survey*. Lethbridge: Chinook Health Region and University of Lethbridge.

Public Health Agency of Canada. (2002). The key determinants of health. Retrieved July 20, 2007, from **http://www.phac-aspc.gc.ca/canada/regions/atlantic/about/e_2.html**.

Schuller, T. (2001). The complementary roles of human and social capital. *Canadian Journal of Policy Research, 2*(1), 18–24.

Statistics Canada. (2006). July Labour Force Survey. Retrieved July 20, 2007, from **http:// www.stats.gov.nl.ca/Statistics/Labour/LFC_Youth.asp**.

University of Lethbridge. (2003). *Minutes of the Board of Governors open session: June 19, 2003, Non-smoking policy: Amendment*. Lethbridge: Board of Governors, University of Lethbridge

University of Lethbridge. (2004). *Campus smoking policy. Policy and procedures. Administrative manual, health*. Lethbridge: Board of Governors, University of Lethbridge.

Yanicki, S. M. (2005). *Students for Tobacco Reduction: YTRS final evaluation report 2004-05* (pp. 1–30). Lethbridge AB: Yanicki Wellness Consulting.

Internet Resources

http://www.hc-sc.gc.ca/hl-vs/tobac-tabac/youth-jeunes/index_e.html
Youth Zone Tobacco

http://www.ccsa.ca/
Canadian Centre on Substance Abuse

http://www.ciet.org/en/documents/projects/200629173854.asp
Canada: First Nations Youth Enquiry Into Tobacco Use, 1996

http://www.phac-aspc.gc.ca/ph-sp/phdd/pdf/overview_implications/03_inclusion_e.pdf
Social Inclusion as a Determinant of Health

http://www.phac-aspc.gc.ca/canada/regions/atlantic/Publications/Making_case/index.html
Making the Case for Social and Economic Inclusion

http://www.ccsd.ca/cpsd/ccsd/
Children and Youth Crime Prevention Through Social Development

http://www.tgmag.ca/centres/
Centres of Excellence for Children's Well-Being

23

Workplace Health Promotion

ROXANNE FELIX

DONNA PIERRYNOWSKI GALLANT

MARY ANN MURRAY

Chapter Outline

Introduction

Workplace Health Promotion in a Municipal
Government Setting

Responsive Workplace Strategies
for Pandemic Influenza

Summary

Learning Objectives

After studying this chapter, you should be able to:

❖ Understand some of the factors that influence the success of health promotion
interventions in the workplace

❖ Describe formal and informal strategies that can be used for assessment of
workplace health promotion settings

❖ Identify the influence of power on participatory processes in workplace health
promotion

❖ Discuss the imperative for population-based influenza immunization

❖ Debate the merits of health care worker immunization as an ethical imperative

Introduction

In Canada, a survey of work sites found that approximately 30% of
workplaces have some type of health promotion program that offers educational,
organizational, or behavioural interventions designed to support positive health
maintenance activities (Macdonald et al., 2006). Workplaces are considered an ideal
setting for health promotion and primary prevention initiatives because they provide access to a large number of people, and this population is most often stable,
which can facilitate sustainability (Harden et al., 1999).

Human service delivery settings (such as health care institutions, schools, clinics) are workplaces for large numbers of employees. These settings can be used to provide disease prevention services to segments of the population. For instance, when a severe communicable disease such as influenza circulates, these workplaces can be decimated if employees are not available to provide service. Influenza vaccination can prevent employees from becoming ill and can further prevent the transmission of influenza to their clientele. Using the Ottawa Charter as a frame Vollman, Thurston, and Anderson (1999) defined each strategy and provided examples of workplace initiatives that can address each (Table 23-1).

To achieve the goals of workplace wellness, employees and managers must come together in a spirit of equity in diversity to participate in partnerships that strive to achieve health in the workplace community. Hancock (1993) suggests that a healthy community is convivial, livable, and sustainable, with equal concern for the environment and economic productivity. Racher (2005) calls for participatory action that moves people in an organization (community) from being to becoming to belonging through their active involvement in the life of the organization.

In the first story, *Workplace Health Promotion in a Municipal Government Setting*, Felix demonstrates how a workplace wellness program in a large city can make a health difference for employees. In the second story, *Responsive Workplace Strategies for Pandemic Influenza*, Pierrynowski Gallant and Murray present an argument for influenza vaccination in health care institutions as a means to protect the public from pandemic influenza.

WORKPLACE HEALTH PROMOTION IN A MUNICIPAL GOVERNMENT SETTING

This case story focuses on the elements of the assessment process within the community-as-partner model for a workplace health promotion program. It also identifies practical factors that can facilitate or impede the development of appropriate health promotion programs in the workplace.

Context of Workplace Health Promotion

Workplace health promotion can be defined as "an approach to protecting and enhancing the health of employees that relies and builds upon the efforts of employers to create a supportive management under and upon the efforts of employees to care for their own well-being" (Shain & Suurvali, 2001, p. 2). What implications need to be considered when planning and implementing a health promotion program based on this definition? Two critical implications relate to expectations and power.

UNDERSTANDING EXPECTATIONS OF OUTCOMES

Unlike other settings, the expected outcomes of workplace health promotion programs are not limited to those within the health sector. While there is an interest

TABLE 23-1

Health Promotion Concepts, Descriptions, and Their Relevance to Workplace Wellness

HEALTH PROMOTION STRATEGIES	DESCRIPTION	WORKPLACE WELLNESS IMPLICATIONS
Creating supportive environments	Supportive environments offer people protection from threats to health and enable people to expand their capabilities and develop self-reliance in health. *Environment* includes where people live, their local community, their home, and where they work and play, including people's access to resources for health and opportunities for empowerment. Both the physical and social environments can be enhanced to be more supportive (Chapter 4).	Peer and supervisor support to take part in health-enhancing behaviours A corporate culture that promotes healthy lifestyles and values its employees Safe buildings, parking, child care Cafeteria and food choice policies
Developing personal skills	Health literacy and empowerment increase the options available to people to improve their health. Personal skills can be developed through information or education that enhances one's abilities for adaptive and positive behaviour. In return, developing such skills allows people to better control and direct their lives in addition to enhancing their capacity to live in or change their environment (Chapter 5).	Programs and services that provide the opportunity to enhance personal coping Balancing work and family responsibilities Providing information on fitness, healthy eating Teaching stress management
Strengthening community action	Community action involves a collective effort of groups of people to increase control over the determinants of health (Chapter 6).	Opportunities for group participation, input, decisions on issues in the workplace
Building healthy public policy	All policy-makers take into account the potential impact of policies on the health and equity of individuals and the population. Healthy policies create and encourage a supportive environment that enables people to lead healthy lifestyles (Chapter 7).	Tobacco policy Procedures and collective agreements Advocacy for change in other sectors that affect employees
Reorienting health services	Involves moving in a health-promoting direction, beyond the traditional provision of clinical and curative services to the creation of health-promoting institutions (Chapter 8).	Focus not only on treating occupational injury and illness but on workplace wellness —healthy and safe workplaces Creating health-promoting institutions that embrace diversity and enhance opportunity for making healthy choices

From Vollman, AR, Thurston, WE & Anderson, D. (1999). An evaluability assessment of the CRHA Workplace Wellness Program. Unpublished report, Calgary AB.

in improving the health status of employees, most employers hope to see this improvement translated to other organizational outcomes such as reduced absenteeism, increased job satisfaction, and even increased profit. The health promotion practitioner has to explicitly outline the linkage between increased social and health capacity of the workforce and its resulting impact on organizational goals.

BOX 23-1

Business Case for Workplace Health Promotion

The following is an excerpt from a business case for workplace health promotion in the City of Edmonton.

Healthy workplaces benefit organizations and individuals alike, resulting in:

1. Cost savings through fewer insurance and worker compensation claims, decreased injuries, decreased absenteeism, reduction in benefit claims; and
2. Employee satisfaction, retention, and recruitment.[1]

The City of Edmonton's workforce fulfils many functions in the municipality that must be done in a productive and safe manner. By investing in the well-being of the workforce, the City of Edmonton would ensure its public is being served in an effective and efficient manner.

A recent review of the cost effectiveness of U.S. workplace health promotion initiatives showed a positive return on investment values up to $8.89 per dollar spent. In Canada, workplace health promotion programs have seen outcomes that provide a $3–$7 return on investment.[2] Most of these monetary benefits are gained through reduced absenteeism.[3]

If a healthy work organization can be created where its culture, climate and practices create an environment that promotes employee health and safety, which in turn improve organizational effectiveness,[4] health and performance stop being competing agendas, and instead become mutually reinforcing.

From Felix, R. (2006). *Corporate Health Promotion Program, City of Edmonton*. Edmonton, Alberta.
[1] The Health Communication Unit (2004). *An introduction to comprehensive workplace health promotion*. Centre for Health Promotion. Toronto, ON: University of Toronto. Version 1.1 Info-pak. Available: **www.theu.ca.**
[2] The Health Communication Unit (2004). Ibid.
[3] Lowe, G. (2003). *Healthy workplaces and productivity: A discussion paper*. Ottawa, ON: Health Canada.
[4] Lim, S. Y., & Murphy, L. R. (1999). The relationship of organizational factors to employee health and overall effectiveness. *American Journal of Industrial Medicine, Supplement May*, 64–65.

The importance of these outcomes will vary depending on the type of workplace setting involved. Corporations might look for specific changes in customer satisfaction or workforce productivity. A government workplace setting, because it is publicly funded, would likely be more interested in outcomes such as increased efficiency or employee retention. It can be expected, however, that in most workplace settings, there would be a high value placed on evaluating the investment put into a health promotion program. Most corporations, public or private, will examine the costs and benefits of any program directed to its internal employees (Box 23-1).

UNDERSTANDING POWER RELATIONSHIPS

In any setting, it is wise to try to understand relationships of power between and among different stakeholders. In a workplace setting, it is essential that these power relationships are explicitly identified and understood; specifically, we need to recognize that employees are dependent on managers for their income and financial sustainability. How this relationship is formally and informally established will affect employee engagement in a health promotion program. For example, if the workforce perceives that managers are supporting health promotion initiatives simply to increase productivity and health promotion professionals are perceived as being aligned with management, it is unlikely that employees will engage in any of the planning, implementation, or evaluation processes necessary to make the program successful. In addition, if the workplace is a unionized environment, understanding the relationship between the union, management, and employees is vital to planning participation strategies.

Another important aspect of power in workplace settings lies in the definition of *health promotion:* "the process of enabling people to increase control over, and to improve, their health" (World Health Organization, 1986). In essence, health promotion seeks to enhance people's ability to exercise control over their environmental and behavioural conditions that affect their quality of life. The impact of worker personal / collective empowerment regarding workplace health issues may be perceived negatively in the corporate boardroom.

For most employers, there is a widespread misconception that health promotion programming involves mostly health education strategies. Do most employers recognize that comprehensive health promotion actually seeks to mobilize its workforce? And, if they did, would they support it? Even though human resource management research points to the contribution of employee involvement to productivity (Leckie et al., 2001), few employers understand the link between participation, locus of control, health status, and subsequent employee productivity. Given such, using research from across the fields of health promotion, organizational science, and human resource management to demonstrate these links is helpful. Case studies are particularly valued, as employers value practical evidence of the effectiveness of participatory approaches.

The issues of power as it relates to employee participation and definition of successful outcomes need to be understood before undertaking the assessment and planning process of health promotion programming.

Assessment

This section will outline the assessment process used in the development of a health promotion strategy for the City of Edmonton workforce. In addition to identifying the community core, lines of defence, and lines of resistance, this section will discuss how assessment can be handled in a larger organization and what issues regarding participation need to be considered.

COMMUNITY CORE

The City of Edmonton employs nearly 10,000 employees in a variety of different sectors of work, including planning and development, transportation, transit, maintenance of parks and city buildings, recreation and community services (e.g., fire, police, and emergency services), waste management, drainage, and infrastructure services to the organization itself (e.g., law, computer technical services, and human resources). The City of Edmonton had a wellness program in the past that focused on providing incentives for employees to be physically active. However, a comprehensive health promotion strategy for employees had not been developed.

Using a setting as a focus for health promotion programs can provide insight into a community's traditions, values, and circumstances. However, in a very large and diverse organization, the nature of "community" and "setting" is very different. There is not a set of shared values, interests, or even geographical location; the common factor is simply the employer, which poses some problems to assessing the population's needs.

However, given that an organization like the City of Edmonton has a large infrastructure to serve its human resource functions, some of the data necessary to understand the community core was readily available. The human resources branch provided information on age, sex, and marital status of its workforce. All members of this community were employed. Other useful information was also available, such as salary range, level of employee satisfaction with their working environment, and ethnicity. However, in order to utilize this information, the linkages between health and its underlying determinants needed to be explicitly outlined.

In a situation where an organization is very diverse, it would be ideal to administer a survey to collect more information about the population. Realistically, however, surveys are not always an option, depending on the resources available to the health promotion program and the importance of health promotion to senior managers. Even if a survey could be developed, how would this type of instrument accurately identify community values, beliefs, and history?

Some strategies used to collect information about the community core in a large workplace setting, without access to survey data, include:

- *Aligning with Others.* There are many people in a large organization who would know about health concerns and issues that may not necessarily be involved in the health field. These individuals, through their own job functions, are aware of employee concerns and could provide insight into the workplace culture, values, and history. We spoke with stakeholders formally and informally to gather intelligence about the population.
- *File Review.* We reviewed historical files that explained successful and failed health promotion efforts. We learned about how and why the current health promotion program was established, who the initiators / supporters are, and what barriers might be in place.
- *Interviews and Site Visits.* Interviews done with interested managers and employees can provide a breadth of expectations for a health promotion program. When possible, we held these interviews at the interviewee's work location. The physical location can provide an understanding of the environment, accessibility to different types of services, and the interconnectedness of employees at the work site. Questions on the interview guide asked about the interviewee's perception

---

BOX 23-2

Stakeholders in a Workplace Setting

Occupational health and safety professionals
Disability management professionals
Chaplains and counsellors
Human resources professionals
Union representatives
Office of the Ombudsman
Training and continuing education professionals
Diversity and inclusion professionals
Employee and family assistance services
Building maintenance professionals

---

of health promotion and opinions about success conditions for a health promotion strategy. Both informal and formal methods were used to identify key informants. Informal mechanisms included identification of interested stakeholders through conversations with colleagues. Formal mechanisms included letters of introduction to key stakeholders (i.e., union leaders, managers) and presentations at management meetings.

◆ *Visibility and Communication.* Taking a community development approach, individuals at every level in the organization need to be aware of the existence and goals of the health promotion program. Communicating the goals and processes of workplace health promotion will need to be a strategy unto itself during the first 3 years of implementation. Often, conversations in elevators and lunchrooms can end up being quite informative about the target population and the community (Box 23-2).

LINES OF DEFENCE

As outlined previously, there were no resources or staff to do a formal health assessment of the employees. Information on the health status, prevalence of disease, injury, and risk factors was not available. As well, employee experience with a previous health survey indicated that many employees had concerns about confidentiality of data. Such data are especially contentious because it reflects the health status and lifestyles of employees whose salaries are paid through public funds. Even if a survey could be implemented, we felt that the likelihood of employee participation in a survey at this point in the health promotion program development would be low.

However, other data sources were used to provide some indication of the "health" of the target population. For these purposes, information on absentee rates, use of employment and family (counselling) services, and types of drugs being claimed on employees' benefits plans provided some insight into the health issues of the target population. For example, drugs being used for circulatory medical conditions were most commonly prescribed for this target population. While such data can be helpful, it is not perfect. For example, absentee rates tell you about employees who are not at work, but they do not provide information on how many employees are at work but not functioning at full capacity (referred to as "presenteeism").

Another source of data on health status that we used was prepared by the regional health authority. Data were available for Edmontonians on morbidity, mortality, and risk factor prevalence; we used this information to make inferences about city employees.

LINES OF RESISTANCE

As part of health promotion programming, it is important to identify community assets that can contribute to the community engaging in the health promotion process. We used key informant interviews, observations, and site visits to identify current strengths in the community, or as identified in the community-as-partner model, the lines of resistance. This approach, identifying assets and community capacity, provided us a great starting point for dialogue with members of the community on how we should proceed with our planning efforts.

For the purposes of working with the City of Edmonton on workplace wellness, we categorized its assets into four areas based on the action strategies of the Ottawa Charter for Health Promotion (World Health Organization, 1986): developing personal skills, creating supportive environments, strengthening department capacity, and demonstrating corporate commitment (i.e., healthy policy). A number of activities, policies, and structures were found that contributed to a healthy working environment and could also serve as natural starting points for future health promotion programming efforts (Box 23-3).

BOX 23-3

City of Edmonton Workforce—Lines of Resistance

Developing personal skills	Lunch N' Learns available on health and leadership development topics; Training Library available
Creating healthy environments	Change rooms, showers, and bike lockers available at some sites; Teambuilding and Effective Management Programs; Working Relationship Agreement between Unions and Management
Strengthening department capacity	Health promotion committees; critical incident stress management peer groups
Demonstrating corporate commitment	50% discount for employees to use city recreational facilities; flex time available to some employees

Practical Factors in Assessment

MULTILEVEL ASSESSMENT

Previously, we described how assessment was handled for the City of Edmonton organization as a whole. However, an organization has many different departments, and if feasible, the assessment process can be repeated to collect more in-depth information for smaller subsections within the workplace setting.

While the information collected in the assessment process was probably complete enough to provide a planning framework for a corporate health promotion strategy, some departments chose to engage in more detailed assessments in order to arrive at a health promotion strategy for their specific employee health needs. In these instances, health surveys and environmental health assessments were undertaken. As well, the assessment process at this level also allows the employees and managers to be more engaged in the assessment process, which leads to a more participatory (and therefore more flexible and relevant) assessment process.

PARTICIPATORY PROCESSES IN ASSESSMENT

It was a challenge to make the assessment process truly participatory for a workplace that was very large and diverse. As well, there were resource and time line restrictions that limited the participatory nature of this process. However, it was clear that a participatory process was necessary if the planning and implementation of a health promotion program was to be successful. In order to ensure that employees and managers were engaged as partners in this process, it was identified early on that an advisory committee at both the corporate and department levels would need to be established. While such a mechanism begins to lay the foundation for formal participatory processes, informal processes can also be established.

The building of relationships during the assessment process is fundamental to establishing health promotion programming that is responsive to the needs of the community. While there might not be the readiness or understanding of the formal declaration of participatory activity, the health promotion professional can certainly create a cultural understanding of this process informally by one's actions and informal interactions. It is important that this responsiveness extends to managers, in addition to the employees. Building trust with the managers and understanding their context and stressors will ultimately lead to a better relationship with their staff and front-line employees.

PRACTICAL CONSIDERATIONS

Some practical factors need to be considered in the assessment process for workplace settings:

◆ *Ensure that you are not perceived as being aligned with either management or front-line employees.* The health promotion program should be perceived as a bridge between the interests of both parties, supporting the maintenance of a resource (health) that can bring benefit to both managers (decreased absenteeism rates) and employees (increased quality of life). If you are a practitioner external to the organization, this neutrality is easier to maintain. However, if you are a practitioner internal to the organization, there might be increased buy-in from employees because the program is perceived as being a priority of the organization, as opposed to a one-time intervention, and is more likely to be sustained over time.

◆ *While it is important to mobilize employees to participate in the assessment process, recognize that equally important is the support of management.* Engagement of employees in the assessment process can lead to the development of social capital in the workplace and other outcomes (i.e., employee satisfaction, increased work morale, etc.); however, this process is nearly impossible without management support. A review of effective workplace health promotion programs has found that achieving a balance between employee ownership and giving employees support through management is a promising strategy for increasing effectiveness (Harden et al., 1999).

◆ *Develop relationships and respect experiential knowledge.* A health promotion practitioner has knowledge to offer, but its usefulness is limited without an understanding of community context and history. Trust the advice given to you by employees, and develop and refine your consultation skills. Be aware that health promotion practitioners are not perceived in the general public as having a set of specialized skills or knowledge. Few people know that research has been done on best practices in health promotion and that health promotion is not just "common sense." Consequently, recommendations about health promotion program development will likely need to be accompanied with the building of a trusting relationship and attentiveness to the organization's evolving needs and unique situation.

◆ Finally, *be creative about finding opportunities for participation.* It does not necessarily need to carry the label of a "participatory" process. If the process is working, it will take on a life of its own and be accepted by stakeholders as an important component of the assessment, planning, and implementation process.

In summary, assessment is one of the most important components of the community-as-partner model. Understanding this process requires the allotment of appropriate time and resources to this process. Assessment as one stage in the development of a health promotion strategy for the City of Edmonton took nearly 6 months to complete. It is a lengthy process but one that is worth time and investment. It can lead to important longer term outcomes like employee and management engagement in health promotion planning and evaluation processes.

RESPONSIVE WORKPLACE STRATEGIES FOR PANDEMIC INFLUENZA

Influenza is a deadly virus (World Health Organization [WHO], 1999); according to the WHO, three influenza pandemics have occurred in the 20th century—1918, 1957, and 1968—killing approximately thirty to fifty thousand Canadians and twenty to forty million people worldwide (Public Health Agency of Canada [PHAC], 2005). Many infectious diseases specialists and researchers believe that another global influenza pandemic is imminent. However, many people are unaware of the potential impact of influenza on global health and lack personal engagement with the issue. For instance, while vaccination is effective and highly protective for health care professionals and others, current low rates of influenza vaccine uptake indicate a general lack of influenza response readiness (Pierrynowski-Gallant & Robinson Vollman, 2004).

While there are limits in our knowledge concerning influenza pathology and vaccination uptake behaviours, we do know that health care is a partnership among individuals, care providers, and larger organizational structures (Gladwell, 2002). Effective influenza prevention and management requires a holistic approach where people work together to achieve practical results. Understanding how to separate and share responsibility for minimizing influenza impact on individuals, the community, and the broader population requires consideration of the relationships among different providers, their diversity, their shared environment, organizational infrastructure, and the sociopolitical contexts that act as facilitators or barriers to influenza-vaccination uptake.

While impractical to think that influenza can be eradicated globally, pragmatic goals and objectives to address the prospect of pandemic influenza and its sequelae can be implemented at the local level. This section addresses implications for influenza response by exploring the epidemiology of the problem. Vaccination as a key strategy to impact flu transmission and control is examined from multiple perspectives. Finally, a multiple intervention approach targeting a variety of strategies and stakeholders is discussed.

A Review of the Landscape

Influenza, an acute viral disease of the respiratory tract, typically manifests with fever, headache, myalgia, exhaustion, rhinitis, sore throat, and cough. Symptoms last about 3 to 4 days with the possibility of cough and fatigue persisting for 1 to 2 weeks. Influenza is associated with serious complications, notably viral and bacterial pneumonia; bacterial pneumonia is the most common complication and can be fatal. Children, adults over the age of 65, and those suffering from chronic medical conditions (respiratory, cardiac, or kidney disease; diabetes; or depressed immune system) are at a higher risk for experiencing complications (Chin, 2000). On average, about 4,000 Canadians die of influenza and related complications each year; in severe seasons, the number of deaths may be as high as 8,000 (PHAC, 2005). Influenza occurs in seasonal epidemics due to changes in the viral antigenic proteins, a phenomenon known as antigenic drift. Antigenic drift refers to changes in the surface of the virus. In temperate climates, the flu season occurs between November and March; in the tropical and subtropical climates of the Southern Hemisphere, from May to September (WHO, 1999).

Take Note

Three types of influenza virus have been identified as part of the genus *Orthomyxovirus:* Types A, B, and C.

Type A is the most common, appearing every year, and is associated with widespread epidemics and pandemics. It infects people, birds, pigs, horses, seals, and whales, with wild birds acting as natural hosts for the virus. Influenza A viruses are grouped into antigen subtypes differentiated by two surface proteins: Haemagglutinin (H) and neuraminidase (N). These proteins are responsible for the antigenic changes in influenza viruses. Currently, there are 16 different H subtypes and 9 different N subtypes. Three haemagglutinin subtypes (H1, H2, and H3) and two neuraminidase (N1, N2) subtypes most commonly cause widespread human disease.

Type B influenza is normally found only in humans, and although generally causing a milder illness, it may be more severe in the elderly. Influenza B can cause human epidemics but has not caused pandemics.

Type C generally causes mild or asymptomatic disease and is typically local in nature.

As an airborne virus, influenza is particularly infectious in crowded enclosed spaces. A short incubation of 2 to 3 days coupled with high titres of the virus, long periods of virus shedding, and the small amount of the virus needed to create infection explains the occurrence of fulminating epidemics. Influenza also presents as worldwide epidemics, or *pandemics*. Pandemics are not influenced by the season, are caused by an extreme antigenic shift in the virus, and are associated with severe morbidity and mortality. The antigenic changes occur so quickly that people do not carry immunity against the new virus and vaccines cannot be developed in time to prevent widespread infection. With a new subtype, everyone is equally susceptible, except for those exposed to an earlier epidemic caused by a similar subtype (Chin, 2000). Being infected produces immunity to that specific virus, but the duration and type of immunity depends on the extent of antigenic drift and the number of previous infections that one has had. In Figure 23-1, the deadly effects that pandemics and epidemics have had on the world since 1580 are summarized.

Of recent concern is the appearance of avian influenza outbreaks and infections among humans (Strain H5N1) and the ongoing widespread cases of avian influenza among poultry in Asia (Centers for Disease Control and Prevention [CDC], 2005). This concern is coupled with the fact that increased pace and frequency of worldwide travel quickens transmission risk (Knobler et al., 2005). At present, H5N1 rarely spreads from person to person (CDC, 2005), yet each additional human case

Conclusion: A future pandemic is inevitable. The **World Health Organization** continues to develop contingency plans to ensure effective response.

Current: A vaccine is being developed in response to the recent avian outbreak. Concern about transmission from birds to people.

Current: Surveillance network has 110 national influenza centres in 83 countries.

1980: License of first surface vaccine in the United Kingdom.

1997: Outbreak of **A/H5N1** influenza occurs, avian in nature, begins in Hong Kong. Virus moves directly from chickens to people; 1.5 million chickens slaughtered; no new human infections found after slaughter.

1999: Two children infected with **H9N2,** which usually affects birds.

1918: J.S. Koen of Fort Dodge, Iowa, discovers the influenza virus from studies on animal disease, specifically pigs.

1928: C.N. McBride successfully transmits influenza from a sick pig to a healthy pig; fails at inoculating through a bacterial filter.

1931: Richard Shoppe repeats McBride's study under strict experimental conditions. It is the first reliable experiment that displays proof that influenza is caused by a virus, becoming the basis for future research.

1933: C. Andrews and W. Smith isolate influenza A in humans.

1935: W. Smith discovers that the influenza virus can be cultivated by inoculating it into a developing chick embryo.

1936: Variants of **Type A** virus found to exist.

1940: Type B influenza virus is isolated.

1941: Hemagglutination of red blood cells discovered by **Hirst,** provides a new way of assaying for the virus.

1943: Killed vaccine is developed and shown to be effective.

1945: Vaccination of U.S. Army shows consistent protection.

1947: Influenza C is isolated. An international network for influenza surveillance is envisioned.

1948: The **World Health Organization** becomes responsible for administration of the surveillance of vaccine.

1955: Avian influenza is recognized.

1957:
Neuraminidase and **interferon** are discovered.

Asian pandemic begins with infection first seen in school children, which coincides with the opening of school in winter.

Asian pandemic, a new subtype (**H2N2**) emerges in Southwest China in February. This virus results from a dual infection with human and avian influenza.

Deaths are mostly due to secondary bacterial pneumonia. The majority affected are the very old and very young; total deaths probably exceed one million.

Vaccine against the Asian flu is approved in July 1957. It was developed late, so only seven million receive the benefit of the vaccine.

1963: Amantadine hydrochloride, the first drug active *in vivo* against influenza, is developed.

1968: Hong Kong Pandemic — A new subtype emerges (**H3N2**): starts in Southeast China in July and claims 700,000 lives worldwide.

1971: Hybridization demonstrated in live animals.

1972: Influenza is found to occur frequently in wild birds.

1976: New influenza virus from pigs causes human infections and severe illness. Persons over age 50 have antibodies to the new variant that is similar to one identified in 1920.

PREDISCOVERY

Canada in 1918: Some 50,000 lives lost when virus crosses the Atlantic to Canada via troopship, with Canadian soldiers; survivors left with heart and respiratory weakness.

Across Canada: Once influenza begins to spread throughout the country, its control becomes a provincial responsibility.

1918: Spanish influenza pandemic occurs: (**A/H1N1**) swinelike virus emerges during final months of the Great War in Europe.

Origin of Spanish influenza: Unknown, but possibly started in the United States and transmitted to France by troopships. High infection rates due to closed quarters.

Effects of 1918: About half the world's population is affected; total mortality is 40 to 50 million. Many die due to complications of bacterial pneumonia.

1918: Younger generation severely affected: Attack rate highest in the age group 0–35; half of deaths occur in the age group 20–40.

Hippocrates: First describes the disease in **412 BC.**

Influenza: The word comes from the Italian world "influence" or "influence of the stars," in **1504.**

1580–1889: Epidemics and pandemics are reported, with high rates of morbidity and mortality.

1889–1890: Germ theory of infectious disease is accepted. In Germany, **Richard Pfeiffer** identifies Pfeiffer's bacillus in the throats of people with influenza.

FIGURE 23-1 ◆ Influenza: A growing discovery. (Reproduced with permission from Pierrynowski-Gallant, D.M. & Robinson Vollman, A. (2004). Influenza vaccination choices. *Canadian Nurse, 100*(2), 16–21.

provides an opportunity to improve virus transmissibility in humans and contributes to the development of a pandemic strain. While neither the timing nor the severity of the next pandemic can be predicted, the probability of a pandemic is increasing.

Lessons Learned From Past Pandemics

The 1918 pandemic had serious consequences and caused significant social chaos. Since then, several advantages against the disease have been gained through (1) experience from previous pandemics, (2) better knowledge about the influenza virus, (3) improved ability to create vaccines and antiviral drugs, and (4) improved ability to identify the viral components that cause virulence (Knobler et al., 2005). As well, we know now that the genetic characteristics of pandemic viruses typically attack younger adults. In 1918, individuals younger than 65 years of age accounted for more than 99% of all influenza-related deaths (Simonsen et al., 1998). Predictions for future pandemics suggest that between 20 and 500 deaths per 100,000 people will occur and that individuals under the age of 65 will account for the majority of these deaths (Knobler et al., 2005).

There is evidence that the mortality impact from the pandemic is not always immediate and that there are often warning signs (Knobler et al., 2005). Ongoing surveillance of age-related mortality statistics and constantly updating influenza vaccines can provide the world with lead time to respond to a pandemic. Lessons about communication strategies are also apparent. During the 1918 pandemic, which coincided with the end of World War I, officials were reluctant to distribute information about the pandemic's arrival, severity, scope, and probable geographic trajectory. Public trust waned as people witnessed firsthand the illness and death of young adults. The need for clear and truthful communications in a public health emergency was an important lesson learned.

To date, Canada has been developing comprehensive plans to mitigate the impact of a pandemic to minimize illness and death and to reduce social disruption (PHAC, 2004). The plan involves surveillance, vaccine programs, use of antiviral drugs, mobilization of health services, emergency services, public health measures, and communications. However, there are specific knowledge gaps and questions to be asked about current Canadian pandemic planning. For instance, what are the effects of school and public facility closures and masks on disease containment, and what are the relationships between animal and human viruses and the typical virus shedding patterns of infected persons and the pathways of transmission to susceptible contacts?

Initially, in a pandemic, most people will need to rely on disease avoidance to minimize infection risk due to limited supplies of antiviral drugs and delayed availability of the pandemic vaccine (Canadian Institutes of Health Research [CIHR], 2005). Thus, more knowledge about nonpharmacological interventions to curtail exposure and infection is needed. Also, in a pandemic situation, demand on health care facilities will occur at an unparalleled scale, as we learned from the 2003 severe acute respiratory syndrome (SARS) experience in Toronto, ON. To date, we know that the most effective public health intervention to address the influenza pandemic is immunization and, to a lesser extent, antiviral drugs.

Current Trends in Influenza Immunity

One century ago, infectious diseases were the leading cause of death worldwide. Today, due largely to the availability of immunization programs, infectious diseases account for less than 5% of all Canadian deaths. Immunization, discovered in the 18th century, can protect an entire population by preventing infection spread between individuals, increasing individual immunity, and in certain instances, decreasing amounts of circulating organisms.

Low uptake of the influenza vaccine leads to inadequate community (herd) immunity. If immunization programs do not achieve threshold coverage, the spread of disease and the number of susceptible individuals increases (Diodati, 1999). Generally, a 70% vaccine coverage rate is required to break the chain of disease transmission (National Advisory Committee on Immunization [NACI], 2002). However, influenza vaccination programs typically aim for a 90% coverage rate (NACI, 2006). Despite these immunization goals, only 70% to 91% of long-term care facility (LTCF) residents and 20% to 40% of adults and children with medical conditions receive the vaccine annually (Russell, 2001; Squires, Macey, & Tam, 2001; Stevenson et al., 2001). As well, recent studies of health care workers in hospitals and LTCFs have shown vaccination rates as low as 26% (Russell, 2001; Stevenson et al., 2001).

Empirical evidence confirms that the risk associated with acquiring influenza far outweighs the risk associated with vaccination. However, despite proven protection at both the individual and community level, debate about vaccination acceptability exists. Complacency exists in part due to the success of vaccines in preventing communicable diseases. Hesitancy or refusal of vaccination may be attributed to religious or philosophic objections, perceptions that mandatory vaccination (as an employment condition) infringes on rights, belief that vaccination is a personal decision, concerns about vaccine safety and efficacy, and/or belief that vaccine-preventable diseases do not pose a serious health risk. Some also believe that immunizations are "not natural" (Public Health Agency of Canada [PHAC] 1997).

Specific reasons for refusal of influenza vaccination include fear of side effects (e.g., Guillain-Barré syndrome and soreness at the vaccination site) (O'Rorke, Bourke, & Bedford, 2003), belief in the body's own defence systems (Begue & Gee, 1998), doubts about vaccine efficacy (Harbarth et al., 1998), not wanting to get sick (Begue & Gee, 1998), and not liking needles (Heimberger et al., 1995). Lack of ready access to vaccination has also been reported as a barrier. Specifically, issues such as lack of information on how to get the vaccine, cost, limited hours of vaccination clinics, and lack of time to get the vaccine have been cited as additional barriers to influenza vaccination (Harbarth et al., 1998).

A Focus on Health Care Workers

Providers of health care are capable of acquiring influenza and then transmitting the virus to clients who are at high risk and susceptible to infection. For example, 25% of all health providers in British Columbia were infected with influenza during the 1998–1999 winter months (Skowronski, Parker, & Strang, 2000). In response to this and similar data (Potter, Stott, & Roberts, 1997), influenza immunization of health providers has been recommended as a means of protecting high-risk clients by the NACI in Canada and the Centers for Disease Control and Prevention (CDC) and the Advisory Committee on Immunization Practices (ACIP) in the United States. There is also some discussion in the literature that health care workers have a duty to actively promote, implement, and comply with influenza immunization recommendations to reduce risk in vulnerable populations for whom they provide care (Orr, 2000). We could extend that argument to other human service personnel such as school teachers, social workers, and others who provide service to community citizens.

Assessment and Planning

Every year, long term care facility (LTCF) residents are exposed to influenza and suffer significant morbidity and mortality. Nevertheless, many LTCF residents and LTCF employees decide *not* to obtain influenza vaccination despite strong evidence of the clinical and economic effectiveness of vaccination. Initial meetings confirmed interest in developing a specific influenza decision aid that could be a helpful tool in one LTCF. Given the impact of health care workers as potential transmission vectors and their important role in the education of residents and their families, nurses and support staff were identified as the target for intervention.

A sequential, planned action approach guided program development and implementation. Information, insights, and evidence gained at each stage informed subsequent steps. Steps included (1) overall gap analysis; (2) survey of nurses and support staff decision making needs; (3) development of an influenza vaccination decision aid; (4) decision aid piloting; (5) an implementation trial including process and outcomes evaluation; and (6) plans for dissemination of findings and, if effective, tools and lessons learned to the larger community.

Gap analysis procedures included literature review, an environmental scan using salient policy and planning documents, and interviews with key informants. A standardized template was adapted to elicit providers' decision-making needs related to influenza vaccination.

A Need for Multiple Interventions

Evidence suggests that combined intervention programs are associated with better vaccination coverage (Russell, 2001; Shefer et al., 1999). Single strategy programs are too simplistic to address the complex challenges inherent in improving influenza-vaccination uptake. A multilevel strategy, delivered through a variety of channels, in conjunction with an interdisciplinary research agenda is required.

Several key areas related to vaccination are amenable to multiple intervention approaches. For example, it is important to win support from opinion leaders. These 'champions' can influence people's decisions through the strength of their personality and commitment to the cause (Pierrynowski-Gallant, 2005). They are influential in workplace administration and political structures, so they can affect influenza vaccine policy at multiple levels and can cultivate buy-in from others.

Those involved in developing health care messages for the public and health care providers also need to be involved in vaccination programs. Public health promotion campaigns need to target multiple age groups and social strata. The post-secondary education setting presents an important opportunity to acquaint students across professional disciplines with current evidence and to correct misperceptions related to vaccination issues and infection control (Pelly et al., 2006). As well, continuing education is a good strategy for updating clinicians on emerging evidence on influenza and best practices in vaccination.

Empiric evidence suggests that collaborative practice improves patient outcomes in populations (Oandasan et al., 2004). Bringing members of different disciplines together encourages 'expansive learning' as team members challenge each other's profession specific cognitive map. Debating, negotiating, and hybridizing different perspectives foster a common vision with collective ownership of the problem and solutions (Engestrom, 2000). While further study is required to evaluate care processes to better understand links between interventions and outcomes, interdisciplinary care is emphasized within most public health care teams. Leveraging interdisciplinary problem-solving and communication is a sound strategy to optimize vaccination programs.

On a broader level, the media, professional regulatory bodies, the NACI, the PHAC, and other professional associations can be involved in widely disseminating supportive messages on vaccination (Pierrynowski Gallant, 2005). Focused efforts by public health program planners, administrators, educators, and health care providers mediated through collective action can create a synergy that will influence attitudes, beliefs, and behaviour related to influenza-vaccination uptake (Gladwell, 2002).

People engage in an internal dialogue as they consider their decision to accept or refuse an influenza vaccine; the diverse factors that shape their decisions must be recognized in order to develop interventions that can be tailored to meet their decision-making needs. Influenza vaccination decision-making should be considered holistically with a focus on population health promotion, allowing for changing social values and structures (Pierrynowski-Gallant, 2005). To do this, framing the issue as an action taken on behalf of others who may be at high risk for acquiring and suffering from influenza (whether those others are patients, family, or friends) may have merit. Clarifying issues and consensus-building could then take place at individual and collective levels.

A Multiple Intervention Vaccination Program Plan

A logic model illustrating key targets to further develop, refine, and synergize vaccination uptake programs within a population based model is illustrated in Figure 23-2. Specific strategies include:

1. A *capacity-building strategy* aimed at informing, influencing, and assisting providers and organizations to gain confidence and competence in providing quality health promoting vaccination programs.
2. A *regulatory strategy* aimed at embedding indicators of vaccination uptake in legislation and policy.
3. A *research strategy* designed to identify indicators of quality vaccination programs relevant to diverse population needs, and application and evaluation of infection control knowledge in clinical practice.
4. A *health efficiency strategy* to balance the cost, accessibility, effectiveness, and sustainability of vaccination programs.

In summary, despite evidence confirming the benefits of vaccination to the individual and community, many people do not participate in annual influenza immunization. Health care providers and human services personnel need to be aware of issues surrounding the immunization debate and of current evidence related to influenza risk, impact, prevention, and management. Use of systematic, evidence-based, planned action approaches to help identify actionable messages, craft context-sensitive dissemination strategies, and guide measures of change are required. Collaborative action and dedicated resources are needed to leverage opportunities and build success potential in responding to population health needs for influenza pandemic planning and response. Health care providers have a pivotal role in ensuring that Canada is ready to meet the challenges inherent in influenza prevention and management.

SUMMARY

Workplaces can be sites for health promotion activity for many reasons: There are inherent risks in certain workplaces; a healthy workforce is a productive workforce; and workers represent a target population for injury prevention, risk and harm reduction, and health protection. One health protective measure for health care and human service workers is immunization against influenza in these prepandemic times. Health and human service workers represent the "front lines" if and when pandemic influenza strikes; further, they can be vectors for the infection. The two stories presented in this chapter offer some important lessons to the health promotion planner: Assessment is an important activity not only to understand needs but also to determine the acceptability of approaches under consideration, multiple interventions are more effective than one-shot approaches, and it is important to evaluate formatively so that plans can be modified to address emerging concerns and issues.

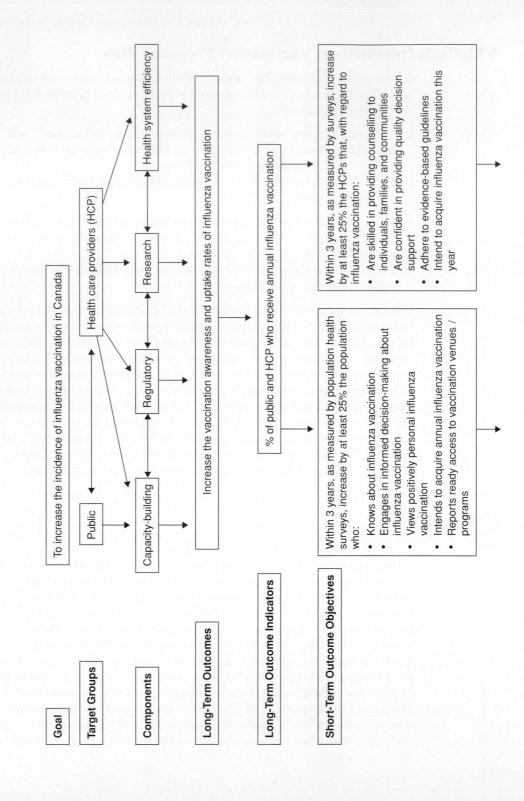

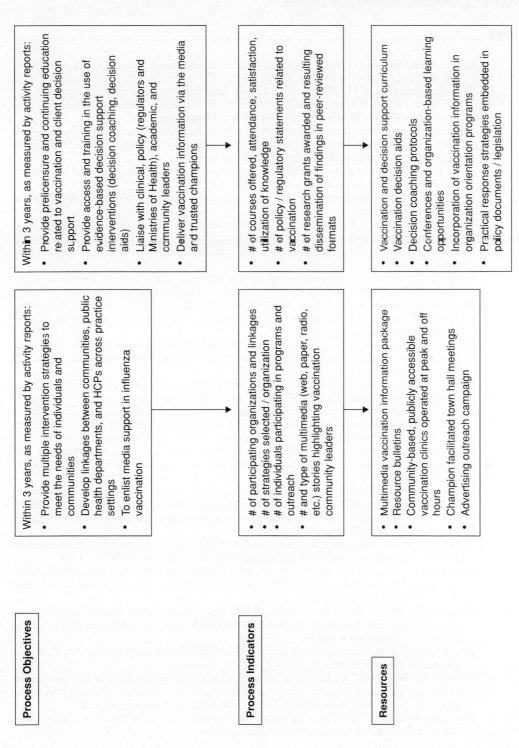

FIGURE 23-2 ◆ Vaccination Uptake Program Logic Model.

References

Begue, R., & Gee, S. (1998). Improving influenza immunization among health-care workers. *Infection Control and Hospital Epidemiology, 19*(7), 518–520.

Canadian Institutes of Health Research. (2005). Proceedings of the influenza research priorities workshop. Institute of Infection and Immunity (III). Retrieved August 8, 2006, from **http://www.cihr-irsc.gc.ca/e/30967.html#summary.**

Centers for Disease Control and Prevention. (2005). Key facts about avian influenza (Bird Flu) and Avian Influenza A (H5N1) Virus. Retrieved August 21, 2005, from **http://www.cdc.gov/flu/avian/gen-info/facts.htm.**

Chin, J. (2000). *Control of communicable diseases manual* (17th ed.). Washington, DC: American Public Health Association.

Diodati, C. (1999). *Immunization: History, ethics, law and health.* Windsor, ON: Integral Aspects Incorporated.

Engestrom, Y. (2000). Activity theory as a framework for analyzing and redesigning work. *Ergonomics, 43,* 960–974.

Gladwell, M. (2002). *The tipping point: How little things can make a big difference.* Boston: Little Brown.

Harbarth, S., Siegrist, C., Schira, J., et al. (1998). Influenza immunization: Improving compliance of health-care workers. *Infection Control and Hospital Epidemiology, 19*(5), 337–342.

Harden, A., Peersman, G., Oliver, S., Mauthner, M., & Oakley, A. (1999). A systematic review of the effectiveness of health promotion interventions in the workplace. *Occupational Medicine, 49*(8), 540–548.

Heimberger, T., Chang, H., Shaikh, M., et al. (1995). Knowledge and attitudes of health-care workers about influenza: Why are they not getting vaccinated? *Infectious Control and Hospital Epidemiology, 14,* 412–415.

Knobler, S., Mack, A., Mahmoud, A., et al. (2005). *The threat of pandemic influenza. Are we ready yet?* Washington, DC: The National Academies Press.

Leckie, N., Leonard, A., Turcotte, J., & Wallace, D. (2001). *Employer and employee perspectives on human resource practices.* The Evolving Workplace Series (Cat. No. 71-584-MPE No. 1). Ottawa: Statistics Canada and Human Resources Development Canada.

Macdonald, S., Csiernik, R., Durand, P., Rylett, M., & Wild, T. C. (2006). Prevalence and factors related to Canadian workplace health programs. *Canadian Journal of Public Health, 97*(2), 121–125.

National Advisory Committee on Immunization. (2002, August 1). Statement on influenza vaccination for the 2002-2003 season. Canada Communicable Disease Report, 28 (ACS-5). Retrieved August 21, 2006, from **http://www.phac-aspc.gc.ca/publicat/ccdr-rmtc/02vol28/28sup/acs5.html.**

National Advisory Committee for Immunization. (2006). Statement of influenza vaccination for the 2006-2007 season. *Canada Communicable Disease Report, 32*(AC-7), 1–28.

Oandasan, I., D'Aour, D., Zwarenstein, M., et al. (2004). *Interprofessional education for collaborative patient-centred practice research report: Environmental scan and systematic literature review.* Ottawa: Health Canada.

O'Rorke, C., Bourke, W., & Bedford, D. (2003). Uptake of influenza vaccine by health care workers in an acute hospital in Ireland. *Irish Medical Journal, 96*(7). Retrieved October 14, 2003, from **http://www.imj.ie**.

Orr, P. (2000). Influenza vaccination for health-care workers: A duty of care. *The Canadian Journal of Infectious Diseases, 11*(5), 1–5.

Pelly, L. A., McNeil, S. A., Halperin, B., et al. (2006, December). *Canada wide curriculum review and assessment of vaccine knowledge and attitudes among trainees in health professional programs.* Seventh Canadian Immunization Conference, Winnipeg, Canada.

Pierrynowski-Gallant, D. (2005). Influenza vaccination: A personal decision. Unpublished doctoral dissertation, University of Calgary, Alberta.

Pierrynowski-Gallant, D., & Robinson Vollman, A. (2004). Influenza vaccine choices. *The Canadian Nurse, 100*(2), 16–22.

Potter, J., Stott, D., & Roberts, M. (1997). Influenza vaccination of health-care workers in long term care hospitals reduces the mortality of elderly patients. *Journal of Infectious Diseases, 175,* 1–6.

Public Health Agency of Canada [PHAC]. (1997). Addressing concerns regarding immunization and vaccines. Canada Communicable Disease Report (CCDR), 2354. Available at: **www.phac-aspc.gc.ca/publicat/ccdr-rmtc/97vol23/2354/2354a-e.html.**

Public Health Agency of Canada. (2004). Canadian Pandemic Influenza Plan. Retrieved August 8, 2006, from **http://www.phac-aspc.gc.ca/cpip-pclcpi.**

Public Health Agency of Canada. (2005). Understanding influenza. Retrieved August 8, 2006, from **http://www.phac-aspc.gc.ca/influenza/influenza-undrstnd-e.html.**

Russell, M. (2001). Influenza vaccination in Alberta long term care facilities. *Canadian Medical Association Journal, 164*(10), 1423–1427.

Shain, M., & Suurvali, H. (2001). *Investing in comprehensive workplace health promotion* (p. 2). Toronto: National Quality Institute.

Shefer, A., Briss, P., Rodewald, L., et al. (1999). Improving immunization coverage rates: An evidence based review of the literature. *Epidemiological Review, 21*(1), 96–142.

Simonsen, L., Clarke, M., Schonberger, L., et al. (1998). Pandemic versus epidemic influenza mortality: A pattern of changing age distribution. *Journal of Infectious Diseases, 178,* 53–60.

Skowronski, D., Parker, R., & Strang, R. (2000). The importance of influenza immunization for health-care workers. *British Columbia Medical Journal, 42*(2), 91–93.

Squires, S., Macey, J., & Tam, T. (2001). Progress towards Canadian target coverage rates for influenza and pneumococcal immunization. *CCDR, 27*(10), 1–12.

Stevenson, C., McArthur, M., Naus, M., et al. (2001). Prevention of influenza and pneumococcal pneumonia in Canadian long term facilities: How are we doing? *Canadian Medical Association Journal, 164*(10), 1413–1419.

World Health Organization. (1986). *Ottawa Charter for Health Promotion.* Geneva, Switzerland: Author.

World Health Organization. (1999, February). Influenza (Fact Sheet No. 211). Retrieved July, 23, 2007, from **http://www.who.int/mediacentre/factsheets/fs211/en/index.html.**

Suggested Readings: Workplace Health

Dugdill, L., & Springett, J. (2001). Evaluating health promotion programmes in the workplace. In I. Rootman, M. Goodstadt, B. Hyndman, et al. (Eds.), *Evaluation in health promotion. Principles and perspectives* (pp. 285–308). WHO Regional Publications, European Series No. 92.

Duxbury, L., & Higgins, C. (2003). *Work-life conflict in Canada in the new millennium: A status report.* Prepared for Healthy Community Division, Health Canada.

Lowe, G. (2004). *Healthy workplace strategies: Creating change and achieving results.* Prepared for the Workplace Health Strategies Bureau, Health Canada.

The Health Communication Unit. (2004). *An introduction to comprehensive workplace health promotion.* Toronto: University of Toronto.

Internet Resources

http://www.thcu.ca/Workplace/Workplace.html
The Health Communication Unit, Workplace Health Promotion Project

www.nqi.ca
National Quality Institute

http://www.hc-sc.gc.ca/ewh-semt/pubs/occup-travail/work-travail/index_e.html
Health Canada—Workplace Health

http://www.ccohs.ca/
Canadian Centre for Occupational Health and Safety

www.canadian-health-network.ca
Canadian Health Network—Workplace Health

http://www.phac-aspc.gc.ca/fluwatch/index.html
FluWatch

http://www.phac-aspc.gc.ca/naci-ccni/index.html
National Advisory Committee on Immunization

http://www.acoem.org/guidelines.aspx?id=730
American College of Occupational and Environmental Medicine

24

Promoting the Health of Vulnerable Populations

JIM FRANKISH

CATHERINE M. SCOTT

WILFREDA E. THURSTON

Chapter Outline

Introduction

Working With Vulnerable Populations
in Urban Settings

Women's Perspectives on Poverty:
Photovoice as a Tool for Social
Change

Summary

Learning Objectives

After studying this chapter, you should be able to:

❖ Appreciate the basic nature of work with vulnerable groups

❖ Understand the use of quality-of-life data as a tool for assessment and community diagnosis

❖ Discuss how you would use this information as a foundation for developing and evaluating potential interventions with marginalized groups

❖ Discuss the links between participatory research processes and social capital

❖ Discuss the benefits and challenges of engaging in participatory research

Introduction

There is strong evidence that disparities in health quality of life are not equally distributed in Canadian society. Within Canadian cities, there are growing problems with homelessness and an increase in marginalized populations. Researchers, practitioners, and policy-makers are increasingly interested in working with vulnerable groups, including the poor and homeless, persons with disabilities, immigrants, seniors, and First Nations. These groups present special challenges and opportunities in work involving research, training, or capacity building.

493

The first part of this chapter presents a project with people who are homeless (and at risk) in Vancouver, British Columbia. This project used a case study design to guide the project. Case study designs are useful for work in a relatively unstudied area of inquiry (such as health literacy) where there is little literature; they offer rich descriptive information and can stimulate insights and hypotheses. A case study can be based on a mix of qualitative and quantitative methods and measures; the main limitation of a case study design is the difficulty in generalizing patterns to other populations and settings.

In the first case study, *Working With Vulnerable Populations in Urban Settings*, Frankish focuses on the assessment and community diagnosis components of the community-as-partner process (Fig. 12-4) and demonstrates how this information can inform the planning, implementation, and evaluation of relevant interventions with communities. A survey approach was used to collect quantitative information from people living in poverty in an inner-city context. This is an example of "assessment as intervention," since the participatory nature of the community assessment process had positive outcomes for the population of interest that built capacity for the next steps in the process.

In the second case study, *Women's Perspectives on Poverty: Photovoice as a Tool for Social Change*, Scott and Thurston tell of women living in poverty in an urban setting using a photographic story method to give voice to their experiences using a qualitative participatory process that is founded on a critical social perspective. The intervention is a roaming gallery exhibit that entertains artistically while informing the public about the experiences of women living in poverty with a view to increasing general awareness and influencing decision makers. In both cases, the authors underscore the importance of examining not only the barriers to health but also the assets and strengths inherent in the populations of interest that can be utilized when developing programs to address disparities.

WORKING WITH VULNERABLE POPULATIONS IN URBAN SETTINGS

One in five Canadians lives in low-income circumstances, and income inequality is increasing. Poverty is tied to poor health, activity limitations, and reduced access to services. Increased homelessness—'absolute' homelessness as well as persons at risk for homelessness—is manifesting in Canada as a tangible marker of poverty and related social and economic ills.

Homelessness is linked with substance use, mental illness, infections, and difficulty in accessing services (Chilvers, Macdonald & Hayes, 2002). A lack of safe, affordable housing leads to physical/mental health issues; negative health behaviours; and increased illness, injury, and disability (Frankish, Hwang & Quantz, 2005). These realities may result in greater use of hospital emergency services, shelters, supportive housing, and correctional institutions (Frankish, Moulton,

Quantz et al., 2005). Increasingly, clientele of these services are becoming more complex in their physical, social, and cultural needs. First Nations status, immigrants, refugees, and persons with mental illness are of particular concern. Insufficient information exists regarding the patterns and levels of use of social or health services in homeless (and at-risk) persons.

The literature linking homelessness, shelters, health, and quality of life is both limited and diverse. There is a growing literature on shelters and transitional housing to address homelessness. Shelters/supportive housing have a positive impact on mental health, physical health, and risk behaviours of clientele (Chilvers et al., 2002). They create a window of opportunity to intervene on behavioural issues (e.g., nutrition, medication management, substance use/abuse). Such facilities may also experience issues including tuberculosis, infections/infestations, and crime. Less is known about the quality of life of the homeless.

Assessment

Our project focuses on a marginalized, vulnerable population—homeless and at-risk clients in the facilities of the Lookout Emergency Aid Society (Lookout) in Vancouver, BC. Lookout operates three shelters, transitional housing, and longer-term supportive housing to provide housing and services to homeless adults. Typical clients are poor with mental illness, addictions, and health issues (e.g., HIV/AIDS).

Our approach to community assessment and diagnosis was grounded in the use of a participatory research philosophy and approach. Seminal work undertaken by our team has defined *participatory research* as "systematic inquiry with the collaboration of those affected by the issue being studied for purposes of education and taking action or effecting social change" (Green et al., 1995). It seems logical from both a philosophical and methodological viewpoint to employ a participatory stance in research with vulnerable populations. Participatory research is not a specific method or design for research that replaces other methods. Used with other methods, it helps make research questions more relevant to the community, methods more acceptable, and results more meaningful. Each activity (and stage in the model) would be developed, implemented, and evaluated using a collaborative approach, with community partners playing an integral role in all aspects. Its purpose is threefold: to create knowledge, to increase community capacity (Kwan, Frankish & Quantz et al., 2003), and to produce meaningful change. The participatory approach incorporated the knowledge of community participants in the planning and implementation of data collection and in the evaluation of results. The research facilitated learning among community participants about resources for participation in health decisions.

For our project research, students at the University of British Columbia (UBC) who were involved in community-service learning collected the data. Community-service learning is intended to engage university students in community-based activities that foster and maintain the creation of healthy communities and a more civil society. Our community assessment involved a brief, face-to-face survey that had demographic information, Likert-type questions (possible responses ranged from 1 = Strongly Disagree, 2 = Disagree, 3 = Agree, and 4 = Strongly Agree), fill-in-the-blanks, and open-ended questions. It asked participants about their experiences at Lookout, relations with staff, perceptions of facilities, the neighbourhood, perceived health, and quality of life. The UBC Behavioural Research Ethics Board approved the procedures.

Our data were evenly drawn from six of Lookout's facilities. Seventy-three residents/attendees participated in the surveys. They ranged in age from 23 to 83 years, with an average age of 46 years, and 78% were male. Participants had been in the area for an average of 9 years and thus represented a relatively stable community. The majority were Caucasian (74%), with the remainder from diverse ethnic (8%) and First Nations (8%) backgrounds. Not surprisingly, 88% were on social assistance/disability.

Responses to each question were listed and then sorted in general categories. The first question asked, *Just before coming to [Lookout], where did you live?* Sixty people reported living in Greater Vancouver. Twelve people were from other parts of Canada, and one was from Israel. Six people mentioned coming from prison.

The top two or three things *that were most liked about the staff* were that they were friendly, helpful, available, respectful, and competent. Several people highlighted their perception that the staff generally treated all residents in an equitable manner. The top two or three things that were *least liked about the staff* were food service, noise problems, and occasional lack of availability. The majority of participants reported no significant problems with staff.

Survey participants were asked, *Have you participated on the residence advisory committee? If not, why?* The reasons for not participating included the following: too busy, not informed, and don't like volunteering. The *top two or three things most liked about the facility* were safety, quiet, security, staff and people, food, and location. The *top two or three things least liked about the facilities* were noise, substance abusers, and security rules. The majority of participants reported no problems with the facilities. Participants were provided an opportunity to identify activities that they wished to see. The most common responses were games, community outings, and skills training.

The *top two or three things most liked about the neighbourhood* were accessibility, people, convenience, and acceptance. The *top two or three things least liked about the neighbourhood* were drug users, crime, and violence. Respondents were asked if they could change *one or two things in the neighbourhood, what would they be?* Common responses included get rid of drugs/crime, more housing, aesthetics (i.e., flowers, parks), and more drop-in facilities.

Most participants expressed a strong desire to stay at a Lookout facility for an extended period. In parallel, they expressed a strong desire for greater independence. Respondents were very diverse in their perceived *readiness* to move to independent housing. Many expressed a level of uncertainty about such a move. A significant number said that they were happy where they were. For those who wished to move, the two most common choices were a personal apartment or supportive housing. Participants were asked *how do you typically spend your day?* and *what kinds of things do you do?* Common responses were visiting friends, watching TV, looking for jobs, and going out in the community.

Finally, participants were asked, *in what ways has your health changed since being at [Lookout]?* The most common responses were feeling calmer, management of medications and health problems, better routine (food), and feeling cleaner.

Analysis

Lookout delivers a variety of services/programs to its clients. It is challenged by funders and policy-makers to be accountable for a wide range of health, social, and quality-of-life–related outcomes. Our assessment provided self-report data on perceptions of staff, facilities, neighbourhoods, participation in activities, and health/quality of life. We recognize that the exploratory questions, the sample size, and self-report all suggest caution in interpreting the meaning or generalizability of our findings to other settings. Within these limitations, our assessment is intended to provide a foundation for future program and policy interventions. Aggregated information will be provided to Lookout staff and residents, and together we will work with them to formulate diagnoses that they as a community agree are meaningful. Then, once consensus has been achieved and priorities have been set, we will work with them to plan actions to meet their desired goals.

We adapted the Precede-Proceed model (Green & Kreuter, 2004) as a foundation framework for analysis and the application of the results of our assessment to planning. The Precede model grows out of the science and practice of health promotion. Often applied to health behaviours at an individual level, the model performs equally well in group- or community-type situations and is an excellent framework around which to organize policies and programs with vulnerable groups. The model can be used to describe the practice of homelessness research. The outcomes of interest are more effective homelessness policies, programs, and practices.

Planning

Our planning processes were grounded in a basic logic model founded on the broader Precede model. We recognized that underlying each program is a set of assumptions regarding how the program works and what its impact(s) will be. These assumptions form a "logic model." Our project logic model had three assumptions: The first is that shelters do not work in a vacuum; all work/activities take place in a societal environment. Second, the model flows from inputs to activities to outputs to impacts to outcomes. Third, the effects of shelter programs and activities can manifest at different levels including *intraindividual*, *interindividual*, *organizational*, and *structural* effects.

The success (or failure) of a program, services, or activity can be judged by monitoring indicators of *success*. Each shelter must state how it will define *success*, that is, what measures it will track *and* where it will *"set the bar"* (i.e., what *standards* it will use to decide if a given level of *success* is a worthy return on its investment of resources).

It is specific, observable, and measurable change that shows a program is making progress toward achieving specified outcomes.

This project focused mainly on the assessment and analysis/diagnosis aspects of the community-as-partner model. The following information provides an example of how diagnostic information can inform planning, intervention(s), and evaluation. In keeping with the Precede-Proceed approach, we focused largely on what we term *antecedents*. We define *antecedents* as the "things that people bring to the table." They include age, sex, education, culture, health status, and the like. The antecedents may manifest at intraindividual, interindividual, organizational, and structural levels. They can be measured to provide a *baseline*—a preprogram measurement of important variables that can be tracked over time.

Subsequent stages of our adapted logic model were also examined:

◆ *Inputs.* The fiscal, human, and/or infrastructure resources that go into a shelter's programs or activities.
◆ *Programs or activities.* The work done by a shelter (*what/how* things are done, not their effects).
◆ *Outputs.* Immediate, short-term products of activities.
◆ *Impacts.* Direct (and possibly indirect) intermediate effects of activities on individuals (e.g., improved knowledge, attitudes, behaviours) and their relations with others. Impacts also include changes in the organizational and/or broader structural (societal) environment and may comprise changes in policies, procedures, and resource allocations.
◆ *Outcomes.* The direct (possibly indirect) long-term effects of activities on individuals (e.g., changes in health status, morbidity, mortality) and their long-term, sustained relations with others. They include also long-term, sustained changes in the organizational/societal environment (i.e., enduring changes in policies, procedures, resources).

Over the long term, the assessment/diagnostic data from the project will be used to inform the *outcomes* of programs and policies. In this project, we examined what the clients at Lookout's facilities brought to the table and what their perceptions and expectations were of Lookout's services and programs.

Assessment as Intervention

We conducted our project with a marginalized, vulnerable population—homeless and at-risk adults in Vancouver, BC. Our findings from a sample of people using Lookout's facilities suggest a stable community and highlight a need for more research on the mobility/migration of the homeless. Similar American research also suggests that the homeless population is not homogenous; our work indicates a need for more research with other groups in Canada.

Further, our assessment results note that the Lookout facilities and staff were seen as offering a highly supportive and valuable set of services, suggesting that it is possible to staff shelters and supportive housing facilities with competent, caring staff. Other research shows that such facilities are also reasonably inexpensive to operate. On the other hand, our project showed that many clients are not actively engaged in facility-related (or outside) activities and that much more work remains to more fully engage and challenge the population to participate in activities that can have an effect on their quality of life.

Our final set of questions provided useful and interesting data on participants' self-reported quality of life. Most agreed that their physical health, happiness, life satisfaction, and sense of independence had improved since being at Lookout. Participants reported feeling calmer, having better management of medications, fewer health problems, and better daily routines (food, personal hygiene). Our results point to strengths on which to build stronger programs and policies. There is a caution, however, in that a significant portion of the sample (20% to 25%) reported experiencing more difficulties; reported self-care was diverse and warrants further investigation.

It is encouraging that 80% of survey respondents reported greater life satisfaction. The other 20%, however, requires attention and probably represents a segment of the homeless population that is harder to reach and harder to support or treat. Finally, it is positive that the rating of overall health had a mean and mode (n = 12) of 7.0 out of 10. This result was somewhat of a surprise and may seem counterintuitive given the self-evident health, social, and economic issues associated with homelessness. While we take the result with caution, we also take it as a testament to the aspirations and hope of our sample respondents.

The above assessment information was presented to Lookout staff and service providers. It informs the potential refinement of current programs, policies, and practices with the target community of vulnerable homeless (and at-risk) individuals.

Evaluation

Taken together, the assessment suggests that shelter/supportive housing can have a positive impact on the mental/physical health, social relations, and quality of life of a highly vulnerable population. The extent and durability of such benefits remains to be more fully documented. However, strong anecdotal evidence, common sense, and reports from front-line service providers support the positive tenor of our findings.

Overall, our approach was successful and would not require major changes for future use. Several possible lessons were learned in the process. First, we learned that there is a need for a diversity of recruitment strategies in work with vulnerable groups. Not all individuals are equally predisposed or motivated to take part in assessment research. Second, there is an equal need for use of strategies that *enable* vulnerable groups to take part in a meaningful way in community-based research. We learned that although opportunities to take part in project research may be *available*, they may not be *accessible*. Accessibility to participation in research may manifest in psychological, social, economic, cultural, and geographic aspects. For example, the location of our data collection mattered, as did the ways in which the research was explained and presented. Third, we learned that there must be an appropriate, proportional incentive, reward, or pay-off for vulnerable individuals who take part in this form of project research. There is an important ethical-practical tension in the provision of any incentives; they should not be coercive and should be proportional to the work involved.

Project Summary

Health is created and lived by people within the settings of their everyday life, where they live, learn, work, play, pray, and love. Health is created by caring for oneself and others, by being able to make decisions and have control over one's life circumstances, and by ensuring that the society one lives in creates conditions that allow the attainment of health by all its members. This suggests that clients, community partners, and Lookout staff alike should be involved in each phase of the planning, implementation, and evaluation of any new services or programs (Judd, Frankish & Moulton, 2001). They should also have a fundamental role in any research on Lookout's programs or services.

Policy-makers, health professionals, and service providers should be supported in their efforts to design, implement, and evaluate services like those offered by the Lookout Emergency Aid Society. In keeping with Ottawa Charter for Health Promotion (World Health Organization, 1986), these services would develop clients' personal skills, create supportive environments for health, strengthen community action, and potentially reorient health services. It is clear that much remains to be done in meeting the needs of vulnerable groups.

From this project, we learned several important points. The use of a community diagnosis (as described in the community-as-partner model) provided the opportunity to collect important information and insights into the perceptions and experiences of a marginalized population. When properly supported, participants were able to provide useful data regarding their experiences and factors affecting their self-reported quality of life. This data fit well with a background planning model (Precede) and a logic model that flowed from inputs to activities to outputs to impacts and to outcomes.

Community-based health promotion, like that in our project, often emphasizes elements of empowerment, participation, multidisciplinary collaboration, capacity-building, and equity. The emphasis of our project on *community* diagnosis may be viewed as being in opposition with equally powerful notions of evidence-based decision-making and accountability. These tensions may be fuelled when community practitioners and lay participants feel that researchers and policy-makers do not appreciate the uniqueness of their community and their inherent abilities to report in practical and useful ways on their experiences.

Our project suggests that community participants can identify useful 'objects of interest' (i.e., foci for evaluation). Our work also highlights the fact that no research is value-neutral; it supports the need for a clear, values-based stance for health promotion that promotes a salutogenic, health-enhancing orientation as a foundation for evaluation of community-based health promotion. Policy-makers and funders must be more supportive of evaluation designs that fit with community realities;

community stakeholders are more capable of, and consistent in, evaluating community-based health promotion programs and policies.

While there is an evident need for more research, we end by quoting Sir Austin Bradford Hill (1965) who said, "*Incomplete scientific evidence does give us the freedom to ignore the knowledge we already have, or to postpone the action that it demands.*" Our project focuses on homelessness—a social and health phenomenon that is rapidly becoming a national Canadian embarrassment. It is an embarrassment that demands immediate and substantial action by all levels of government and all sectors of Canadian society.

WOMEN'S PERSPECTIVES ON POVERTY: PHOTOVOICE AS A TOOL FOR SOCIAL CHANGE

Context and Background

In the late 1990s, seeds were sown for the Women's Perspectives on Poverty project. In 1998 and 1999, the Calgary Status of Women Action Committee conducted focus groups with women living in poverty in southern Alberta. The report generated from that work, *Watering Down the Milk: Women Coping on Alberta's Minimum Wage* (Calgary Status of Women Action Committee [CSWAC], 1999), clearly described the extreme circumstances of women living on the lowest minimum wage in Canada in the wealthiest province in the country. In 2002, a small group of women who had been involved in the *Watering Down the Milk* project decided that it was time to update the report. We wanted to see if life had improved for low-income women in the intervening years given the Alberta government's gradual increase in the minimum wage and other changes in social assistance projects.

Action Process

In early 2003, we formed the Women and a Fair Income Working Group, which comprised women who were living in poverty, community agency representatives, City social workers, and university researchers.[1] At the second meeting, women who were living in poverty said quite clearly that they did not want to write another report that would gather dust on a shelf. They wanted to do something that gave their experiences more voice, something that would have an impact on people who knew nothing about poverty. The idea of photovoice as a research tool was presented to the group and accepted with enthusiasm. (More detail on this method is located in Chapter 19.)

---

[1] We would like to acknowledge all members of the Women and a Fair Income Working Group. Current members: Joan Farkas, Susan Gillies, Fan Guindon, Beryl Kootenay, Lynda Laughlin, Donna McPhee, Maggie Pompeo, Cathie Scott, Wilfreda Thurston, and Erica Welsh. Past members: Julie Black, Lisa Lorenzetti, Lillian Parent, Pam Parry, Pascal Ujuok, and Patricia Vanbeselaere.

Members of the Working Group went out into their communities to recruit women to participate in the project. In the summer of 2003, we held two training sessions, during which 12 women were trained in photographic techniques by a professional photographer and were engaged in discussions of ethics. Over a 3-month period, photographers took pictures to assist in developing and analyzing the impact of living on low income. Together, we reviewed the pictures, related the stories behind the images, analyzed their meaning, and created a powerful advocacy tool. Initially, we thought that we would do a comprehensive thematic analysis of the stories, but we soon realized that the power of the voice was diminished when it was removed from the overall story of the photographer. While common themes cut across the pictures (e.g., housing and homelessness, lack of nutritious food, health, childhood development), when on display, the pictures and stories remain grouped by photographer. Since that time, we have acquired funding to mount the photographs in a gallery-ready format and take the exhibit on the road. Each time the exhibit travels to outlying communities, Working Group members work with community representatives to engage the broader community in the development of action strategies against poverty. Wherever the exhibit travels, there is always at least one photographer present. Three of the photographers, in collaboration with the Working Group, developed a report that is available from the website **www.fp.ucalgary.ca/wafi**. Working Group members have also developed a popular education tool that uses pictures, stories, and statistics to combat myths about poverty. Since 2003, the photographs have been on display at numerous community sites, conference venues, and university classes.

Making Space for Voices

Every woman has a story. Too few have a safe place to tell it. (Laughlin, 2004)

The above quote is on the cover of our report and reflects the wisdom of one of the members of the group. One of the explicit purposes of our project was to give women who were living in poverty a safe place to talk. To a certain extent we managed to do this, but it was not always the case. The photographers were able to take pictures that conveyed some of their experiences, but at times, they hesitated to tell too much of their stories. One section of the report speaks of pictures that were not taken and the stories that were not told, "For many of us, the picture we wanted to take would have put someone at risk of embarrassment, harassment or loss of support" (WAFI, 2004, p. 4). Despite the gaps, the stories that were told present insights into the lives of women who are living in poverty, exposing aspects of poverty that have, out of shame, been kept secret and often hidden. The photographers who were members of the Working Group have been active participants in the design, implementation, and dissemination of the project. At least one of the photographers is actively involved in presenting each time the exhibit travels to a new community or venue. Over the past 2 years, photographers have responded to requests for information about the project and have spoken openly about their experiences of living in poverty and their experiences with the project.

A recent comment by one of the photographers when speaking to a university class exemplifies the impact that this work has had. When the class thanked her for sharing her perspectives with them, she said, "If it hadn't been for this project I would not be here. Two years ago, I would not have had the confidence to speak in public and I would have continued to wonder whether anyone cared about my poverty. Now I know there are many people who care. I also know that there are many people who are living on the edge like me—this isn't an isolated experience. I know I have to speak out." This sentiment is reiterated in the report, "We say it's time to come forward as people who live in our shared community and who deserve human rights and quality of life" (WAFI, 2004, p. 4).

Multiple Constituencies

Members of the Working Group shared a common passion for the project; we were committed to raising public awareness about realities of living in poverty and advocating for social change to reduce poverty. Despite this commitment, it was unrealistic to assume that there would be no conflict among a diverse group of women working across multiple constituencies. We anticipated some areas of potential conflict [e.g., tensions associated with differing needs of university-based researchers and community agency representatives (Seifer & Calleson, 2004; Stoecker, 2002); power differences that could arise between people with access to resources (i.e., professionals and researchers) and those who had limited access (i.e., women who were living in poverty)], but we had limited discussion of strategies to address such conflicts should they arise.

Naively, we did not anticipate conflict among the Working Group members to the extent that it would undermine the project. We assumed that a common experience of poverty for some members of the group and a common passion for social action against poverty would be enough to overcome such obstacles. This assumption proved to be detrimental to the project, as dealing with conflicts among the photographers, among the professionals, and between professionals and women living in poverty required unanticipated expenditure of resources of time and emotional energy. Some of us had worked together before, and we wrongly made many assumptions about the ease of working together again. We made assumptions about the type of communication and governance strategies that would work in this context.

In order to compensate photographers for their unique skills and expertise, honoraria were allotted for attendance at meetings. Photographers also earned $10 per hour for their time at public presentations and workshops. Despite this, there remained pay inequities among members of the group, (i.e., the hourly wages paid to the professional members of the Working Group were greater than the hourly rate allowed through funding agencies). While we were able to advocate for more compensation for the photographers than was typically granted through such programs, pay inequities remained. Some members felt that the differences in compensation between professionals and photographers contributed to the ongoing power issues that we faced.

Challenges and Impacts

From the outset, our aims had been to promote public dialogue and engage decision-makers. At the end of the first year, we had accomplished this to a limited extent. There was energy and commitment within the group to do more, but our original grant of $5,000 could not be stretched much further. As support began to grow and funding applications were successful, it became difficult to envision an end to the project. When asked, members of the Working Group continued to support taking next steps to share the project results, but in reality, there were fissures among members, and it was difficult to sustain the effort required to engage in all of the activities. It was at this point that some of the funding was used to hire a part-time project coordinator, and this position has continued to be funded.

The project faced several challenges: membership, roles and status, trust and control, and conflict resolution. Membership issues included confusion about who were members of the Working Group and the status of members within the group. Some women who had taken photos were interested in remaining involved in decision making regarding the next stages of the project. Some of the Working Group members preferred to keep the group to its original number while others did not. Without design, the Working Group has remained small; erosion of personal relationships between photographers resulted in one person withdrawing from the Working Group, and other photographers could not continue the commitment due to time constraints.

Within the Working Group, there was confusion also around roles and status. The four who began to talk about the project assumed that we would implement joint leadership structure with the women who were living in poverty, but this was not specifically discussed. Professionals within the group made explicit efforts to avoid the appearance of taking control or leading, but institutionalized relationships of professional "power over" were not so easily overcome; members of the group who were living in poverty initially expected professionals to take control. It was quite some time before there was sufficient trust among all Working Group members to permit a rotating chair system to work. Hesitancy about taking control was a characteristic of the early stages of the project when processes and activities were still evolving. More recently, meetings have become more focused on the accomplishment of set tasks, and processes have become more directive with all members of the Working Group taking leadership roles related to different tasks. From that point on, meetings were chaired on a rotating basis, and minutes were taken by different people most of the time. Frustrations also arose from instituting consensus decision making without critical reflection regarding when, and if, such processes were appropriate.

Negotiation of roles and multiple constructions of power required ongoing attention to formal and informal communication strategies. Tensions related to communication took many forms. Photovoice is based on the premise that photographers will find a safe place to talk about their stories. While this was true for our group, it was unrealistic to expect that we could create a climate in which full disclosure could take place. Photographers openly talked about fear of loss of income support if information shared in meetings was shared with providers of social support and fear of sharing personal information with other photographers. Methods of communication also proved to be a challenge. The academics and agency people preferred to use e-mail for some types of communication (e.g., convening meetings, updates regarding progress), whereas the majority of the photographers did not have regular access to e-mail. Differing styles of communication were quite evident at the face-to-face meetings. Some members of the Working Group were more comfortable with consensus processes, while others preferred more directive strategies. When conflict arose during meetings, it was not always handled well. At one point, we had a facilitator assist with working through communication issues, focusing explicitly on how we deal with power and conflict.

Based on this description, it might appear that this project was not a success. This is not the case. All members of the Working Group continue to play an active role and continue to talk openly of the incredible achievements that we have made. Perhaps one of the major things that we have all learned is that creating supportive communities requires that all participants acknowledge conflict and its resolution as a fundamental characteristic of successful collaboration.

Project Summary

Creating environments in which women living in poverty can give voice to their frustrations, challenges, and triumphs is not simple and requires ongoing negotiation. Engaging in participatory, community-based research means that all of the people who participate make a long-term commitment to one another and to the goals that they jointly set. In Chapter 4, Table 4-1, the phases (i.e., developing the vision, identifying potential participants, understanding context, developing ground rules, obtaining commitment, implementing, maintaining, and winding down) and associated considerations for a participatory project such as this were outlined. Listing these phases as we have greatly oversimplifies the complexity of the process. Through this case description, we have attempted to provide a more detailed picture of how community-based participatory projects evolve and succeed.

Many of the women who participated in this project were well versed in the art of handling disappointment, and I believe that they entered the project with low expectations of what we could achieve as a group. As time passed and we were able to create a space where we trusted one another, the power of the group was phenomenal and the achievements were monumental. For a short time, this small group of women worked together to draw attention to the injustice of poverty and to dispel myths that constrain their lives.

SUMMARY

The Ottawa Charter (WHO, 1986) calls for the participation of the public, specifically those people/communities toward which interventions are directed, if we hope to build capacity, enable empowerment, and enhance the potential for sucessful interventions. Regardless of the apparent lack of capacity and/or interest of the population, those working in communities must recognize the moral imperative to work also *with* the members of those communities. The two examples detailed in this chapter indicate that the effort to overcome the inherent challenges are indeed worthwhile.

ACKNOWLEDGMENTS

The Photovoice case described in this chapter was a participatory research project. I would like to thank all members of the Women and a Fair Income Working Group for making this project the success that it was. I would also like to thank Dr. Anne Hofmeyer for her insightful feedback and for helping us to strengthen the discussion of social capital.

References

Calgary Status of Women Action Committee (CSWAC). (1999). *Watering down the milk: Women coping on Alberta's minimum wage*. Calgary, AB. Available: www.fp.ucalgary.ca/waf.

Chilvers, R., Macdonald, G., & Hayes, A. (2002). Supported housing for people with severe mental disorders. *Cochrane Database of Systematic Reviews*, (2), CD000453.

Frankish, J., Hwang, S., & Quantz, D. (2005). Synthesis paper: Lessons in the prevention and treatment of homelessness in Canada. *Canadian Journal of Public Health, 96*, S23–S30.

Frankish, J., Moulton, G., Quantz, D., Carson, A. J., Casebeer, A. L., Eyles, J. D., et al. (2007). Addressing the non-medical determinants of health: A survey of Canada's health regions. *Canadian Journal of Public Health 98*(1), 41–47.

Green, L., & Kreuter, M. (2004). *Health program planning: An educational and ecological approach*. New York: McGraw-Hill.

Green, L., George, A., Daniel, M., et al. (1995). *Participatory research in health promotion*. Ottawa: Royal Society of Canada.

Hill, A. (1965). The environment and disease: Association or causation? *Proceedings of the Royal Society of Medicine, 58*, 295–300.

Judd, J., Frankish, J., & Moulton, G. (2001). A unifying approach to setting standards in the evaluation of community-based health promotion programs. *Health Promotion International, 16*(4), 367–380.

Kwan, B., Frankish, J., Quantz, D., et al. (2003). *A synthesis paper on the conceptualization and measurement of community capacity*. Report to Health Policy Research Program, Health Canada.

Laughlin, L. (2004). Personal communication. Cited in *Women's perspectives on poverty: Photos and stories by women on low income in Calgary*. Calgary, AB: Women and a Fair Income Working Group.

Seifer, S., & Calleson, D. (2004). Health professional faculty perspectives on community-based research: Implications for policy and practice. *Journal of Interprofessional Care, 18*(4), 416–427.

Stoecker, R. (2002). Practices and challenges of community-based research. *Journal of Public Affairs Supplement*, *1*(6), 219–239.

WAFI. (2004). *Women's perspectives on poverty: Photos and stories by women on low income in Calgary*. Calgary, AB: Women and a Fair Income Working Group.

World Health Organization. (1986). *Ottawa Charter for Health Promotion*. Ottawa, Canada: Author.

Suggested Readings

Frankish, J., Green, L., Ratner, P., et al. (1996). Health impact assessment as a tool for healthy public policy. WHO Series on Evaluating Health Promotion. Geneva: WHO.

Frankish, J., Kwan, B., Larsen, C., et al. (2002). Challenges of community participation in health-system decision making. *Social Science and Medicine*, *54*(10), 1471–1480.

Frankish, J., Larsen, C., Ratner, P., et al. (2002). Social and political factors influencing the functioning of regional health boards in British Columbia (Canada). *Health Policy*, *61*(2), 125–151.

Hwang, S. (2001). Homelessness and health. *Canadian Medical Association Journal*, *164*(2), 229–233.

Internet Resources

http://policyresearch.gc.ca/page.asp?pagenm=v7n2_art_09
Research Brief: Canada's Working Poor, Social Development Canada

http://www.toronto.ca/socialservices/pdf/singleparentsurvey.pdf
Social Assistance and Social Exclusion, Toronto Community and Neighbourhood Services

http://www.cdnwomen.org/eng/3/3i.asp
Canadian Women's Foundation

http://www.swc-cfc.gc.ca/pubs/pubspr/0662281594/index_e.html
The Dynamics of Women's Poverty in Canada

http://www.hc-sc.gc.ca/dc-ma/aids-sida/index_e.html
HIV and AIDS in Canada

http://www.leadingtogether.ca/602_act.html
Leading Together: Canada Takes Action on HIV/AIDS

http://pubs.cpha.ca/PDF/P14/20673.pdf
Social Marketing for Health

http://www.cmaj.ca/cgi/reprint/164/2/214
Commentary: Inner City Health

25

Using Technology to Promote the Health of Homebound Seniors

ANTONIA ARNAERT

Chapter Outline

Introduction
Background
TELESENIOR: A Tele-Homecare Project

Evaluation
Lessons Learned
Summary

Learning Objectives

After studying this chapter, you should be able to:

❖ Appreciate the challenges facing homebound senior citizens

❖ Describe the use of e-health technology with a vulnerable population

Introduction

As early as 1992, the European Union sponsored the RACE (Research and Development of Advanced Communications in Europe) TeleCommunity program with the aim of using video-telephony (VT) in the care and support of elderly people and people with disabilities in their own homes or within the community. This chapter presents a tele-homecare project in Belgium, called TELESENIOR, a part of the RACE TeleCommunity program. The project was a joint community-oriented initiative by the city of Kortrijk and its municipal welfare centre, the cable-television company, and the nonprofit organization Open Net. The aim of this project was to investigate to what degree elderly people at home can be helped and supported by means of individual video-communication, to what extent health and social care services can be delivered through VT, and to identify the characteristics of groups of homebound elderly whose functioning would significantly improve following tele-nursing care. TELESENIOR involved a group of dedicated community members who sincerely wanted to improve the health and quality of life of the elderly via the delivery of tailored, holistic tele-nursing care.

BACKGROUND

As people age, accumulated and continuing changes and losses occur in health, emotional, mental, social, and functional status. Without appropriate care and support, the interactions of these multiple aspects place elderly people at risk for adverse health outcomes, including mortality, falls, institutionalization, and hospitalization (Fried et al., 2001). Caring for the elderly with complex needs continues to be a challenge for health care systems. In recent years, health policies have promoted community-based care, as it offers the prospect of considering cost savings as well as improved care (Johri, Béland, & Bergman, 2003). The home space is arguably the most important site for the provision of community services, as most elderly people hope to live at home for as long as possible. This requires that health and social care programs be "client-centred" and respond to the needs and preferences of the care recipients in a holistic way (Chapman, Keating, & Eales, 2003). However, these services are still fragmented; various health providers are involved, with little apparent coordination. Some health care reform initiatives in geriatric care, such as a single entry-point system with case management, have been implemented successfully (Johri et al., 2003). However, the challenge remains to develop complementary evidence-based models of integrated care that provide tailored care and better health outcomes for the homebound elderly (Shaul, 2000).

Increasingly, multiple forms of technologies are being used to deliver health care to patients in their home. The availability of health care when needed is one of the key benefits of *tele-homecare*, which has been defined as the use of information, communications, measurement, and monitoring technologies to evaluate health status and deliver health care from a distance to patients at home (Celler, Lovell, & Chan, 1999). Tele-homecare trials for the elderly have shown that the delivery of interventions focused on monitoring, teaching, communication, support, and care improve their health, autonomy, and quality of life (Bowles & Dansky, 2002; Savenstedt, Zingmark, & Sandman, 2003). The tele-care delivery model makes it feasible, through the deployment of telecommunication networks, to target packages of care in response to assessed needs. It would promote the delivery of targeted health and social services and improve cost control, which is of interest to governments everywhere. Young (2003) believes that the efficacy of community services has been hard to demonstrate due to lack of targeting, which dilutes the effect of the interventions over a broad and diverse elderly population. Identifying groups of elderly at particular risk for certain outcomes is an important step in addressing their needs, expectations, and preferences. Developing a better profile of the characteristics of the homebound elderly will assist in developing strategies that personalize treatment at the point of care and improve health outcomes.

TELESENIOR: A TELE-HOMECARE PROJECT

Description

The concept "video-telephone" has been used to refer to an audio-visual technological tool for interactive, real time, interpersonal communication. The tele-service centre, located in one of the residential homes of the public welfare centre of Kortrijk, was set up in a region with about 74,601 residents of whom 20% were older than 65 years. It was served by a cable-television network that serviced up to 95% of the homes in the area. The centre was equipped with a VT, document camera, public switched telephone network (PSTN) alarm centre, and line adapter unit connected to a maximum of three telephone lines (Fig. 25-1). The unit allowed the tele-nurse to switch the voice connection among three simultaneous calls, based on urgency. Audio and video signals were transmitted bidirectionally using a PSTN channel and an analog broadcast television channel.

Clients were able to use four services—VT, telephone, television, and alarm system—with one integrated terminal consisting of a PSTN alarm station, telephone, television, colour camera, and necklace transmitter with four buttons. It had the following functions: A = *Make a call to the tele-service centre;* E = *View your own image on the television screen;* C = *Switch on the camera;* U = *Disconnect the VT call* (Fig. 25-2). The system was set up in such a way that it was only the client who could decide to transmit his or her picture, by using the control necklace. In case of a normal call, the client could preview what his or her picture would look like before transmitting it to the service centre. In case of emergency, the client could pull the necklace transmitter to switch on the camera automatically. The camera,

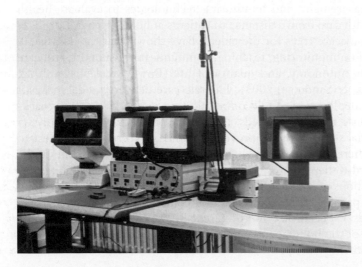

FIGURE 25-1 ◆ The centre was equipped with a VT, a document camera, a PSTN alarm centre, and a line adapter unit connected to a maximum of three telephone lines.

FIGURE 25-2 ◆ A necklace transmitter with four buttons had the following functions: A = *Make a call to the tele-service centre;* E = *View your own image on the television screen;* C = *Switch on the camera;* U = *Disconnect the VT call.*

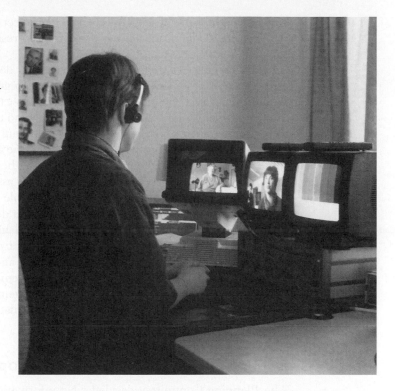

which could be covered for privacy if so desired, gave the tele-nurse a moderately wide-angle view of the client sitting in his or her preferred position for television viewing. Every client participated without any obligation or fee. During the project, the equipment and VT communications were free. Some clients received additional benefits: an updated television set and a free telephone or a television cable connection. Finally, each client paid only 50% for all the telephone and cable television services beyond the limits of the VT project. The tele-nurses delivered psychosocial support and educational interventions, which were based on three principles: contact and communication, safety and protection, and care mediation.

Building Participatory Relationships

About a year before project implementation, a Steering Committee, comprising stakeholders of key agencies representing various interests in this VT project and the project coordinator, had been convened to guide the strategic planning of TELESENIOR. The financial accountability, part of the strategic planning, also rested with the Steering Committee. It provided ongoing, wide-based support to the Planning Committee, an interprofessional core group of community workers employed by the public welfare centre. The project evaluator was also a member of the Planning Committee since a project-based research model was used, making research an integral part of the project.

The Planning Committee was responsible for designing and organizing the VT nursing services. At the outset, it was critical to generate enthusiasm and energy around the project, as some common constraints existed among the group of community workers, such as a lack of staff, money, and time. Actually, these constraints were used to develop a well-thought-out "community-focused plan" with goals and concrete steps for action. As part of the plan, the Planning Committee discussed some process and related outcome objectives in their monthly meetings. Examples of process issues were how to conduct a needs assessment, how to organize the opening hours of the centre, how to define the role of the nurses as case-managers, how to recruit potential clients, when to set up a demonstration site, how to publicize the project, and when to have the official launch. The Planning Committee also recruited, at the start of the planning stage, two community nurses with professional experience in the field of elderly care and basic know-how in handling computer technology to provide the VT interventions. These nurses were given 2 days of training, by the Communication Management Department of a local high school, to become familiar with VT (e.g., articulation, face and voice expression, speed of speech, clothing, etc).

Needs Assessment: Discovering the Elderly Population

The Planning Committee decided *what* information was needed from our "core people" to meet the objectives and *how* it would be collected. Approximately 6 months before the start of the project, they developed a questionnaire to collect data from all potential clients (n = 88) about their use of support services from lay and professional caregivers. Additional demographic data on age, sex, level of education, marital status, and family situation were also collected. The social worker, a member of the Planning Committee, collected the information during his regular home visits. A summary is provided in Table 25-1.

During the project, client functioning was measured on three dates at 6-month intervals, using eight reliable and valid assessment scales selected from the literature: Loneliness Scale (de Jong-Gierveld & Kamphuis, 1985), Geriatric Depression Scale SF-15 (Burke, Roccaforta, & Wengel, 1991), Lubben Social Network Scale (Lubben, 1998), Activities of Daily Living (Katz & Apkom, 1976), Instrumental Activities of Daily Living (Lawton & Brody, 1969), Medical Outcome Study SF-36 (Ware et al., 1993), Philadelphia Geriatric Center Morale Scale (Lawton, 1975), and the Mini-Mental State Examination (Folstein, Folstein, & McHugh, 1975).

Data on the type and frequency of the VT nursing interventions were gathered by the tele-nurses. After each VT conversation, they classified the type of VT care into 11 categories: contact, recreation, physical health, psychological health, social health, living, financial, elderly care services, social administration, leisure activities, and other care. A software program was used that automatically generated, for

TABLE 25-1

Sociodemographic Data and Support Services

CHARACTERISTICS	n = 88	%
Sex		
male	37	42.0
female	51	57.9
Age		
Mean age	72 (SD = 8.8)	
56–60	9	10.2
61–65	14	15.9
66–70	19	21.6
71–75	17	19.3
76–80	12	13.6
81–85	11	12.5
86–90	5	5.7
90+	1	1.1
Civil State		
married	23	26.1
single	8	9.1
divorced/separated	20	22.7
widowed	35	39.8
live together	20	2.3
Family Situation		
living alone	60	68.2
with husband/wife	22	25.0
with partner	4	4.5
with child	2	2.3
Education		
preschool age	2	2.3
lower secondary	64	72.7
higher secondary	16	18.2
high school	4	4.5
unknown	2	2.3
Informal Care		
husband/wife/partner	15	17.0
child living at home	2	2.3
child not living at home	27	30.7
grandchild	1	1.1
brother/sister	6	6.8
friend/neighbour	8	9.1
volunteer	1	1.1
unknown	28	31.8
Formal Care		
yes	62	70.4
no	25	28.4
unknown	1	1.1

each incoming call, the client's name, the date, and the beginning and end time of the call. The tele-nurses manually entered data about sound and picture quality of the VT call. Appropriate descriptive and inferential statistical techniques were used to analyze, evaluate, and interpret the process and outcome of VT care, in view of improving home care management of the elderly.

Implementation

Due to technical limitations, the VT project was only accessible in three areas of the city with high concentrations of potential clients. All senior citizens in these areas were invited to participate in the project on a voluntary basis. A town hall meeting with the mayor and the public welfare president was organized to present the project to the community, to overcome prevailing mistrust, and to assure the elderly people that the project was completely free. The public forum was held on a Sunday afternoon in the cafeteria of the residential home of the public welfare centre, with coffee and cake offered for comfort and to provide a positive atmosphere. All potential clients and their family members received a pamphlet with detailed information about the project. For the wider public, there was a series of newspaper articles and an announcement from the public welfare president on the local television channel. Participating elderly (n = 71) gave their informed consent and signed a contract, which stated that all VT equipment was free during the project. With the agreement in place, the tele-nurse and an engineer from the cable company visited each client's home to install the VT equipment in an area preferred by the client. They tested the VT equipment, explained fully how to use the system, and provided contact information in case of technical problems. This in-person visit was extremely important in order to foster a relationship of confidentiality and trust between the client and nurse.

The service hours fluctuated in line with the number of connected clients. At the outset, when only seven clients were connected, the centre was open from 9:00 AM until noon. Later, when the number of clients increased, the opening hours were extended to include the afternoon, from 1:00 until 4:00 PM. In the evening, at night, and during the weekend, clients were linked by telephone to the caretaker on duty for the public welfare sheltered houses for emergency care only.

EVALUATION

The Steering and Planning committees were both convinced that effective community practice requires an integrated approach to evaluation. Hence, from the onset of the project, the project evaluator was part of the Planning Committee. In collaboration with the tele-nurses, she provided the committee with regular feedback on the results of the formative process evaluation, which led to revisions of the planned actions and interventions stipulated in the community-focused plan.

Process Evaluation

The tele-nurses recorded a total of 11,209 VT calls with 21,013 VT interventions (one call could contain a number of interventions). At the start of the project, the average duration of VT calls was about 24 minutes. Later on, when the number of clients increased, the average length decreased to approximately 10 minutes. The number of VT calls fluctuated; during July and August the number decreased. During those months, the majority of the clients had more contact with their neighbours and did not feel a need to call the tele-nurse. Clients called the nurse mainly for social contact and communication (35%); being alone most of the time, they wanted to chat and tell their story. Each nurse–client interaction was based on relationships and authentic communication. Nurses were "active listeners" and fully present for their clients in each communication. While giving comfort and encouragement, the nurses delivered physical (17%) and social (15%) health support as well. Calls included, for example, requests regarding information about medications prescribed by their family physician, advice about how to pursue a medical complaint, instructions on how to complete a form to obtain meals-on-wheels, advice on problems with their pension plan, support in filling out their income tax forms, and the like. If necessary, after the VT call, nurses might contact the client's family physician, a volunteer group, or a family member (e.g., in case of a quarrel). Most (79%) of the VT calls were of good sound quality, and 59% had good picture quality. In many cases, the picture was blurred or disturbed, and in 39% of calls, there was no picture at all. Overall, the VT calls ended normally, meaning that the client and nurse ended the conversation together. In a few cases, the nurse ended the conversation because of an incoming VT call, meetings, or visitors at the centre.

Client Outcomes

At the end of the project, 69% of the clients reported that contact via VT was as personal as face-to-face contact. Only one woman saw the use of the headphone by the tele-nurse as impersonal; it distracted her when she wanted to speak about her personal problems, concerns, and worries. Although they all ranked face-to-face encounters highest, according to the clients, VT certainly has the potential to become an electronic substitute for homebound elderly. It gave them a feeling of being connected, despite some perceptions of jerkiness, delay, and asynchrony while talking via VT. In fact, the majority (69%) wanted to keep the VT and buy it if the price was affordable. Only four female clients were still sceptical at the end of project, as they did not understand the value of the VT medium for their age group.

The research showed that tailored VT nursing care led to significant improvements in overall health functioning, levels of social activity, memory function, and positive self-perception as well as a reduction in feelings of melancholy and social and emotional loneliness. It also led to improved social contact and the maintenance of a network of friends for groups of homebound elderly. The results revealed that for certain groups of elderly people, an improvement in one domain of functioning is likely to have a spill-over effect on another. Moreover, those elderly who are older, widowed, lived alone, had financial problems, and used several health and social care services showed positive changes in feelings of social isolation. The mechanism behind this improvement may be that the VT intervention provided them with a network of relationships in which they felt accepted; shared common interests and concerns; and found help, advice, and support. These elderly asked to be connected through the VT to their children who lived far away and to other clients of the tele-care centre. Characteristically, the elderly spent time watching television and listening to the radio from early in the morning until late in the evening. It was noted that they used their television as a focal point around which they structured their daily routines. It served as a "window to the outside world" and may have been a substitute for primary interpersonal communication and relationships, offering companionship, information, and entertainment. This study also showed that VT care may have had an indirect effect on the self-perception of the group of elderly. The study suggests that even leisure activities provided by the VT medium, such as playing party games or just having a chat or sharing a joke with the tele-nurse, improved their levels of social activity and memory. An argument can be made that these leisure activities and the use of VT equipment may provide more memory training for some. The group of younger elderly who had general physical and mental health problems, a low level of life satisfaction, and reduced levels of social activity showed decreased feelings of emotional loneliness following VT care. This group also showed a positive change in feelings of melancholy. Studies have reported the importance of isolation from friends or family or a decline in the social support network as precipitants of depressed feelings related to a low level of life satisfaction (Minardi & Blanchard, 2004). Meaningful social relationships included having a good friend with whom to talk, providing a sense of security, and offering opportunities for companionship and intimacy that improve life satisfaction in old age.

This study revealed no positive improvements for elderly clients in change in activities of daily living and change in instrumental activities of daily living despite the external help for housekeeping, such as laundry and food preparation, arranged by the tele-nurse. It may also be that the elderly accepted the inevitability of their deteriorating daily living functioning, which resulted in a positive change of their self-perception rather than a positive change in daily living functioning.

LESSONS LEARNED

Setting up and evaluating a community-oriented program is a constant challenge. The most important lesson we learned in this tele-homecare project is that community practice requires "joint action" among all stakeholders and community members. This means not only with the health providers who serve the elderly people in the community but also with the elderly themselves. It is essential in community work that members of the population of interest be part of the team to ensure a smooth process. In this project, the collaborative approach would have likely enhanced the implementation process, as the team encountered some barriers during the entry phase, such as fear on the part of some elderly about having VT in their homes. Probably, some elders would have perceived their participation on the team as a privileged position.

At the beginning of this tele-homecare project, all the prospective VT clients were motivated and encouraged to participate in the program. Some homebound elderly really enjoyed using VT, as they had, in addition, many visitors at their home for a demonstration, including the media, health policy-makers, and health professionals. Also, participation in this project was free of charge and offered additional benefits, including an updated television set and free telephone and television cable connection. We learned that the extra attention the elderly received may have contributed to changes in self perception and loneliness, especially for those with high social needs.

SUMMARY

This tele-homecare project was designed in collaboration with different stakeholders and community members with the purpose of addressing the health needs of the homebound elderly in the community. It was a community-oriented project, driven by the need of homebound elderly for support and friendship to combat the effects of loneliness and isolation. Combating feelings of loneliness among elderly people in this study had a spill-over effect on other domains of functioning related to their quality of life. The evidence indicates that there are benefits to providing care via VT for groups of homebound elderly who are widowed, live alone, have a limited network of friends, have financial problems, and use several health and social care services. Tele-care is an alternative care model that could be integrated to existing home care services to provide elderly people with integrated health and social services. Additional studies need to be done in other localities, cultures, and health care systems to identify those patients who could benefit from tele-care.

ACKNOWLEDGMENTS

We thank the European Union, the city of Kortrijk (Belgium) and its municipal welfare centre, the cable-TV company, and the nonprofit organization Open Net for funding this tele-homecare project.

References

Bowles, K. H., & Dansky, K. H. (2002). Teaching self-management of diabetes via tele-homecare. *Home Healthcare Nurse, 20,* 36–42.

Burke, W. J., Roccaforta, W. H., & Wengel, S. P. (1991). The short-form of the geriatric depression scale: A comparison with the 30-item form. *Journal of Geriatric Psychiatry and Neurology, 4,* 173–178.

Celler, B. G., Lovell, N. H., & Chan, D. K. Y. (1999). The potential impact of home tele-care on clinical practice. *The Medical Journal of Australia, 171,* 518–521.

Chapman, S. A., Keating, N., & Eales, J. (2003). Client-centred, community-based care for frail seniors. *Health and Social Care in the Community, 11,* 253–261.

de Jong-Gierveld, J., & Kamphuis, F. (1985). The development of a Rash-type loneliness scale. *Applied Psychological Measurement, 9,* 289–299.

Folstein, M., Folstein, S. E., & McHugh, P. R. (1975). 'Mini-mental state': A practical method for grading the cognitive state of patients for the clinician. *Journal of Psychiatric Research, 12,* 211–218.

Fried, L. P., Tangen, C. M., Walston, J., et al. (2001). Frailty in older adults: Evidence for a phenotype. *Journal of Gerontology: Medical Sciences, 56A,* M146–M156.

Johri, M., Béland, F., & Bergman, H. (2003). International experiments in integrated care for the elderly: A synthesis of evidence. *International Journal of Geriatric Psychiatry, 18,* 222–235.

Katz, S., & Apkom, C. A. (1976). A measure of primary socio-biological functions. *International Journal of Health Services, 6,* 493–507.

Lawton, M. P. (1975). The Philadelphia geriatric center morale scale: A revision. *Journal of Gerontology, 30,* 85–89.

Lawton, M. P., & Brody, E. M. (1969). Assessment of older people: Self-maintaining and instrumental activities of daily living. *Gerontologist, 9,* 179–186.

Lubben, J. E. (1988). Assessing social networks among elderly populations. *Family and Community Health, 11*(3), 42–52.

Minardi, H. A., & Blanchard, M. (2004). Older people with depression: Pilot study. *Journal of Advanced Nursing, 46,* 23–32.

Savenstedt, S., Zingmark, K., & Sandman, P. O. (2003). Video-phone communication with cognitively impaired elderly patients. *Journal of Telemedicine and Telecare, 2,* S52–S54.

Shaul, M. P. (2000). What you should know before embarking on telehome health: Lessons learned from a pilot study. *Home Healthcare Nurse, 18,* 470–475.

Ware, J. E., Snow, K. K., Kosinski, M., et al. (1993). *SF-36 health survey: Manual and interpretation guide.* Boston, MA: The Health Institute, New England Medical Centre.

Young, H. M. (2003). Challenges and solutions for care of frail older adults. *Online Journal of Issues in Nursing, 8.* Retrieved October 12, 2005, from **www.nursingworld.org/ojin/topic21/tpc21_4.htm.**

Suggested Readings

Arnaert, A., & Delesie, L. (2001). Telenursing for the elderly—The case of care via videotelephony. *Journal of Telemedicine and Telecare, 7*(6), 311–316.

Arnaert, A., & Delesie, L. (2005). Information visualization: A holistic tool to discover knowledge. Case study: What video-telephone care? What elderly? *Knowledge Management Research & Practice, 3,* 3–9.

Internet Resources

http://www.hc-sc.gc.ca/fnih-spni/services/ehealth-esante/index_e.html
e-Health in First Nations & Inuit Health

http://www.internet-health.org/ehi200214.html
The Promise of e-Health: A Canadian Perspective

http://www.hc-sc.gc.ca/hl-vs/seniors-aines/index_e.html
Healthy Living: Seniors

http://www.cda-adc.ca/jcda/vol-67/issue-9/504.html
Access to Care for Seniors—Dental Concerns

A Model Assessment Guide for Nursing in Industry

COMPONENTS	QUESTIONS TO ASK
The Company	
Historical development	How, why, and by whom was the company founded?
Organizational chart	What is the formal order of the system, and to whom are the health providers responsible?
Company policies	Is there a policy manual? Are the workers aware of the existence of the manual?
Length of the work week	How many days a week does the industry operate?
Length of the work time	Are there several shifts? How many breaks? Is there paid vacation?
Sick leave/Parental leave	Is there a clear policy, and do the workers know it?
Safety and fire provisions	Is management aware of situations or substances in the plant that represent a potential danger? Are there organized fire drills? (The *Federal Register* is the source of information for federal standards and serves as a helpful guide.)
Support services (benefits)	
Insurance programs	Is there a system for health insurance and life insurance, and is it compulsory? Does the company pay all or part? Who fills out the necessary forms?
Retirement program	Are the benefits realistic?
Educational support	Can the workers further their education? Will the company help financially?
Safety committee	If there is no committee, do certain people routinely handle emergencies? The Red Cross First Aid Course through programmed instruction is excellent (for information consult your local Red Cross).
Recreation committee	Do the workers have any communication with or interest in each other outside the work setting?
Employee relations Gender and equity	Are there problems in employee relations? (This is difficult information to get, but it is important to get a sense of how employees feel generally about management and vice versa.)

COMPONENTS	QUESTIONS TO ASK

The Plant

General physical setting	What is the overall appearance?
The construction	What is the size and general condition of buildings and grounds?
Parking facilities and public transportation stops	How far does the worker have to walk to get inside? Are parking areas well lighted at night? Are there escorts for women/others that work shifts?
Entrances and exits	How many people must use them? How accessible are they?
Physical environment	What conditions exist in the physical environment? (Comment on heating, air-conditioning, lighting, glare, drafts, and so forth)
Communication facilities	Are there bulletin boards and newsletters?
Housekeeping	Is the physical setting maintained adequately?
Interior decoration	Are the surroundings conducive to work? Are they pleasing?
Work areas	
Space	Are workers isolated or crowded?
Heights: workplace and supply areas	Is there a chance of workers falling or being injured by falling objects? (Falls and falling objects are dangerous and costly to industry.)
Stimulation	Is the worker too bored to pay attention?
Safety signs and markings	Are dangerous areas well marked?
Standing and sitting facilities	Are chairs safe and comfortable? Are there platforms to stand on, especially for wet processes?
Safety equipment	Do the workers make use of hard hats, safety glasses, face masks, radiation badges, and so forth? Do they know the safety devices that the OSHA regulations require?
Nonwork areas	
Lockers	If the work is dirty, workers should be able to change clothes. Are they accidentally carrying toxic substances home on their clothes?
Hand-washing facilities	If facilities and supplies are available, do workers know how and when to wash their hands?
Rest rooms	How accessible are they, and what condition are they in?
Drinking water	Can workers leave their jobs long enough to get a drink of water when they want to?
Recreation and rest facilities	Can a worker who is not feeling well/pregnant lie down? Do workers feel free to use the facilities?
Telephones	Can a worker receive or make a call? Does a working mother have to stay home for a call because she can't be reached at work?

COMPONENTS	QUESTIONS TO ASK

The Plant

Ashtrays	Are people allowed to smoke in designated areas? Are they safe areas?

The Working Population: Include workers and management, but separate data for comparison

General characteristics	(Be as accurate as possible, but estimate when necessary.)
Total number of employees	(Usually, if an industry has 500 or more employees, full-time nursing services are necessary.)
General appearance	Are there records of heights, weights, cleanliness, and so forth? Ask to see them.
Age and sex distribution	What are the proportions of the different groups? (Certain screening programs are specific for young adults, whereas others are more for the elderly. Some programs are more for women; others are more for men.) Is there any difference between day and evening shift populations? Are the problems of the minority sex unattended?
Race distribution	Does one race predominate? How does this compare with the general community?
Socioeconomic distribution	Are there great differences in worker salaries? (This can sometimes cause problems.)
Religious distribution	Does one religion predominate? Are religious holidays observed?
Ethnic distribution	Is there a language barrier?
Marital status	What proportion of the workers are widowed, single, or divorced? (These groups often have different needs.)
Educational backgrounds	Can all teaching be done at approximately the same level?
Lifestyles practiced	Is there disapproval of certain lifestyles?
Types of employment offered	
Background necessary	What education level is required? Skilled versus unskilled?
Work demands on physical condition	What level of strength is needed? Is the work sedentary or active?
Work status	How many employees work full-time? Part-time? Is there overtime?
Absenteeism	Is there a record kept? By whom? Why?
Causes	What are the five most common reasons for absence?

COMPONENTS	QUESTIONS TO ASK

The Working Population: Include workers and management, but separate data for comparison (cont'd.)

Length	What are the patterns of absences? (Absenteeism is costly to the employer. There is some difference between one 10-day absence and 10 one-day absences by the same person.)
People with disability	Does the company have a policy about hiring people with disability?
Number employed	Where do they work? What do they do?
Extent of disability	Are they specially trained? Are they in a special program? Do they use prosthetic devices?
Personnel on medication	What medication do employees take?
Personnel with chronic illness	What chronic illnesses are prevalent? What are the impacts of these illnesses on work ability? Do work protocols need to be adapted to accommodate?

The Industrial Process: What does the company produce and how?

Equipment used	Is the equipment portable or fixed? Light or heavy?
General description of placement	Ask to have each piece of large equipment marked on a scale map.
Type of equipment	Fans, blowers, fast moving, wet, or dry?
Nature of the operation	Ask for a brief description of each stage of the process so that you can compare the needs and abilities of the worker with the needs of the job.
Raw materials used	What are they and how dangerous are they? Are they properly stored? Check the provincial guidelines on storage.
Nature of the final product	Can the workers take pride in the final product or do they make parts?
Description of the jobs	Who does what? Where? (Label the map.)
Waste products produced	What is the system for waste disposal? Are the pollution-control devices in place and functioning?
Exposure to toxic substances	To which toxins are the workers exposed? What is the extent of exposure? (Include physical and emotional hazards. Remember that chronic effects of industrial exposure are subtle; a person often gets used to having mild symptoms and won't report them. The Provincial Occupational Health Acts contain specifications for exposure to toxins, and some provinces issue standards.)

COMPONENTS	QUESTIONS TO ASK

The Health Program: Outline what is actually in existence as well as what employees perceive to be in existence

Existing policies	Are there informal, unwritten policies?
Objectives of the program	Are they clear?
Preemployment physicals	Are they required? Are they paid for by the company? Is the information used to select?
First aid facilities	What is available? What is not available?
Standing orders	Is there a company physician who is responsible for first aid or emergency policy? (If so, work closely with him or her in planning nursing services.)
Job descriptions for health personnel	Are they in writing? (If there are no guidelines to be followed, write some.)
Existing facilities and resources	Sometimes an industry that denies having a health program has more of a system than it realizes.
Trained personnel	Who responds in an emergency?
Space	Where is the sick worker taken? Where is the emergency equipment kept?
Supplies	What are they? Where are they kept? (Make a list and describe the condition of each item.)
Records and reports	What exists? (Occupational Health and Safety Regulations require that employers keep three types of records: a log of occupational injuries and illnesses, a supplemental record of certain illnesses or injuries, and an annual summary. Good records provide data for good planning.)
Services rendered in the past year	Describe as specifically as possible.
Care needed	Chronic or acute? Why?
Screening done	Where? By whom? Why?
Referrals made	By whom? To whom? Why?
Counseling done	Formal or informal? (Often informal counseling goes unnoticed.)
Health education	What individual or group education was offered by the company?
Accidents in the past year	During working hours? After hours? (Include those that occur after work hours; some may be directly or indirectly work related.)
Reasons why employees sought health care	What are the five major reasons?

COMPONENTS	QUESTIONS TO ASK
Stressors	
As identified by employees	What pressures are felt on the job?
As identified by health providers	What problems do they perceive?

Adapted from Serafini, P. (1976). Nursing assessment in industry: A model. *American Journal of Public Health*, *66*(8), 755–760.

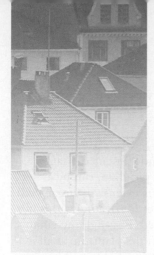

APPENDIX B

Assessment of an Industry

COMPONENTS	DESCRIPTION

The Company

Name and location	The AAB Chemical Company Hampton Industrial Complex Located west of State Highway 519 and Loop 177
Historical development	The AAB Chemical Company separated from the AAB Refinery in 1957, and the present plant was completed in 1961. The parent company is a major oil company with headquarters in Chicago. The plant is today the most complex and versatile in the AAB system.
Organizational chart	A formal organizational chart was not available. However, by observation and interview, a structure consisting of a plant manager, with a supervisor in charge of each production area, safety, and maintenance was noted. There are overseers for each area of operation for each shift. The medical staff, which consists of one doctor and one nurse, are not hired by the plant personnel department but by the parent company in Chicago.
Company policies	The plant operations are never shut down. There are shifts around the clock for operators and craftspeople. Employees such as clerical, administrative, and medical staff work 8-hour days, 40-hour weeks. Breaks are provided during the work period. Employees are eligible for 2 weeks of paid vacation per year after working 1 year. This increases in 5-year increments. A 20-year employee is eligible for 5 weeks of vacation. Employees are eligible for sick leave after 6 months of service. Parental leave is provided for birth, adoption and child emergencies. Benefits vary with length of service. All benefits are published in an employee handbook, distributed to all employees.

COMPONENTS	DESCRIPTION

The Company (cont'd.)

Company policies	Management is well aware of situations and substances that pose danger to the workers. The safety program, run by a safety supervisor and a safety engineer, is extensive. Organized fire drills are held frequently. Procedures for dealing with spills and other hazards are also well organized. Fire-fighting equipment and an ambulance are available on the plant site at all times. Certain employees are trained as firefighters. There are EMTs available inside the plant in addition to the nurse. Fire extinguishers are placed throughout the plant in strategic locations.
Support services	A comprehensive medical expense plan is compulsory for all employees. In addition, disability up to 40 weeks owing to occupational illness or injury is provided to all employees regardless of length of service. Term life insurance under a group plan is available at a low rate. A long-term disability plan is available to employees covered under the basic life insurance plan. A retirement plan is provided at complete cost to the company. A savings plan in which employees may invest in company stock is also available. Employees are offered an educational assistance program and are encouraged to advance their careers. On-line-job training is provided to help employees advance.
Employee relations	The workers are affiliated with the Oil, Chemical and Atomic Workers International Union, a part of the AFL-CIO. It was difficult to perceive how management and labour relate to each other. However, several workers mentioned the family-like atmosphere among employees, and hopefully, this bridges the gap between labor and management. The last strike occurred approximately 2 years ago. Pay equity policies govern salaries to minimize gaps in wages between men and women.

The Plant

General physical setting	The appearance of the plant is best described as an intimidating maze of pipes, towers, and vessels. The main building, in which the clinic is located, is modern and attractive, with well-tended grounds. Ample parking is available, with areas provided for the handicapped. The building is air conditioned, spacious, and clean, with a pleasing interior.

COMPONENTS	DESCRIPTION

The Plant

	The grounds and buildings inside the plant are also neat and well maintained. Scattered through the plant in strategic locations are eye-bubbling devices for flushing the eyes and showers for removing irritants from the skin. Danger areas are clearly marked with yellow paint and warning signs. Employees working in areas where hydrofluoric acid is used are provided with complete protective covering, and they shower immediately upon leaving the area. Earplugs and earmuffs are required in high-noise areas. Compliance in use of safety devices is good, and workers are aware of Occupational Health and Safety (OH&S) regulations.
Work areas	Some work areas, especially where craftspeople are involved, are cramped and close, owing to the physical structure of the myriad pipes and lines. Some areas are also elevated in height. One problem noted by the plant nurse is occasional heat stress during summer months when employees are working in these areas on equipment that reflects heat. Another problem noted was the stress, manifested in muscle and joint discomfort, of working in cramped quarters, especially when employees work a lot of overtime. Occasionally employees are injured by falling objects, such as heavy wrenches. Burns are the most common type of injuries. Operators who work in the processing units and monitor the gauges and flow rates are in stressful jobs because a mistake could be costly and dangerous.
Nonwork areas	Each work area has a kitchen area, restrooms, and water fountains that are easily accessible. Lockers and showers are also available. Communication by phone is possible in all areas of the plant. Facilities are available in the clinic so that workers who are ill may lie down. However, in some areas, repeated visits to the clinic are discouraged. Employees are instructed regarding handwashing and prompt attention to small wounds by the nurse as part of new employee orientation. Smoking is permitted only in specifically designated parts of the fenced area of the plant, the docks, and warehouses.

COMPONENTS	DESCRIPTION

The Working Population

General characteristics	AAB Chemicals employs approximately 500 people. Age and sex distribution data were not available. However, the plant nurse stated that employees range in age from age 18 to retirement at age 65, and that male employees outnumber female employees. The nurse also stated that some women were moving into previously male-dominated jobs. Race distribution data were not available. By observation, the distribution appeared to be predominantly white, followed by Asian and then Arabic employees, which is in line with the population distribution in the community. Data regarding religious and marital status were not available. Wages and salaries are commensurate with education, qualifications, and years of service. Educational backgrounds range from high school graduates to advanced degrees in engineering and the sciences. Therefore, health teaching must be geared to match the educational level of the group being instructed.
Type of employment offered	Types of employment include skilled craftspeople, operators, lab analysts, chemists, engineers, clerical and administrative personnel, and a nurse and a physician. The background required for each area varies with the complexity and nature of the job. Most employees are full-time and work overtime as required.
Absenteeism	Records of absences are kept in the employee's work unit. The nurse keeps records on illness- or injury-related absences. An employee who has been absent owing to an extended or serious illness, an injury, or surgery must report to the medical department before returning to work and must supply a statement from a doctor regarding the nature of his or her disability and the limitations, if any, on permissible work. The medical department then determines the physical condition of the employee and notifies his or her supervisor regarding the employee's return to work. Strict record keeping also is done for OH&S requirements. According to the nurse, the most common reasons for absence are not occupationally related. They are most often for upper-respiratory infections and other common health problems or for accidents that occurred away from the plant.

COMPONENTS	DESCRIPTION
The Working Population	
People with disability	The AAB Company is an equal opportunity employer. Information regarding employees with disabilities, the nature of their handicaps, and the jobs they fill was not available.
Personnel on medication Personnel with chronic illness	The nurse keeps records of employees on medication. This information is confidential. The confidentiality of employees' medical records is strictly enforced.
The Industrial Process	
Equipment used Nature of the plant operation	The basic job of the plant is to produce specialty chemicals and petrochemical intermediates for manufacture of products that range from boats and surfboards to carpets and furniture. Production of these chemicals involves moving raw materials (called "feedstock") from AAB's Hampton Refinery and another chemical plant and mixing them with xylenes and benzenes. Some of the chemicals produced are propylene, styrene, paraxylene, metazylene, aromatic solvents, oil-recovering chemicals, oil-producing chemicals, and polybutenes. The equipment used involves miles of pipes and many towers and vessels. Process units are designed to be energy efficient, and in many instances, energy-producing hydrocarbons are a by-product of a process. These are then recovered and used as fuel in other operations. Flammability and danger of explosion are major concerns when dealing with the above-named chemicals. Proper storage is essential and is carried out with care in this plant. The final product of the production process is barrels of chemicals. Workers take pride in turning out a certain number of barrels in a time period and in keeping the plant operating efficiently. The treatment of wastewater is through an effluent water-control system that is one of the most sophisticated in the industry. The facility handles wastewater not only from AAB Chemical but also from the AAB Refinery and another chemical plant in the area. Air-pollution control is done in two steps: first by eliminating potential contaminants whenever possible and then through the use of devices such as scrubbers, filters, cyclone separators, and a flare system to burn up the waste hydrocarbons.

COMPONENTS	DESCRIPTION

The Industrial Process (cont'd.)

Exposure to toxic substances	The major substances of concern are benzene and xylene. Benzene is a colorless, flammable, volatile liquid. The major hazard with this chemical is chronic poisoning by inhalation of small amounts over a long time. It is one of the most dangerous organic solvents in common use. Benzene acts primarily on the blood-forming organs. Skin contact also is to be avoided. Benzene is suspected of being carcinogenic. Xylene resembles benzene in many chemical and physical properties but is not involved in causing chronic blood diseases. It has a narcotic effect and can cause dermatitis with repeated contact. Benzene screening is done on all employees on a yearly basis.

The Health Program

Existing policies	The objectives of the program are to monitor the status of each employee's health in order to pinpoint problems at an early stage and to provide prompt attention to accidents or emergencies as they occur at the worksite. The employees perceive the second objective more readily than the first. Many of them perceive the yearly physicals as a low priority. Preemployment physicals are done by the nurse and company doctor at no charge to the client and are used as a baseline for future reference. The ambulance kept at the plant is equipped for all emergencies. Injured or ill employees requiring more than initial first aid are taken immediately to the hospital. There is a set of comprehensive standing orders, written through collaborative effort by the nurse and doctor. Yearly physicals include chest x-ray, blood work that includes benzene screening, urinalysis, vision and hearing assessments, and physical exams by the physician. Pregnant women are seen each month by the doctor in addition to their own private doctors. No screening programs alone are done, but they are incorporated into the yearly physical. Health teaching and informal counseling are done on an individual basis by the nurse and doctor. CPR is taught to selected personnel throughout the plant by the nurse.

COMPONENTS	DESCRIPTION
The Health Program	
Existing facilities and resources	The medical department consists of one full-time nurse and a physician who cover this plant and AAB's larger plant near Avina, as well as a part-time secretary. The facilities include the nurse's office, where all medical records are kept and where employees check in when visiting the clinic; a treatment room; a small lab and pharmacy; a radiology room; an exam room; and the physician's office. First aid facilities are extensive and well supplied. ECG equipment and defibrillator are also available. The nurse sees between 12 and 15 clients per day in the clinic. The major reasons employees seek health care are non–occupationally related sicknesses or accidents, stress-related complaints, and minor accidents on the job.
Stressors	
Employees	Job pressure, as with operators who control the process units Overtime hours, when worked frequently Knowledge of potential fire or explosion Shift work that may not be in sync with normal body rhythms Strikes or layoffs
Health care providers	Problems with role definition. Nurse wishes to do more health teaching but feels Safety Department has taken over many of her functions. Feels powerless to change the situation. Feels that physician also perceives her role as limited to specific, traditional areas.

Index

Note: Page numbers followed by f, t, and b indicate figures, tables, and boxed material, respectively.

A

Aboriginal peoples, 165–166, 166t
  Inuit *vs.*, 400
Acculturation, 175–177, 176f
*An Act for the Preservation and Enhancement of
    Multiculturalism in Canada*, 173, 174
Action, public, 79
Action Process for Creating Supportive Environment for
    Health Action Plan (APCSEH), 83–85, 84f, 85b
Activities, program, 318, 319f
Adjusted rates, 61, 61t
Adolescent pregnancy, 17–18
  in Exemplar Health District, 388–390, 389f, 389t,
    390t
Adolescents
  high-risk, 440–441
  school health promotion in, 110–116 (*See also* School
    health promotion, partnership model)
Advocacy, 41. *See also* Ethics
  media, 340–341, 341t
  strengthening, 79
Advocacy coalitions, 144
Age distribution, 258, 258t
  in Exemplar Health District, 375, 375f
Agenda-setting, 141
Agent, 51–52, 52f
Aggregating data, 288
Air quality, 80–81
Alcohol sales, in Exemplar Health District, 383–384, 383t
Alliances, building, 79–80
Alternating rhythms, 36
America Speaks, 118, 119b
American melting pot, 176–177
American Public Health Association Code of Ethics,
    42–43, 43t
Analysis, 281–283
  classification in, 281
  in community-as-partner model, 232
  cost-benefit, 365–366
  cost-effectiveness, 365–366
  gender-based, 141
  interpretation in, 282–283
  issues and strategies in, 284t
  in model to guide practice, 232
  social network, 78–91 (*See also* Supportive environment
    for health)

  of Students for Tobacco Reduction program,
    463, 464t
  summarization in, 282
  validation in, 283
  of vulnerable populations in urban settings, 497
  of women's health program, northern Pakistan,
    426–429, 428t
  of youth engagement in social policy action planning,
    457–458
Analysis sample, 283–298
  aggregating (pooling) data in, 288
  community core in, 284–290, 285t–297t, 287f
  demographics in, 285t
  dependency ratio in, 286–287, 289t
  economics in, 294–298, 295t, 296b, 297t
  health and social services in, 292–294, 293t, 294t
  health status in, 286t
  history in, 285t
  overview of, 283–284
  physical environment in, 290–292, 291b
  population pyramid in, 284–286, 287f,
    288t, 289t
  sex and age in, 284, 288, 288t, 289t
  vital statistics in, 285t
Analytic measures, 62–68
  attributable risk, 65
  attributable risk percent, 65
  cause and association, 65–68
  internal and external risk factors, 62–63
  interpretation of, 64–65, 65t
  odds ratio, 63–64, 64t
  relative risk, 62
*An Inclusion Lens: Workbook for Looking at Social and
    Economic Exclusion and Inclusion*, 180–181
Assessment
  as intervention for vulnerable populations in urban
    settings, 498–499
  needs, for TELESENIOR, 512–514, 513t
Assessment, community, 238–276
  communication in, 273–274, 274t
  in community-as-partner model, 230–232
  community assessment wheel in, 225, 226f, 231f, 239,
    240f, 253
  community core in, 225, 226f, 254–255, 254t, 256t
  data collection methods in, 245–253 (*See also* Data
    collection methods)

535

Assessment, community (*continued*)
  definition of, 238–239
  downtown health facilities in, 262–265, 263f–265f
  downtown social services in, 262–265, 266b
  economics in, 265–269 (*See also* Economics)
  education in, 274–275, 275t
  getting to know community in, 241–243, 243t
  health and social services in, 230, 261–262, 262t,
      292–294, 293t, 294t
  identifying community in, 253
  of influenza pandemic worker strategies, 485
  information needed for, 245
  physical environment in, 260, 261t
  planning of, 243–245
  politics and government in, 272–273
  population description in, 256–259 (*See also* Population
      description)
  purpose of, agreement on, 244–245
  recreation in, 275–276, 276t
  safety in, 269–272, 271t, 272t
  subsystems in, 225–227, 226f, 259–276 (*See also*
      Subsystems)
  team in, 239–241, 241t
  team member role in community in, 242–243, 243t
  transportation in, 272, 272t
  of vulnerable populations in urban settings,
      495–497
  water and sanitation in, 270–271
Assessment, in municipal government workplace health
      promotion, 474–477, 476b
  multilevel, 478
  participatory processes in, 478
  practical considerations in, 478–479
Assessment, of industry, 527–533
  company in, 527–528
  health program in, 532–533
  industrial process in, 531–532
  plant in, 528–529
  stressors in, 533
  working population in, 530–531
Assessment guide for nursing in industry, 521–526
  company in, 521
  health program in, 525
  industrial process in, 524
  plant in, 522–523
  stressors in, 525
  working population in, 523–524
Assets, community, 228
Assimilation, 176–177, 176f
Association, 65–67
Asthma, air quality on, 80
Attributable risk (AR), 65
Attributable risk percent, 65

Attunement, cultural, 182–185, 185b. *See also* Cultural
      attunement
Autonomy, 31
Avian influenza (H5N1), 481–485

B
Bangkok Charter, 13–14
Becoming, 223, 223f
Being, 223, 223f
Belonging, 223, 223f
Beneficence, 31–32
Bias, cultural, 178
Bioethics, 27
Biological hazards, 82
Biomedical model, 151–152, 219
Birth rate, in Exemplar Health District, 375–376
Bisexuals, discrimination against, 105
Body mass index (BMI), 210
Brachycephaly, 426
"BreakFree" campaign, 18–19
British ancestry, 166–168, 167t
Budgeting, in planning process, 324
Building healthy public policies, 138–145. *See also* Public
      policies, healthy
"Building on Values: The Future of Health Care in
      Canada," 160
Built environment, 82
Bureaucracy, 144
Business, 168f, 266–267

C
Calendar chart, for planning activities, 318, 319f
Canada, rural, 432
Canada Health Infoway, 196
Canada Mortgage and Housing Corporation Report,
      2005, 290, 291b
Canadian Charter of Rights and Freedoms, 27, 173–174
Canadian cultural mosaic, 175–177, 176f
Canadian ethnic origin, 167–168, 167t
Canadian Healthy Communities Project (CHCP), 158
Canadian Institutes for Health Research (CIHR), 14
Canadian Multiculturalism Act, 174
Canadian Pandemic Influenza Plan, 206–207, 207b
Capability deprivation, 108
Capacity, nonprofit, 429
Capacity building approach
  to influenza vaccination, 487
  to reorienting health services, 158–159
  to Strengthening Community Action, 115–116, 115b
Capacity Building Framework, 429–430, 429f
Caring, 36

Case study approach, 354–358
  Delphi technique in, 358
  nominal group in, 357
  observation in, 356–357
  usefulness of, 358
  value and content of, 354–356
Categorization, 178
Causation, 65–68
  criteria for determination of, 67–68
  variables and constants in, 66–67
  web of, 53–54, 54f
Census, 68–69
Change, planned, 311–316, 312t–315t. See also Planned
    change
Chemical hazards, 82
Child protection cases, in Exemplar Health District, 382,
    383t
Chlorine, in tap water, 81
Chronic diseases, as emerging threats to community
    health, 210–211
Citizen engagement, nine criteria for sustaining, 119b
Climate description, 260, 261t
Code of ethics
  American Public Health Association, 42–43, 43t
  health promotion, 43–44
  public health, 42–43, 43t
Code of Ethics for Registered Nurses, 35
Collaboration, 124–126. See also Partnerships for health
  definitions of, 124, 124b
  in planning process, 321–323
  in population health approach, 22
Collaborative advantage, 126, 126b
Collaborative inertia, 126, 126b
Collective unit, interaction as, 404–405
Communicable diseases, in Exemplar Health District,
    291t, 390–391
Communication
  in partnership framework, 128t, 129
  in partnerships, strategies of, 134
Community, 225
  in community-as-partner model, 233–234
  core data on, 254, 254t
  definitions of, 114–115, 299
  descriptions of, 255, 256t
  healthy, 225
  policy, 143–144, 143f, 144t
Community action, strengthening. See Strengthening
    Community Action (SCA)
Community analysis. See Analysis
Community-as-client model. See Community-as-partner
    model
Community-as-partner model, 224–235, 226f
  assessment in, 230–232

central factors in, 225, 226f
community assessment wheel in, 225, 226f, 231f, 239,
    240f, 253
community health diagnosis in, 230, 232
community health team goal in, 224
community in, 225
core in, 225, 226f, 254–255, 254t, 256t
degree of reaction in, 229, 229t
ecology and, 227
evaluation in, 234–235, 303–304, 346–366
    (See also Evaluation)
flexible line of defence in, 227–228, 229t, 231f
healthy community in, 225
history of, 224
intervention in, 231f, 232–234
lines of resistance in, 228–229, 229t
normal line of defence in, 227, 229t, 231f
partnership planning and teamwork in, 235–236
stressors in, 229, 229t
subsystems in, 225–227, 226f, 259–276 (See also
    Subsystems, community)
Community assessment, 238–276. See also Assessment,
    community
Community assessment team, 239–241, 241t
Community assessment wheel, 231f, 233, 239, 240f, 253
Community awareness, in cultural attunement, 185b
Community-based research, 116, 117b
Community capacity, building, 115–116, 115b
Community development, 114
  methods of, 116, 117b
  process of, 117–118, 118t, 119b
Community empowerment, 98–99, 98f, 415
Community Health Action Model, 404, 405f
Community health diagnosis. See Diagnosis, community
    health
Community health focus, 331–335
  environmental and cultural support in, 332–333
  levels of practice in, 335
  levels of prevention in, 333–335
  overview of, 331–332
Community health informatics. See Informatics,
    community health
Community practice, reflection and building awareness
    on, 185, 185b
Community practice foundations, 4–7
  Alma Ata Declaration on, 5–7, 5b, 7t, 23, 149–151, 152
  Lalonde Report on, 4–5, 149, 151–152
Community process model, 219
Community profiles
  Exemplar Health District, 373–396 (See also Exemplar
      Health District)
  Inuit women's health, 398–403 (See also Inuit women's
      health)

Community profiles (*continued*)
　Leaf Rapids community, 403–412 (*See also* Photovoice, youth participation via)
　municipal government health promotion, 471–479 (*See also* Municipal government workplace health promotion)
　responsive worker strategies for pandemic influenza, 479–489 (*See also* Influenza pandemic, responsive worker strategies for)
　schoolchildren's health, oral, 432–439 (*See also* Oral Health Programming)
　schoolchildren's health, partnership model, 440–446
　technology in promoting homebound seniors' health, 508–517 (*See also* Technology in promoting homebound seniors' health)
　vulnerable populations in urban settings, 494–501 (*See also* Urban settings, vulnerable populations in)
　women's health, empowering Canadian immigrants in, 415–422 (*See also* Women's health, empowering pregnant Canadian immigrants in)
　women's health, northern Pakistan, 422–430 (*See also* Women's health, northern Pakistan)
　Women's Perspectives in Poverty, Photovoice in, 501–505 (*See also* Women's Perspectives in Poverty, Photovoice in)
　youth engagement in social policy action planning, 450–459
　youth participation through Photovoice, 406–412 (*See also* Photovoice, youth participation via)
Community services, 10
Commuting, 82
Comparative data, 282
Comparison groups, 66
Comprehensive school health model, 156
Conceptual model, 219
Configuration, partnership, 129–130, 130f, 131f
Confounding variables, 66–67
Congenital anomalies, in Exemplar Health District, 387–388, 388f
Consequentialism, 29
Constants, 66
Constraints, in planning process, 323–324
Contaminants
　food-borne, 82
　in natural environment, 80
　outdoor air, 80–81
Context, 19
Control groups, 66
Coordination, 124
Core, community
　in community analysis sample, 284–290, 285t–297t, 287f (*See also* Analysis sample)

in community-as-partner model, 225, 226f, 254–255, 254t, 256t
in community assessment, 225, 226f, 254–255, 254t, 256t
Cost-benefit analysis (CBA), 365–366
Cost-effectiveness analysis (CEA), 365–366
Cost-efficiency, in evaluation, 353
Cree First Nation, 109–110
Crime rates, 270, 271t
Crime statistics, 270
Critical social action theory, 15b
Crude rates, 60, 61t
Cultural attunement, 182–185, 185b
　acknowledging pain of oppression in, 183
　acting with reverence in, 184
　engaging in acts of humility in, 183–184
　engaging in mutuality in, 184
　maintaining "not knowing" position in, 184–185
　overview of, 182–183
Cultural bias, 178
Cultural competence, in community practice, 181–182, 182t
Cultural Competence Continuum, 181–182, 182t
Cultural humility, 186–187, 186b
Cultural identity, 99–100
Cultural imposition, 178
Cultural landscape, Canada, 165–171
　aboriginal peoples, 165–166, 166t
　founding nations, 166–168
　immigrants, 168–171, 169t, 170t
　population by ethnic origin, 167–168, 167t
Cultural pluralism, 172
Cultural power dynamics, 102–106
Cultural relativism, 172
Cultural support, 332–333
Culture and diversity, 164–187, 171
　background on, 164–165
　in Canada, 165–171 (*See also* Cultural landscape, Canada)
　Canadian mosaic *vs.* American melting pot in, 175–177, 176f
　cultural pluralism (relativism) in, 172
　definition of, 171
　ethnicity in, 171
　key concepts in, 171–172
　multiculturalism in, 172
　multiculturalism in, barriers to, 177–180 (*See also* Multiculturalism)
　multiculturalism in, facilitators of, 180–181
　multiculturalism in, in Canada, 172–175 (*See also* Multiculturalism)
　multiculturalism in community practice and, 181–187 (*See also* Multiculturalism in community practice)
　race in, 171
　universal principles in, 172

CYN. *See* Youth engagement in social policy action planning
Cynicism, avoiding, 346

D
Data
  in Exemplar Health District, 393
  non-numerical, 244
  numerical, 243–244
  primary *vs.* secondary, 244
Data collection methods, 245–253
  assessment questions in, 245, 246t
  focus groups in, 251
  information needs and, 245
  key informant interview in, 247, 250
  observation in, 246–247, 248t–249t, 250b
  other assessment strategies in, 252–253
  population data in, 252
  surveys and questionnaires in, 251–252
Data collection methods for evaluation, 354–366
  case-study approach in, 354–358 (*See also* Case-study approach)
  cost-benefit analysis in, 365–366
  cost-effectiveness analysis in, 365–366
  experimental design in, 360–363 (*See also* Experimental design)
  key points for deciding on, 354
  monitoring (process) in, 363–365, 364t
  paradigms for, 354, 355t
  summary of methods of, 366–368, 367t
  surveys in, 358–360
Data gaps, 282, 284, 286t
Data sources, 68–70, 243–244
  census, 68–69
  medical and hospital records, 70
  notifiable disease reports, 70
  social welfare reports, 70
  vital statistics, 69
David Thompson Health Region, 433. *See also* Oral Health Programming
Death, causes of, in Exemplar Health District, 384–386, 385t
Death rate, in Exemplar Health District, 375–376
Decision making, in public policy development, 142
Decision making structure, in Exemplar Health District, 394
Declaration of Alma-Ata on Primary Health Care, 5–7, 5b, 7t, 23, 149–151, 152
Defence, lines of
  flexible, 227–228, 229t, 231f
  in municipal government workplace health promotion, 476–477, 476b
  normal, 227, 229t, 231f
  in Students for Tobacco Reduction program, 463
Degree of reaction, 229

Delphi technique, 358
Democratic racism, 179
Demographic data, in Exemplar Health District, 374–377. *See also specific data*
Demographic measures, 56
Demography, 49, 50. *See also* Epidemiology
Dental caries, 433–434
Dental health. *See also* Oral Health Programming
  in Exemplar Health District, 392, 392f
  promotion of, approaches to, 434–435
  promotion of, in rural Canada, 432–439 (*See also* Oral Health Programming)
  quality of life and, 433–434
Deontology, 29
Dependency ratio (DR), 286–287, 289t, 376
Dependent variables, 66
Deprivation
  capability, 108
  in empowerment terrain, 107–108
  material, 103–104
  in power-culture dynamics, 103
  relative, 103–105
Descriptive measures, 56–61
  demographic, 56
  incidence, 57
  interpretation, 57
  morbidity and mortality, 56–57
  prevalence, 57
  rates, 57–61 (*See also* Rates)
Determinants of health, 16–17, 16f, 18t, 193
  emerging public health issues and, 205
  in Exemplar Health District, 377–384 (*See also* Exemplar Health District)
  in Newfoundland and Labrador youth, 451, 452t
  in youth, 451, 452t
Deworming, maternal, in northern Pakistan, 427–428
Diabetes, relative risk of, 63
Diagnosis, community health, 230, 232, 443–444, 443t
  in community-as-partner model, 232
  definition of, 298
  medical, 298
  in model to guide practice, 232
  nursing, 298
  prioritizing, 310–311, 311t, 312t
  sample of, 298–303 (*See also* Diagnosis sample, community health)
  in school health promotion, partnership model, 443–444, 443t
  in Students for Tobacco Reduction program, 463, 464t
  in vulnerable populations in urban settings, 500
  wellness, 443, 443t
  in women's health project, northern Pakistan, 426–429, 428t

Diagnosis sample, community health, 298–303
  derivation of, 300–301
  in downtown, 299, 301t
  example of, 299, 300b
  focus of, 299
  format of, 298–299
  inference statements in, 299
  inner city survey in, 301–303, 303t
  manifestations in, 299, 299b
  multiple subsystems in, 299–300, 301b, 301t
  signs and symptoms in, 299
  template for, 299, 299b
Discrimination, 105, 179–180
Diversity, 40. *See also* Cultural; Culture and diversity
  ethical (moral), 28
  in public health and community practice, 40
Domain, 127, 128t

E
Ecological perspective, 85–86, 85b, 86f
Ecology, 227
Economics, 265–269
  business in, 168f, 266–267
  in community analysis sample, 294–298, 295t, 296b, 297t
  in community-as-partner model, 234
  household structure in, 269
  indicators and sources of information in, 266, 267t
  labour force in, 268–269
  in power-culture dynamics, 103
  scope of, 265
  of seniors and children in poverty, 266, 267t
  shelter in, 269, 269t, 270t
Education
  in community assessment, 274–275, 275t
  health, 335–337
  level of, in Exemplar Health District, 378, 378f
Effectiveness, 353
e-Health, 198–201
  factors preventing uptake and increasing attrition in use of, 200b, 201
  implications and scope of, 198
  literacy competencies in, 198, 199t
  usefulness of, 198–199
Electronic health records, 196
Emergency housing, 290–291
Emerging threats to community health, 204–213, 207
  chronic diseases in, 210–211
  environmental health in, 207–208
  identification of, 205–206
  infectious diseases in, 208–210
  influenza pandemic in, 206–207, 207b
  mental health in, 211–213

Employment characteristics, in community analysis sample, 295, 295t
Employment rate, 379, 379t
Employment-to-population ratio, 379, 379t
Empowerment, 40, 94–110
  actualizing, 96
  community, 98–99, 98f, 415
  critical postmodern approach to, 108, 109b
  globalization on, 95–96
  health and, 99–100
  health promotion example of, 108–110, 109b
  income inequalities and, 96
  literacy in, 100–102, 101f
  meanings of, 96
  in Ottawa Charter for Health Promotion, 94, 95
  personal, in context, 97–99, 98f
  power-culture dynamics in, 102–106 (*See also* Power-culture dynamics)
  of pregnant Canadian immigrant women, 415–422 (*See also* LOV Parc-Extension program; Women's health, empowering pregnant Canadian immigrants in)
  psychological, 98
  youth, 451
Empowerment terrain, 106–108, 107t
  deprivations within, 107–108
  external, 106–107, 107t
  internal, 106, 107t
Enabling communities, 79–80
Enforcement, 342
Engineering, 340–342, 341t
  enforcement in, 342
  media advocacy in, 340–341, 341t
  policy formulation in, 341
Environment, 19, 51–53, 85b, 86–87
  built, 82
  in community-as-partner model, 234
  definition of, 85b, 223
  healthy, 9–10
  in integrated model of health, 153–154
  in intervention, 232–234
  natural, 80
  physical (*See* Physical environment)
  risk, 105–106
  supportive, for health, 78–91 (*See also* Supportive environment for health)
Environmental health, 207–208
Environmental support, in implementation, 332–333
Epidemics, 49–50. *See also* Influenza pandemic
Epidemiologic triad, 50–53, 51f
  agent in, 51–52, 52f
  environment in, 51–53
  host in, 51, 52

Epidemiological research, 50–55
  epidemiologic triad in, 50–53 (*See also* Epidemiologic
    triad)
  Haddon matrix in, 54, 55f
  person–place–time model in, 53
  web of causation in, 53–54, 54f
Epidemiology, 49–74
  analytic measures in, 62–68 (*See also* Analytic measures)
  in contemporary community health, 50
  current health status in, 205
  data sources in, 68–70
  definition of, 49
  descriptive measures in, 56–61 (*See also* Descriptive
    measures)
  history of, 49–50
  outbreak management in, 73–74
  prevention and, 55–56
  screening in, 70–72, 72t
Epp Framework, 7–11
Equity, 79
Ethical advances, 42–44, 43t
  communal dialogue in, 44
  health promotion code of ethics in, 43–44
  public health code of ethics in, 42–43, 43t
Ethical Foundations of Public Health and Community Practice,
    181. *See also* Ethics
Ethical pluralism, 28
Ethical principles, 27
Ethical principlism, 29–35, 39t. *See also* Rule ethics
Ethical relativism, 28
Ethical theories, 29–38, 39t
  feminist ethics, 36–38, 39t
  rule ethics (ethical principlism), 29–35, 39t (*See also*
    Rule ethics)
  virtue ethics (moral virtues), 35–36, 39t
Ethics, 26–45
  bioethics, 27
  challenges in, 44, 45b
  definition of, 27
  diversity in, 28
  key concepts in, 27–28
  overview of, 26–27
  professional, 27
Ethics, in public health and community practice, 39–41
  advocacy, 41
  diversity, 40
  empowerment, 40
  inclusion, 39–40
  interdependence, 41
  participation, 40
  social justice, 41
Ethnicity, 171
Ethnocentrism, 178

Evaluability, program, 351–352
Evaluation, 346–366
  approaches to, 347
  in community-as-partner model, 233, 304–306, 348
  community health time in, 347
  community involvement in, 347
  components of, 352–354
  cost-efficiency in, 353
  data collection methods for, 354–366 (*See also* Data
    collection methods)
  definition and scope of, 347–348
  effectiveness in, 353
  evaluability of program in, 351–352
  example of, 303–304
  formative, 350t, 351
  impact, 350t, 353
  of implementation, 342, 343t
  importance of, 349
  of LOV Parc-Extension program, 420–422, 421b
  in model to guide practice, 233, 303–304
  models of, 350, 350t
  outcome, 350t, 351, 354
  policy, 143
  principles of, 349
  process (formative), 350t, 351
  process (formative), in TELESENIOR, 515
  process of, 350–352, 350t
  of program plan and implementation, 342, 343t
  progress in, 353
  in public policy development, 143
  relevancy in, 353
  strategies of, 354
  of Students for Tobacco Reduction program,
    467–468
  summative, 350t, 351
  surveys in, 358–360
  of vulnerable populations in urban settings, 499–500
  of youth engagement in social policy action planning,
    458
Evidence, 22, 195. *See also* Data
Evidence-based practice, 195–196
Exemplar Health District, 373–396
  definition of health in, 374
  demographic data in, 374–377
    age distribution, 375, 375f
    birth and death rates, 375–376
    living status of persons 65+, 377, 377f
    lone parent families, 376
    occupational distribution, 376, 376f
    old age dependency ratio, 377
    population, 374–375, 375f
    young age dependency ratio, 376
  framework for, 374

Exemplar Health District (*continued*)
  health determinants in, 377–384
    alcohol sales, 383–384, 383t
    child protection cases, 382, 383t
    income, 377, 378f
    labour force, 378–380, 379t, 380t
    levels of education, 378, 378f
    social allowance, 381, 381t, 382f
  health status, 384–392
    adolescent pregnancy, 388–390, 389f, 389t, 390t
    causes of death, 384–386, 385t
    communicable diseases, 291t, 390–391
    congenital anomalies, 387–388, 388f
    dental health, 392, 392f
    injury deaths and hospitalization, 386, 386f
    low-birth-weight babies, 387, 388f
    potential years of life lost, 386–387, 387t
    sexually transmitted infections, 390t, 391–392, 392t
  observations and recommendations, 392–394
    additional measures, 394
    data, 393
    data interpretation, 393
    decision-making structure, 394
    frameworks and understanding health, 392–393
  regional health indicators, 394, 395t
Experimental design, 360–363
  pretest–posttest one-group design, 361, 361t
  pretest–posttest two-group design, 361–363, 362t
  questions answered by, 360
  selective implementation of, 360
  usefulness of, 363
External risk factors, 62–63
Extra-local relations, 127, 128t

F
Feedback loop, for well-being, 16–17, 16f
Feminist ethics, 36–38, 39t
  application of, 37–38
  critique of, 38
  historic evolution of, 37
  principles of, 36
Fidelity, 31, 33
Fire protection services, 297, 297t
Flexible line of defence, 227–228, 229t, 231f
Fluoridation, of water, 81
Focus groups, 251
Folklorama, 180
Formative evaluation, 350t, 351
Founding nations, 166–168
Framework, 125b
  bilingual, 173
  Capacity Building, 429–430, 429f

Epp, 7–11
  for Exemplar Health District, 374, 392–393
  partnership, 127–129, 128t (*See also* Partnership framework)
  population health promotion, 7–11 (*See also* Population health promotion framework, in Canada)
French ancestry, 166–168, 167t

G
Gender-based analysis (GBA), 141
German ancestry, 166–168, 167t
Global climate change, 208
Global conferences, health promotion, 11–14
  WHO, 1986, 11, 12f
  WHO, 1988, 11
  WHO, 1991, 11–12, 77–80
  WHO, 1997, 13
  WHO, 1999, 13
  WHO, 2005, 13–14
  WHO, 2007, 14
Globalization, 95–96, 209
Goal setting, 330–331
Goals, program, 224, 317–318
Goodness, 35
Government, 272–273. *See also specific agencies and programs*

H
Haddon matrix, 54, 55f
Head Start, 19
Health, 220
  creation of, 500
  definitions of, 219–220, 223, 374
  determinants of (*See* Determinants of health)
  in Epp framework, 8
  population (*See* Population health)
  understanding, in Exemplar Health District, 392–393
Health Canada, 152–153, 329
Health care, primary, 149–151. *See also* Primary health care
Health care reform, 153
Health determinants. *See* Determinants of health
Health disciplines, mandate of action of, 223
Health education, 335–337
Health facilities, downtown, 262–265, 263f–265f
"Health for All by Year 2000," 23
Health promoting hospital, 154–156, 155b
Health promoting universities, 156–157, 157t
Health promotion, 15b, 118–119
  community-based, 500
  definition of, 474

in human service delivery settings, 471
population (*See* Population health promotion)
workplace, 470–489 (*See also* Workplace health
    promotion)
Health promotion, youth engagement in, 449–468
postsecondary tobacco reduction in, 459–468 (*See also*
    Students for Tobacco Reduction)
social policy action planning in, 450–459 (*See also* Youth
    engagement in social policy action planning)
Health services, 261–262, 262t
in community analysis sample, 292–294, 293t, 294t
in community assessment, 261–262, 262t, 292–294,
    293t, 294t
reorienting (*See* Reorienting health services)
Health services subsystem
downtown, 262–265, 263f–265f
general, 230, 261–262, 262t
Health status, 193
in Exemplar Health District, 384–392 (*See also specific
    measures*)
Health surveillance, 194–195
Health system decision-making lens, 121–122, 121f
Health systems, 149
Health team, 3
Health worker, 3
Healthy Cities movement
in Canada, 14
WHO, 19
Healthy community, 88, 225
Healthy community approach, 157–158
Healthy environment, 9–10
Healthy public policies, 10–11, 341
building, 138–145 (*See also* Public policies, healthy)
formulation of, 341
Heritage enhancement, 174
Homebound seniors, technology in promoting health of,
    508–517. *See also* Technology in promoting
    homebound seniors' health
Homelessness, 212, 290, 494–495. *See also* Urban settings,
    vulnerable populations in
Homosexuals
discrimination against, 105
homelessness and, 105
Hospital, health-promoting, 154–156, 155b
Hospital records, 70
Household structure, 269
Housing
disparities in, 104, 104t
emergency and transitional, 290–291
rental, 290, 291b
Humility
cultural, 186–187, 186b
engaging in acts of, 183–184

I
Immigrant population, 168–171, 169t, 170t
Immigrants, to Canada
culture of, 168–171, 169t, 170t
health of, 416–417
population of, 168–171, 169t, 170t, 416–417
pregnancy in health of, 417–418 (*See also* LOV Parc-
    Extension program)
pregnant, empowerment of, 415–422 (*See also* Women's
    health, empowering pregnant Canadian
    immigrants in)
Impact evaluation, 350t, 353
Implementation, 327–345. *See also specific models and
    programs*
community health focus in, 331–335 (*See also*
    Community health focus)
community interventions in, 335–342 (*See also*
    Interventions, community)
engineering in, 340–342, 341t (*See also* Engineering)
environmental and cultural support in, 332–333
evaluation of, 342, 343t
goal setting in, 330–331
health education in, 335–337
levels of practice in, 335
levels of prevention in, 333–335
overview of, 331–332
participation checklist for, 342, 343t
promoting community ownership in, 328–329
of public policy, 143
selective, 360
social marketing in, 337–340, 337f, 338t
of TELESENIOR, 514
of unified program, 330
Imposition, cultural, 178
Incidence, 57
Inclusion, 39–40
in *An Inclusion Lens: Workbook for Looking at Social and
    Economic Exclusion and Inclusion*, 180–181
in public health and community practice, 39–40
social, 258–259, 259t
Income
in Exemplar Health District, 377, 378f
inequalities in, 96
Income, low (poverty), 494
in community analysis sample, 295–296, 296b
low-income cut off for, 295
Women and a Fair Income Working Group and,
    501–502 (*See also* Women's Perspectives in
    Poverty)
Independent variables, 66
Indigenous medicine, 100
Individual patient/client care lens, 122, 122f
Indoor air quality, 81

Industry, assessment of, 527–533
  company in, 527–528
  health program in, 532–533
  industrial process in, 531–532
  plant in, 528–529
  stressors in, 533
  working population in, 530–531
Industry, model assessment guide for nursing in, 521–526.
  See also Assessment guide for nursing in industry
Infant mortality rate, 58–59, 59t
  interpretation of, 59–60, 60b
  pneumonia and, in northern Pakistan, 426–427
Infectious diseases
  as emerging threats to community health, 208–210
  influenza (*See* Influenza)
  parasitic, in northern Pakistan women, 427
  sexually transmitted (*See* Sexually transmitted infections
    [STIs])
Inference statements, 299
Influenza
  avian (H5N1), 481–485
  disease aspects of, 479
  epidemiology of, 479
  infectivity of, 481
  types of, 481
  workplace spread of, 471
Influenza pandemic
  Canadian Pandemic Influenza Plan for, 206–207, 207b,
    483
  exposure and infection prevention in, 483–484
  historical perspective on, 479–480, 482f
  immunization and immunity to, 484
  lessons learned from, 483–484
  mortality impact of, 483
Influenza pandemic, responsive worker strategies for,
    483–489. *See also* Influenza; Influenza pandemic
  assessment and planning in, 485
  exposure and infection prevention in, 483–484
  in health care workers, 485
  immunization and immunity in, 484
  multiple intervention vaccination program plan in, 487,
    488f–489f
  multiple interventions in, 485–486
Influenza vaccination, 471, 484–487, 488f–489f
  combined intervention with, 485–486
  current trends in, 484
  of health care workers, 485
  multiple intervention plan for, 487, 488f–489f
  refusal of, 484, 486
Informant interview, key, 247, 250
Informatics, community health, 190–201
  conceptual model for, 191, 192f
  e-Health in, 198–201, 199t, 200b (*See also* e-Health)
  electronic health records in, 196
  evidence-based practice and research dissemination in,
    195–196
  health status in, 193
  health surveillance and performance measurement in,
    194–195
  information and service access in, 197–198
  key word search on, 190–191, 191t
  knowledge, understanding, and skills for, 197–198
  policy development in, 193
  technology infrastructure for, 197
Information and communication technology literacy, 198
Informed consent, 31
Injury deaths and hospitalization, in Exemplar Health
    District, 386, 386f
Inner City Family Resource Centre Network (ICFRN),
    301–303, 303t
Inner city survey, 301–303, 303t
Integrated model of health, 151–154
  vs. biomedical model, 151–152
  challenges in, 152
  constituent demands in, 153
  core strategies for, 152–153
  health care reform in, 153
  history of, 152
  sociopolitical and environmental approaches in,
    153–154
Integration, 176, 176f
  multicultural, 174
Interaction, as collective unit, 404–405
Interactiveness, in observation, 357
Interdependence, 41
Internal risk factors, 62–63
International Conference on Health Promotion, WHO.
    See WHO International Conference on Health
    Promotion
Interpretation, 57
  in analysis, 282–283
  of analytic measures, 64–65, 65t
  of data, in Exemplar Health District, 393
  of infant mortality rates, 59–60, 60b
  of odds ratio, 64–65, 65t
  of rates, 59–60, 60b
  of relative risk ratio, 64–65, 65t
Intervention, in community-as-partner model, 231f,
    232–234
  community assessment wheel in, 231f, 232, 239, 240f,
    253
  community in, 230–234
  economy in, 234
  environment in, 234
  outcome desired in, 232
  prevention in, 232–233

Interventions, community, 335–342
    engineering in, 340–342, 341t (*See also* Engineering)
    health education in, 335–337
    social marketing in, 337–340, 337f, 338t
Inuit women's health, 398–403
    assessment of, 400–401
    demographics of, 400
    history of, 399–400, 399f
    insight into, 402–403
    issue identification in, 401–402, 403
    main themes in, 402
    research on, 400

J

Jakarta Declaration on Leading Health Promotions into the
    21st Century, 13
Journey Forward, 228t
Justice, 32
Justice, social, 41

K

Kantianism, 30
Key informant interview, 247, 250

L

Labonté model, 220–221, 221f
Labour force, 268–269
    in Exemplar Health District, 378–380, 379t, 380t
Labrador
    map of, 453f
    youth engagement in social policy action planning in,
        450–459 (*See also* Youth engagement in social
        policy action planning)
Ladder of participation, 122–123, 123f
Lalonde Report
    on community practice foundations, 4–5, 149, 151–152
    four health fields in, 15, 17
Leadership, 126b, 128
Leaf Rapids community crisis, 403–412. *See also*
        Photovoice, youth participation via
    Community Health Action Model for, 404, 405f
    engaging youth expression in, 405–406
    interaction as collective unit in, 404–405
    Leaf Rapids community crisis and, 403–404
    Photovoice for youth participation in, 406–412
        (*See also* Photovoice, youth participation via)
Lenses, three, 120–122, 120f–122f
Lessons learned
    in influenza pandemic planning, 483–484

    in Oral Health Programming, 438, 439t
    in school health promotion, partnership model,
        445–446
    in TELESENIOR, 516–517
    in youth participation via Photovoice, 412
Levels, 3
Lewin's stages of planned change, 312–313, 313t
Lifestyle, 222
Lines of defence
    flexible, 227–228, 229t
    in municipal government workplace health promotion,
        476–477, 476b
    normal, 227, 229t, 231f
    in Students for Tobacco Reduction program, 463
Lines of resistance, 228–229, 229t
    in municipal government workplace health promotion,
        477, 477b
    in Students for Tobacco Reduction program, 463
Lines of strength, 463
Literacy, 100–102, 101f
    e-Health, 198, 199t
    information and communication technology, 198
Living status of persons 65+, in Exemplar Health
        District, 377, 377f
Lone parent families, in Exemplar Health District, 376
LOV Parc-Extension program
    as adaptation of provincial program, 418
    circle of empowerment in, 420
    empowering interdisciplinary work in, 418
    evaluation of, 420–422, 421b
    group meetings in, 419–420
    history and origin of, 417–418
    individual meetings in, 419
    model for, 415, 415f, 419t
    professional and leader meetings in, 420
Low-birth-weight babies, in Exemplar Health District,
        387, 388f
Low-income cut off (LICO), 295

M

Malnutrition, 211
Mandala of Health model, 221–223, 222f
Marginalization, 176, 176f
Material deprivation, 103–104
Media, 105
Media advocacy, 340–341, 341t
Mediating, 80
Medical model, 151–152, 219
Medical records, 70
Mental illness, 211–213
    populations with higher levels of, 104
    racism and, 105

Minority population, visible, 168
Model, 125b, 151–152
Model to guide practice, 218–236
    analysis, diagnosis, and planning in, 232
    assessment in, 230–232
    community-as-partner, 224–230, 226f (*See also*
        Community-as-partner model)
    community process, 219
    conceptual, 219
    essential elements of, 219–220, 220t
    evaluation in, 234–235, 303–304
    intervention in, 231f, 232–234 (*See also* Intervention, in
        community-as-partner model)
    Labonté, 220–221, 221f
    Mandala of Health, 221–223, 222f
    medical (biomedical), 151–152, 219
    partnership planning and teamwork in, 235
    professional practice in, 224
    Rural Development Institute, 223, 223f
Models of evaluation, 350, 350t. *See also specific models*
Monitoring charts, 364–365, 364t
Monitoring (process), 363–365, 364t
Moral diversity, 28
Moral virtues, 35–36, 39t
Morality. *See* Ethics
Morbidity, 56–57
Mortality, 56–57
Motor vehicle mortality, 18
Multiculturalism, 172
    barriers to, 177–180
    community and organizational initiatives on, 180–181
    definition of, 172
    ethnocentrism as barrier to, 178
    facilitators of, 180–181
    government programs and policies on, 180
    prejudice as barrier to, 177–178
    professional and individual responsibilities for, 181
    racism as barrier to, 179–180
    stereotyping as barrier to, 178–179
Multiculturalism in Canada, 172–175
    benefits of, 174–175
    within bilingual framework, 173
    Canadian Charter of Rights and Freedoms and,
        173–174
    Canadian Multiculturalism Act and, 174
    history of, 172–173
Multiculturalism in community practice, 181–187
    cultural attunement in, 182–185, 185b (*See also* Cultural
        attunement)
    cultural competence in, 181–182, 182t
    cultural humility in, 186–187, 186b
Municipal government workplace health promotion,
        471–479
    assessment in, 474–477, 476b
    assessment in, multilevel, 478
    assessment in, participatory processes in, 478
    assessment in, practical considerations in, 478–479
    community core in, 474–476
    context of, 471–474
    expectations of outcomes in, 471–473, 473b
    lines of defence in, 476–477, 476b
    lines of resistance in, 477, 477b
    power relationships in, 473–474
    stakeholders in, 476, 476b
Mutual aid, 9
Mutuality, engaging in, 184

N
Natural disasters, in infectious diseases, 209
Natural environment, 80
Networks, policy, 144f, 145
Newfoundland
    map of, 453f
    youth engagement in social policy action planning in,
        450–459 (*See also* Youth engagement in social
        policy action planning)
Nobody's Perfect program logic model, 19, 321, 322t
Nominal group technique, 357
Nonmaleficence, 32
Nonprofit capacity, 429
Normal line of defence (NLD), 227, 229t, 231f
Notifiable disease reports, 70
"Not knowing" position, maintaining, 184–185
Nunavut, 399–400, 399f. *See also* Inuit women's
        health
Nursing in industry, model assessment guide for,
        521–526. *See also* Assessment guide for
        nursing in industry

O
Obesity, 210–211
Objectives, program, 318–321, 322t
Observation
    in case-study approach to evaluation, 356–357
    in data collection, 246–247, 248t–249t, 250b
    in Exemplar Health District, 392–394
Occupational distribution, in Exemplar Health District,
        376, 376f
Odds ratio (OR), 63–64, 64t
Odds ratio (OR) interpretation, 64–65, 65t
Old age dependency ratio (OADR), 377
OLO program, 417–418
Operations, in partnership framework, 128t
Oppression, acknowledging pain of, 183

Oral health
    in Exemplar Health District, 392, 392f
    promotion of, approaches to, 434–435
    promotion of, in rural Canada, 432–439
    quality of life and, 433–434
Oral Health Programming, 432–439
    approaches to oral health promotion in, 434–435
    community assessment in, 435–436, 436t
    determining target schools in, 437
    evaluating intervention in, 438–439
    implementing oral health initiative in, 437–438, 438t,
        439t
    lessons learned from, 438, 439t
    oral health goals in, 435, 436t
    program planning in, 437
    quality of life and dental health in, 433–434
Organizational awareness, in cultural attunement,
    185b
Ottawa Charter for Health Promotion, 11, 12f, 20,
    23, 94, 95
Outbreak management, 73–74
Outcome
    desired, in community-as-partner model, 233
    expectations of, in workplace health promotion,
        471–473, 473b
    in school health promotion, partnership model, 444
    in TELESENIOR, 515–516
Outcome evaluation, 350t, 351, 354
Ownership, promoting community, 328–329

P

Pandemic, influenza. See Influenza pandemic
Pan West Community Futures Network, 180
Parasitic infections, in northern Pakistan, 427
Parc-Extension (See LOV Parc-Extension program)
    sociodemographic characteristics of, 416
Participation, 40
    community, 328–329
    ladder of, 122–123, 123f
    public, 10
    public, in health, 118–123 (See also Public participation
        in health)
    youth, via Photovoice, 406–412 (See also Youth
        participation via Photovoice)
Participation checklist, for program implementation, 342,
    343t
Participation rate, 379, 379t
Participatory Action Research (PAR), 117b.
        See also Photovoice
    on Inuit's women's health, 401
Participatory democracy, in youth empowerment
        programs, 451

Participatory research, 495
Partner characteristics, 127–129, 128t
Partner identification, 134
Partnership, 124–126
    across levels, 3
    across sectors, 3
    definitions of, 124, 124b
    failure to include essential elements in, 130, 130f
    in healthy public policies, 145 (See also Public policies,
        healthy)
    improper configuration of elements in, 130, 131f
    inclusion of nonessential elements in, 130, 130f
    overview of, 3–4
Partnership characteristics, 128t, 129, 134
Partnership configuration, 129–130, 130f, 131f
Partnership development, process model of, 131–133, 133f
Partnership framework, 127–129, 128t
    communication in, 128t, 129
    domain in, 127, 128t
    extra-local relations in, 127, 128t
    operations in, 128t
    partner characteristics in, 127–129, 128t
    partnership characteristics in, 128t, 129
    for school health promotion, 440–446 (See also School
        health promotion, partnership model)
Partnership organization, 131, 132f
Partnership planning, in practice models, 235
Partnerships for health, 123–137
    application of tools for, 133–135
    characteristics of, 134
    collaboration and partnerships in, 123–126
    communication strategies in, 134
    configuration of, 129–130, 130f, 131f
    framework of, 127–129, 129t (See also Partnership
        framework)
    guiding principles in, 135
    organization of, 131, 132f
    partner identification in, 134
    process model of development of, 131–133, 133f
Perception, selective, in observation, 356–357
Performance measurement, 194–195
Personal skills development. See Empowerment
Person-mapping exercise, 454, 455f
Person–place–time model, 53
Photovoice
    premise of, 505
    in Women's Perspectives in Poverty, 501–505 (See also
        Women's Perspectives in Poverty, Photovoice in)
    youth participation via, 406–412 (See also Youth
        participation via Photovoice)
Physical environment, 80–83, 230, 260–261, 261t
    air quality, 80–81
    built environment, 82

Physical environment (*continued*)
    chemical and biological hazards, 82
    in community analysis sample, 290–292, 291b
    in community assessment, 260, 261t
    natural environment, 80
    risk assessment, 83
    water quality, 81–82
Place, in social marketing, 338
Plagiocephaly, 426
Planned change, 311–316
    definition and scope of, 311–312
    developing program logic model for, 317–325
        (*See also* Program logic model development)
    Lewin's stages of, 312–313, 313t
    Reinkemeyers stages of, 312, 312t
    transtheoretical model of, 313, 314t, 315t
Planned change in community planning, 313–316
    stage 1, 314
    stage 2, 314–315
    stage 3, 315–316
    stage 4, 316
    stage 5, 328
    stage 6, 328
    stage 7, 368
Planning
    of assessment, 243–245
    in community-as-partner model, 231, 235
    for influenza pandemic, responsive worker strategies in, 485
    in model to guide practice, 230
    in Oral Health Programming, 437
    in school health promotion, partnership model, 441–442, 444
    for vulnerable populations in urban settings, 497–498
Planning, community health program, 306–326
    in partnership with community, 208f, 307–310
    planned change in, 311–316, 312t–315t
        (*See also* Planned change)
    populations at risk in, 309
    prioritizing community diagnoses in, 310–311, 311t, 312t
    team members in, 309–310
Pluralism, 108
    cultural, 172
    ethical, 28
Pneumonia in infants/children, in northern Pakistan, 426–427
Policy communities, 143–144, 143f, 144t
Policy evaluation, 143
Policy formulation, 141–142, 341
Policy, healthy public, 10–11
Policy implementation, 143
Policy networks, 144f, 145
Policy stream, 141–142

Policy window, 142
Politics, 272–273
Pooling data, 288
Population
    in Exemplar Health District, 374–375, 375f
    source, 379
    total, 256–257, 257f, 257t
Population data, 252
Population description, 256–259
    age distribution in, 258, 258t
    social inclusion in, 258–259, 259t
    total population in, 256–257, 257f, 257t
Population health, 14–19
    definition and scope of, 14–15, 15b
    definition of, 15b
    determinants of health in, 16–17, 16f, 18t
    vs. health promotion, 14–16, 15b
    history of, 14
    key elements of, 22–23
    settings in, 19
    target populations in, 17–19
Population health promotion, 2–23
    Alma Ata Declaration on, 5–7, 5b, 7t, 23, 149–151, 152
    definition of, 15b
    "doing with" in, 3–4
    foundations of community practice in, 4–7
    health worker and health team in, 3
    history of, 2–3
    implications for "community as partner" of, 23
    Lalonde Report on, 4–5, 149, 151–152
    model for, 20–21, 20f
    partnerships in, 3–4
    population health approach in, 22–23
    population health in, 14–19 (*See also* Population health)
Population health promotion framework, in Canada, 7–11
    aim of, 8–9
    challenges in, 9
    community services in, 10
    context of, 7–8
    definition of health in, 8
    healthy environment in, 9–10
    healthy public policy in, 10–11
    mutual aid in, 9
    public participation in, 10
    self-care in, 9
Population health promotion global conferences, 11–14
    WHO International Conference, 1986, 11, 12f
    WHO International Conference, 1988, 11
    WHO International Conference, 1991, 11–12, 77–80
    WHO International Conference, 1997, 13
    WHO International Conference, 1999, 13
    WHO International Conference, 2005, 13–14
    WHO International Conference, 2007, 14

Population health promotion lens, 121, 121f
Population Health Promotion (PHP) model, 114
Populations at risk, planning for, 309
Potential years of life lost, in Exemplar Health District, 386–387, 387t
Poverty, 494. *See also* Urban settings, vulnerable populations in
  in community analysis sample, 295–296, 296b
  Women's Perspectives in, 501–505 (*See also* Women's Perspectives in Poverty, Photovoice in)
Power, 415
Power-culture dynamics, 102–106
  definition of, 103b
  deprivation in, 103
  example of, 108, 109b
  for homosexuals and bisexuals, 105
  housing disparities in, 104, 104t
  media in, 105
  poor mental health in, 104
  risk environments and behaviors in, 105–106
  socioeconomics in, 103
Power relationships, 473–474
Practical ethics, 27
Practice, levels of, 335
Precede-Proceed model, 497
Pregnancy
  adolescent, in Exemplar Health District, 388–390, 389f, 389t, 390t
  challenges of, for immigrant women, 416–418
  empowering Canadian immigrants during, 415–422 (*See also* Women's health, empowering pregnant Canadian immigrants in)
  health promotion in, Pakistan, 426 (*See also* Women's health, northern Pakistan)
  maternal deworming in, northern Pakistan, 427–428
Pregnant immigrant women, challenges of, 416–418
Prejudice, 177–178
Pretest–posttest one-group design, 361, 361t
Pretest–posttest two-group design, 361–363, 362t
Prevalence, 57
Preventing Disease Through Healthy Environments—Towards an Estimate of the Environmental Burden of Disease, 207–208
Prevention, 55–56
  levels of, 333–335
  primary, 55, 232, 333–334
  screening in, 70–72, 72t
  secondary, 56, 233, 334
  tertiary, 56, 233, 334
Primary health care, 149–151
  definition of, 15b
  essential services in, 150–151
  patient–public health care relationship in, 150

  principles of, 149–150
  strategic imperatives for, 151
  systems level of, 149–151
Primary prevention, 55, 230–232, 333–334
Principles, ethical, 27
Principles of Biomedical Ethics, 30
Principles of the Ethical Practice of Public Health, 42–43, 43t
Principlism, 30
Process evaluation, 350t, 351
  in TELESENIOR, 515
Process model of partnership development, 131–133, 133f
Product, in social marketing, 338
Professional ethics, 27
Professional practice, 224
Program activities, 318, 319f
Program goals, 317–318
Program logic model development, 317–325
  budgeting in, 324
  collaboration in, 321–323
  constraints in, 323–324
  "Nobody's Perfect" program logic model in, 321, 322t
  overview of, 317
  program activities in, 318, 319f
  program goals in, 317–318
  program objectives in, 318–321, 322t
  recording in, 324–325
  resources in, 323
  revised plans in, 324
Program logic model, for Students for Tobacco Reduction, 464, 465f
Program objectives, 318–321, 322t
Progress, in evaluation, 353
Promotion, in social marketing, 338
Proportions, 57–58
Public action, 79
Public Health Agency of Canada (PHAC), health promotion info from, 329
Public participation, 10
Public participation in health, 118–123
  benefits of, 122
  health system decision-making lens in, 121–122, 121f
  history of, 118–119
  individual patient/client care lens in, 122, 122f
  population health promotion lens in, 121, 121f
  public participation spectrum in, 122–123, 123f
  range of activities in, 119–120
  three lenses of, 120–122, 120f–122f
Public participation spectrum, 122–123, 123f
Public policies, healthy, 138–145
  definition of, 138–139
  development of, 139–143 (*See also* Public policy development)
  partnerships in, 145

Public policies, healthy (*continued*)
  policy communities in, 143–144, 143f, 144t
  policy networks in, 144f, 145
Public policy, 139
Public policy development, 139–143
  agenda-setting in, 141
  decision-making in, 142
  five aspects of, 139–140, 140f
  health informatics and, 193
  implementation and evaluation in, 143
  policy formulation in, 141–142

Q
Questionnaires, 251–252

R
Race, 171
RACE TeleCommunity program, 508
Racism, 179–180
  democratic, 179
  mental illness and, 105
  systemic, 179
Rakaposhi Viewing Point, 423, 423f
Rates, 57–61
  adjusted, 61, 61t
  calculation of, 58
  commonly used, 60, 61t
  crude, 60
  definition and use of, 57–58
  example of, 58–59, 59t
  interpretation of, 59–60, 60b
  vs. proportions, 57–58
  specific, 60–61, 61t
Reaction, degree of, 229
Recording, in planning process, 324–325
Records
  electronic health, 196
  hospital, 70
  medical, 70
Recreational opportunities, in community analysis
    sample, 298
Referent organization, 124b
Regional health authority, public participation with,
    144–145, 144t
Regional health indicators, in Exemplar Health District,
    394, 395t
Reinkemeyers stages of planned change, 312, 312t
Relative deprivation, 103–105
Relative risk (RR) ratio, 62
Relative risk (RR) ratio interpretation, 64–65, 65t
Relativism, cultural, 172

Relevancy, in evaluation, 353
Reliability, 71
Rental accommodations, 290, 291b
Reorienting health services, 148–160
  capacity building in, 158–159
  health care reform in, 153
  health sector reform in, 159–160
  integrated model of health in, 151–154 (*See also*
    Integrated model of health)
  overview of, 149
  primary health care in, 149–151 (*See also* Primary
    health care)
  settings approach in, 154–158 (*See also* Settings approach)
  sociopolitical and environmental approaches in,
    153–154
Report on the Health of Canadians, 330
Request for information (RFI), 197
Request for proposal (RFP), 197
Research
  community-based, 116, 117b
  participatory action, 117b
  in population health approach, 22
Research-based evidence, 195–196
Research dissemination, 195–196
Resilient community, 88, 227–228
Resistance, lines of, 228–229, 229t
  in municipal government workplace health promotion,
    477, 477b
  in Students for Tobacco Reduction program, 463
Resources
  for data comparison, 282–283
  in planning process, 323
Respect for persons, 33
Reverence, acting with, 184
Revised plans, in planning process, 324
Rightness, 29
Risk assessment, 83
Risk behaviours, 105–106
Risk communication, 83
Risk conditions, 21
Risk environments, 105–106
Risk factors, 21, 62–63
Risk perception, 83
Rule ethics, 29–35, 39t
  autonomy in, 31
  beneficence in, 31–32
  critique of, 34
  fidelity in, 31, 33
  historical evolution of, 29, 30t
  justice in, 32
  method in, 31
  nonmaleficence in, 32
  prima facie vs. a priori, 31

principles for practice of, 30–34
respect for persons in, 33
sanctity of life in, 33
schools of, 29–30
veracity in, 31, 33–34
Rural Communities Impacting Policy (RCIP) Project, 88
issue in, 89
keys to success in, 91
overview of, 88
policy change strategy in, 90–91
Upper Bay of Fundy Wharf Pilot Project in, 89–90
Rural Development Institute (RDI) model, 223, 223f

S
Safe community approach, 158
Safety, 269–272, 271t, 272t
in community analysis sample, 297, 297t
protection services in, 270, 272t
Sanctity of life, 33
Sanitation, 270–271
SARS outbreak, 73–74, 209
Saskatchewan Cree First Nation, 109–110
School health promotion, 156–157, 157t
oral, 432–449 (See also Oral Health Programming)
School health promotion, partnership model, 440–446
alternative school setting for, 440–441
assessment and analysis in, 441–442
diagnosis in, 443–444, 443t
lessons learned in, 445–446
outcome in, 444
planning in, 441–442, 444
Schools, in community analysis sample, 296–297
Screening, 70–73, 72t
decision making in, 72–73
definition of, 70–71
purpose of, 71
reliability of, 71
validity of, 71–72, 72t
Secondary prevention, 56, 233, 334
Sectors, 3
Selective implementation, 360
Selective perception, in observation, 356–357
Self-awareness, in cultural attunement, 184–185, 185b
Self-care, 9
Self-efficacy, in empowerment, 98
Self-esteem, in empowerment, 98
Self-exploration, in cultural attunement, 184–185
Seniors, technology in promoting health of, 508–517.
See also Technology in promoting homebound
seniors' health
Senses, in interviewing, 247, 250b
Sensitivity, 71–72, 72t

Separation, 176, 176f
Settings, 85b, 86–87
for population health, 19
Settings approach, 154–158
health-promoting hospital movement, 154–156, 155b
healthy and safe communities, 157–158
school health promotion, 156–157, 157t
scope of, 154
Sexually transmitted infections (STIs), in Exemplar
Health District, 390t, 391–392, 392t
Shelter, 269, 269t, 270t
Silk Road. See Women's health, northern Pakistan
Smoking reduction, youth, 18–19
Social allowance, in Exemplar Health District, 381, 381t,
382f
Social capital, 85b, 87–88
Social inclusion, 258–259, 259t
Social justice, 41
Social marketing, 337–340, 337f, 338t
Social network analysis, 78–91. See also Supportive
environment for health
Social networks, 85b, 87–88
Social policy action planning, youth engagement in,
450–459. See also Youth engagement in social
policy action planning
Social safety net, 261
Social services, 261–262, 262t
in community analysis sample, 292–294, 293t
in community assessment, 261–262, 262t
downtown, 262–265, 266b
Social services subsystem, downtown, 262–265, 266b
Social support, in school health, 156
Social welfare reports, 70
Societal adaptation, 174
Societal factors, in public health, 205–206
Sociodemographic characteristics, 258–259, 259t
Socioeconomics, 103
Source population, 379
Specificity, 71–72, 72t
Specific rates, 60–61, 61t
Spectrum of public participation, 122–123, 123f
Stereotyping, 178–179
Strategies for Population Health: Investing in the Health of
Canadians, 17
Strength, lines of, 463
Strengthening Community Action (SCA), 113–137
collaboration and partnerships in, 123–126
community capacity in, building, 115–116, 115b
community development in, 114
community development methods in, 116
community development process in, 117–118, 118t, 119b
partnerships for health in, 123–137 (See also
Partnerships for health)

Strengthening Community Action (SCA) (*continued*)
  public participation in health in, 118–123 (*See also*
    Public participation in health)
Strengthening Community Health Project (SCHP), 158
Stress, 211
Stressors, in community-as-partner model, 229, 229t
Students for Tobacco Reduction, 459–468
  analysis and diagnosis in, 463, 464t
  assessment in, awareness of tobacco industry tactics,
    461–462
  assessment in, policy text, 462–463
  assessment in, tobacco use in young adults, 461, 462b
  evaluation in, 467–468
  history of, 459–460
  interventions and innovation in, 466–467
  mobilization in, 460–461
  partnerships with purpose in, 464–466
  project development, roles and responsibilities in, 464,
    465f
Subsystems, community, 259–276
  communication, 273–274, 274t
  in community-as-partner model, 225–227, 226f
  downtown health facilities and social services, 262–265,
    263f–265f, 266b
  economics, 265–269 (*See also* Economics)
  education, 274–275, 275t
  health and social services, 230, 261–262, 262t, 292–294,
    293t, 294t
  physical environment, 80–83, 230, 260–261, 261t
    (*See also* Physical environment)
  politics and government, 272–273
  recreation, 275–276, 276t
  safety and transportation, 269–272, 271t, 272t
  value of, 259–260
Suicide, 211
Summative evaluation, 350t, 351
Sundsvall conference, 78–79
Sundsvall statement, 79–80
Superbugs, 209
Supportive environment for health, 78–91. *See also* Social
    network analysis
  Action Process for Creating Supportive Environment
    for Health Action Plan, 83–85, 84f, 85b
  actions for creation of, 79–80
  case study on, 88–91 (*See also* Rural Communities
    Impacting Policy [RCIP] Project)
  dimensions of, 78–79, 79b
  ecological perspective on, 85–86, 85b, 86f
  environments and settings for, 85b, 86–87
  physical environment in, 80–83
  social capital and social networks in, 85b, 87–88
  Sundsvall conference and statement on, 78–80, 79b
Suraj Health Network, 424

Suraj Health Network Health Promotion Program, 424
Surveillance, health, 194–195
Surveys, 251–252, 358–359
  in evaluation, 358–360
Systemic racism, 179

T
Target populations, 17–19
TEACH, 336
Team building process, 244–245
Team development process, 240, 241t
Teamwork, in practice models, 235
Technology infrastructure, for community health
    informatics, 197
Technology in promoting homebound seniors' health,
    508–517
  background on, 509
  building participatory relationships in, 511–512
  description of, 510–511, 510f, 511f
  evaluation of, 514–516
  history of, 508–509
  implementation of, 514
  lessons learned in, 516–517
  needs assessment for, 512–514, 513t
  sociodemographic data on, 512, 513t
  support services for, 513t
Tele-homecare, 509. *See also* Technology in promoting
    homebound seniors' health
Teleology, 29
TELESENIOR, 508–515. *See also* Technology in
    promoting homebound seniors' health
Tertiary prevention, 56, 233, 334
"The Health of Canadians—The Federal Role,"
    159–160
Threats to community health, emerging. *See* Emerging
    threats to community health
Three lenses, 120–122, 120f–122f
Tobacco industry tactics, awareness of, 461–462
Tobacco policies, 141b, 462–463
Tobacco reduction, youth, 18–19, 459–468. *See also*
    Students for Tobacco Reduction
Tobacco use, in young adults, 461, 462b
Total population, 256–257, 257f, 257t
Towards a Healthy Future, 330
Transitional housing, 290–291
Transportation, 272, 272t
Transtheoretical model of stages of change, 313, 314t, 315t

U
Ultraviolet (UV) radiation, 81
Unemployment rate, 378–379, 379t

Unified program, implementation of, 330. *See also* Implementation
Universal principles, of moral action, 172
Universities, health promoting, 156–157, 157t
Upper Bay of Fundy Wharf Pilot Project, 89–90
Urban settings, vulnerable populations in, 494–501
  analysis of, 497
  assessment as intervention in, 498–499
  assessment of, 495–497
  background on, 494–495
  evaluation in, 499–500
  objects of interest in, 500–501
  planning for, 497–498
  project summary for, 500–501
  statistics on, 494
Utilitarianism, 29

V
Vaccination, influenza, 484–487, 488f–489f. *See also* Influenza vaccination
Validity, 71–72, 72t
Values, 27
Variables, 66
  confounding, 66–67
  dependent, 66
  independent, 66
Variety of strategies, in population health approach, 22
Veracity, 31, 33–34
Virtue ethics, 35–36, 39t
Virtues
  definition of, 27–28, 35
  moral, 35–36
Visible minority population, 168
Vital statistics, 69
Voices and Choices: Health and Participation, 156
Vulnerable populations in urban settings, 494–501. *See also* Urban settings, vulnerable populations in

W
Water, 270–271
Water quality, 81–82
Water treatment devices, home, 82
Watering Down the Milk, 501
Web of causation, 53–54, 54f
Well-being
  in community analysis sample, 298
  feedback loop for, 16–17, 16f
Wellness diagnosis, 443, 443t
WHO International Conference on Health Promotion
  1986, 11, 12f
  1988, 11

  1991, 11–12, 77–80
  1997, 13
  1999, 13
  2005, 13–14
  2007, 14
Windshield/walking survey, 247, 248t–249t, 297
Women and a Fair Income Working Group, 501–502. *See also* Women's Perspectives in Poverty, Photovoice in
Women's health, empowering pregnant Canadian immigrants in, 415–422
  challenges of pregnant, 416–418
  empowerment model in, 415
  LOV Parc-Extension program in, 415, 415f, 418–422 (*See also* LOV Parc-Extension program)
  sociodemographic characteristics in, 416
Women's health, Inuit, 398–403. *See also* Inuit women's health
Women's health, northern Pakistan, 422–430
  analysis and diagnosis in, 426–429, 428t
  assessment in, 424
  building capacity in, 429–430, 429f
  community overview in, 422–423, 423f
  health promotion in pregnancy and postpartum in, 426
  maternal deworming in, 427–428
  messages relating to illness prevention in, 425, 425b
  method in, 424
  parasitic infections in, 427
  pneumonia prevention in, 426–427
  professional support during breast-feeding period in, 427
  recommendations for changes to Health Promotion Program in, 428–429
  results in, 424–425
  Suraj Health Network and, 424
Women's Perspectives in Poverty
  action process in, 501–502
  context and background on, 501
Women's Perspectives in Poverty, Photovoice in, 501–505
  challenges and impacts in, 504–505
  making space for voices in, 502–503
  multiple constituencies in, 503–504
  project summary for, 505
Workplace health promotion, 470–489
  business case for, 473b
  concepts, descriptions and relevance in, 471, 472t
  context of, 471–474
  definition of, 471
  expectations of outcomes in, 471–473, 473b
  in municipal government setting, 471–479 (*See also* Municipal government workplace health promotion)
  power relationships in, 473–474
  prevalence of, 470

Workplace health promotion (*continued*)
   responsive worker strategies for Influenza pandemic in,
     483–489 (*See also* Influenza pandemic, responsive
     worker strategies for)
Worldviews, 99–100

Y
Young age dependency ratio (YADR), 376
Youth
   determinants of health in, 451, 452t
   tobacco use in, 461, 462b
Youth engagement in health promotion, 450
Youth engagement in social policy action planning,
     450–459
   accomplishments and reflections in, 458
   background and context of, 451, 452t
   evaluation of, 458
   overview of, 450–451
   planning/methodology of, 451–456, 453f
   planning/methodology of, development and
     monitoring, 456
   planning/methodology of, development of
     training and action plan workshops,
     452–454

   planning/methodology of, presentation of training and
     action plan workshops, 454–456, 455f
   planning/methodology of, principles of, 451
   project analysis in, 457–458
   project data on, 456–457
   themes in, successful, 457
   themes in, unsuccessful, 457–458
Youth expression, engaging, 405–406
Youth participation via Photovoice, 406–412
   benefits of, 406–407
   cameras in, 408, 408b
   consent in, 407, 408b
   distribution and discussing photographs in, 408–409
   learning from photographs/photologs in, 409–411,
     409b, 410f, 411f
   lessons learned in, 412
   logistics of, 407
   method in, 406
   photo logs in, 409, 409b
   project initiation in, 407–408
   sharing photographs with community in, 411–412
   themes in, 409–411
   youth on community action in, 412
Youth tobacco reduction, 18–19, 459–468
     (*See also* Students for Tobacco Reduction)